CATAMOUNT SURGEONS

SURGERY AND SURGICAL EDUCATION
AT THE
UNIVERSITY OF VERMONT
1804-2008

DAVID B. PILCHER, MD

WITH

MICHAEL G. CURRAN, MD

UNIVERSITY OF VERMONT
COLLEGE OF MEDICINE
DEPARTMENT OF SURGERY

Copyright ©2010 by the
University of Vermont and Michael G. Curran

All rights reserved.
Printed in the USA by
Queen City Printers Inc., Burlington, VT 05401

First edition, first printing.
ISBN 978-1-4507-0170-9

THANKS TO
JOAN AND JULIUS H. JACOBSON II, MD

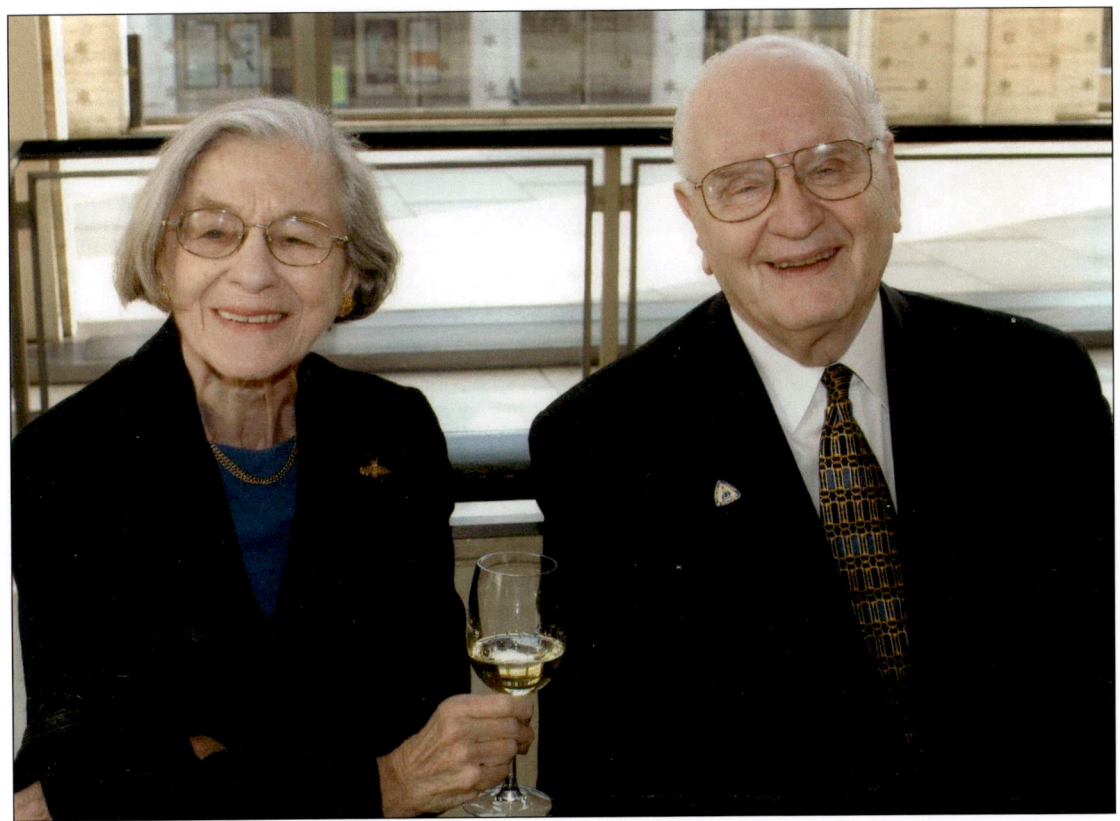

The Department of Surgery and the authors express their deep appreciation to the Jacobson's for their support and encouragement which has helped make this publication possible. (Courtesy of JH Jacobson II, MD)

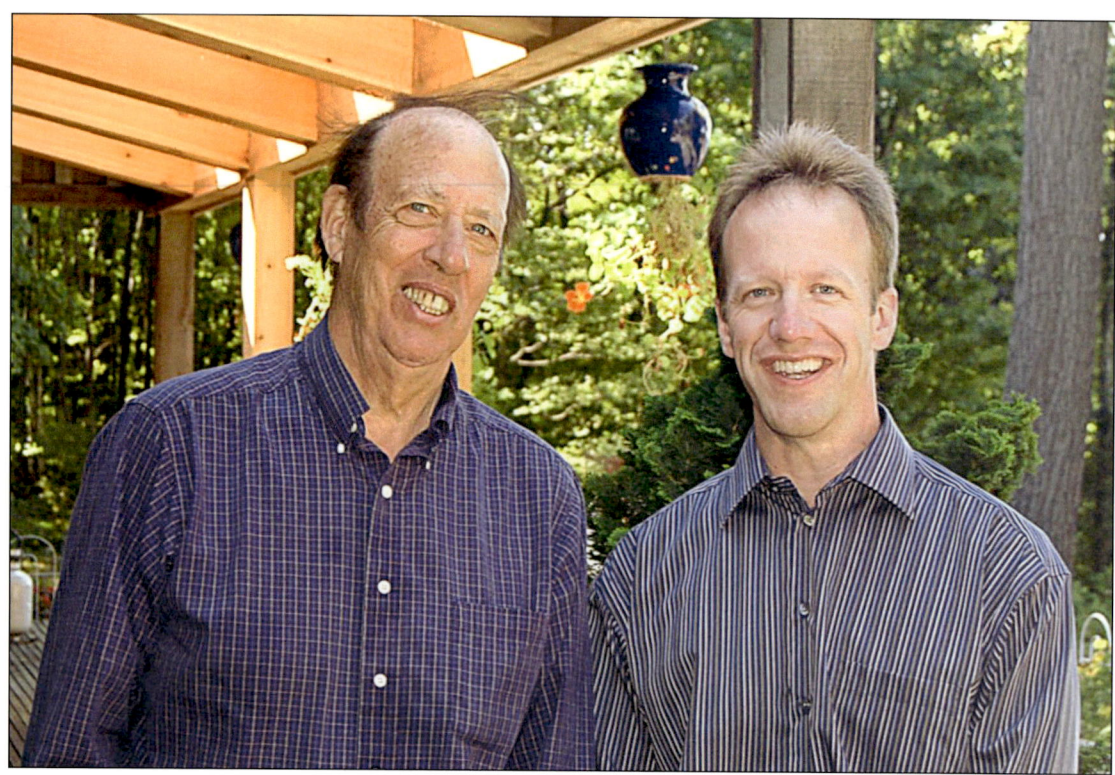

David B. Pilcher and Michael G. Curran stressed out from working on the book in 2008. (Photography by the author, DBP)

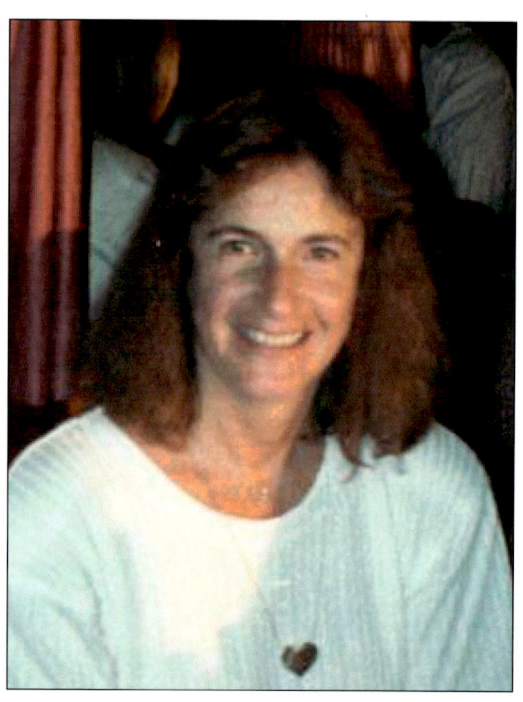

Suzanne Wulff Pilcher, who read and improved the manuscript many times (Photography by the author, DBP)

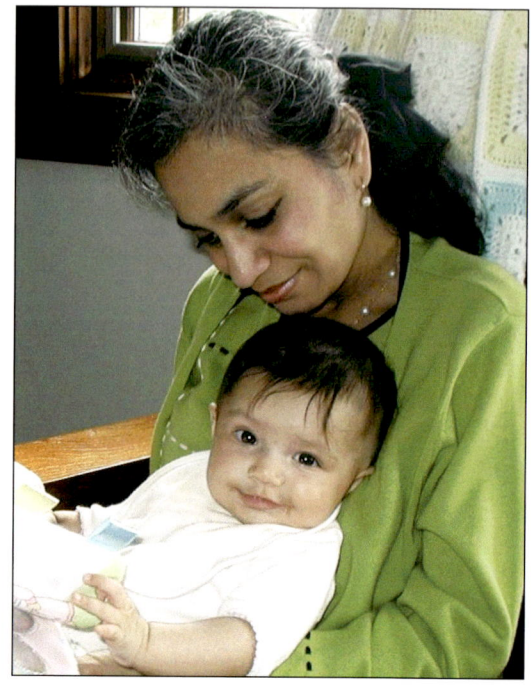

Manisha Patel (Curran) MD and Meghana Maeve Curran
Thanks to Meghana for waiting to come until after Dad had done much of his prodigious work (Photography by the author, MGC)

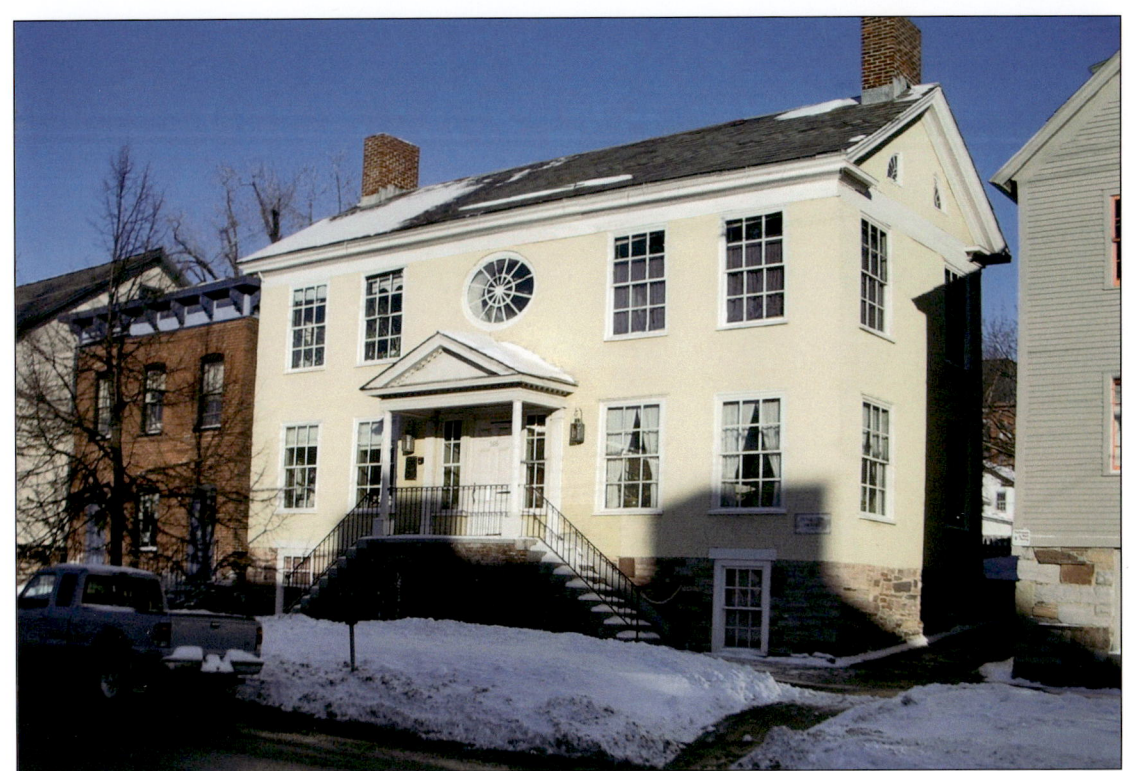

1804 Medical "Classroom" on Battery Street in Burlington (Pomeroy's House) (Photography by the author, DBP)

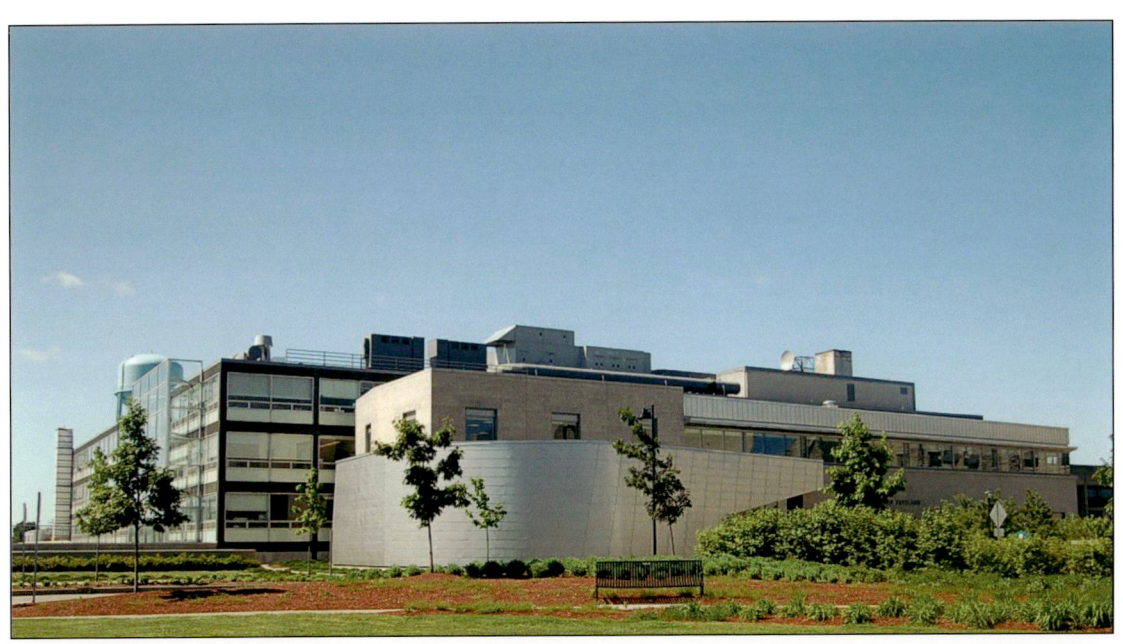

2008 UVM Medical Education Pavilion, with 1962 Given Building in background (Photography by the author, DBP)

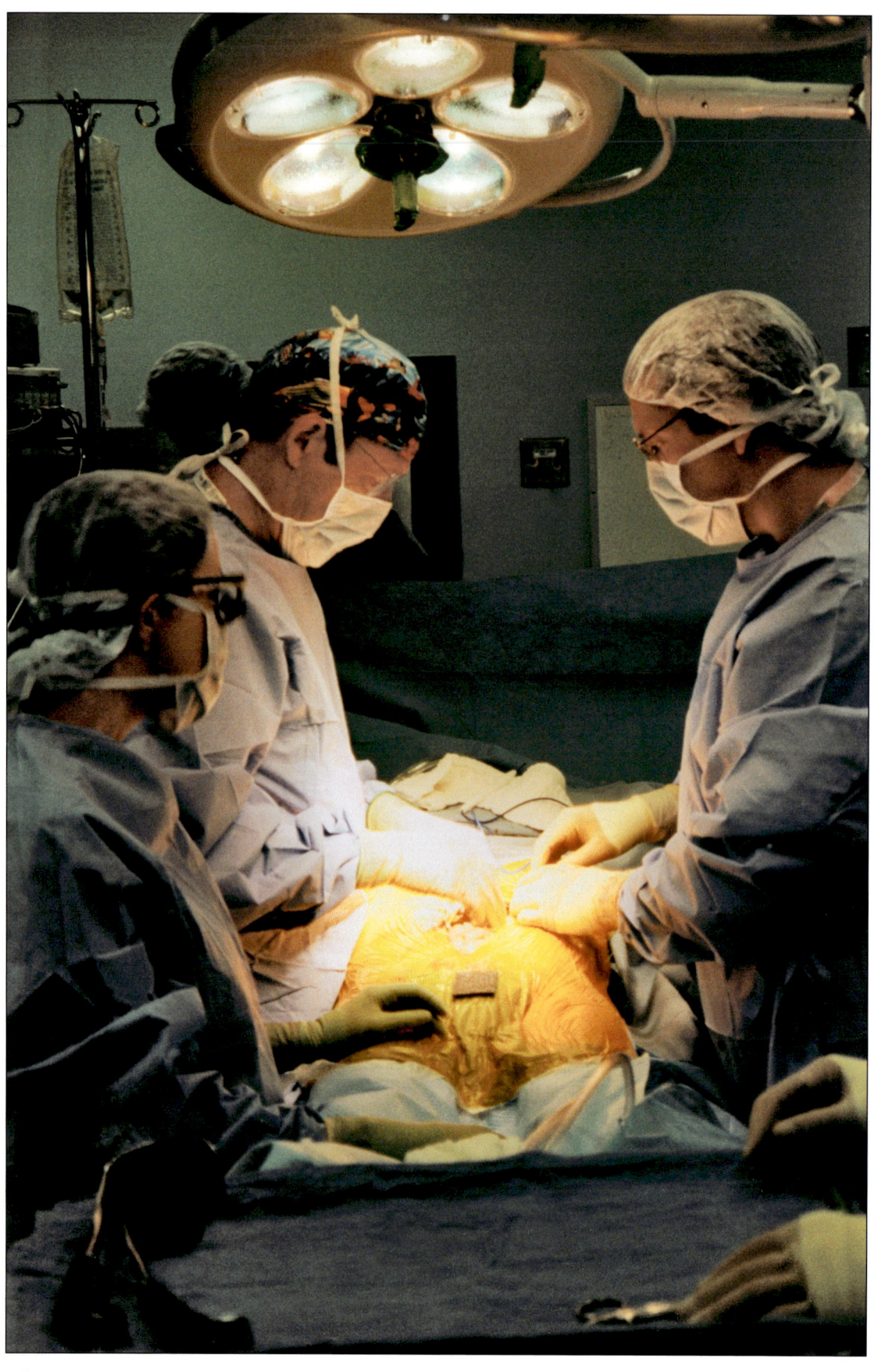

The author (DBP) left, operating with his medical student son, Jonathan Pilcher, in 1998. Julie Adams surgical resident, and later vascular attending at UVM, assisting. (Courtesy of: Douglas Halporn MD, UVM 2000.)

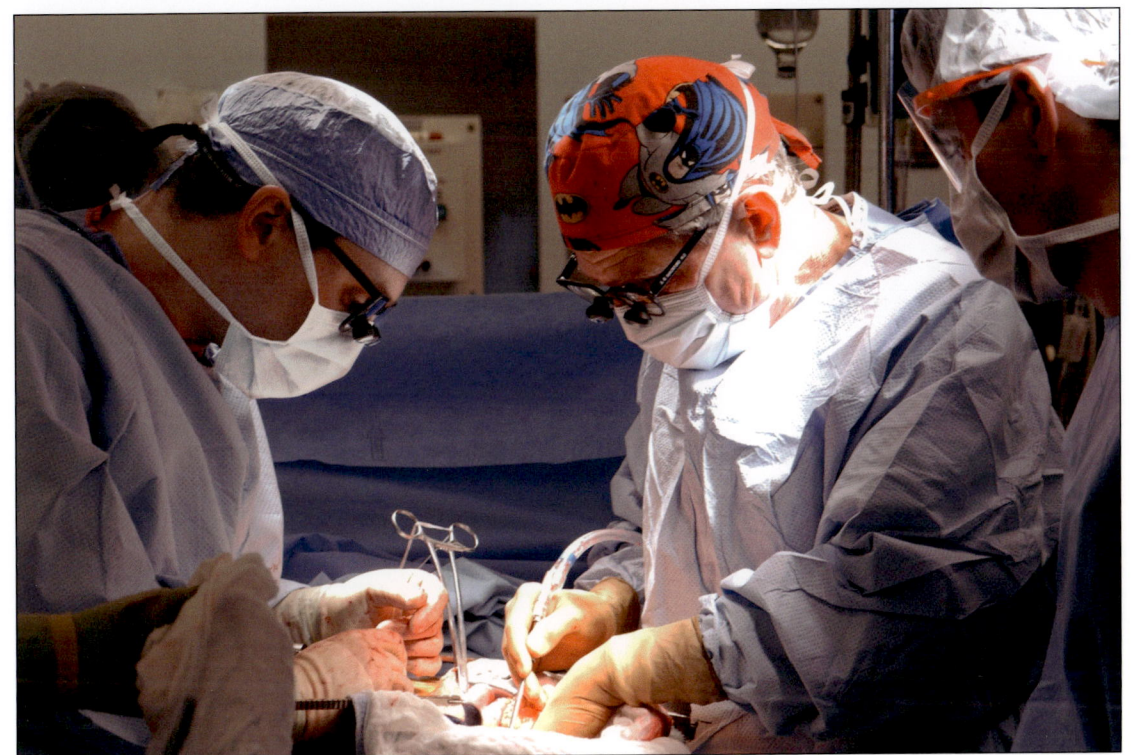

Steven Shackford (Chief of Surgery 1989-2006) operating with resident Brad Jimmo. (Courtesy of UVM Medical Photography)

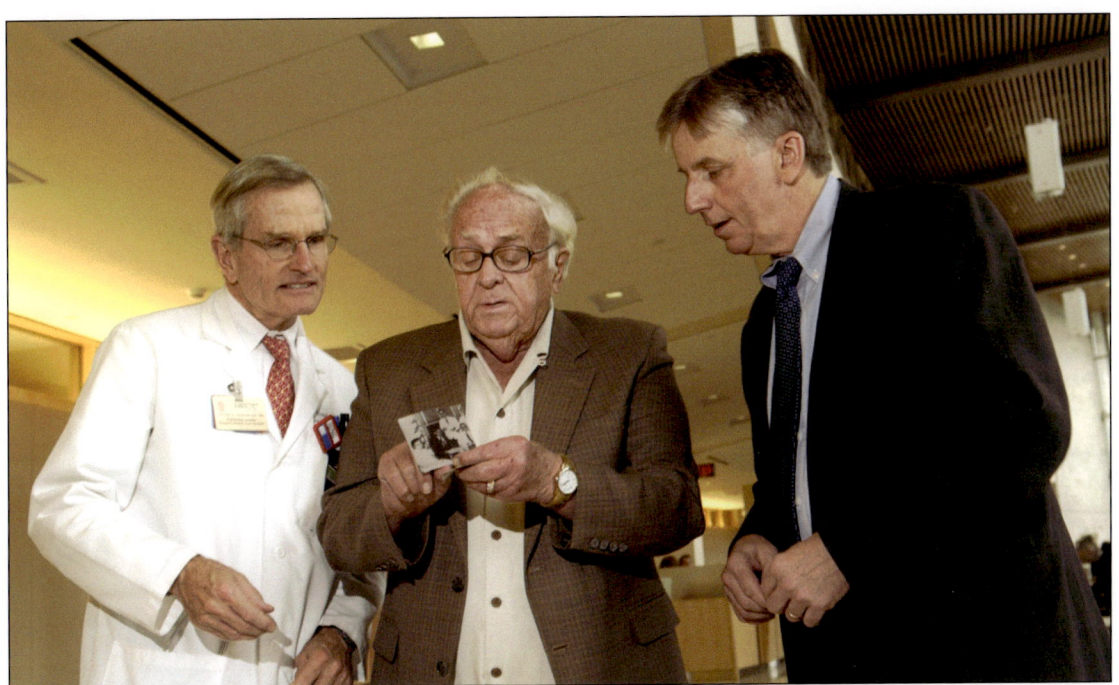

H. Gordon Page reminisces with Steven Shackford, and James Hebert on the occasion of the dedication of the Albert G. Mackay, MD, '32 and H. Gordon Page, MD, '45 Professorship of Surgery in 2005. (Courtesy of UVM Medical Photography)

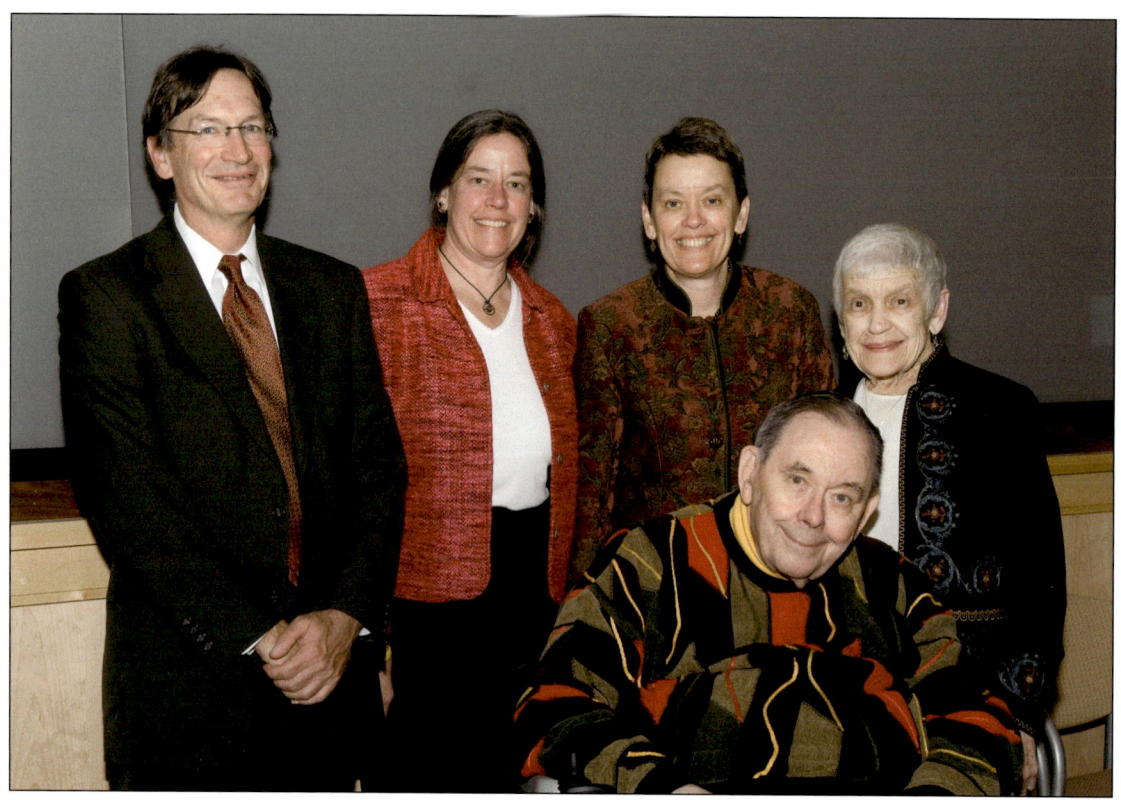

John Davis with his past resident William Cioffi (now Chair of the Department of Surgery at Brown Medical School), and L to R: daughters Halle Davis, Wendy Davis and wife Peg Davis in 2007. (Courtesy of UVM Medical Photography)

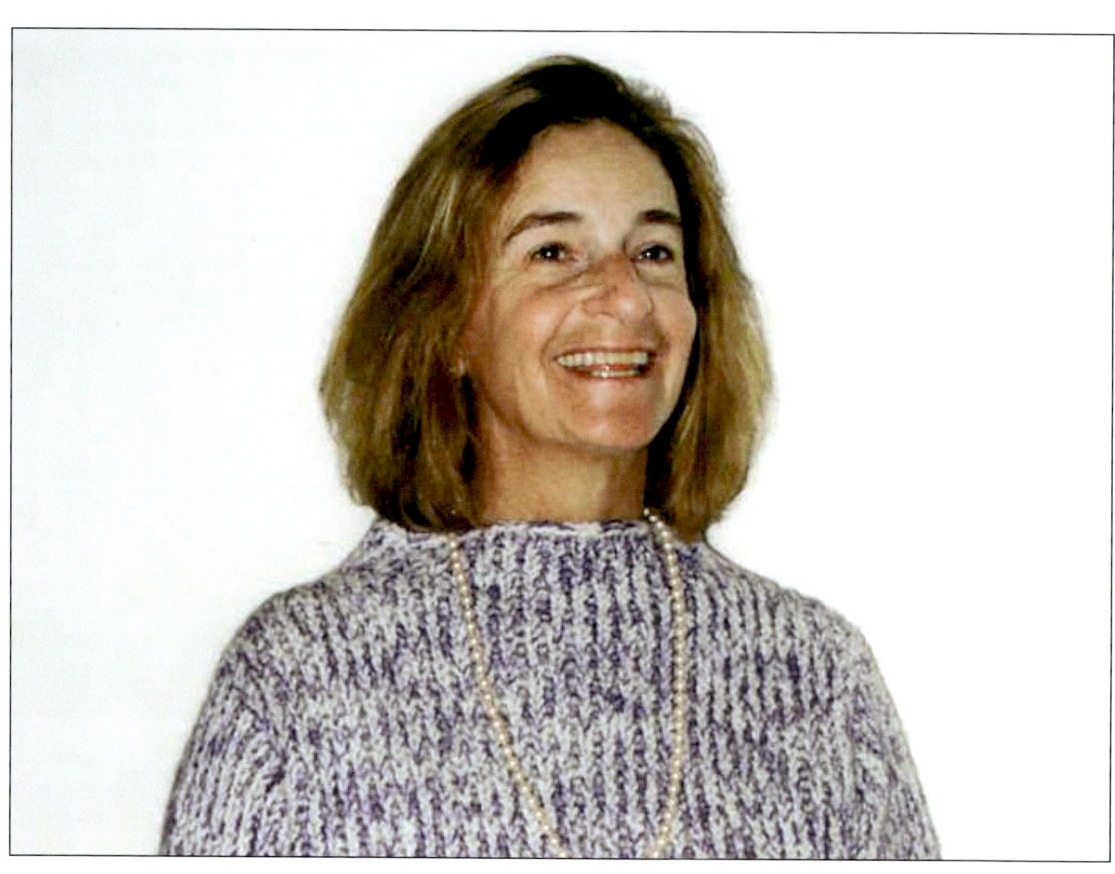

My most lifesaving procedure was tying the knot with Suzanne. (Photography by the author, DBP)

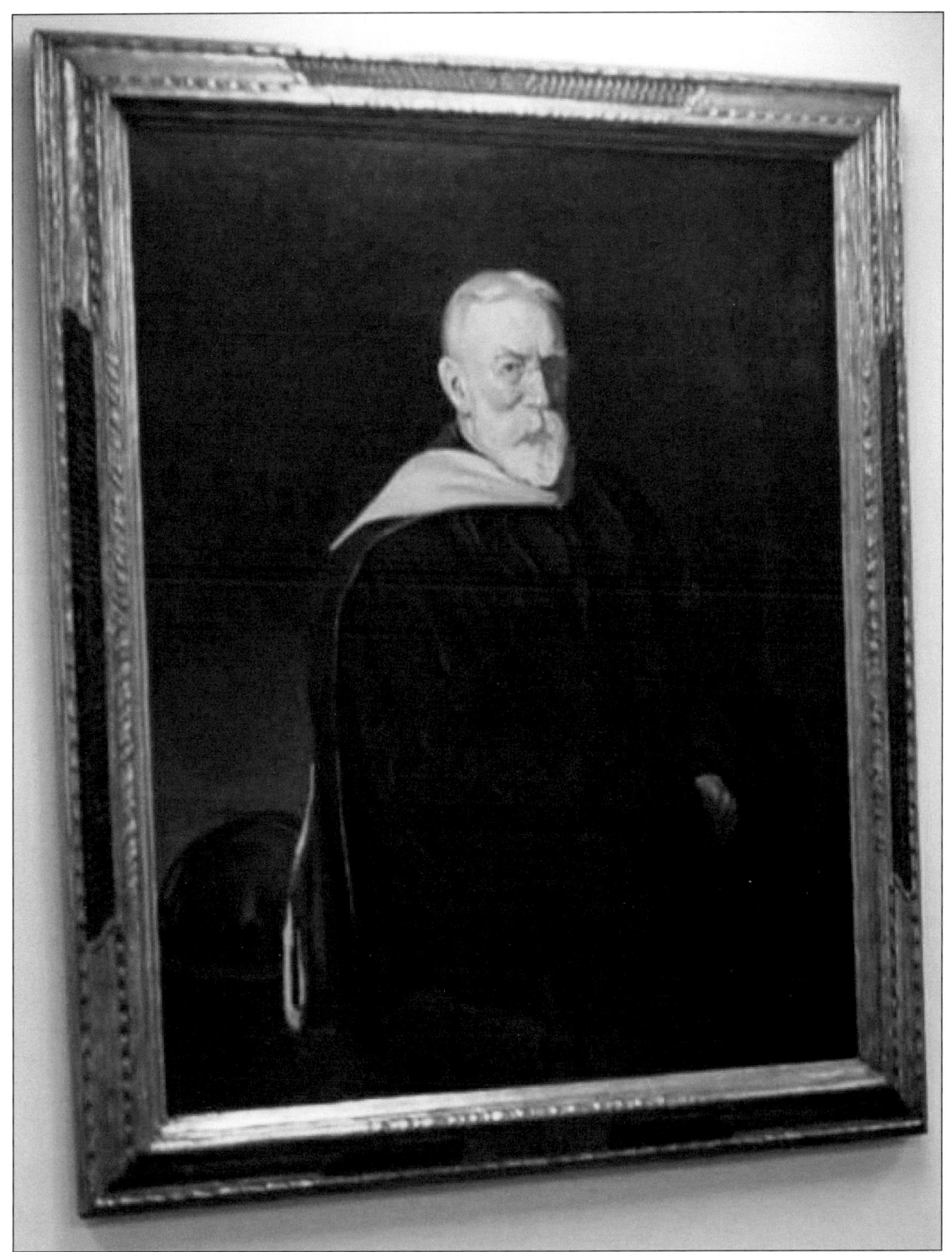

JOHN BROOKS WHEELER
PROFESSOR OF SURGERY, UVM 1900-1924
*Portrait commissioned by the class of 1927
located in the Abrams Library, UVM. (Courtesy of Surgical Archives,
Fletcher Allen Health Care, and UVM College of Medicine)*

Author's Preface and Acknowledgements

Dr. Who? I asked, as my mentors recounted tales of unfamiliar surgeons before my time. The same query was asked of me when I talked of my teachers and compatriots to newer doctors at UVM and elsewhere. Now in my retirement calling through to the hospital operator: "This is Dr. Pilcher, could I be connected to the operating room?" elicits the familiar response: "Dr. Who?"

My experiences at UVM started as a summer medical student fellow in 1959 visiting from Rochester NY, and now in 2009, I participate in teaching conferences and examinations as an emeritus professor. I thought this uniquely qualified me to compile the history prior to and after my own experiences. Surgery has changed dramatically over the years that UVM has participated in medical education. I have attempted to capture these changes in surgery elsewhere as well as to relate unique aspects of its development in Vermont. I realize that some of the anecdotes and details are mainly of interest to the participants and their friends and relatives, but after having read many sterile histories, I have attempted to keep this a little more lively and personal.

Julius Jacobson was my first inspirational role model in surgery at UVM and mentored me in that summer of 1959. He has been a friend and supporter ever since though we have been geographically separated. When this book was stalled getting off the ground, Julius and his wife Joan stepped up and supported the book and me.

The UVM medical community is comprised of full time and part time attending physicians. The part time attendings contribute significantly to the practice of medicine and education at UVM College of Medicine. I realize they have not been fully included, and apologize for any omissions of these physicians. Much else has been omitted, and much forgotten.

My own disorganization and writing style have been well compensated for by the amazing and prodigious assistance of Michael G. Curran, MD. Michael lived in Cincinnati, Ohio during the writing of this book, yet was able to dig out dates, facts, and references and organize and restructure beyond my own abilities. The entire book has been vastly improved by his Herculean efforts.

Michael's wife Manisha Patel, a surgeon trained at UVM, lent her support and insightful critiques to us both.

Developments in the divisions of surgery and the Departments of Anesthesia and Orthopaedics sometimes coincided with those in the Department of Surgery as a whole. Each division has its own chapter, and this led to partial duplication in recounting the overall history. The author apologizes for any confusion, as in reality it was all one story.

My wife Suzanne, read every word (several times) and corrected my train of thought as well as my grammar, and her support and encouragement have been a wonderment.

Joan Young, MS, who was editorial associate for the Journal of Trauma for many years when it was edited at UVM, helped with copy editing, as did my daughter Wendie Wulff, PhD ... whose assistance and suggestions far exceeded copy editing and developmental editing.

John Frymoyer re-wrote and edited the Orthopaedic chapter, helping me, instead of writing the history of his department independently; as he had seriously considered before our collaboration. Joe Kreutz in anesthesia contributed knowledge, text and photos as well as encouragement.

I was assisted by present and retired staff, families and friends of surgeons and the Department of Surgery who participated in interviews and contributed written and photographic memoirs, as well as encouragement. Suzanne Ferland provided valuable information. The librarian staff at UVM's Wilbur Collection of historical documents, The Dana Medical Library Archives, and the Fanny Allen Archives housed at Saint Michael's College have all been most helpful.

The people at Queen City Printers Inc. were exceedingly helpful and professional. In particular, Phil Gramling provided publishing suggestions beyond that of a printer.

Thank you to all the above.

I would never have thought writing this book would take over four years.

I hope you enjoy the story.

David B. Pilcher, MD
Burlington, Vermont
2009

Author's Note:

This book is largely based on material found in archives, and on personal interviews and recollections of people featured in the book or associated with the material. To the extent it is based on individuals' recollections, it should be understood as a memorialization of this oral history, preserved before more information could be lost to posterity on account of death or further erosion of memory. I apologize to anyone I have left out, and to anyone who may have experienced this history from a different and unrepresented perspective.

This was a huge undertaking and I realize people and events could have slipped by me, but such omissions were not made on purpose.

This book is donated to the University of Vermont with no remuneration to its authors.

About the Authors

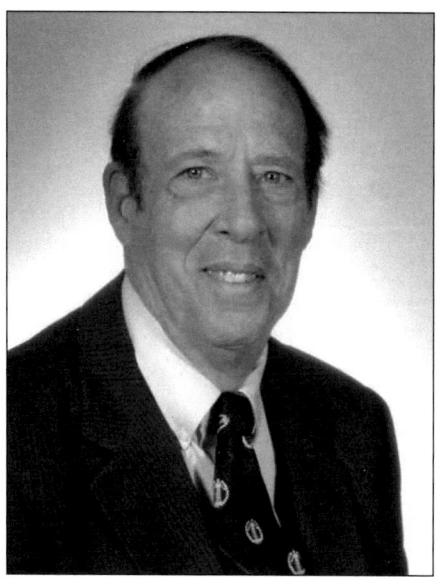

David B. Pilcher, MD, is Professor Emeritus of Surgery at UVM having first visited there in 1959 as a student fellow visiting from Rochester (NY) School of Medicine and Dentistry. He finished his surgical residency at UVM in 1966. He then spent two years as a surgeon in the army, the second of which was in Vietnam. A peripheral vascular fellowship at UCLA preceded joining the faculty at UVM.

Dr. Pilcher was an active member of the surgical faculty for 34 years, before retiring from practice in 2003. During these years he practiced Vascular Surgery, was the Chief of the Vascular Division, the Director of the Emergency Department, and the founder and first Director of the Non-Invasive Vascular Laboratory at UVM. He was President of the New England Society for Vascular Surgery, and Vice President of the New England Surgical Society. He was deputy Editor of the Journal of Trauma for 22 years, and Medical Advisor to the Smugglers Notch Ski Patrol for 30 years. He taught and upgraded Emergency Medical Services for New England as well as Vermont. He has published over 50 articles and book chapters. He lives with his wife Suzanne in Colchester, VT, and occasionally in Florida.

Michael G. Curran, MD, finished his surgical residency at UVM in 1999. He practiced surgery in Barre, VT at the Central Vermont Hospital before moving to Cincinnati, Ohio where he currently resides with his wife surgeon Manisha Patel, who also trained at UVM. Luckily Michael was able to help with the book, before his lovely daughter Meghana Maeve Curran arrived to usurp all of his free time. Michael's revisions were always thoughtful and accurate. The bibliography was carefully researched.

Dedication

This book is dedicated to all the physicians who have practiced surgery and its specialties everywhere.

This book is also dedicated to those who share their lives with surgeons on a daily basis: family, spouses, significant others and colleagues at work. This includes other health care professionals, support staff, nurses and secretaries. The debt is beyond repaying.

If surgeons seem at times not to acknowledge or appreciate this help, it only reflects that we fail to show our gratitude, not that we deny its existence.

"There are tales to be told here of epic struggles for survival and supremacy, giant egos in collision and collusion, dreams attained, hopes dashed, and talents squandered, talents recognized and encouraged, battles won and lost ...The archives are few and time is fleeting ... these remembrances will be collected in a history of the department of surgery to be written later."

(Prophetically) E. Douglas McSweeney Jr., MD, UVM Surgery newsletter, October 1992

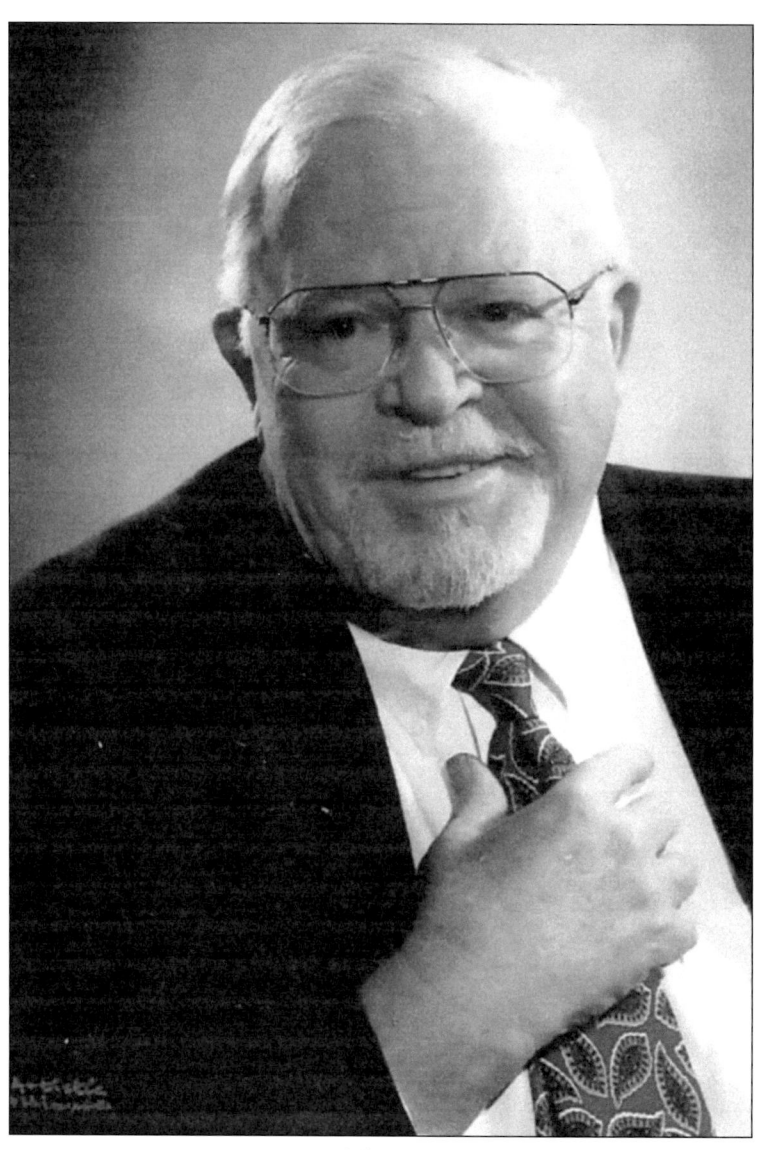

(photo courtesy of Marilyn McSweeney)

CATAMOUNT SURGEONS
Surgery and Surgical Education at the University of Vermont 1804–2008

TABLE OF CONTENTS

Introduction: Catamount Surgeons
Prelude: From Bunker Hill to Burlington

I. START AND STOP (1804-1837)
1. Pomeroy's Medical School: A Teacher Without a School
   Apprenticeship Makes a Surgeon   3
   Burlington Beckons   4
   Pomeroy Helps Establish UVM and Becomes its Second Faculty Member   5
   Pomeroy Institutes Professional Standards for Doctors   6
   UVM Grants its First Medical Degrees   7
   William Beaumont — Vermont's First Famous Research Surgeon?   8
   UVM's Fortunes Take a Turn for the Worse During the War of 1812   9
   The Most Remarkable Journal of Erastus Root   10
   Pomeroy's Hard Work Hits a Roadblock   12

2. A Medical School Without a Structure
   The College of Medicine Formally Incorporates   13
   Nathan Smith "The Johnny Appleseed of American Medicine"   13
   Smith Founds Schools at Yale, and Then Bowdoin   16
   UVM Catches Smith's Attention   16
   Pomeroy is Left Out of the New College of Medicine   17
   Smith Gets UVM Off to a Good Start   18
   Attempting to Fill Nathan Smith's Shoes   19
   Fate Brings Death of the Chief of Surgery and Fire to UVM   20
   Fortune Totally Deserts the College of Medicine   22

3. Setback: Competing Proprietary Medical Schools Take Over
   The Proprietary Medical System   23
   UVM Constructs its First Strictly Medical Building   24
   Benjamin Lincoln's Preparation to Lead UVM College of Medicine   24
   The Darker Side of Anatomy and Dissection is Revealed   26
   Lincoln "Reforms" the College of Medicine   27
   The Battle with Castleton Escalates   28
   Lincoln Runs a One Man Medical School   29
   The Fight With Castleton Comes to a Head   29
   Lincoln Struggles for Improved Medical Education   29

        The College of Medicine Fails to Revive After Lincoln's Death   31
        Edward Phelps and the "Man With a Hole in His Head"   32
        Unable to Compete, the UVM College of Medicine Closes   33

II. THE CLINICIAN TEACHING ADVENTURE BEGINS (1853-1900)

4.   The College of Medicine Reopens
        Surgery Undergoes Revolutionary Changes   37
        The College of Medicine is Re-established   38
        The Professor of Surgery Absconds With the Funds   39
        The Carpenter Surgeon   40
        UVM and the War of the Rebellion   41
        A. B. Crosby and His "Pavilion Plan" Hospital   42
        Henry Janes' Civil War Medical Journal   43
        The Professor of Surgery Becomes a Medical Innovator   48

5.   New Facilities Breathe Life Into the Program
        Surgical Techniques Change After the Civil War   51
        Lister Declares War on Pasteur's Bacteria   52
        James L. Little, the Big Surgeon   53
        The College of Medicine's First Hospital   56
        The College Gets a New Medical Building   62
        UVM's Less Than Advanced Academics   63
        A New Chairman and a New Controversy   64
        The Secret Service Surgeon   64
        An Orthopod in General Surgeon's Clothing   66
        Progress in Academic Advancement   66
        The End of the Proprietary Era   67

III. ADVERSITY AND ADAPTATION (1900-1942)

6.   Trouble at the Turn of the Century
        John Brooks Wheeler Becomes Professor of Surgery   71
        Antisepsis Gives Rise to Asepsis   74
        The Academic Clinician   74
        Fire Destroys the Second Medical Building   76
        The "Other" Professor of Surgery   79
        The Flexner Report Suggests Closing the Medical College (1910)   80
        The College of Medicine Fights Back   81
        Frances Margaret Allen and Her Hôtel-Dieu   83
        The College of Medicine Retains Its Class A Status   87

7.   New Leaders and New Hospitals Fail to Solve Old Problems
        Wheeler Relinquishes the Chair of Surgery After 25 Years   89
        Homegrown Chairman   89

Back in Trouble   92
The Bishop DeGoesbriand Hospital Opens   93
Surgery Becomes an In-hospital Specialty   95
The Nascent Department Grows   97
Vermont's First Colo-Rectal Specialist   98
The AMA Returns   99

IV. WAR AND ITS AFTERMATH (1942-1969)

8. World War II Brings Dramatic Changes to Surgery at UVM
   The Mary Fletcher Hospital Sits Proudly on the Hill   105
   The Department Continues to Grow   106
   UVM's Future Chief of Surgery Grows Up in Peacham, Vermont   107
   The Catholic Hospitals' First Surgical Instructors   110
   A Jewish Surgical Leader for the Catholic Hospital in Town   111
   Medical Education is Accelerated as a Part of the War Effort   112
   Mackay Mans the Home Front Virtually Alone   113
   Crandall's Unit was the Forerunner of the MASH   114
   A.G. Mackay is Appointed Chief of Surgery   115
   Jay Keller is the First to Return From the War   117

9. The Need for Growth
   Sub-Specialization Follows World War II   119
   UVM's First Residents Stay On as Attending Surgeons   121
   Page Becomes the Second-Busiest Surgeon in Burlington   124
   Surgical Residency During the 1950s and 60s   128
   David B. Pilcher Prepares to Become a Resident Under Mackay at UVM   128
   Gaining Acceptance at Medical School in the 1950s   129
   The Demands of Medical School (1956-1961)   130
   Surgical House Officer Years in Boston (1961-1963)   131
   Vermont Beckons (1963-1966)   132
   Mackay Tries to Embrace Academia   134
   Julius Jacobson Brings Surgical Research to UVM (1959)   135
   UVM's Early Attempts at Cardiac Revascularization   138
   Jacobson and Donaghy Join Forces   139
   Surgical Research Decelerates After Jacobson Leaves   140
   Formation of a Full Time Group Fails to Revitalize Surgery   141
   Mackay Seeks a New Leader for Surgery   142

V. MATURATION INTO ACADEMIA: THE DAVIS YEARS (1969-1989)

10. Resurrection of the Department of Surgery
    Mackay Steps Down After 27 Years as Chief of Surgery   145
    The Formation of the Medical Center Hospital of Vermont (MCHV)   147
    John Herschel Davis, Chairman for Rebirth   149

A Full-time Chief of Surgery Arrives From Out of State   150
Jerome Sanford Abrams, Vice Chair Complementary to Davis   151
Roger Sherman Foster, Oncologic Surgeon   151
David B. Pilcher, Vascular and Trauma Surgeon, Returns to Vermont   153
Amalgamation Into a Full-time Group   154
The University Health Center   156
The New Fanny Allen Hospital   156
Pagers and the Answering Service   158
Koplewitz Emigrates From St. Albans to Burlington   158
Moonlight(ing) in Vermont and Other Tales of Residency   159
The Journal of Trauma and Additional Research Come to UVM   160
Richard L. Gamelli Joins the UVM Surgery Staff   161
James C. Hebert Continues Research and Becomes the Surgeon for All Jobs   161
A Resident's View of Training in the 1980s at UVM   162
Paralysis Strikes the Chief of Surgery   164

VI. THE SHACKFORD YEARS AND BEYOND: 1989-2007

11. Tragedy and Transition: Rebirth of the Department
    The Search for a New Chair Proceeds   171
    The Surgery Staff Turns Over   173
    A Vascular Surgeon Embraces Change   173
    Shackford Recruits New Troops   174
    Financial and Administrative Reorganization   175
    Rejuvenating Research   175
    Reforming Curricula and Recognizing Academia   176
    Surgical Outcomes and Complications   178
    Non-Clinical Innovations   179
    The Great Ice Storm of 1998   182
    Fletcher Allen Health Care   184
    The World of the 80-Hour Work Week   185
    Shackford Steps Down at His Peak   186

12. The Future Will Be History

VII. THE DIVISIONS OF THE DEPARTMENT OF SURGERY

13. Anesthesia
    Anesthetics Arise During the 19th Century   193
    UVM's Original Anesthetists   194
    John Abajian Recruited as Chief of Anesthesia   195
    Abajian Goes to War With Patton   196
    Anesthesia After the War   197

        The Shift to Regional Anesthesia 198
        UVM Leads the Nation In Halothane Administration 199
        John Mazuzan, the Division's "De Facto Chief" 200
        Research Remains a Part of Abajian's Division 201
        UVM Finally Gets an ICU and a Recovery Room 202
        A New Chief and Department In Name Only 203
        UVM Leads the Nation in Pediatric Spinal Anesthesia 204
        Music in the Operating Room 205
        The New Department Nearly Falls Apart 206
        Howard Schapiro Rebuilds the Department 207

14. Orthopaedic Division/Department
        Orthopaedists Are Found in Vermont in the 19th Century 209
        The First Spine Fusion by a Vermont Orthopaedist? 210
        David Bosworth Starts a 47 Year Career as a Teacher at UVM College of Medicine 211
        Orthopaedic Handicapped Children's Clinics 213
        The First Recognized Ruptured Disc Removal 214
        Vermont Gets Orthopaedists after WW II 215
        Orthopaedics Seeks Departmental Status 217
        The New Chief of Orthopaedics Starts Out by Taking a Sabbatical Year 217
        John W. Frymoyer, First Orthopaedic Resident at UVM 218
        Sports Medicine Assumes Priority and Prominence at UVM 220
        Scoliosis Becomes a Vermont Focus 221
        Physicians' Assistants Start at UVM in Orthopaedics 222
        Hoaglund Takes a Second Sabbatical 222
        UVM Forays Into Foot and Ankle Surgery 223
        Frymoyer Takes a Sabbatical to Begin Spine Research 224
        Frymoyer Returns From Sabbatical With UVM in Crisis 224
        Research Grows at UVM 225
        Trauma Finds a New Leader in Thomas Kristiansen 229
        Sports Medicine Continues to Grow at UVM 229
        Frymoyer Moves Up to Be CEO of UHC 229
        Howe Steps Down as Chair of Orthopaedics and Nichols Takes Over 230
        Knee Arthroscopy Comes to Vermont 231
        Rebirth of an Orthopaedic Hand Section 232
        Struggles to Restart Foot and Ankle Surgery 232
        Orthopaedic Research Continues 233

15. Cardiothoracic Surgery Division
        Thoracic Injuries Were Treated By Surgeons for Years 235
        Cardiac Surgery Begins at UVM in the 1950s 236
        Cardiac Surgery is Halted Twice at UVM 239

UVM Gets a New Cardiac Leader and Transiently a Thoracic Surgery
    Residency   239
Double-Teaming Cardiac Surgery   241
UVM's Future Cardiac Surgery Leader Emerges   242
UVM Requires a Couple of Transfusions   243
Leavitt Leads a New England Registry and Learns a French Valve Repair   246
Physicians Assistants   247
1997 Brings a New Face to Cardiac Surgery   248
Schmoker Adds Research and New Talents to the Cardiac Program   248
New Frontiers   249

16. Dentistry, Oral and Maxillofacial Surgery Division
    Dentists Are Supplanted by Oral and Maxillofacial Surgeons   251
    UVM's General Dental Residency   251
    The Faculty Grows During the 1970s   253
    Relocation and Adaptation   254

17. Emergency Medicine Division
    Early Emergency Room Care   255
    The Medical Society's Bright Idea   256
    Multiple Emergency Rooms Eventually Merge   257
    Beside the Lake in the Winter of 1970   257
    Surgery Teams with Epidemiologist Julian Waller   258
    Ambulance Movies and M&Ms   259
    Burlington Fire Department Ambulance and College Student Ambulance
        Services   261
    Advanced EMT Training at UVM   262
    Vermont EMT Course Has an Animal Cardiac Model   262
    Emergency Room Physicians Arrive at UVM   263
    The Vermont Amtrak Disaster: Spring 1984   264
    1985 Emergency Room Remodeling   265
    Clinicians Perform Trauma Ultrasounds   266
    Helicopter Ambulances in Vermont   267
    A New Emergency Room and a Changing of the Guard   268

18. Colorectal/Bariatric/Minimally Invasive Surgery Division
    UVM's First Colorectal Surgeons   269
    Gladstone and Koplewitz Join Forces   271
    Hyman and Cataldo Usher in a New Era   272
    The Community Surgeon Connection   273
    Bariatric Surgery Section Slowly Grows   274
    Minimally Invasive Surgery Comes to UVM   275
    The Next Generation   276

19. Oncology Surgery Division
  UVM's Early Breast Cancer Research 279
  The Sentinel Node Ignites UVM 280
  Help Arrives Just in Time 282
  Surgical Oncology Adopts Ultrasound 283
  Oncology Surgeons Tackle Liver Resections 283
  New Faculty and New Frontiers 284

20. Trauma and Critical Care Division
  Trauma Surgery Lags at UVM 287
  The Division of Trauma and Critical Care 288
  Burn Care at UVM 288
  Davis Promotes Trauma Research 291
  The Pilcher-Moore Shunt 292
  Advanced Trauma Life Support (ATLS) Courses Come to Vermont 292
  Vermont ACS Chapter Meetings 294
  Critical Care Matures at UVM 295
  New Faculty Recruited for Trauma and Critical Care 297
  Research Strengthens Under Shackford 299
  UVM Achieves a Level I Trauma Center First 299
  Today's Critical Care Staff 300

21. Neurosurgery Division
  Diseases of the Mind and Nervous System 301
  R.M.P. Donaghy: In the Beginning 301
  Research on a Shoestring Budget 303
  The Yasargil Connection and EC/IC 304
  Beyond Microvascular Neurosurgery 307
  Henry Schmidek Builds a Department and Then Leaves 307
  Cordell Gross Becomes Chief of a Phantom Division 309
  Tranmer Resuscitates the Division 310

22. Opthalmology Division
  Ophthalmology is Originally Combined With ENT 313
  The Twitchells of UVM 315
  A New Department Looks Into Research 316
  Opthalmology Briefly Attempts a Residency Program 317
  UVM Recruits Full-time Ophthalmologists 317
  Cataract Surgery Evolves to Intraocular Lenses 318
  1980: Happy Times and Harmony 318
  1987: The First Exodus 319
  1994: The Second Exodus 320
  An Unlikely Ophthalmologist Prepares to Come to Vermont 320

    2005: The Third Exodus 323
    A New Division at UVM 324

23. Otolaryngology Division
    Horace Green: Vermont ENT Pioneer 325
    UVM's Early Otolaryngologists 326
    The First Chief of ENT 327
    An "Un-needed" Surgeon is Put in Charge 329
    Sofferman Assumes Control Three Years Out of Fellowship 329
    Challenges Arise During the 1990s 331
    A New Era Unfolds 332

24. Pediatric Surgery Division
    Mackay Builds UVM's Program with a Pediatric Surgeon 335
    UVM's Second Pediatric Surgeon 337
    Dennis Vane Fills the Pediatric Surgery Void 337
    UVM Needs Two Pediatric Surgeons 338
    Pediatric Trauma: How Old is Too Old? 339
    Back to Basics 340

25. Plastic Surgery Division
    Early Plastic Surgery at UVM 341
    Plastic Surgery Comes to Vermont in 1955 342
    Linton Arrives in Burlington 343
    A Unique Search Committee Hires a Plastic Surgeon 344
    The Plastic Surgeons Engage in Outreach Programs 345
    Trabulsy Walks into Plastic Surgery 345
    Vignettes of Microvascular Plastic Surgery in Three Decades 347
    What Would You Do if You Contracted Hepatitis C? 349
    Another New Plastic Surgeon is Hired 351
    The Division's Approach to Breast Reconstruction 352
    The Future 353

26. Transplant and Immunology Division
    The Recent Rise of Transplantation 355
    Kidney Transplantation Arrives at UVM in 1971 355
    Organ Procurement Then and Now 357
    The Legionnaire's Epidemic of 1977 358
    Low Urine Output Isn't Always Rejection 358
    UVM Recruits Fellowship Trained Transplant Surgeons 359
    The Montreal Transplant Connection 360

27. Urology Division
    Stone Crushers Become Skilled Specialists   363
    Visiting Professors Become Part-Time Staff   364
    Urology Residency Starts After World War II   365
    A New Chief of Urology is Recruited From the MGH   366
    The Calm Before the Storm   368
    The Perfect Storm   369
    After the Storm   369
    Urology Research Shifts Into High Gear   370
    New Horizons   370

28. Vascular Surgery Division
    Vascular Surgery has a Long Legacy   373
    Vascular Surgery Comes to UVM in the 1950s   374
    UVM's First Fellowship Trained Vascular Surgeons   375
    "Quite a Piece of Surgery"   377
    Davis Brings Vascular Specialists and Innovation to UVM   377
    It's a Vascular Team, Not a Division   379
    The Non-Invasive Vascular Laboratory   379
    Making Movies and Teaching Residents   380
    Vascular Surgery at UVM's Referral Hospitals   381
    Davis Hires a New Vascular Surgeon but Forgets to Tell the Dean   381
    Shackford Takes Over Thoracic Outlet Syndrome Care   383
    Ultrasound Comes to Vascular Surgery via the Caribbean   384
    The Dawn of the Endograft Era   385
    Vascular Surgery Partners With a Podiatrist   387
    New Blood Arrives at UVM as Communities do Fewer Vascular Cases   388
    The Vascular Study Group of Northern New England   390
    The Present Faculty Comes Together   390

29. UVM Frontline Surgeons and the Evolution of Forward Surgical Hospitals
    The Evolution of Frontline Surgical Hospitals   393
    William I. Shea: 30th Portable Surgical Hospital: Pacific Theater, 1944-45   394
    Albert J. Crandall: 1st American Airborne Surgical Team: European
      Theater, 1944   396
    Crandall's Team is Operational in France Before the D-Day Invasion   397
    John H. Davis: 8209th Mobile Army Surgical Hospital: Korea, 1951   400
    David B. Pilcher: 48th Medical Detachment (KA Team): Vietnam, 1967-68   403
    A Patient From Vietnam Reconnects   405
    Matthew A. Conway: 947th Forward Surgical Team: Afghanistan, 2002
      and Iraq, 2003   406
    Gino T. Trevisani: 691st Forward Surgical Team: Afghanistan, 2003-04
      and Iraq, 2008   407

Michael A. Ricci: 158th Medical Group: Iraq, 2006-07   408
A Legacy of Service to Vermont   410

Appendices
- A. Chiefs of Surgery at UVM College of Medicine   430
- B. Graduates of the Residency Programs
  1. General Surgery   431
  2. Anesthesiology   434
  3. Orthopaedic Surgery   438
  4. Neurosurgery   440
  5. Otolaryngology   441
  6. Urology   441
- C. General Surgery Teacher of the Year as Selected by the Residents   442
- D. Orthopaedic Teacher of the Year as Selected by the Residents   442
- E. Major Donors to UVM Department of Surgery   443

Introduction: Catamount[1] Surgeons

Vermont is a way of life, at times inexplicably divergent and following the path less traveled. The metamorphosis of learning and teaching surgery took place despite seemingly insurmountable obstacles of size and place.

This story begins with and in the state of Vermont. To understand what is about to unfold, some understanding of "the state of Vermont" will be helpful. In 1791 UVM was chartered and the state of Vermont was admitted to the union as the 14th state. Vermont was barely settled, and known for the ingenuity and independence of her people. Today, some 200 years later, Vermont is still a small and rural state, whose people, if given the chance, still prefer to do things by themselves, with their own resources, in their own way. Giving credit to Vermont's popular adopted poet, Robert Frost: Vermont is a way of life, at times inexplicably divergent and following the path less traveled.[2]

In Vermont, the metamorphosis of learning and teaching surgery from hands-on apprenticeship, often at the scenes of crises, into institutionalized accredited education drawing on formal lectures, textbooks and experiences took place despite seemingly insurmountable obstacles of size and place. Some sudden changes of course failed. There were some spectacular successes. Some paths proved to be dead ends. Evolutionary change brought varied results.

But, in the end, surgery and surgical education in Vermont — with The University of Vermont's College of Medicine's Department of Surgery in the leadership role, grew to become a well respected consortium of surgical sub-specialists.

This book highlights selected, historical excerpts from the Department's journey. It begins with early surgical preceptors who somehow successfully practiced surgery while teaching those who were to become new surgeons in other, more distant rural communities. It ends by shedding light on selected contemporary surgeons and educators from selected sub-specialties. Individuals, settings, and events are portrayed as pertinent to the metamorphosis.

The transformation to academia faltered and at times fell back, but the department has entered the 21st century with quality surgical education and significant contributions on the national scene.

The Vermont way of achieving these changes has at times been uniquely Vermont, at times leading, in the mainstream of, or behind surgical transformation in general. The story may not be universally applicable, but then, it is uniquely Vermont.

---

[1] The Catamount is the mascot of the University of Vermont.

[2] With apologies to Robert Frost and his poem "The road not taken" Frost R. Mountain interval. (New York: Henry Holt, 1916).

Prelude: From Bunker Hill to Burlington.

It is well known that the University of Vermont sits on land donated by Ethan Allen's brother Ira. What may come as a surprise, though, is that the University's affiliated teaching hospitals, the College of Medicine, and the Department of Surgery, can also trace their roots back to Allen's Green Mountain Boys and their fellow veterans from Ticonderoga, Bunker Hill, and the Siege of Boston.

Following the Battles of Lexington and Concord, Colonial leaders scrambled to obtain supplies and fortify strategic locations. Their attention soon turned to Fort Ticonderoga on the western edge of Lake Champlain. Ethan Allen, a military veteran with extensive knowledge of the region, was dispatched to take the citadel and the heavy weaponry it contained.

Allen, in conjunction with his brothers Ira and Heman, Eleazer Claghorn, and Noah Phelps, assembled over one hundred of his Green Mountain Boys for the attack. Shortly after midnight on May 10, 1775, the "Boys" stormed through a gap in the fort's crumbling ramparts. Ethan roused the outpost's commander from bed and demanded an immediate surrender. The startled officer, pants still in hand, complied.[1]

Back in Boston, the British were backed into a corner. If the Colonists could fortify Bunker Hill to the north or Dorchester Heights to the south, the English Army would have to evacuate the city. The Americans, however, mistakenly dug in on nearby Breed's Hill.

On June 17, 1775, the Redcoats charged the Patriot positions. The Rebels held firm, but eventually withdrew after running out of ammunition. Surgeons Thomas Kittredge and John Warren tended to the wounded militiamen well into the night.

A stalemate ensued over the next several months. The British were afraid of suffering more casualties and the Americans did not have the resources to support an assault. General Benjamin Lincoln organized and drilled the Colonial troops as the Siege wore on, while surgeon's mates James Bradish, John Thomas, and Josiah Waterous helped treat the increasing numbers of ill and injured soldiers.

That December, a crew of men retrieved Ethan Allen's spoils from Ticonderoga. The sixty tons of weaponry were floated across Lake Champlain and then dragged over the Berkshires during the dead of winter. Shortly after reaching Boston, the fifty-nine big guns were positioned on Dorchester Heights. The British launched one futile attack, but came up short. Under mutual agreement, the Americans let the Tories retreat in peace; the British, in turn, did not raze Boston to the ground as they left.[2]

The resolution of the Siege of Boston on March 17, 1776 marked not only the end of major hostilities in New England, but also the beginning of the end of British rule over the thirteen colonies. Ticonderoga's cannons had clearly tipped the scales in the Patriots' favor. The ability of the Vermonters to act independently and take the lead in a worthwhile fight proved crucial to the American cause.

Several years later, the same small group of Green Mountain Boys, New England Militiamen, and their descendents proved crucial to another cause — the establishment of surgical training at the University of Vermont. Ira Allen donated the land upon which the University is situated. Heman Allen's heirs settled the site now occupied by the Mary Fletcher Hospital. Ethan Allen's daughter, Fanny, provided the inspiration for the nearby institution that bears her name. And the soldiers, surgeons, and commanders mentioned above trained and influenced the College of Medicine's founders and its earliest professors of surgery. Each of these professors, in turn, played a vital role in the metamorphosis of the small school into a nationally known center for surgical research and patient care.

References, Prelude
[1] Davis KS. "In the name of the Great Jehovah and the Continental Congress!" American Heritage Magazine, 1963; 14: 65-77.
[2] Hamilton EP, Fort Ticonderoga: Key to a continent. (Boston: Little, Brown & Co., 1964): 129-131.

PART I
START AND STOP
1804-1837

CHAPTER 1

Pomeroy's Medical School: A Teacher Without a School

A 15 year-old farm boy turned surgeon's mate began a lifelong career in medicine during the midst of the Revolutionary War. Twenty-five years later, he became the first professor of surgery at the University of Vermont.

John Pomeroy strove to legitimize medical education and develop a model of preceptorship and physician peer review over a period of two decades. Unfortunately, he lacked the infrastructure and finances to support his efforts.

In the end although he had worked hard to develop a medical school and witnessed his efforts come to fruition, he was left out of the results. He was a successful teacher without a school.

Apprenticeship Makes a Surgeon

Revolutionary War surgeons, more often than not, were self-proclaimed "doctors" trained under the time-honored but inconsistent apprenticeship method. They were assisted in their treatments by a "surgeon's mate." The mate was usually an industrious soldier with a steady hand, a calm stomach, and an interest in medicine.[1] John Pomeroy of Middleboro, Massachusetts was one such soldier turned mate. He had left the family farm at age 15 in 1779 to join the 9th Massachusetts Regiment. Within three months, he had become the regiment's mate beneath surgeon John Thomas.[2] Pomeroy resumed farming following his military service, but devoted all of his spare time to the acquisition of knowledge. In 1784, he apprenticed himself to one of Thomas' surgical colleagues from the Siege of Boston, James Bradish of Cummington, Massachusetts.[3, 4]

Pomeroy lived and studied with Bradish for three years. As a typical apprentice of the time, he assisted Bradish with all medical chores, organized his office, took care of his horses, collected his bills, and performed any other duties deemed necessary. He not only accompanied Bradish on calls to see patients, but also visited them by himself if his mentor was indisposed. In return, Pomeroy received appropriate instruction from Bradish and permission to read his books. He participated in dissections if and when cadavers were available. In addition, Pomeroy was given meals and a place to stay.[5] The system was relatively adequate as long as the preceptor was well trained and had an interest in teaching. Luckily for Pomeroy, this was the case.

After completing his apprenticeship in 1787, Pomeroy moved to the recently chartered town of Cambridge, Vermont. There he started what soon became a large and lucrative practice.[6] But the remote setting presented many logistical challenges. During one spring thaw, Pomeroy was summoned to help with a difficult pregnancy. The patient lived deep in the woods near a stream, three miles from her nearest neighbor. By the time Pomeroy reached the brook, it had risen so high that his horse could barely cross it. The patient's house, in the meantime, had been engulfed by the torrent and was filling with water. With the help of the woman's husband and a nurse already on the scene, the industrious physician built a temporary shelter on higher ground where he conducted the delivery.[7]

Burlington Beckons

Although Cambridge was no smaller than any other Vermont town of the time, relative isolation and poor soil limited its potential for future growth. Perhaps sensing this, Pomeroy decided it was time to make another move. He relocated to Burlington, a town of 332 residents, in 1792. Access by stagecoach was limited and the arrival of the railroad was still 56 years away! But as a lumber port on the Lake Champlain inland waterway, the city soon benefited from increased trade and travel. Pomeroy's business immediately flourished. In 1797 he built the town's first brick house on Water Street. Shortly thereafter, he began to attract students who knew of his scholarly approach and teaching excellence. His home, the site of his medical lectures, had an extensive library of medical texts. Apprentices came from all over the state to study with him. "University degrees were not necessary for the practice of medicine and were indeed looked upon as a pleasant but not indispensable part of a physician's equipment."[8]

Pomeroy was described as "a man of robust constitution and great energy of character." The following three excerpts are illustrative:

"In a case of white swelling [tuberculosis] in the knee-joint, the doctor, regardless of the doctrine or dogma of the time that no opening of the joint and consequent discharge of the synovia could be tolerated, opened the swelling and discharged a large quantity, and all of the fluid in the joint, with dozens of secretions in the form and appearance of small white beans — and the patient recovered the full use of his limb." [9]

"He performed double amputation in the lower third of the femur upon a patient whose condition was most critical at the time and who had been pronounced incurable by associate physicians. Only one of those who had examined the case consented to be present at the operation, and he, even refusing to share the responsibility, being simply willing to grace the occasion by his presence. The doctor ... resolute in his conviction of the feasibility of the operation, decided to do it, and the result fully attested the correctness of his judgment. When we remember that anesthetics were unknown at this time, that no Esmarch had arisen to prevent hemorrhage, no Lister had furnished an antidote to septic germs ... we should be surprised to learn of his patient's complete recovery." [10]

"On one occasion he was summoned to attend a case of laryngitis and found the patient asphyxiated, on a rude bed in the hold of a vessel anchored at the dock. Comprehending the gravity of the situation and in opposition to violent resistance on the part of friends of the

patient, he performed laryngotomy, inserting a quill into the opening, through which the patient peacefully breathed and life was restored. It was the first operation of this nature he had ever seen and had the patient died, lynch law would doubtless have been employed to prevent in the future surgical interference in such cases."[11]

Pomeroy Helps Establish UVM and Becomes its Second Faculty Member

The progressive 1777 Constitution of the Republic of Vermont called for the creation of a university. Green Mountain Boy veteran Ira Allen — seeking to improve the value of his nearby real estate — pledged fifty acres of land and £3,000 towards the school if it were to be located in Burlington. The University of Vermont finally received its charter in November 1791, eight months after the state was admitted to the Union. The land was allocated, but Allen was unable to provide the promised funds. As a result, the University could not begin classes.[12, 13]

Burlington was in need of both a minister and a church when, in 1799, the Unitarian church in nearby Vergennes relieved its pastor, the Reverend Daniel Clarke Sanders, of his duties. Upon hearing the news, Pomeroy and an associate rode south and persuaded the reverend to come to town. The two agreed to pay his wages for the next year. They also suggested that he take an academic appointment at the new school.[14]

Although Sanders, a Harvard graduate, started preaching in the county courthouse the next year, his real interest lay in the establishment of the University. He was elected its president and sole professor within months of his arrival. Meanwhile, Pomeroy helped conduct a

FIGURE 1-1.
Medicine and surgery were taught in UVM's original 1804 College Building from 1815 until 1824, when it was destroyed by arson.

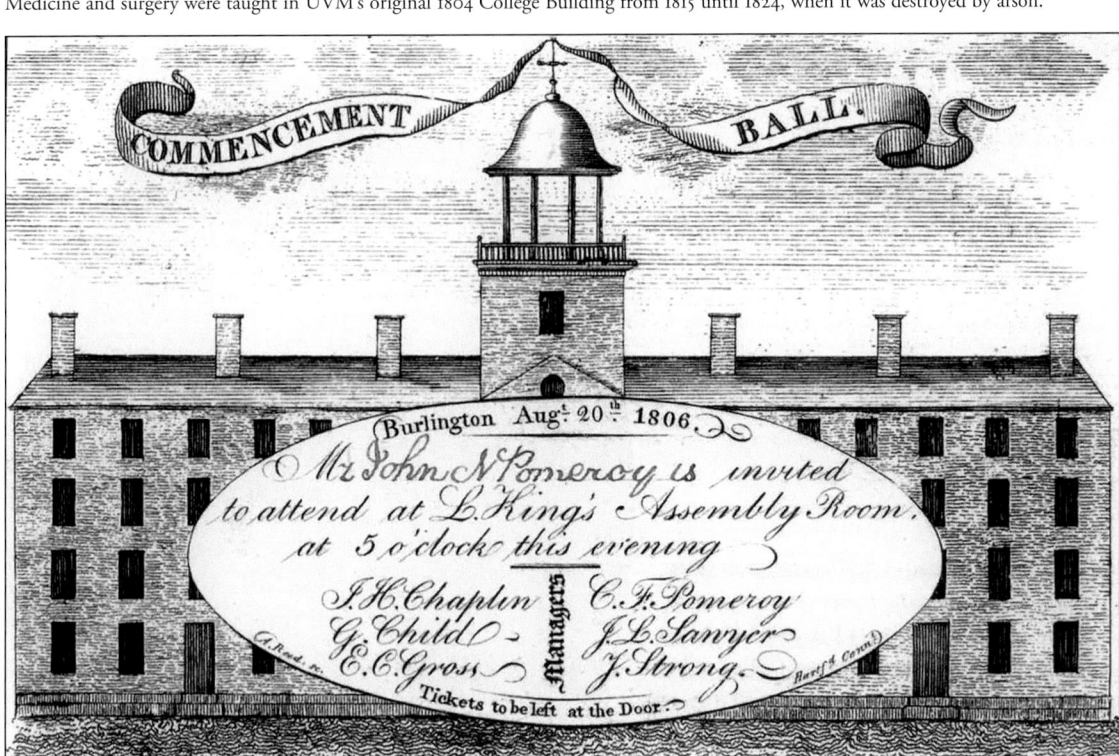

Chapter One: Pomeroy's Medical School

public campaign that raised $2,300 for the purchase of building materials, books, and other supplies. In addition, he supported an endowment to cover the president's salary for the next three years. Reverend Sanders pitched in by clearing trees from the site of the future College Building (completed in 1804) and by holding the school's first classes in his house in 1800.[15, 16]

Pomeroy was conducting classes of a sort at the same time. Having been in practice for more than a dozen years, he had started teaching pupils the basics of medical and surgical care. Some stayed only a few days or weeks, but others completed months of training. Pomeroy took pleasure in giving lessons and his students appreciated his efforts. His actions were not undertaken for financial gain, as "it was considered extravagant on the part of the students to pay and undignified on the part of the professors to receive."[17]

Pomeroy's next step was to bring some legitimacy to his medical instruction. He approached the University's board of trustees in 1804 and presented his case. His argument must have been persuasive, since the trustees unanimously voted to make Pomeroy the school's second faculty member. As lecturer in "chirurgerie and physic" (surgery and medicine), he was expected to give a course in both subjects once a year.[18] Like Sanders, Pomeroy continued to teach in his own home. Unlike the president though, the doctor did not receive a salary. Instead, he was partially supported by voluntary contributions from students.[19]

Pomeroy Institutes Professional Standards for Doctors

There were no educational or licensing requirements regarding the actual practice of medicine during this period. Only a handful of physicians could afford to study at the great universities of England, Scotland, Germany and Austria. And even though medical schools had opened in Philadelphia, New York, Boston, Hanover, NH, and Lexington, KY by 1800, possession of a degree was still unusual. In fact, fewer than 400 physicians had medical degrees at the time.[20] A diploma may have given a doctor a little added prestige in the community, but it did not provide an advantage when it came to treating patients. Most physicians and surgeons still obtained their entire education by apprenticing with other practitioners. Some hung out a shingle after undergoing little or no training at all!

Pomeroy was distressed that the community was unable to differentiate between incompetent "quacks" and skilled physicians. In response, he founded the "Third Medical Society" in 1803. The Society recognized properly trained doctors living in the greater Burlington area by awarding them a license to practice. Potential members were examined by "censors" and expected to know "the theory of anatomy, animal functions in their natural and diseased state, and of the remedies in general use both simple and compound."[21] The idea was "to regulate medical practice by drawing a distinction between the qualified physicians, who were admitted to the society, and the 'empirics' [quacks], who continued to treat the ill."[22]

A decade later, through Pomeroy's efforts, the regional medical societies were consolidated into the Vermont State Medical Society. This society assumed the role of a licensing agency. Students were expected to pass a "strict examination" in order to secure a license. Applicants were to study from a list of books that included Benjamin Bell's 1791 six-volume masterpiece, A System of Surgery.[23]

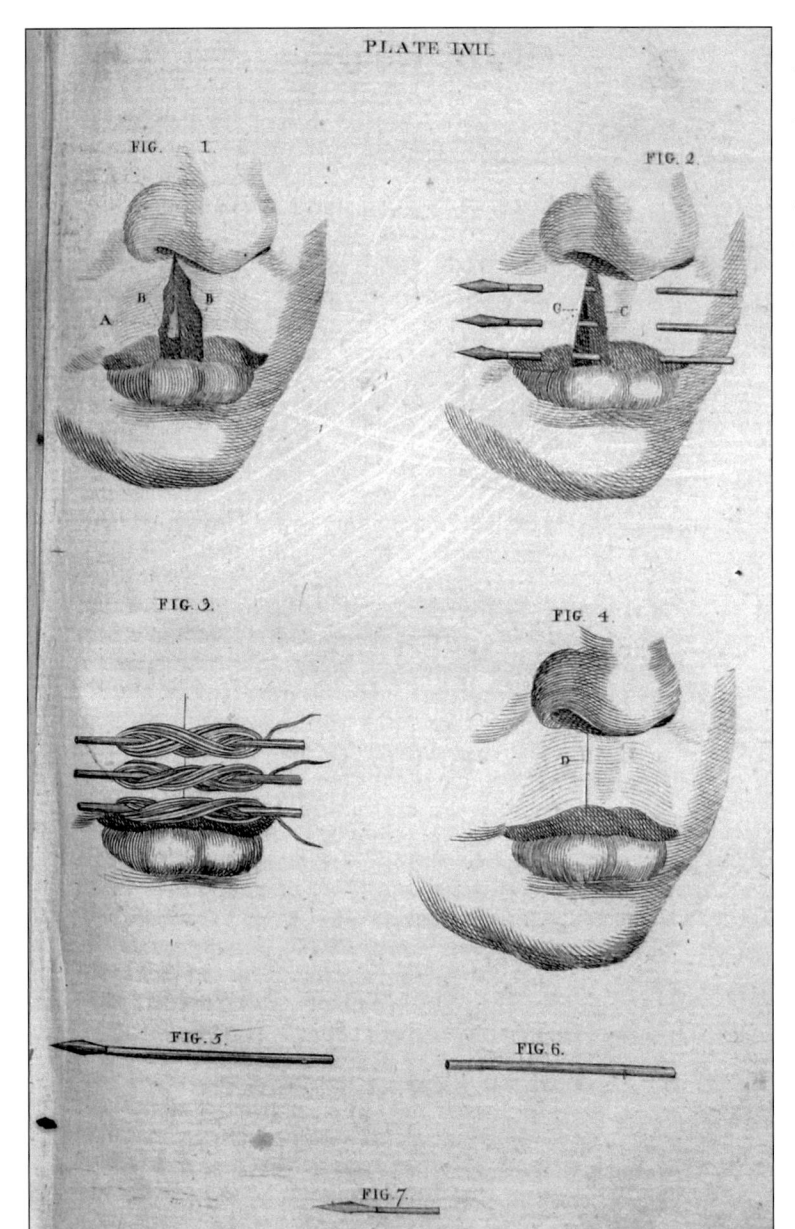

FIGURE 1-2. Among the texts in Pomeroy's library was Benjamin Bell's 1796 edition of, A System of Surgery. Teachers and students alike studied this illustration of "Hare Lip" reconstruction. Pomeroy and Nathan Smith both performed such operations in the early 19th century.

UVM Grants its First Medical Degrees

One of Pomeroy's students, Truman Powell, delivered a dissertation before the board of trustees in August of 1809 "on the use and action of Mercury on the human system."[24] Impressed with the presentation, the trustees conferred a Bachelor of Medicine degree on Powell. Pomeroy was promoted from lecturer to full professor of "anatomy and surgery, and of the theory and practice of physic." More notably, he was given an honorary Doctorate of Medicine — his first degree of higher education! The day after Powell's talk, the board voted to bestow a "Bachelor of Physic" degree on "any person who has been licensed to practice physic by any Medical Society established by law, and has attended two courses of lectures delivered by the professor of medicine."[25]

The University of Vermont was quite progressive in one respect. By making a license from a medical society a prerequisite, the University (and by extension, Pomeroy) ensured that its ing medical degrees at most other institutions did not necessarily know or even care if a student had received an adequate education. Pomeroy's idea that physicians should license other physicians and determine the adequacy of their training was somewhat advanced for his day.

Not long after Pomeroy received his honorary MD degree in 1809, Edinburgh-trained Ephraim McDowell of Danville, Kentucky became the first surgeon in the United States to successfully remove an ovarian cyst. As McDowell later wrote: *"The intestines as soon as the opening was made, ran out upon the table, remained out for thirty minutes, and being upon Christmas day, they became so cold that I thought proper to bathe them in tepid water previous to my replacing them; I then returned them, stitched up the wound, and she was perfectly well in twenty-five days."* Even though McDowell excised the twenty-pound cyst with his bare hands on a kitchen table, the patient lived for another thirty-one years.[26]

Despite the triumph of McDowell's operation, abdominal surgery remained unsafe prior to the advent of anesthesia and antiseptic technique and was not performed in this country by others. Abdominal wounds were largely fatal during this period. Patients either succumbed within hours from hemorrhage, or within days from infection.

William Beaumont — Vermont's First Famous Research Surgeon?

In 1811, Truman Powell, UVM's first medical graduate, moved thirty miles north to take a job with Benjamin Chandler of St. Albans. A distinguished physician in his own right, Chandler had been the recipient of the University of Vermont's second honorary MD in 1810. Powell arrived to find an apprentice in his new partner's charge named William Beaumont. The former grade school teacher had been preparing himself for a career in medicine since 1806 by reading books he had borrowed from Pomeroy. Beaumont worked under Chandler and Powell's supervision until June 1812. Upon satisfactorily completing his studies, he received a license from the Third Medical Society signed by Pomeroy, its president.[27]

Beaumont left his preceptor, moved across the lake to New York, and joined the army. He served as a surgeon's mate in the 6th infantry at the Battles of Little York and Plattsburgh during the War of 1812. After resigning his commission in January 1813, he opened an office in Plattsburgh. His license to practice was still that of the Third Medical Society of Vermont.[28]

Beaumont re-enlisted in 1819 and was sent to Fort Mackinac in Michigan. It was there, in 1822, that French-Canadian voyageur Alexis St. Martin (in Beaumont's words) *"was most dan-*

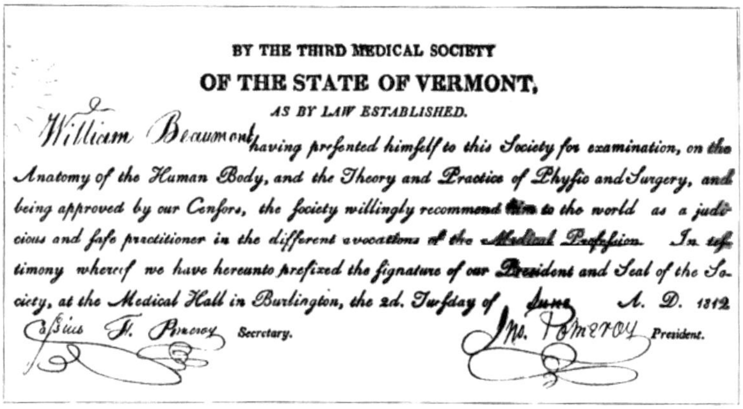
BY THE THIRD MEDICAL SOCIETY
OF THE STATE OF VERMONT,
AS BY LAW ESTABLISHED.

William Beaumont having prefented himfelf to this Society for examination, on the Anatomy of the Human Body, and the Theory and Practice of Phyfic and Surgery, and being approved by our Cenfors, the fociety willingly recommend him to the world as a judicious and fafe practitioner in the different avocations of the Medical Profeffion. In teftimony whereof we have hereunto prefixed the fignature of our Prefident and Seal of the Society, at the Medical Hall in Burlington, the 2d. Tuefday of June A. D. 1812

Caſsius F. Pomeroy Secretary.
Jno. Pomeroy President.

FIGURE 1-3. William Beaumont's license from the Third Medical Society, signed by John and Cassius Pomeroy.

gerously wounded by the accidental discharge of a heavily loaded musket. The wound was received just under the left breast, and supposed at the time to have been mortal. A large portion of the side was blown off, the ribs fractured, and openings made into the cavities of the chest and abdomen, through which protruded portions of the lungs and stomach, much lacerated and burnt, exhibiting altogether an appalling and hopeless case. The diaphragm was lacerated, and a perforation made directly into the cavity of the stomach, through which food was escaping at the time." [29]

During an era when abdominal wounds were usually lethal, St. Martin's survival was unexpected. Beaumont studied the workings of the human stomach through his patient's gastrocutaneous fistula over the next decade. In 1833, he published his findings and conclusions in the book *Experiments and observations on the gastric juice and the physiology of digestion*. The work was a landmark in experimental physiology that contributed greatly to the science of gastric digestion.[30] Although his research was conducted a decade after he left the state, his roots were from Vermont. Perhaps he can be considered Vermont's first surgical researcher.

UVM's Fortunes Take a Turn For the Worse During the War of 1812

The United States, thinking that an attack from the British Army stationed in Canada was imminent, declared war against Great Britain in 1812. Burlington, with around 1,000 inhabitants, became a site of strategic interest. The Army built an earthen battery at the north end of Water (now Battery) Street shortly after the war began. A cantonment containing a guardhouse, an armory, a powder magazine, storehouses, soldier's barracks, officer's quarters, and a hospital was constructed within a few months. The site was home to 4,000 troops by the end of the year.[31]

The hospital, Burlington's first ever, overflowed with patients suffering from infectious diseases such as smallpox, measles, and dysentery. In addition, a highly lethal form of influenza, known as *peripneumonia notha*, was running rampant through the town. At least 500 soldiers and civilians died that winter. Pomeroy's son Cassius , who had been studying medicine in Philadelphia, came home to help fight the epidemic. But within weeks of his return, he too fell victim to the scourge and died.[32]

In an effort to overcome his sorrow, Pomeroy threw himself back into the business of teaching. The trustees had established a professorship of chemistry and mineralogy in 1811, but had been unable to fill the position. Pomeroy started his own search, reasoning that a suitable candidate could also teach medical chemistry and pharmacology. In mid-1813, he convinced Jairus Kennan, a member of UVM's first graduating class, to leave New York City and take the job. The two-person faculty delivered the expanded series of medical and surgical lectures that fall.[33]

In March 1814, the Army looked to the University for housing. The trustees agreed to "rent" the College Building to the Federal government for $5,000 a year. Classes were suspended and "all the members of the institution relinquished their relationships with her [the college] and were provided with honorable dismissions to other seminaries."[34] Soldiers occupied the building for the next thirteen months. The government eventually paid the "rent," but the damage done by the troops cost $6,000 to repair — a net loss of $1,000 to the school.[35]

Pomeroy, still giving lectures in his house, was largely unaffected by the situation at the College Building. But in the fall of 1814, a logistical problem arose when twelve students — his largest group ever — signed up for classes. Pomeroy solved it by renting a nearby empty store and converting it into a classroom. Just before the session began, however, Jairus Kennan wrote to say that he could not continue to fulfill his obligations after all. At the last minute, Pomeroy asked his second son, John Norton Pomeroy (who had assisted Kennan the year before), to give the chemistry lectures. Although he did an admirable job, John Norton decided against pursuing a career with the University. He read law and became an attorney instead.[36]

Kennan resumed his position as professor of chemistry in 1815. The trustees allowed him a total salary of $500. Part of this sum was to be funded by student fees; the rest was to be paid by Pomeroy. The trustees also granted the faculty the use of four rooms in the College Building, thus marking the first time that medical lectures were held on campus.[37]

The Most Remarkable Journal of Erastus Root

One of Pomeroy's students during the fall of 1815 was Erastus Root. He had obtained his bachelor's degree from UVM in 1811 and then apprenticed with Willard Arms of Brattleboro. He returned several years later to study with Pomeroy on Arms' recommendation. Root kept a detailed diary from October 10, 1815 to February 10, 1816 that chronicled his time in northern Vermont.[38] Excerpts from 1815 give an insight into the nature of Pomeroy's instruction at UVM:

> *"Thursday, October 12, 1815*
> *Two study rooms in the upper story [of the college building] have been converted into a medical hall, a chemical hall, museum, etc."*

> *"Monday, October 16, 1815*
> *Introduced to Dr. Pomeroy this morning and agreed to put myself under his instruction. He is a man of much vivacity; his appearance manifests a strong mind and a penetrating genius. I was much impressed by this remarkable man."*

> *"Thursday, October 19, 1815*
> *Attended the reduction of a fractured thigh bone by Dr. Pomeroy. The subject was a boy about 12 years of age who had fallen from a horse and fractured his thigh. It was very handsomely reduced according to Benjamin Bell's principles. Five splints and the nine tailed bandage were used."*

> *"Friday, October 27, 1815*
> *Finished reading of Dobson's 'Edinburgh System of Anatomy.' (Andrew Fyfe's Compendious System of Anatomy, in Six Volumes published by Thomas Dobson in 1792)"*

> *"Monday, October 30, 1815*
> *I perused Cooper on the joints (Samuel Cooper's Treatise on the Diseases of the Joints, 1808.)"*

"*Tuesday, October 31, 1815*

Professor Pomeroy gave us a very eloquent and reasonable lecture on the diseases of the joints; and his remarks were demonstrated by practical observations. His pathology of those parts does not differ materially from authors on the subject; but his method of treatment may be said to differ from the practice of surgeons of the present day. After pursuing the discutient [non-operative] plan with the utmost vigor together with blistering without success, and perceiving matter to have collected in the joint, he then proceeded to foment, and never fails to make an incision thro' the capsular ligament, and cleanse the whole joint from noxious matter and even raising the patella and with the finger probe under it and inject tepid water. Dr. Pomeroy declares positively from experience in these cases that he is in no fear of an inflammation of the ligament from the incision, and different from most surgeons, he fears not the admission of air to this or any other wound, as a promoter of inflammation; but considers it rather as an healthy medicine, though he neither endeavors to admit nor prevent the access of air to wounds and ulcers.

His reasons for supposing the ligaments of the joints are not more easily inflamed than other parts, are firstly from observation. The Doctor says that in his practice, he has never seen but few instances of inflammation in the ligaments from incision, where the treatment was good and carefully attended to, though his cases in the diseases of the knee have been numerous. Secondly, the ligaments are not more highly organized, or more vascular than other organs, namely the brain, eyes, lungs, heart, etc., and everyone knows these are the organs most subject to inflammation, yet wounds in these parts recover from inflammation."

"*Wednesday, November 8, 1815*

Dr. Pomeroy returned from a patient in Westford who had fallen from her horse and fractured badly both the tibia and fibula ... it is both compound and comminuted, and several ulcers have formed. Dr. Pomeroy says he shall amputate the leg tomorrow or the next day."

"*Friday, November 10, 1815*

The medical students with Dr. Pomeroy started by 6 o'clock ... our journey [one way, was] 18 miles ... though we had paid a dollar each, we had to walk half the way ... we did not arrive until 2 o'clock.

All things were ready for the operation in a few minutes. Dr. Pomeroy then performed it in less than three minutes. The limb was off, and neatly dressed in five minutes more. We returned to Burlington the same evening, we arrived about half past eleven."

After completing the six-week course, Root took a job as a schoolmaster in Grand Isle, where he worked as a doctor also, and continued his diary. He traveled the twenty-six miles back to Burlington one day to get Pomeroy's help with a difficult case:

"*Saturday, December 16, 1815*

Phelps girl ... age three years, who had by accident got a buckshot into the trachea or wind pipe and had sank down as far as the bronchus. The patient's breath appeared some obstructed, considerable cough and evacuation of blood from the nose. Mr. Phelps engaged me to go to Burlington and advise with Dr. Pomeroy."

> *"Sunday, December 17, 1815*
>
> *He [Pomeroy] concluded that there was no other way to give relief than by suspending the patient by the feet, with the head downwards, compressing the thorax and exciting a cough; as the specific gravity and very globular body, might probably fall out and relieve her. If this did not succeed ... bronchostomy may need to be tried, if it fails ... it will probably bring on the consumption."*

> *"Friday, December 22, 1815*
>
> *I heard this evening that the experiment of suspending the child by the feet to extricate the buckshot was without effect."*

> *"Saturday, December 23, 1815*
>
> *This evening I called on Mr. Phelps' little girl, and found her much relieved, for this afternoon in a violent fit of coughing she had thrown out the shot from the trachea."*[39]

Root returned to study at UVM in January 1816. Two weeks later, tragedy befell the University again when Jairus Kennan, the professor of chemistry, died of "a pulmonary complaint."[40] Since the school could no longer offer lectures in Chemistry, Root left to complete his M.D. degree at Dartmouth.

Pomeroy's Hard Work Hits a Roadblock

In early January of 1818, after years of neglect, the trustees decided "as speedily as possible to perfect the medical establishment attached to the University, and to render it so respectable as to invite the attention of medical students in this part of the country."[41] The declaration, however, came too late. The financial drain from the War of 1812 had led to changes in leadership at the University's highest levels. The new administration was unsympathetic to Pomeroy's monetary and material needs. The recently hired Professor of Anatomy John Le Conte Cazier left shortly thereafter to join the competing medical school sixty miles to the south in Castleton.[42]

Pomeroy was at a loss. He had developed professorships of surgery and medicine, chemistry, and anatomy for the school. He had conducted a structured, biannual six-week course of lectures based on accepted principles and practical experience. And he had eventually held his classes in the College Building. But in the end, he could not continue without the financial support of the University. He suspended classes in the fall of 1818. Medical lectures would not be announced again in the local newspapers for the next three years.[43]

The Castleton Medical Academy, on the other hand, got off to a good start. It had ample upfront funding and used aggressive advertising. It also let students defer their tuition payments. The school soon became a force to be reckoned with, as its attendance from 1823-26 was greater than that of any other medical institution in New England.[44] Pomeroy, meanwhile, continued his waterfront practice and bided his time.

CHAPTER 2

A Medical School Without a Structure

After UVM formally incorporated its medical school in 1821, surgeons other than Pomeroy were the new leaders. Nathan Smith, the founder of the Dartmouth Medical School, brought his talents and reputation to UVM. He could not sustain his role as UVM's leader, due to his prior obligations to Yale. True structure and effective leadership were lacking. The school almost closed due to multiple leadership changes.

UVM did not seem to be on the right road to successfully prevail over competing proprietary medical schools.

The College of Medicine Formally Incorporates

The success of the Castleton Medical Academy did not go unnoticed in Burlington. Although the town's population had doubled over the past ten years to 2,111, attendance at the University of Vermont had dramatically declined. In an effort to attract more students, the trustees asked several local physicians to form a medical school. After four agreed to participate, the College of Medicine was formally incorporated on March 22, 1821.[1] Some might argue, of course, that UVM had been sanctioning a medical school since 1804!

John Pomeroy was named professor of surgery. At age 57, he was the oldest and most experienced appointee, but he was also the only one without an earned medical degree. Nathan Ryno Smith was elected professor of anatomy and physiology. The 23 year old, Ryno, as he was known had just moved to Burlington the year before.

The trustees hoped that by naming Ryno to the faculty they might also lure his father, the eminent educator and surgeon Nathan Smith, to the new College. The ploy worked. When it came time to deliver the first set of surgical lectures in 1822, it was the elder Smith, not Pomeroy, facing the class.

Nathan Smith "The Johnny Appleseed of American Medicine"

By the time he lectured in Burlington, Nathan Smith was well on his way to becoming "the Johnny Appleseed of American Medicine."[2] He had single-handedly founded the Medical Department of Dartmouth College in 1797. He had also played a major role in the creation of the Medical Institute of Yale College in 1813 and the Medical School of Maine at Bowdoin College in 1820. He had petitioned for funding grants, testified in favor of anato-

FIGURE 2-1. Nathan Smith founded Dartmouth, Bowdoin and Yale Medical Schools, and played a major role in the UVM College of Medicine startup.

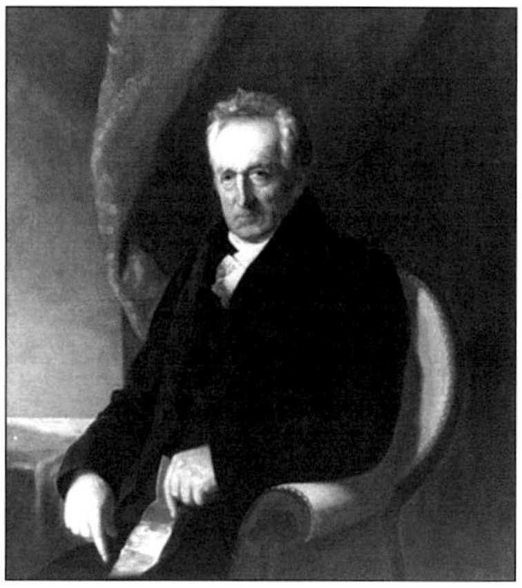

my law reform, and proposed physician-licensing guidelines. He was well known and widely respected. UVM's new school would achieve instant recognition if Nathan Smith were on board.

The senior Smith was born on September 13, 1762, in the town of Rehoboth, near Fall River, Massachusetts. He and his parents moved to Chester, Vermont, in 1772. As a young man, he assisted a local surgeon named Josiah Goodhue with a leg amputation. Goodhue had been a student at Harvard during the Battle of Bunker Hill, but left Harvard due to a "white swelling of the knee." Goodhue had been treated by Thomas Kittredge, one of the surgeons at the Battle, and then became Kittredge's student.[3]

Smith was transformed upon watching Goodhue operate. He decided at once to become a doctor. Following preparatory studies, Smith apprenticed under Goodhue for the next three years. At the end of his training, he started a practice across the river in Cornish, New Hampshire.[4]

One night, a few of the locals decided to have some fun at Smith's expense. He was called to see a patient in urgent need of his services. He raced to the local tavern to find a goose with a broken leg laid out on a bed. Smith assessed the situation, reduced the fracture, and bound the limb. He told the innkeeper to keep the bird off its feet for a week and to feed it cornmeal and water. "There was not much laughter when the doctor went away, though thus far all had gone well enough; but the next day the joke really became serious, when a good round *bill for professional services* came around to the landlord, which he found himself obliged to pay."[5]

After a few years of practice, Smith felt that he had reached the limits of his capabilities. On Goodhue's recommendation, he enrolled at the recently formed Medical School of Harvard College. There he trained under John Warren, another Bunker Hill veteran. Warren had been in charge of the main camp hospital during the Siege and was considered the foremost surgeon in the region. Smith ended up being better prepared than he realized; he completed two years worth of courses in just seven months. On July 5, 1790, he became the fifth person to receive a Bachelor of Medicine degree from Harvard (it was reissued as a Doctor of Medicine in 1811, as were prior Bachelor of Medicine degrees from Dartmouth).[6, 7]

In short order, Smith took on his own apprentices in Cornish, NH, much in the same way John Pomeroy did in Vermont. He discovered that he had an ability to teach and enjoyed it. But he had difficulty securing books and cadavers. His students could not afford to acquire their formal degrees at Harvard as he had done. As a result, Smith decided to affiliate himself with an institution of higher learning. In August 1796, he approached the "Board of Trust" at Dartmouth — the only college in northern New England at the time and proposed the creation of a medical school.[8]

The trustees agreed with the idea in principle, but first required Smith to spend nine months studying in Glasgow, Edinburgh, and London at his own expense. Lectures were then held *near* Dartmouth in November 1797. The school and Smith's professorship were officially approved in the fall of 1798 and the first two medical degrees were issued. Smith moved his classes into Dartmouth Hall the next year. There he taught every subject himself — with the occasional exception of chemistry — for the next decade.[9]

Smith was a prolific surgeon. He operated on cataracts, bladder stones, cancers, fractures and infected bones. He also performed trepanations, hernia repairs, and amputations. In addition, he was one of the first surgeons in America to repair a cleft palate, amputate at the knee joint, and invent a useful posterior leg splint.[10] He also fabricated instruments to both dilate the esophagus and remove foreign bodies from it. And although Ephraim McDowell of Kentucky had pioneered the removal of ovarian cysts in 1809, Smith was the second in this country to publish an account of a similar procedure he had performed in July of 1821.[11, 12, 13]

He also created an inadvertent but ultimately functional colostomy in a patient with "breach and stoppage following the ingestion of Vermont plums, stones and all." Smith "cut above the groin and found the intestine broken; he got out the stones and relieved him, but could not heal the ruptured intestine, so his excremental discharges always afterward passed out of the aperture made by the doctor. By wearing a belt and cloth over the aperture he was made quite comfortable, and able to work for some several years."[14]

Smith's most famous operative patient, perhaps, was only a child when the two first met. A typhoid fever epidemic had spread through the Connecticut River valley in 1813. While recovering from the disease, a seven-year old boy developed pain and swelling over his left lower leg. Two attempts were made to drain the infection, but both failed. When the chief surgeon recommended amputation, the boy's mother asked for another opinion. Smith, "the only physician in the United States who aggressively and successfully operated for osteomyelitis," was summoned. He bored into alternate sides of the youngster's tibia and removed the diseased portions of bone. The lad walked with crutches for three years thereafter, but eventually made a full recovery. We are thus left to wonder, would the boy, Joseph Smith (no relation), still have gone on to found the Church of Jesus Christ of Latter Day Saints if he had been an amputee?[15, 16]

Word of Smith's abilities spread and he eventually lectured to well over one hundred students at a time. By 1811, he had secured the appointment of two additional professors and arranged for a "New Medical House" to be built with funding from the State of New Hampshire. But his administrative duties became taxing. The battle over whether Dartmouth should remain a college or become a university was tiring. The money from the state came with political headaches. And land speculation losses and construction cost overruns had left him deeply in debt.[17]

Smith lived most of his life on the edge of financial solvency. He made a considerable amount of money as a busy practitioner. But he usually put the interests of his patients, students, and school ahead of his own. In one case, "an explosion had taken place, so shattering a poor man's leg as to require its amputation. The $50 fee demanded by the doctor having been collected from the crowd of sympathizing bystanders, the operation was performed. At its close Dr. Smith handed the patient the money, duly counted, and rode away."[18]

Smith Founds Schools at Yale, and Then Bowdoin

Smith felt "the conduct of people and parties has cooled my ardor for laboring in my avocation in this place, and determined me to sell my talents in physic and surgery to the highest bidder."[19] So in July 1813, at the height of his educational success, Smith accepted a position at Yale's new medical school, although not resigning totally from Dartmouth. Yale had the money and stability Dartmouth lacked. Smith became professor of the theory and practice of medicine, surgery, and obstetrics — half the curricula for which he had previously been responsible. His salary was tripled and his new employer assumed some of his debts.[20]

But after a few years, Yale posed its own problems for Smith. The conservative religious atmosphere was stifling. Class sizes were smaller than expected. And some of the students were not diligent in their studies. One somewhat thick pupil wondered if it were "possible to transfer living, sentient brains from one head to another." Smith politely replied that, "if the gentleman who puts the question could make a discovery of this nature, it might prove of great advantage to himself."[21]

In addition, Connecticut's anatomy laws were restrictive regarding cadaver procurement. Private practice revenue fell short when patients did not pay their bills. His wife and children still lived in New Hampshire. Smith taught one more term at Dartmouth, but was bothered by the campus politics. After Yale doubled his salary in 1817, he agreed to move his family to New Haven and teach there exclusively.[22] But two years later he wrote, "I am not satisfied with my situation and contemplate a removal but do not know yet whether it will be towards the North or South. Medical science will never flourish in Connecticut; the soil is too dry."[23]

The "removal" was to Brunswick, Maine. Bowdoin College had asked for Smith's help when it started planning its own medical school. Maine was newly independent from Massachusetts and a state free of political turmoil and religious fervor. An appointment would give Smith an opportunity to travel (which he enjoyed) and promised to augment his Yale salary by two-thirds. With permission from Yale's trustees, Smith taught as a "lecturer" in medicine, anatomy, and surgery at Bowdoin in March 1821. This did not translate into personal financial success though, because students paid with promissory notes.[24] But by proving he could teach at New Haven in the winter and Brunswick in the spring, the stage was set for Smith to find a spot at a fall school.

UVM Catches Smith's Attention

Smith made it known, through his son Ryno, that he was interested in joining the faculty in Burlington. UVM's trustees used the same tactic as Bowdoin to appease Yale (perhaps at Smith's suggestion) by naming him a "lecturer" instead of a professor in March of 1822.[25] Smith was optimistic about the situation, comparing it favorably with conditions at New Haven and Brunswick. "Burlington has one advantage over the others & that is good rooms & accommodations for medical purposes ... [the] College too will soon be in funds sufficient to aid the school."[26]

Smith may have taken the job because he needed the money, but he truly was devoted to teaching. He wrote, "A medical school does more toward ameliorating conditions of mankind than any other institution, as the knowledge acquired in them is of more practical importance."[27] But his economic woes were not solved in Burlington either. The faculty did not receive a salary. Incomes were derived from lecture ticket sales, which were again often paid with promissory notes.[28]

The trustees supplied the new venture with a grand total of thirty-five dollars. The funds were used to renovate two rooms in the College Building "for the accommodation of the chemical apparatus [instruments]."[29] In addition, the board gave UVM's president "discriminating power to confer medical degrees on such persons as shall attend the medical lectures and are recommended by the medical professors and lecturers of the University."[30]

Pomeroy is Left Out of the New College of Medicine

In July of 1822, the following announcement appeared in a local newspaper:

"MEDICAL LECTURES, UNIVERSITY OF VERMONT [BURLINGTON]
The Medical Lectures in the University of Vermont will commence on the first Monday of September next and continue twelve weeks. Nathan Smith, M.D. (Professor of Practice of Physic and Surgery in Yale College) Practice of Physic and Surgery; Nathan R. Smith, M.D. Anatomy and Physiology; Arthur L. Porter, M.D. Chemistry and Pharmacy; William Paddock, M.D. Botany and Materia Medica; James Dean, A.M., A.A. Natural and Experimental Philosophy; Students may obtain good board from $1.00 to $1.25 per week. Rooms may be had in the College building free of expenses. The ticket to the lectures: $40.00. There will average four lectures on each day."[31]

Notably absent from the announcement was the name of John Pomeroy. As president of the local medical society, it was his responsibility to determine which students were qualified to receive diplomas. It did not sit well with him that the president was bypassing his peer review system. And having witnessed poor financial planning in the past, he also disapproved of the plan to fund the new College through ticket sales.

The arrival of Nathan Smith probably caused some resentment as well. Given their similarities in age and experience, Pomeroy likely felt that Smith's appointment had been unnecessary. A feud with Smith's son Ryno must have completely undermined their relationship. A faction of the county medical society (encouraged by Pomeroy) had seceded from the state society. Ryno (now president of the "official" county society) publicized the fact that none of the secessionists had "received instruction at public seminaries." Pomeroy's group, in turn, maintained that training under a preceptor was just as good as training at a college.[32]

Pomeroy now held an untenable position. He could not be the head of a medical society that disputed the need for higher education and be a professor at the same time. He questioned the University's authority to grant degrees, had religious differences with the president, disagreed with the trustees over monetary policy, and viewed Nathan Smith's presence with suspicion. Although still officially on the faculty, Pomeroy did not teach during the inaugural set of classes. He let his term on the board of trustees expire and, in July 1823, he either left of his own accord or was removed. The board accepted his "official" resignation the next month.[33]

Pomeroy continued to conduct a busy practice from his lakeside office until 1834. He enjoyed several years of retirement, but in 1839 experienced an episode of "nervous prostration" that "made him a patient and confined him to his house." He died on February 19, 1844 at the age of 79.[34] More than one hundred years later, in 1950, UVM finally recognized Pomeroy's contributions to the College of Medicine. Although he had never set foot in the school's first medical building (it was completed in 1828, five years after he stepped down), it was renamed Pomeroy Hall in his honor.[35]

Smith Gets UVM Off to a Good Start

Smith remained enthusiastic, despite Pomeroy's acrimonious departure. In the fall of 1822, he wrote that "Our medical school flourishes well. So far we have a class of 24 all good and true men which is a greater number than any other medical school in the United States has commenced with."[36] His first set of lectures was given before a total of 53 students. He presented material from the leading textbooks of the day and, like his predecessor, augmented it with practical advice. The following selections are typical of his instruction during the early 1820's:

With respect to hernias versus other scrotal masses:

> *"A man must be a great bungler not to be able to distinguish between these diseases. An enlarged testicle can generally be very readily distinguished from hernia. You can feel above the enlargement. An enlargement of the veins of the spermatic cord can be distinguished from hernia by several circumstances."*[37]

On other common conditions, like breast cancer:

> *"A tumor in the breast will sometimes be accompanied with a tumor in the axilla; but sometimes the disease remains a long time before these take place. The breast is sometimes much enlarged. I performed the operation on a breast that weighed nine pounds. The wound soon healed after the operation. A few years after another tumor appeared which was removed and this also was healed."*[38]

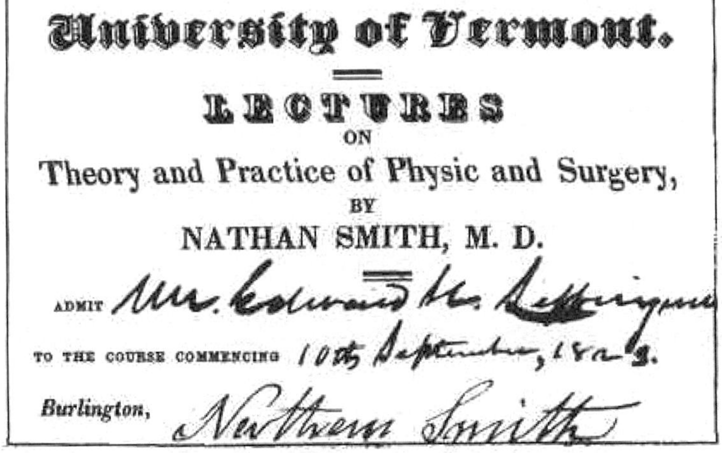
University of Vermont.
LECTURES
ON
Theory and Practice of Physic and Surgery,
BY
NATHAN SMITH, M. D.
ADMIT
TO THE COURSE COMMENCING
Burlington,

FIGURE 2-2.
An admission ticket to one of Nathan Smith's surgery lectures at UVM.

"If the breast has contracted itself and the surface falls in I believe we ought never to operate. If white lines are to be discovered extending over the whole breast it is not best to operate because it will generally return again. It should be a rule never to operate unless you can operate so as to be sure you cut off all the cancer."[39]

In the treatment of dislocations of the upper and lower extremities:

"In almost every instance you can use the limb as a lever with advantage and reduce it easier than by pulling directly ... In dislocation of the shoulder you must not depend entirely on pulling. When the accident has frequently happened I can generally reduce a luxation without an assistant. Seat the patient low and use your knee as a fulcrum."[40]

Even mundane topics, such as placing sutures, were covered:

"Several kinds of sutures are used. There has been a good deal of quibbling as to the kind ... It is better to have them waxed because they will slide better ... All the sutures should be passed that are necessary and then tied with the surgeon's knot. It will remain firm enough by turning the thread two or three times over without tying the second knot ... Some recommend silks, some linen and some leather ... All that is necessary is that it should be a small string, the smaller the better if of sufficient strength, and it should be drawn so tight as to destroy the vitality of the end of the artery."[41]

Smith lectured to an average of 50 students a year through 1825. But he continued to have academic responsibilities at both Bowdoin and Yale. He had neither the time nor the approval from the trustees in New Haven to hold another full professorship in Burlington. Someone else had to assume a leadership role.

Attempting to Fill Nathan Smith's Shoes

The trustees decided that the faculty member with the most education and experience among those remaining was the Professor of Midwifery, James K. Platt. He appeared to be the ideal person for the job of Professor of Surgery.[42]

Platt came from a distinguished and affluent family. His uncle, Benjamin Mooers, had served at Ticonderoga.[43] James himself graduated from Middlebury College in 1812. He went to Yale as a graduate student around the same time that Nathan Smith was organizing the college's Medical Institute.[44]

Perhaps Smith's activities inspired Platt to read medicine over the next three years. He attended medical lectures in Philadelphia and then earned an MD from New York's College of Physicians and Surgeons in 1816. Supported by his family's resources, he spent another two years of study in London under the brilliant surgeon and inguinal anatomist, Sir Astley Paston Cooper.[45]

Platt was present in 1817 when Cooper became the first surgeon to intentionally ligate the abdominal aorta. The patient was a thirty-eight year old man with a leaking post-traumatic, external iliac artery aneurysm. Cooper had successfully treated *chronic* aneurysms of the common carotid and femoral arteries several years earlier using a similar technique.[46]

Platt described the case in a letter to a former teacher in New York:

> *"Mr. Cooper tied the aorta just above its bifurcation, in a man who was labouring under an immense aneurismal tumour of the left external iliac artery. The aneurism was too high and large to admit either of the external or common iliac being secured, and as the sac had sloughed and haemorrhage had begun, it was thought justifiable to pass a ligature around the aorta itself. It was dangerous, but it was a dernier [last] resort."*[47]

After outlining the procedure step by step, Platt continued:

> *"The operation did not produce any extraordinary pain. The man lived two days after it — on dissection ... nothing, besides the aneurismal tumour, appeared unnatural within the cavity of the abdomen. It may be proposed as a question, what was the immediate cause of the man's death? Mr. Cooper suggested no explanation. The patient seemed in tolerable good health previous to the operation. I do not know how we shall account for his sinking so suddenly, unless we call in the aid of the old doctrine of sympathy. According to that, the general system received so violent a shock from the operation that it was unable to rally its vital forces; it made an attempt at resistance, but finding itself unequal to the task, it sunk under the effort."*[48]

Cooper, of course, later acknowledged that the patient's death was "owing to the want of circulation in the aneurismal limb," which was "cold and lacking in sensibility."[49] Full appreciation for the effects of aneurysm ligation in the absence of collateral circulation would have to wait until the twentieth century.

After becoming a Fellow of the Royal College of Surgeons in 1818, Platt returned to upstate New York. Ill health drove him to the West Indies shortly thereafter, but he did not benefit from the change in climate. Following his return home, Platt was asked to become the first Professor of Midwifery at the UVM College of Medicine. He accepted the position and gave his initial series of lectures in the fall of 1822. The talks were "spoken of in terms of the highest commendation."[50]

Fate Brings Death to the Chief of Surgery and Fire to UVM

In the spring of 1823, Nathan Smith wrote, "The next year will decide the fate of the school in Burlington. We made a very good beginning last year, and if no untoward circumstances occur I think it will live."[51] On August 14, the first four M.D. degrees were issued. That fall, Platt taught the surgical courses with Smith's assistance. But then an "untoward circumstance" did occur as Platt's chronic illness worsened. The effort of teaching "was too great, and the pulmonary disease with which he had so long struggled with developed itself with fatal rapidity, and in a few weeks terminated his earthly career."[52] He died on April 4, 1824, at the age of 32.

After less than a year, the trustees had to search for yet another professor of surgery. But a suitable candidate would not be found before the next set of lectures began, even though there was a lead-time of several months. This was because the very continuation of the school was threatened when the College Building was destroyed by arson on May 27, 1824. Ironically, the culprit turned out to be the president's "servant girl."[53]

The few pieces of property belonging to the College of Medicine were not seriously damaged and temporary quarters were erected in time for fall classes.[54] Nathan Smith gave another set of surgical lectures in 1824, but again could not assume the professorship on account of his other obligations. The situation seemed to improve in 1825, however, when Henry S. Waterhouse was chosen as the next professor.[55]

Waterhouse was born in northern Connecticut on February 20, 1783. He moved to Vermont at the age of eight with his father, Josiah Waterous, a former surgeon's mate who had served at the Siege of Boston.[56] Henry later lived with his uncle, Eleazer Claghorn, a Green Mountain Boy who had helped Ethan Allen take Fort Ticonderoga.[57]

Waterhouse, like the great majority of physicians of the day, did not have the extensive medical training of his immediate predecessor. Instead, he studied on his own and then apprenticed with John Horton of Salisbury, Vermont. After practicing in Salisbury for a few years, he moved across the lake to Malone, New York.[58] During the War of 1812, he gained additional operative experience as an assistant hospital surgeon for the 42nd infantry brigade.[59]

Even though Waterhouse had run a successful practice for almost 15 years, his lack of formal medical instruction weighed heavily upon his mind. So he moved back to Vermont and attended classes at the College of Medicine. A year later, in 1824, he was awarded an honorary medical degree.[60]

That same year, he published an early account of external cardiopulmonary resuscitation. A reviewer reported:

> *"Dr. Waterhouse relates a very interesting case of a child, who, while eating some watermelon, drew one of the seeds into her windpipe. The consequence may be readily imagined. Coughing, strangling, convulsive efforts continued for several months. At length, Dr. W. being called determined on tracheotomy. There was no little difficulty exhibited during the operation. The distance from the angle formed by the meeting of the skin of the chin, with that of the neck, and the upper extremity of the sternum was only one inch. The hæmorrhage was dreadful, and ligatures could not be used. Compression with a sponge was the only resource. The scene was appalling in the extreme, owing to the hæmorrhage, and the struggles and screaming of the child. After the operation was completed, the little sufferer seemed to have lost her life. Every attempt to reanimate her was used. The child was suspended by the heels, and while in this position, repeated pressure to the abdomen, with support to its back, had recourse to imitate the act of respiration. It was a long time before resuscitation took place — but the child recovered. Dr. W. deserves much praise for his persevering efforts. The recovery of his patient is his best reward."*[61]

Waterhouse's serious, studious nature and previous practical experience drew him to the attention of the trustees. He was described as "an avid reader and a learned man ... with a sallow complexion and cadaverous expression. The contours of his mouth were altered by an ill-fitting set of false teeth, which he assured his friends were manufactured from the tusk of a hippopotamus. His erudition and flawless diction earned him the nickname of Dr. Syntax."[62]

Fortune Totally Deserts the College of Medicine

After his appointment to the professorship, Waterhouse lectured alongside Nathan Smith in 1825 and then on his own in the autumns of 1826 and 1827. But he too contracted a pulmonary condition [felt to be tuberculosis] and had to resign his position. He relocated to the Florida Keys where he gradually regained his health. But his good fortune ran out on January 17, 1835 when his boat capsized during a violent squall and he drowned.[63]

Deaths and resignations were not limited to professors of surgery. In fact, all of the College's original instructors had left by 1828.[64] Nathan Smith discontinued his involvement with UVM and Bowdoin after 1825. He prophetically wrote: "I think the four schools which I have been concerned in bringing forward will, in addition to Harvard, be as much as New England will bear, and I think these will not be too many. Every state should have one medical school and no more."[65] Unfortunately, Smith did not live to see the fruits of his labors ripen; he suffered a stroke in July 1829 and died shortly thereafter.

His son, Nathan Ryno Smith, left in May 1825 for Philadelphia's newly established Jefferson Medical College. Two years later, he took a position at the University of Maryland School of Medicine, which he kept for the next forty years.[66]

The College of Medicine had gone through three surgical professors and one "lecturer" during its first six years. The stability provided by John Pomeroy over the previous two decades had disappeared. Nathan Smith filled the seats twelve weeks a year, but was otherwise unavailable to the students or the school. Smith's two successors showed promise but were still years away from matching his skills. Platt was short on clinical experience and Waterhouse was deficient in scientific knowledge. If the College was to successfully compete with the proprietary schools spreading across New England, the next professor of surgery would have to be a dynamic, well versed, visionary.

CHAPTER 3

Setback: Competing Proprietary Medical Schools Take Over

Benjamin Lincoln ran the medical program single-handedly during his time at UVM, just as Nathan Smith had done at Dartmouth. Both men dedicated themselves and their schools to the provision of high quality medical education.

Competing proprietary medical schools offering inexpensive, assembly line "degrees" doomed Lincoln's attempts to upgrade UVM's curriculum. As a result, the College of Medicine folded in 1837.

The Proprietary Medical System

The typical unaffiliated medical school of the 1820-30s was a for-profit venture. Students paid fees in order to enter, to attend lectures, and to graduate. Professors collected the money, paid the overhead and pocketed the rest. By setting the admission requirements low and forming large classes, these institutions became quite profitable. Faculty members, in turn, augmented their incomes by lecturing at multiple establishments each year. Such facilities thrived in the absence of accepted standards and regulations.[1] An affiliation with a University was not a requirement. As Castleton and the newly established school in Woodstock flourished, UVM fell behind.

While better than the apprenticeship method, the proprietary system was still subject to abuse. Fees were paid with four-year promissory notes. Lectures were given over a twelve-week period and then repeated almost verbatim the next year. Operative surgery was demonstrated on cadavers, as there were no clinical cases presented to the students. Graduation usually required attendance at two series of sessions. Different schools conducted courses at various times of the year, often giving credit for classes taken at other locations. Some students "earned" their degrees in as little as nine months.[2]

To be fair, university-affiliated programs such as at UVM were not materially different in their requirements and goals. Fees were collected in a similar manner, as the College of Medicine's schedule for 1825 demonstrates:

Dean's Fee:	$ 3
Anatomy and Physiology:	$ 14
Surgery and Obstetrics:	$ 10

Chemistry and Natural Philosophy:	$ 10
Theory and Materia Medica:	$ 10
Graduate's Fee:	$ 8
Total Cost for Two Terms:	$100[3]

Inconsistent education led to irregular delivery of care. A doctor taught in older "heroic" methods might give massive amounts of purgatives or bleed someone to the point of unconsciousness. Practitioners with rudimentary knowledge, on the other hand, regularly did too little or too much in the face of an uncomplicated illness. As a result, patients often viewed physicians with suspicion.[4]

UVM Constructs its First Strictly Medical Building

Inadequate medical training and its repercussions were just two of the problems confronting Waterhouse's successor at UVM. The University was still trying to recover from the effects of the 1824 fire. The College of Medicine suffered from a shortage of lecture space, instructional materials, and teachers. As the undergraduate professor of chemistry George Benedict later recalled:

"I came here in May, 1825 ... I was shown a few baskets full of books of a very motley character, which were said to have been snatched from the fire. In another place one or two old bits of cheap philosophical apparatus [instruments] were saved in a like manner. That was all the material part of the institution as far as it was visible to my eyes."[5]

There was some cause for optimism, however. William Sweetser, Jr., the professor of the theory and practice of medicine (and the College of Medicine's only other employee after Waterhouse's departure), had begun raising funds for the construction of a new "Medical House."[6] During the winter of 1826, he charged fifty cents a head to "deliver to such Ladies and Gentlemen of Burlington, who may feel disposed to attend, a short popular course of Lectures on Physiology, the special object of which is to aid in obtaining means for erecting a suitable building for Medical Lectures, which is now absolutely demanded to place the Medical Institution on a sure and respectable foundation."[7]

Benedict and the board of trustees secured additional capital from businesses and individuals, raising $8,362.50 in the process. Land at the south end of the campus was donated for the purpose. Master carpenter John Johnson, builder of the "Old Mill", proceeded to erect what has persisted as Pomeroy Hall in the summer of 1828. Originally a two story gabled Federal-style brick building, it bore little resemblance to today's cupola topped three-story structure. The exterior was completed in August, just in time for the arrival of Benjamin Lincoln, the new professor of surgery.[8]

Benjamin Lincoln's Preparation to Lead UVM College of Medicine

Lincoln was born on October 11, 1802, in the town of Dennysville, in the far eastern part of what is now Maine. He was named after his grandfather, General Benjamin Lincoln, one of George Washington's key aides during the Siege of Boston. He enrolled at Bowdoin

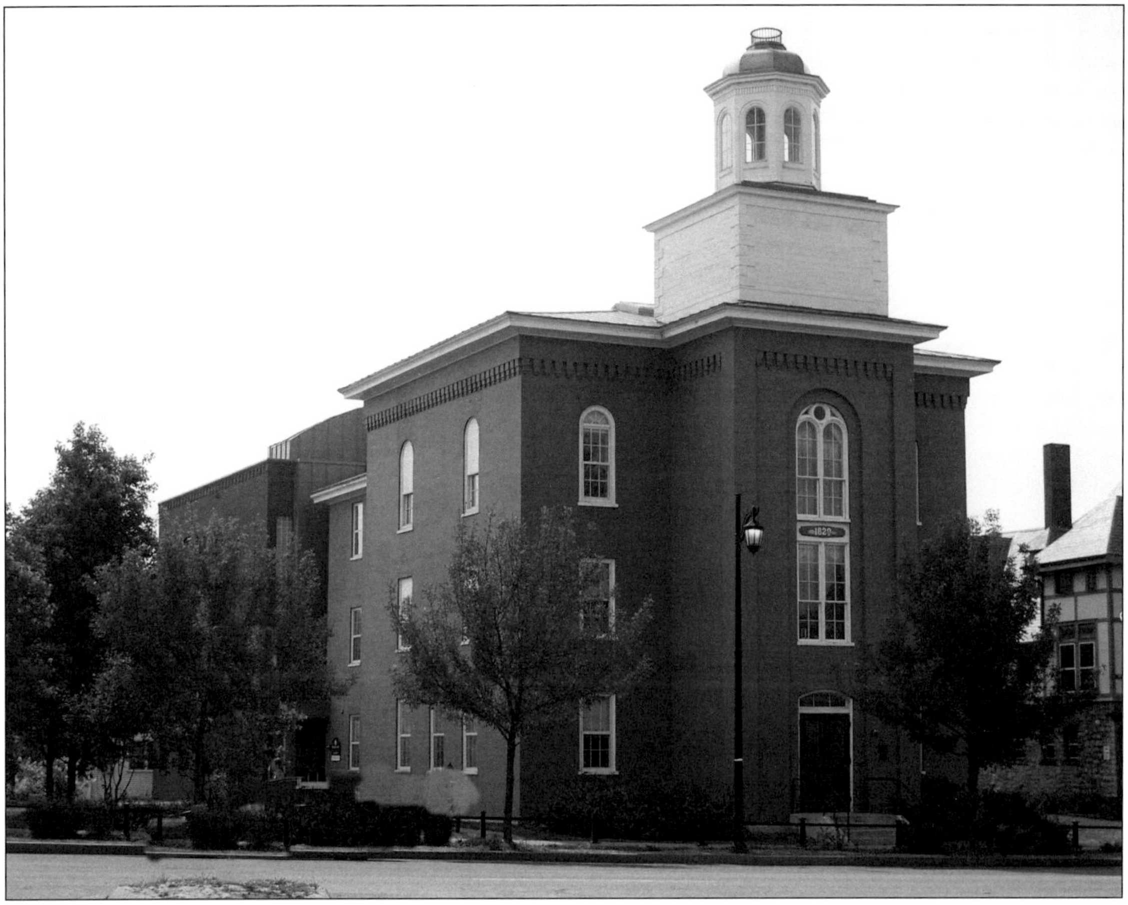

FIGURE 3-1.
UVM's first Medical Building, later renamed "Pomeroy Hall", was completed in 1829. Originally it was only two stories high. The third story and cupola tower were added in 1855, to resemble the present day building in this photograph.

College after completing a classical preparatory education. Lincoln contracted what is thought to have been rheumatic fever at age twenty, but recovered enough to graduate with a Bachelor of Arts in 1823.[9]

He then worked with Nathan Smith as a demonstrator of anatomy at Bowdoin's newly established medical school. This was followed by an apprenticeship with George Shattuck in Boston.[10] Shattuck, another of Smith's early students at Dartmouth, was professor of medicine at Harvard for over twenty years and dean of its medical school for an additional five.[11]

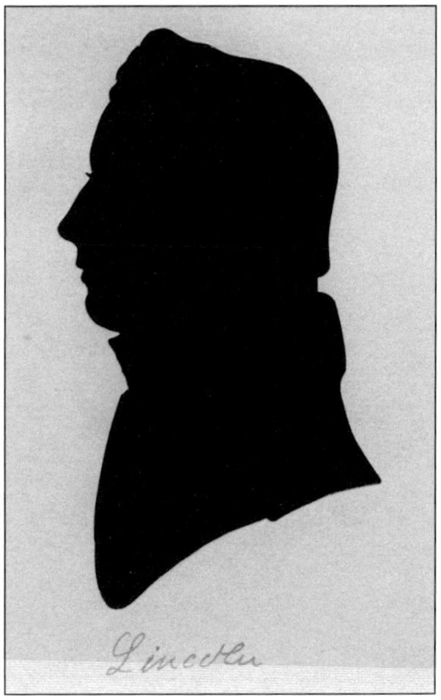

A silhouette of Lincoln from 1823 captures his handsome features.[12] Over the course of the next few years though, he developed a severe curvature of the upper spine. "From being a model of delicate, elegant and manly beauty, he gradually bent under the rigid contraction of muscular rheumatism."[13] Prolonged periods spent dissecting and operating probably worsened his condition. The deformity

FIGURE 3-2.
Silhouette of Lincoln in 1823

Chapter Three: Setback: Competing Proprietary Medical Schools Take Over

"bent his elegant frame almost into a circle"[14] but it did not affect his ability to work.

Lincoln returned to Bowdoin in 1825, attended medical school, and resumed his duties as demonstrator of anatomy. He received his degree from the Medical School of Maine in 1827 and started a local practice. Aware of his accomplishments, the trustees in Burlington invited him to deliver a course of lectures on anatomy and physiology in 1828.

The proficiency and clarity with which Lincoln presented his lectures had an immediate impact upon the students and faculty. He further endeared himself to the school by donating "some preparations of bones" to the student-run anatomical cabinet.[15] His impressive performance resulted in an appointment to the professorship of anatomy and surgery in 1829, at UVM.[16]

The Darker Side of Anatomy and Dissection is Revealed

The new professor's approach to anatomy was more academic than pragmatic. This may have been due to his limited operative experience. Lincoln held the enlightened view that operations should be performed only after acquiring a thorough understanding of human structure. But anatomical textbooks, such as Charles Bell's *System of Dissections* (1801), John Syng Dorsey's *Elements of Surgery* (1813), Astley Cooper's *Surgical Essays* (1819), and William Gibson's *Institutes and Practice of Surgery* (1824), were hard to come by, especially for the College.[17]

Thus, the most effective way to learn anatomy was by tissue dissection and careful study of the finished product. The absence of reliable embalming techniques, however, led to difficulty preserving specimens. In an effort to overcome this obstacle, Lincoln paid a medical student to help with dissections. The student was sent to New York, Philadelphia, and Washington, D.C. to procure material. After running out of options in those cities, he finally met with success in Baltimore. He collected two cadavers from a "resurrection man," stuffed them into barrels, and took them by stage and boat back to Vermont.[18]

Lincoln had been wise to acquire his subjects in other states. Grave robbing was not only deemed immoral, it was also highly illegal. State legislators passed laws "against disturbing the remains of the dead" that carried heavy penalties.[19] Nevertheless, Vermont cemeteries were still violated. The most notorious incident occurred in Hubbardton, sixty miles south of Burlington, in November 1830.

Following the desecration of a fresh grave, a mob descended upon the medical school in nearby Castleton and demanded an immediate search of the premises. As the dean fumbled with the keys, a student waded through the crowd carrying a bundle under his coat. After the throng burst into the building and pulled up some loose floorboards, it discovered the corpse of a recently decapitated woman. Despite the hastily performed mutilation, her remains were quickly identified. And so, after the sheriff assured the dean that charges would not be filed if the body were reburied intact, the same student returned with the woman's head.[20]

Prior to this episode, Lincoln had actually written a series of anonymous letters to the editor defending body snatching. While admitting the manner of procurement was "improper," he condoned the practice for the sake of medical education. Without a supply of cadavers, he argued, society would suffer from the "effects of ignorance of anatomy." The dilemma could be

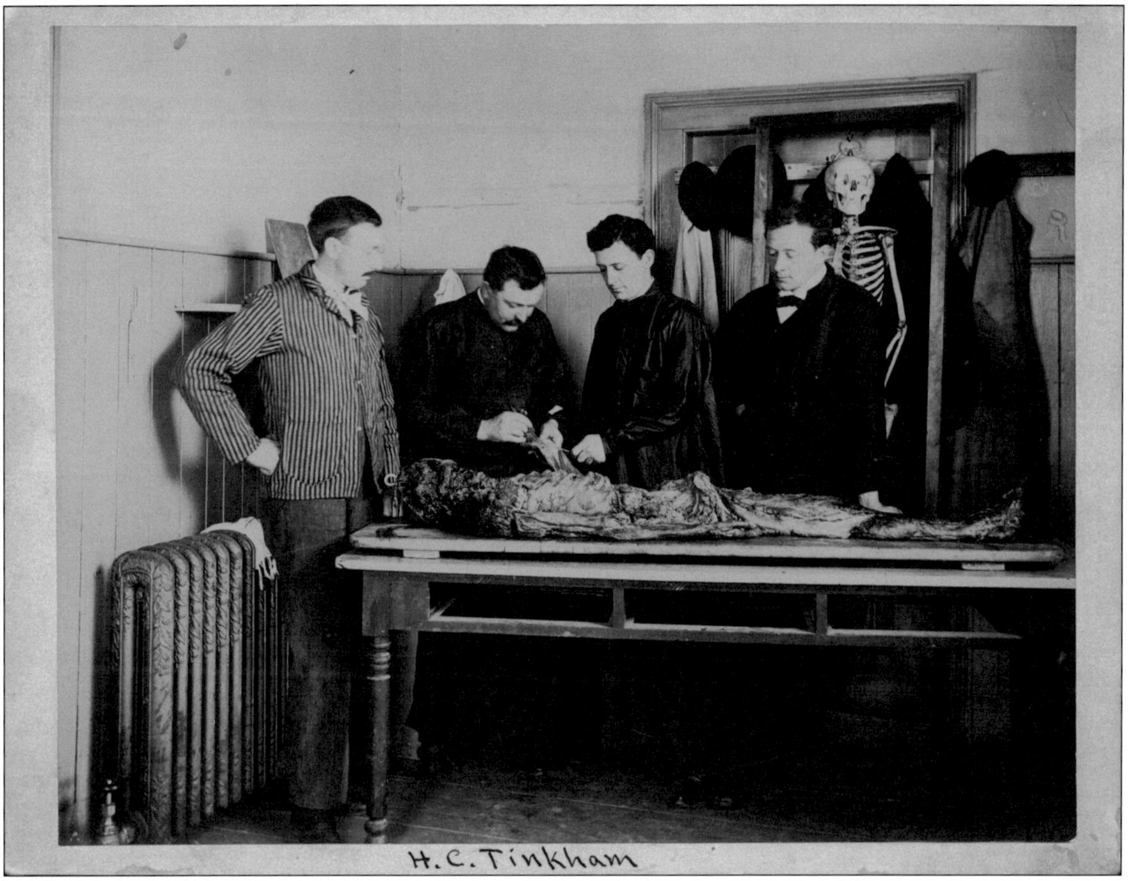

FIGURE 3-3.
Anatomy and techniques of operative surgery were taught using cadavers. Embalming was not perfected until the Civil War, and procurement of fresh cadavers was problematic. Here future Dean Henry Tinkham (2nd from left) conducts a dissection during the 1890s.

resolved, he proposed, by supplying medical schools with the bodies of paupers and criminals.[21]

Lincoln went public with his cause in March 1830 by giving a series of free anatomical lectures. The talks served to demonstrate the usefulness of dissection and dispel commonly held myths about the handling of dead bodies.[22] Although the citizenry welcomed the effort, the laws were not changed. Lincoln himself did little to improve anatomists' reputations during an inquest into the death of a woman following an abortion. He confirmed that the defendant — one of his medical students — had sold him a fetus for use as a specimen shortly after the victim's demise.[23]

Lincoln "Reforms" the College of Medicine

John Wells, Lincoln's former instructor, died in 1830. Lincoln gave the surgical lectures in his place at Bowdoin that year and at the University of Maryland in Baltimore the next, in addition to performing his duties at UVM. Both institutions immediately offered him professorships, but he turned them down in order to develop his own progressive school in Vermont. As UVM President John Wheeler stated, "He hoped to realize, he cared not on how small a scale, if it were but done, his idea of a medical school in this University, without the hindrance of encrusted organic remains from old formations."[24]

Lincoln used the three thousand dollars he made in Baltimore to buy books, anatomical preparations, and illustrated color plates. He renovated the demonstration theater and added a storage room next to the specimen museum. He also purchased land abutting the medical school and built a small structure in which to perform dissections.[25]

Around the same time, Lincoln set out to dramatically change the manner in which medical education was conducted. He may have been motivated by his experience at Maryland — an enormous facility of over two hundred students. He wrote to George Shattuck in April 1831:

"I have taken up in arms against what I conceive to be certain abuses in the system of public medical instruction, and that (in my own opinion) I am now in the attitude of a determined reformer ... teachers think too much of their own purses, and they think too much of the means of magnifying their own praise and of inculcating their own particular dogmas. They think too little of the real good of their pupils and think far too lightly of the responsibility which rests on their shoulders as the protectors of the public against quacks." [26]

The plan was to admit qualified students, forego promissory notes, and provide a comprehensive education. Lincoln would then,

"... withhold my name from all diplomas except such as are earned by study instead of money alone ... I have faith enough in the ultimate success of my plan ... Still for the present, the sacrifice is great, and there is a chance of utter failure in the end. We shall require much more of our pupils ... than is required by any other school." [27]

The Battle With Castleton Escalates

Lincoln's regard for the proprietary schools sank even lower that August. Four Canadian medical students approached UVM chemistry professor George Benedict. The quartet had completed courses at McGill University in Montreal, but the school was unable to confer a Doctorate of Medicine. Another school was willing to apply the McGill attendance tickets towards a degree; would the University of Vermont do the same? Benedict agreed to accept the students if McGill could verify its credits were legitimate in London and Edinburgh.[28]

Lincoln met with the four and suggested that they approach Castleton with the same request. Castleton's Dean, Theodore Woodward (yet another of Nathan Smith's pupils),[29] dispatched one of his students with instructions to meet any terms UVM offered. His agent went further though, and promised free tuition for one if the other three enrolled at Castleton. In the end, assurances regarding McGill's legitimacy arrived, and the Canadians, suspicious of Castleton's overtures, matriculated at Burlington.

Lincoln was amazed to hear from one of the new enrollees about Woodward's actions. He was even more astounded to learn that the discounts were offered before the applicants' credentials had even been checked. He became more determined than ever to conduct his school in an aboveboard manner.[30]

Lincoln Runs a One Man Medical School

The concepts of paying in cash, studying diligently, and exhibiting proficiency prior to graduation, unfortunately, were too much for most students to accept. The College of Medicine had been averaging more than forty members a class each year during the 1820s. Following implementation of the reform measures, class sizes dropped into the mid-teens. Only twelve people signed up in 1832. The gross income from the group was just four hundred dollars. This was not enough to cover salaries and operating expenses. William Sweetser resigned later that year. Unable to afford a replacement, Lincoln taught all courses except chemistry himself.[31]

One member of that year's incoming class was George Shattuck, Jr., of Boston. Dispatched specifically to study under his father's former apprentice, the younger Shattuck wrote a number of letters to his family about his experiences in Burlington. He reported on the small classes, which were often attended by local citizens "who took pity in our loneliness and came up from the village." He pointed out that Lincoln was very devoted to education and spent a great deal of time with the students.[32]

Shattuck felt that Lincoln's lectures were better than any offered in Boston. He considered his professor "something superior to what we commonly meet with." On a more ominous note, the younger Shattuck also mentioned that Lincoln was experiencing episodes of bronchial hemorrhage.[33] Lincoln himself wrote the elder Shattuck with the same news, lamenting that he could only conduct recitations for one hour at a time.[34]

Despite the declines in both his health and his class size, Lincoln still felt he ought to continue promoting the need for reform. He did so by sending a series of letters to the newspapers in Burlington, Castleton, and Woodstock. First, he outlined the questionable practices those offending schools used to attract pupils. Then he supported his statements with affidavits and depositions from the Canadian students and other witnesses. Finally, he explained that his exposé was not to be construed as an advertisement for his school, since staffing concerns precluded the College's ability to hold classes.[35]

The Fight With Castleton Comes to a Head

Castleton's Woodward took the matter personally, calling the letters "the smut of a blackguard." He accused Lincoln of destroying the school in Burlington with his incompetence and insinuated that the professor had been rejected at Bowdoin and Maryland. At the same time, he acknowledged all of the charges brought against him without reservation. He ended by saying Lincoln's efforts amounted to "the convulsive struggles of a disappointed, neglected, and evil-minded nincompoop."[36] Nathan Ryno Smith, who had become friends with Lincoln during the latter's time at Maryland, later wrote Lincoln a letter (as a joke) that began "Dear Nincompoop".[37]

Lincoln Struggles for Improved Medical Education

Lincoln wrote a pamphlet that assessed the current state of medical training and made recommendations for its improvement titled "Hints on the Present State of Medical Education and the Influence of Medical Schools in New England." He stressed the importance of a

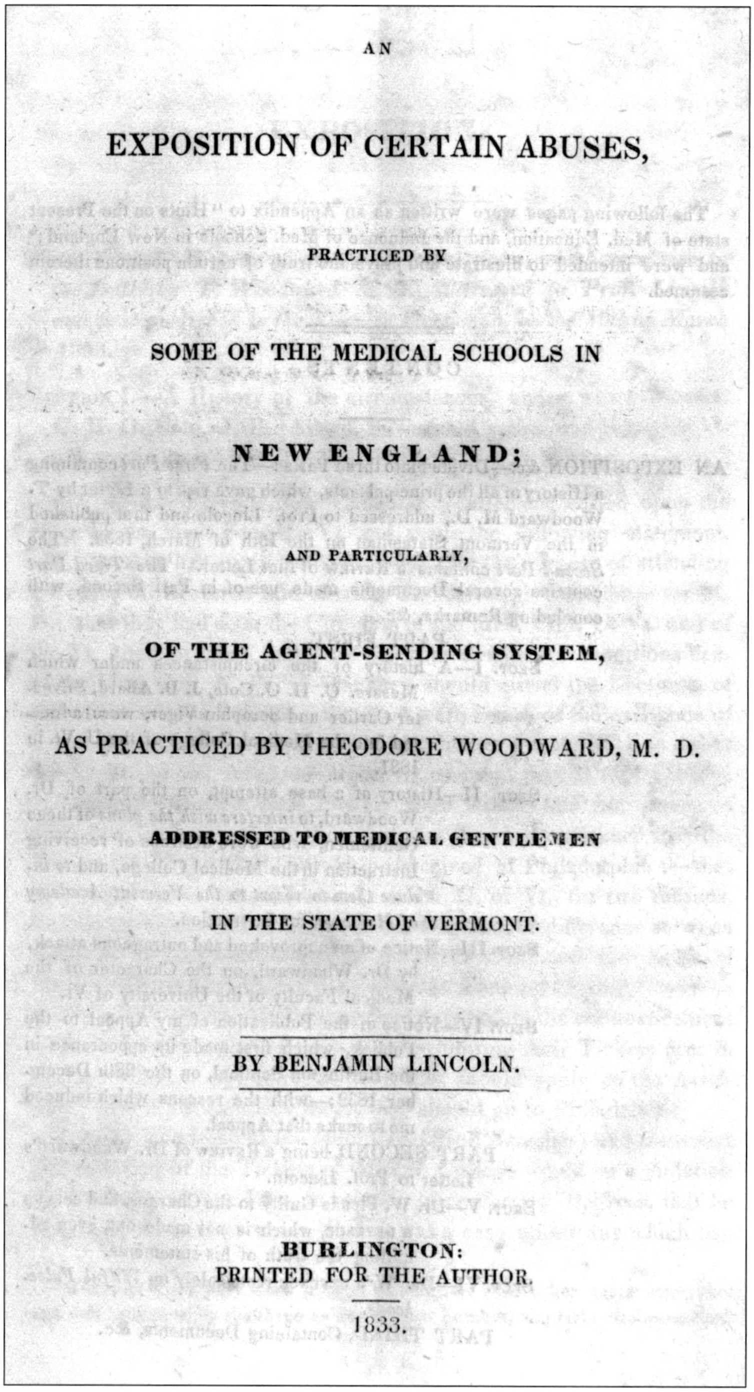

FIGURE 3-4. The title page of Lincoln's ground breaking medical education reform pamphlet.

AN

EXPOSITION OF CERTAIN ABUSES,

PRACTICED BY

SOME OF THE MEDICAL SCHOOLS IN

NEW ENGLAND;

AND PARTICULARLY,

OF THE AGENT-SENDING SYSTEM,

AS PRACTICED BY THEODORE WOODWARD, M. D.

ADDRESSED TO MEDICAL GENTLEMEN

IN THE STATE OF VERMONT.

BY BENJAMIN LINCOLN.

BURLINGTON:
PRINTED FOR THE AUTHOR.

1833.

sound education as it related to the fields of government, business, and specifically medicine. He argued that rigorous medical instruction was in the public's best interest. The process had to begin with qualified students. It was impossible for "those whose whole education is included in being able to read, write, and cipher," to properly process scientific principles. He felt that a preliminary bachelor's degree was essential in order to understand "the Philosophy of Medicine."[38]

He pointed out that acquisition of knowledge and mastery of skills took time. In defending a three year program of study, he noted it was still "less than is required for the apprentice to learn the 'Art and Mystery' of the smith or the joiner (carpenter)." A graded curriculum that began with fundamentals and progressed to more comprehensive material each year was also necessary. Professors ought to have "the right to exclude a student from further attendance if found to be improperly prepared." And, faculty members' salaries needed to be fixed and independent of student fees. "This plan I hope to see in successful operation at one school in New England before many years."[39]

The pamphlet and the points it raised seemed to have a positive effect overall. Instead of canceling classes in the fall of 1833 as anticipated, the College of Medicine found itself with fifteen students. Not a huge improvement, perhaps, but much better than expected. Lincoln continued to run a one-man medical school. A private class of eight was tentatively set for the summer of 1834, reflecting the potential for an even larger group that fall.[40]

But it was not to be. Lincoln's "bleeding from the lungs" worsened in the spring of 1834. After being diagnosed with tuberculosis, he returned to the family homestead in Dennysville for rest. His colleagues "turned away our eyes in sorrow as ... we bid him our last farewell."[41] As George Shattuck, Jr., wrote his father in May 1834, "Never did a man labor with less regard to self than has Dr. Lincoln during his residence in Burlington. His object has been to raise the standard of medical education in this part of the country" but "his strenuous efforts ... have met with little cooperation from those amongst whom his labors have been performed."[42]

Lincoln resigned that June, telling the trustees "in consequence of ill health" it was "improbable that I shall ever be able to resume the duties of the office which I now hold in the University."[43] He kept in touch with Benedict and completed a written account of his anatomical museum in November. But the end finally came on February 26, 1835 when "weighed down by disease and racked with pain,"[44] he died. He was just 32 years old.

The College of Medicine Fails to Revive After Lincoln's Death

When it became clear that Lincoln's health was not going to improve, the trustees turned to Edward E. Phelps of Windsor, Vermont. Phelps had studied under Nathan Smith at Yale around the same time Lincoln was working with Smith at Bowdoin. And he supported Lincoln's ideas for a reformed school.[45] But the trustees feared Phelps might not be able to deliver a good lecture as "he has naturally a very thick tongue."[46] In spite of his perceived lack of oratory skills, Phelps was appointed professor of anatomy and surgery in September 1835 — six months after Lincoln's death.[47]

Phelps was born in Peacham, Vermont, on April 24, 1803. His grandfather, Elkanah Phelps, had performed garrison duty at Ticonderoga and his great uncle, Captain Noah Phelps, as Ethan Allen's spy had helped deliver the Fort.[48] He received his MD from the Medical Institute of Yale College in 1825 under Smith's tutelage. He ultimately relocated in Windsor, VT just South of White River Junction in 1828 and started a practice.[49]

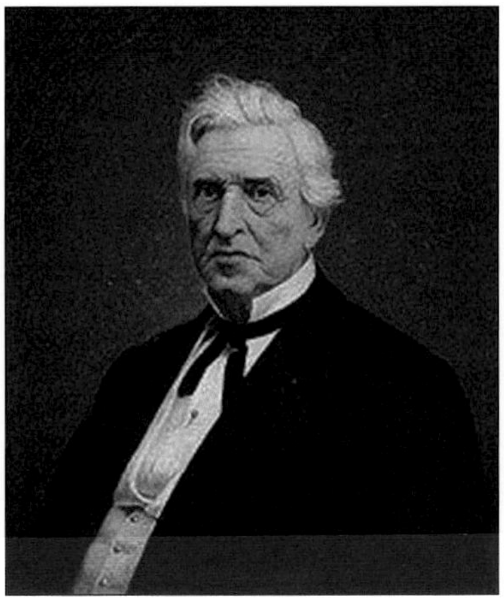

When Phelps arrived in Burlington, he found that medical instruction had not been offered for almost two years. In March 1836, the local papers announced the resumption

FIGURE 3-5. Edward E. Phelps succeeded Lincoln as Professor of Surgery at UVM from 1835 to 1841.

of classes. It is doubtful, though, that the news reached anyone beyond the city. Phelps taught anatomy, surgery, and physiology to just a handful of students. The fall series of lectures were subsequently cancelled as a result of poor enrollment and overall disorganization.[50]

The panic of 1837, and the five-year depression it spawned, sapped the school of what little financial resources it had. Phelps resigned in 1841 to become professor of materia medica and therapeutics at Dartmouth. He remained there until his retirement in 1871.[51]

Edward Phelps and the "Man with a Hole in His Head"

Despite primarily teaching pharmacology at Dartmouth, Phelps continued to see surgical patients. In November 1848, he examined a local railroad worker who had been injured in an industrial accident. The man had been packing blasting powder into a ledge when a spark from his tamping rod set off an explosion. The resulting blast knocked the railman flat on his back. When he got up, he found sizable wounds under his left eye and on the top of his head. The rod, three and a half feet long and an inch and a quarter in diameter, was found nearby, covered with blood and gray matter.[52]

The victim was taken to his boarding house in Cavendish, Vermont and treated by local physician John Harlow. Although expected to die from such a devastating injury, the man recovered in the span of five weeks. He returned home to Lebanon, New Hampshire, and presented himself to Phelps. The professor found the entry and exit sites well granulated and without communication.[53]

Unfortunately, Phelps (unlike William Beaumont) did not take advantage of the research opportunity sitting before him. For even though his injuries healed, the worker "would gradually change from a simple country man to a loudmouthed, boisterous and very profane individual."[54] It was left to Harlow to discover and publish the connection between left frontal lobe injury and personality change twenty years later.[55]

The patient, Phineas P. Gage, made substantial earnings on the circus sideshow circuit for the next several years as "The Only Living Man With a Hole in His Head." The effects of Gage's mishap finally caught up with him in 1860, however, when he died following a series of epileptic seizures. His skull and tamping rod were eventually donated to the Warren Anatomical Museum at Harvard Medical School, where they reside today as reminders of a classic case study in traumatic brain injury.[56]

FIGURE 3-6. An engraving of Phineas Gage's skull as depicted in Henry Bigelow's original case report of 1850.

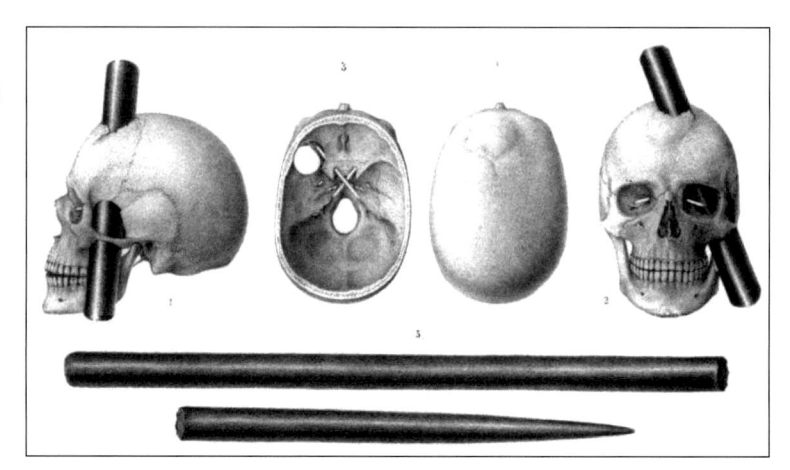

Unable to Compete, the UVM College of Medicine Closes

It was on this note, then, that the first incarnation of the College of Medicine came to a close. One hundred and fourteen earned doctorates, twenty-four courtesy and honorary doctorates, and a single bachelor of medicine degree had been granted.[57] But the persistent decline in enrollment and the subsequent loss of revenue were too much for the fledgling University to absorb. The College of Medicine had survived the deaths of its most promising faculty members, the destruction of its facilities, and the poaching of its students by the proprietary schools. It was unable, however, to realize its honorable yet poorly timed efforts to bring about improvements in medical education.

Formal surgical instruction returned to Burlington within seventeen years, but it was conducted on a for-profit basis with minimal support from the University. The reforms proposed by Lincoln had to wait another half a century for implementation. The dramatic events in medicine and advances in operative and anesthetic technology during this period of closure of the medical school would affect the College in a positive manner. The future leaders of what eventually became the Department of Surgery otherwise kept up with the times, despite the occasional presence of a scoundrel or two within their ranks.

PART II

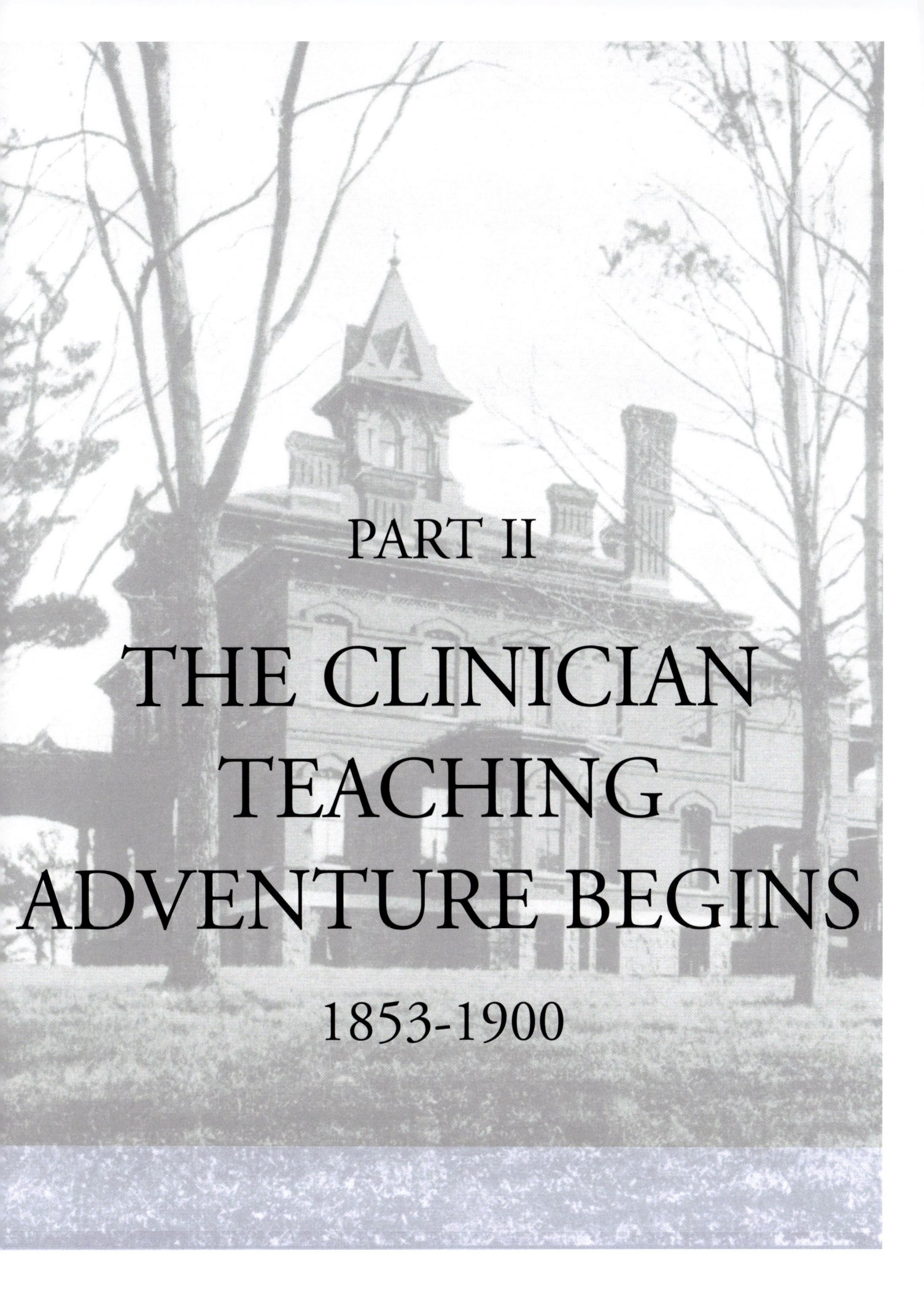

THE CLINICIAN TEACHING ADVENTURE BEGINS

1853-1900

CHAPTER 4

The College of Medicine Reopens

THE discovery of anesthesia revolutionized surgery worldwide overnight. The acceptance of antisepsis, in contrast, took years to achieve.

The sheer volume of complicated cases unleashed by the Civil War transformed American surgery, as did the introduction of sanitary commissions, pavilion plan hospitals, and battlefield ambulances.

As these advancements unfolded, UVM carried on with an unstable non-resident faculty, an inadequate curriculum and no proper teaching hospital.

Surgery Undergoes Revolutionary Changes

During the seventeen years in which the College of Medicine's classrooms lay dormant, the practice of surgery was changed owing to three notable events. The first, in 1845, was the call for a national body dedicated to the improvement of medical education.[1] Although its impact was small at first, the American Medical Association went on to play a major role in the future directions of surgical training — especially at the University of Vermont.

The second, more dramatic development was the "discovery" of inhaled anesthesia. Vermonter Horace Wells, after taking a dose of "laughing gas" at a traveling lecture show, adapted the compound to his Hartford, Connecticut dental practice with great success. In January of 1845, he demonstrated its usage to the medical staff and students of Harvard University. Regrettably, "the gas bag was by mistake withdrawn much too soon" and the patient did not receive the full effect of the nitrous oxide. When it became clear that the subject had felt some pain during his tooth extraction, the affair was dismissed as a "humbug" by the establishment.[2]

Wells discussed his findings with another dentist, William Morton, and a chemist, Charles Jackson. Jackson, having undertaken similar research over the past few years, convinced Morton that sulfuric ether was a better agent due to its liquid properties. Upon confirming its effectiveness, Morton (like Wells) went before Harvard's faculty on October 16, 1846 to present his breakthrough. As the anesthetized patient lay perfectly still, a small vascular tumor was removed from his neck. At the end of the operation, John Collins Warren (son of Nathan Smith's instructor John Warren) softly said to the astonished audience, "Gentlemen, this is no humbug."[3]

In 1847, Scotsman James Simpson found that chloroform delivered an effect similar to that of ether and was less irritating to the eyes and nose.[4] Within a year, inhalation anesthetics were used for nearly all operations. As confidence in the safety and efficacy of anesthesia grew, more and more procedures were performed.

Another advancement during this time was the early appreciation of antisepsis. In March of 1847, Ignaz Semmelweis, a Hungarian obstetrician, found that the death rate from puerperal (childbirth) fever was higher in the ward run by his medical students than in a similar one supervised by midwives. He noted that the midwives' personal hygiene was scrupulous, whereas the students' hands were often contaminated from their cadaveric dissections. Semmelweis demonstrated that rabbits infected with pus from fever victims survived if they were also treated with a solution of chlorinated lime. Deaths from puerperal fever fell from fifteen to one percent after he made every student wash with a similar compound before entering the ward.[5]

Twenty years later, Englishman Joseph Lister found that spraying his surgical field, instruments, sponges, and dressings with diluted carbolic acid led to far fewer wound infections. Although his techniques dramatically reduced the presence of purulence, Lister met with opposition. Surgeons could see the effects of anesthesia and thus understand its benefits. Infection, while ever present, was harder to explain prior to the germ theory of disease. Although Pasteur's germ theory was described during this same time period, most surgeons were not aware of it. It was felt that as long as wounds were left open, "laudable" pus would escape. As a result, antisepsis received limited acceptance.[6]

The College of Medicine is Re-established

Samuel White Thayer had been petitioning the UVM trustees to reopen the College of Medicine. Thayer, the son of a physician, was born in Braintree, Vermont on May 21, 1817. His grandfather (and namesake) had served as a private under General Benjamin Lincoln during the Revolutionary War. Thayer himself had graduated from Woodstock's medical school in 1838 and set up a practice in nearby Northfield. In March of 1853, the board finally took Thayer up on his proposal.[7]

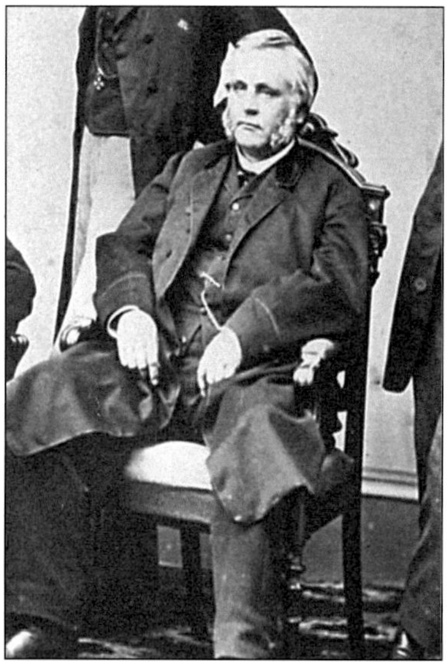

FIGURE 4-1.
Samuel W. Thayer was briefly UVM's Professor of Surgery (1853-1854), but continued as a staff surgeon thereafter. He was Dean of the College of Medicine until 1871. This picture was taken about 1866.

The trustees granted the new College a great deal of latitude. Its professors were allowed complete control over staff, subject material, and salaries as long as they did not "charge the corporation (trustees) with any pecuniary liability whatever."[8] The faculty was given free use of the Medical Building and the equipment it contained, provided that it was kept in good repair. The University was to award degrees upon the receipt of a fee, but the College was to collect the tuition, pay the bills and keep the profits.[9] It became, in essence, a proprietary school, enhanced by its UVM association.

Potential students had to be intelligent, moral and at least twenty-one years old at the time of expected graduation. They had to pay a $5 matriculation fee and a $70 tuition bill for the sixteen-week term. In order to receive an M.D., students had to attend two full courses of lectures [4-6 months each] at either UVM or another medical school, complete three years of study under a preceptor, present a written thesis to the dean, and remit a $25 graduation fee to the University.[10] These somewhat loose requirements remained in place for the next forty years.

Thayer organized the faculty and appointed himself chair of surgery. He asked Horace Henry Nelson to be professor of the theory and practice of medicine. Nelson, a native of Vercheres, Quebec, had obtained his MD from New York University in 1843. He moved to Plattsburgh and started a practice.[11] In January of 1847, he became one of the first surgeons in Canada to operate on an anesthetized patient.[12] Nelson agreed to come to Burlington, but then insisted on teaching surgery instead. Thayer, ever the gentleman, relinquished the chair in his favor.[13]

The Professor of Surgery Absconds With the Funds

Classes got under way in March of 1854. Nelson taught the first term of surgery and Thayer taught anatomy. At the end of the session, Nelson was sent to New York City to buy cadavers. Perhaps feeling that he had been underpaid, he decided to keep the money for himself and go back to Plattsburgh. The College was left with a balance of zero cadavers, zero professors of surgery, and $7.25.[14] Thayer came to the rescue again. He not only gave the surgical lectures in Nelson's place, but he also contributed $250 to the school's coffers. His wife organized a benefit fair and raised another $450 herself.[15] Nelson, meanwhile, had the gall to subsequently advertise himself as *the late* professor of surgery at UVM.[16]

Thayer continued to teach anatomy and physiology for the next eighteen years. He also served as the College of Medicine's first dean during this entire time. Unfortunately, he contracted septicemia in 1867 after performing an amputation. Upon developing diabetes in 1871, he gave up his medical practice, professorship, and deanship. He eventually returned to UVM in 1879 and resumed the role of dean until his death three years later from diabetic gangrene of the foot.[17] An operation was withheld "as at that time there was no known way of making the patient sugar-free."[18]

It was later said that Thayer "was a man of good judgment, and of rare good sense. He was remarkably unselfish, and generous to a fault."[19] This was evidenced by the fact that he "paid absolutely no attention to the financial side of his work. He kept no books and never sent a bill." The resourceful Mrs. Thayer, however, made note of his patient visits and then submitted a charge for what she felt was a fair amount.[20]

Thayer did keep tabs on some bills, though, as an 1891 UVM graduate related:

"Once when he was well along in years his friends made up a purse for him so he could enjoy a vacation in Florida. The hotel presented him a bill including $50.00 for 'Extras,' for use of the golf course, tennis courts, bowling alley etc. Doctor Thayer sent for the manager and said, 'you are charging me fifty dollars for this list of extras, and I have not used one of them. That is not fair.' The manager replied, 'But they were here and available, and you could have had the benefit of them.' The doctor sat down and wrote out a bill against the hotel 'for professional services $50.00.' The manager said, 'We haven't had any professional

services from you.' 'No,' replied Dr. Thayer, 'but I was here and available, and you could have had the benefit of them.' The manager saw the point and cancelled the bill."[21]

The Carpenter Surgeon

Thayer's attempts to find a local physician willing to fill the now vacant chair were unsuccessful. The area's practitioners remained uninterested due to the school's shaky financial situation. He finally convinced professional lecturer David Sloan Conant of New York City to take the position in 1855.[22] Although this seemed an appropriate decision at the time, it established an unfavorable precedent. By choosing reputation over dedication, the College set a revolving door of itinerant surgical educators into motion. Like Nathan Smith before them, the next six chairmen were to be well qualified, prominent surgeons with practices or academic positions elsewhere who came to Burlington only to lecture.

Conant was born on January 21, 1825, in Lyme, New Hampshire. Under pressure from his father, he became a carpenter. He detested the trade, but kept with it until he turned twenty-one. He then embarked on an academic career, paying his way through medical school by building furniture and demonstrating anatomy. After graduating from Bowdoin in 1851, he was appointed demonstrator of anatomy at the New York Medical College. He was put in charge of the city's prestigious Mott Street Cholera Hospital in 1854 and became chief surgeon at the nearby Demilt Dispensary the same year. A few years later, while still at UVM, he also held the professorships of surgery at both Bowdoin and the New York Medical College.[23]

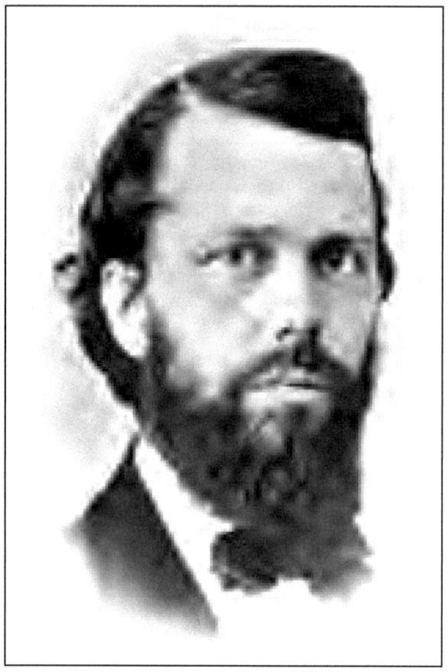

FIGURE 4-2. David S. Conant was Professor of Surgery from 1854-1865, while simultaneously holding the chair at Bowdoin and New York Medical College. This was to be a pattern for many years at UVM.

Conant lectured to an average of 85 students a year during his decade in Burlington.[24] He made use of "Separate bones, parts of all of the skeleton, parts or all of the dead subject, pathological specimens, cases of disease for comparison, manikins, models, plates, photographs, and other illustrations ... to imprint his teachings deeply upon the mind."[25] It was said that, "as a teacher, he was exact, comprehensive and forcible; as a surgeon, bold, courageous and skillful; while as a man he was genial, upright and honorable."[26]

In 1855, the faculty began holding a surgical "clinique" in the Medical Building every Saturday. Students observed amputations, tumor excisions, fracture dressings, laceration repairs, and other operations. The procedures were conducted on charity cases from Vermont, northern New York, and Lower Canada.[27] The overall number of surgeries must have been limited, however, since most operations were still done in patient's homes prior to the existence of hospitals and reliable transportation.

Around the same time, the effects of age and neglect began to take their toll on Benjamin Lincoln's original building (later to be named Pomeroy Hall.) A public fund drive raised $4,000 for renovations. A third story was added, which contained an amphitheater and a dissecting room. The structure was fronted by a new cupola-topped tower and covered with a hipped roof. By September of 1858, the building had finally taken a shape similar to its appearance today.[28]

UVM and the War of the Rebellion

The ensuing four years brought additional changes. Fallout from the financial Panic of 1857 led to the closures of both the Woodstock and Castleton medical schools. Enrollment at the College of Medicine, on the other hand, continued to increase. Within a few years there were more medical students than undergraduates. The school's prosperity continued despite the outbreak of the Civil War.[29]

The College did its part, as over 30 faculty and alumni became military surgeons.[30] Samuel Thayer was appointed chairman of the State Board of Medical Examiners in 1861. Using his organizational skills to the fullest, he helped appoint regimental physicians and secure soldiers' medical care. He also led groups of volunteer surgeons to the front to help overwhelmed battlefield doctors. In recognition of his contributions, he was named Vermont's first Surgeon General in 1864.[31] Former chairman Edward E. Phelps also became involved. He worked alongside Thayer on the Board and reviewed conditions at out-of-state camps.[32] Horace Nelson even made an appearance at a Confederate field hospital.[33]

Conant tried to contribute as well. He became a field surgeon after the Battle of Antietam, but came down with an unspecified gastrointestinal disorder that remained with him for the

FIGURE 4-3.
This matriculation card from 1862 is signed by Dean Thayer, and shows the Medical Building (Pomeroy Hall) after its renovation in 1855, looking remarkably similar to its appearance in the 21st century.

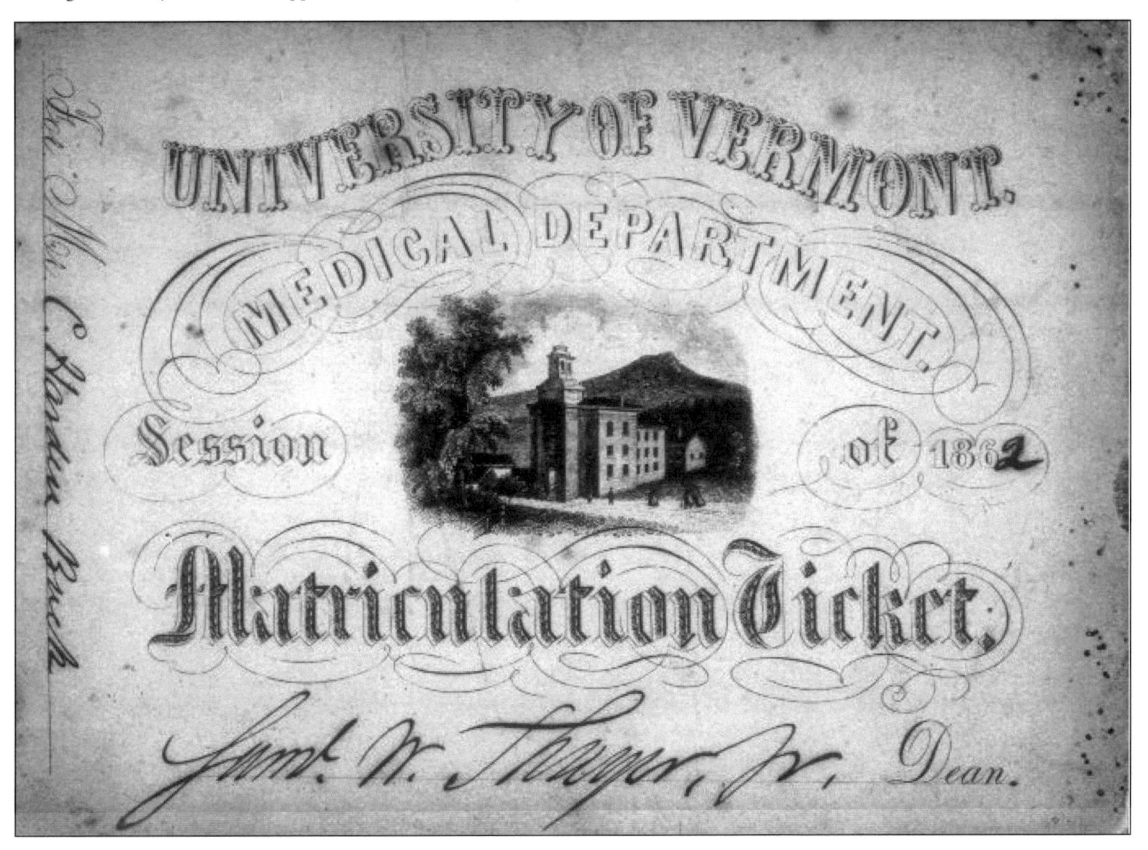

rest of his life.[34] Discharged from duty, he went back to New York and started teaching again. In the fall of 1865, he developed a "small furuncular inflammation on the right side of the nose" after being "repeatedly exposed to an exceedingly offensive, probably exceedingly noxious sick-room air." The abscess, inadequately drained at first, tracked across his face and into his right orbit. It was unroofed two more times without effect. He died from the resulting bacterial meningitis on October 8, 1865.[35]

A.B. Crosby and His "Pavilion Plan" Hospital

The College, looking regionally, invited Dartmouth's Alpheus Benning Crosby to be the next professor of surgery in 1866. Crosby, the son of famous surgical educator Dixi Crosby, was born in Gilmanton, New Hampshire on February 22, 1832. A brilliant student, he assisted his father with operations and the administration of chloroform anesthesia while still a teenager. After obtaining his M.D. from Dartmouth in 1856, he became that school's demonstrator of pathological anatomy.[36]

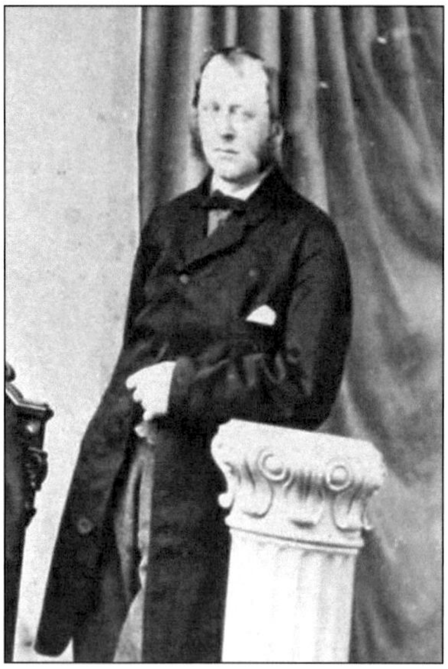

FIGURE 4-4. Alpheus Benning Crosby (Dr. Ben) seasoned by Dartmouth and the Civil War, was UVM's Professor of Surgery from 1866-1872.

Crosby was appointed surgeon to the 1st New Hampshire Volunteers in May of 1861. He was soon promoted to Brigade Surgeon, then Division Surgeon. The new posts came with commands to accommodate and treat scores of wounded soldiers. Familiar with Florence Nightingale's dicta regarding hygiene, spaciousness, and ventilation, and aware of the new French manner of arranging hospital wards, he constructed what many consider to be the first "pavilion plan" hospital in the United States that October.[37]

The compound that arose near Poolesville, Maryland, was quite a departure from the filthy, crowded, multi-story city hospitals of the period. In Crosby's words:

> *"It consisted of a series of one-story buildings, each large enough for a single ward of thirty beds. Each building was made of rough boards, the cracks being battened with strips, and all thoroughly whitewashed, inside and out. There was a window at the head of each bed, suitable ventilators which were always kept open, and a large stove in each ward. The kitchen and offices were in a building by themselves. All these buildings were connected by water sheds, without walls, so that each ward was distinct, and elevated walks were made beneath the sheds. The ground was elevated and dry, and as trenches were dug around each building to receive the droppings from the eaves, the drainage was perfect."*[38]

Endorsed by the U.S. Sanitary Commission, the pavilion model was applied to the majority of military and civilian hospitals built over the next forty years, including Burlington's Mary Fletcher Hospital in 1879.

Crosby was also ahead of his time when it came to antisepsis. He felt that, "Filth in wounds means poison, and poison means death."[39] He explained how he attacked this problem in the following manner:

> "On arriving at the division hospital at Poolesville, a uniform plan of treatment was adopted. The sum and substance of this plan was absolute cleanliness. This was enforced by frequent scourings of the wards, and the instant removal of dejections [bodily waste] and all effete [worn out] matter from them. The bedding was changed as often as it was in the slightest degree soiled. A rough washhouse was extemporized, where four men incessantly boiled, washed and ironed the bedding. The patients' bodies were sponged with warm water; those suffering from surgical fever at shorter intervals."[40]

Crosby then prohibited the customary treatment of packing gunshot wounds with lint and hermetically sealing them with adhesive strips:

> "Every injury was treated as an open wound; a water dressing was applied, which was changed at short intervals, and burned as soon as soiled. All wounds which were offensive were treated with antiseptic and stimulating applications. No wound was drawn together until its surfaces were covered with bright healthy granulations."[41]

The staff halted superficial infections with "a few pounds of copperas" (ferrous sulfate mixed with molasses). The only other medications at their disposal were opium, cinchona (quinine), Epsom salts, and whiskey. The death rate for the entire hospital, including patients already known to be mortally wounded on admission, was ten percent — roughly a third of the rate at the Army's other facilities.[42]

"Dr. Ben", as he was known, resigned his commission in June of 1862. He was named associate professor of surgery at Dartmouth that August, and succeeded his father as full professor in 1870 while still on the staff at UVM. He outdid Conant by holding the Chairs of Surgery at the Long Island Hospital College, the University of Michigan, and Bowdoin, and the chair of anatomy at Bellevue Hospital Medical College simultaneously.[43, 44] "As a lecturer he was a master of his subject — clear and definite in his demonstrations, direct and incisive in his manner, apt in illustration, brimful of good humor and pointed anecdote, and fluent, even to prodigality, in his words, so that his power over students was immense and his classroom was crowded."[45]

He discontinued his associations with every school except Dartmouth and Bellevue in 1872, thereafter teaching at the former in the summer and the latter in the winter. His actions led some to believe that he was overworked. This seemed to be confirmed in August of 1877 when he experienced an abrupt decline in mental function and died a few days later at the age of 45. His autopsy, however, revealed what Crosby, an excellent diagnostician and expert on the subject, had known for years — that he was afflicted with the untreatable (and thus fatal) condition of diabetes mellitus.[46]

Henry Janes' Civil War Medical Journal

Native son Elisha Harris, a co-founder of the U.S. Sanitation Commission, shared Crosby's wartime attitudes regarding patient care. Feeling that Vermont's soldiers should be convalesc-

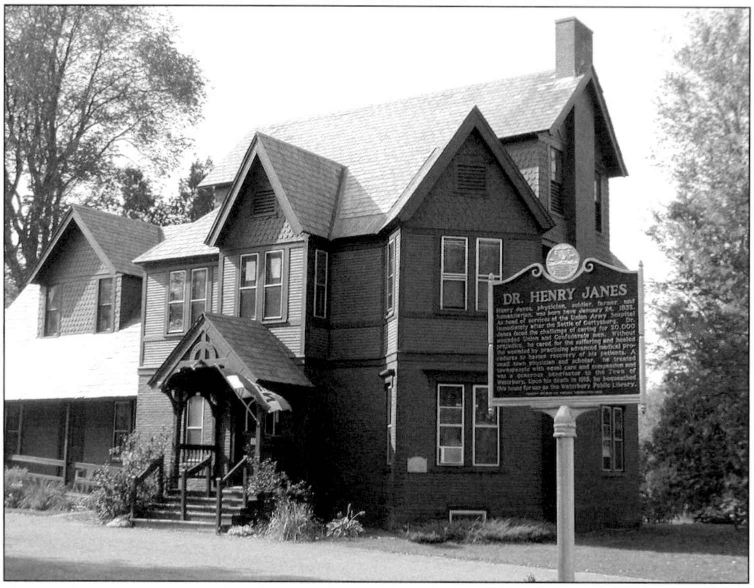

FIGURE 4-5. Henry Janes' house in Waterbury, Vermont is now a library and a museum that contains some of his Civil War treasures.

ing closer to home in cleaner surroundings, he facilitated the construction of three in-state military hospitals. Samuel Thayer ran Burlington's Baxter Hospital, Edward Phelps oversaw Brattleboro's Smith Hospital, and Henry Janes supervised Montpelier's Sloan Hospital.[47] From May of 1862 to December of 1865, the three facilities treated a total of 8,574 soldiers. The overall death rate was just two percent, a figure much better than that of the big city "tent hospitals."[48]

Janes was already a seasoned war surgeon by the time he took control of Sloan Hospital. A lifelong resident of Waterbury, Vermont, he was born on January 24, 1832. At the age of 21, he left home to attend medical schools in Woodstock and New York City. After graduating from the Columbia College of Physicians and Surgeons in 1855, he worked at Bellevue Hospital for a year. Janes returned to Waterbury in 1857 and began his practice. In June of 1861, he joined the 3rd Vermont Volunteer Infantry as a surgeon. Like Crosby, he rapidly rose through the ranks, directing hospitals at Burkettsville, Frederick, and Potomac Creek, Maryland. At the conclusion of the Battle of Gettysburg, Janes was appointed Surgeon-in-Charge of all hospitals in the area, including the massive Letterman General Hospital. The 250 surgeons under his command treated more than 20,000 wounded Union and Confederate troops.[49]

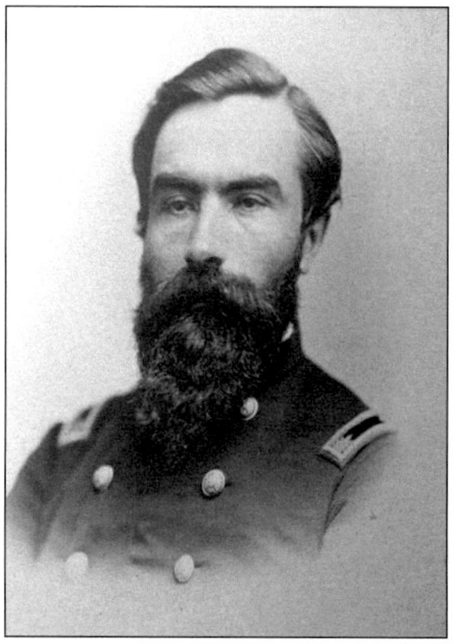

FIGURE 4-6. Henry Janes cared for the wounded of Gettysburg and other Civil War Battles, before returning to practice surgery in Waterbury, and instruct medical students briefly at UVM.

Janes was a humane and versatile surgeon dedicated to his patients' long-term rehabilitation. He kept a handwritten journal filled with hundreds of detailed notes and photographs of injured soldiers and their wounds. The book provides a unique insight into the era's treatment of traumatic injury.[50]

44 CATAMOUNT SURGEONS

Janes categorized the patients he chronicled as follows:

Extremity with amputation:	717
(205 above-knee, 293 below-knee, 150 arm, 45 shoulder)	
Extremity without amputation:	478
(268 upper leg, 136 lower leg, 57 upper arm, 13 forearm)	
Chest:	136 (1 died)
Abdomen:	34 (17 died)
Spinal cord:	2
Skull and brain injury:	9 (4 died)
Other:	532
Total number of cases:	1772

The journal demonstrates that most survivors suffered from extremity wounds, many requiring amputation. The devastating injuries left by Claude Étienne Minié's high-velocity rifle bullets were prone to infection, thus dooming most attempts at limb preservation. In fact, the majority of soldiers hit in the chest and abdomen by these projectiles died long before reaching the evacuation hospital. The excerpts below illustrate some of the problems Janes faced:

"C.E., age 20
Wounded July 3rd [1863] by a minnie ball entering the left side of the thorax, anteriorly between the sixth and seventh ribs, and passing downwards and backwards, made its exit two inches to the left of the first lumbar vertebra, penetrating the lower lobe of the left lung. Sept. 1st took charge of the case. I found the anterior wound healed, while the posterior was discharging healthy pus in small quantities with occasional clots of extravasated blood. There is no cough or expectoration and no difficulty of respiration. There is a consolidation to a considerable extent of the lower lobe of the left lung. Transferred Sept. 12th to Baltimore Convalescent, unfit for field service. March 7th [1864] detached at Patterson Park Hospital, Baltimore."

"W.W., age 27
Wounded July 2nd by a minnie ball passing through the left middle lobe. Patient is very weak and the wounds are discharging copiously. He has been affected with a troublesome diarrhea since Sept. 1st. Air is constantly escaping from the lung through the wound of entrance. Has also been troubled by a constant cough. Died Sept. 24th."

"W.M., age 27
Wounded July 2nd by a minnie ball entering 3 inches below the right nipple and passing obliquely downwards and backwards, made its exit posteriorly near the last rib and about 4 inches from the spine. The patient has expectorated considerable pus Sept. 2nd to 23rd. Improving rapidly. External wounds healed. Transferred Sept. 28th cured."

FIGURE 4-7. Photo of "C.H.S." from Janes' Civil War Casebook.

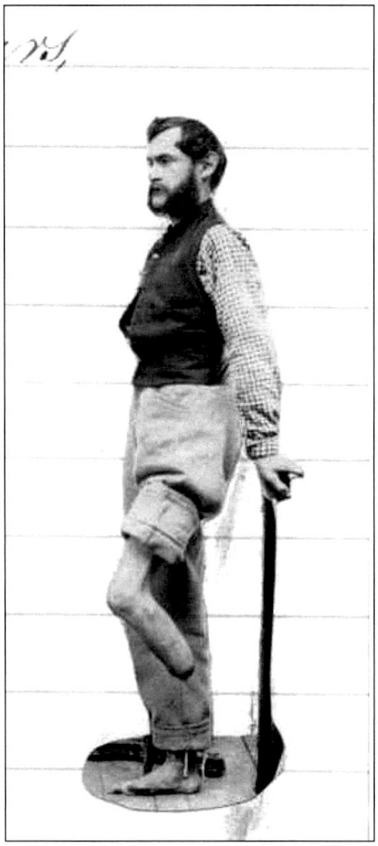

"C.H.S., age 25
Co K 6th Vermont. Admitted Sept 21, 1864, operated Oct 13, Injured Sept 19, 1864. Discharged Sept 11, 1865.

Wounded at Winchester [Virginia] Sept. 19, 1864 by a piece of shell fracturing the left ankle and destroying the right great toe. Toe amputated about the last of Sept. and healed without accident. Oct. 13th the leg amputated at the junction of the middle and lower thirds by the flap operation: five days afterwards flaps sloughed: abscess formed in the front part of the stump: the anterior edge of the tibia necrosed and came away to the length of four inches on the 19th of June 1865. After that, the stump healed rapidly. August 21st transferred from Brattleboro Vt. to Montpelier Vt. Stump healed and flexed upon the thigh at an angle of about 135 degrees. [note that a 135° flexion contracture of the knee prohibits wearing a prosthesis!] General health was good. Sept 11th transferred to New York, for an artificial limb. Not yet able to completely extend the leg: step firm, not at all tender."

"J.S., age 24
Wounded at the Battle of Charleston by a mini-bullet which shattered the left knee. Thigh amputated 3 hours afterwards. He was taken to a field hospital at Sandy Hook until Dec. 1st 1864. Three or four weeks after the operation, the flaps sloughed. Two weeks later, a piece exfoliated from the end of the femur. The wound then healed rapidly until the first of December when another piece of necrosed bone came away ... Feb. 22nd ... he fell and injured the stump ... March 2nd 1865 he was transferred to Montpelier. While at the transit hospital his stump was dressed and he thinks inoculated with gangrenous matter, for in a few hours it began to swell and became painful. When he arrived at Montpelier March 8th there was a gangrenous spot the size of half a dollar. This extended until the whole end of the stump was involved but the bone was not exposed. Nitric acid was applied several times and the gangrene was arrested in the latter part of March. After that time the stump healed rapidly, but it occasionally became inflamed and painful. On the 1st of Sept. it was entirely healed save for a sinus into which a probe could be passed for 4 inches. The discharge amounted to about one ounce a day. The sinus became obstructed and an abscess formed which was opened and a probe inserted for several inches. But no necrosed bone could be reached though it probably existed ... His general health was good. Discharged Oct 5, 1865."

"A.D.D., age 44
Wounded near Lee's Mills Va. [April 16th, 1862] by a musket ball which entered the center of the right patella and lodged in the knee joint. The thigh was amputated in the middle third by the flap method 25 hours after injury by C.M. Chandler 6th Vt. Chloroform was

used as the anesthetic. He remained about three weeks in the Savage Station Field Hospital when the stump was healing nicely. After three weeks he was taken 12 miles to Yorktown over a corduroy road in an army wagon and during the trip the flaps were torn open. Two days afterwards he was taken to Judiciary Square Hospital, Washington D.C. where he remained until July 1st '62 when he was discharged from the service. The ligatures did not come away [until] late Sept. when the stump healed rapidly.

Sept 20th '65: He is in good health. The stump has now broken open and no bone has come away. He has worn a Palmer leg since January '63 and has nearly worn it out. The socket often chafes the stump which has lately diminished in size."

"G.T.A., age 21
Wounded at the Wilderness by a minie bullet which entered the inner side of the right arm about the middle. Fractured the humerus and lodged under the skin on the posterior and outer side from whence it was cut out. No bone was removed with the ball but a fragment 1/4 by 3/4 of an inch came away 4 days afterwards and another 1/4 by 1 inch together with a small piece of the bullet came away 5 months later. No other pieces came away. For the first week no retention apparatus was used, after that an angular splint was applied. Six weeks after injury the wound became gangrenous. The gangrene was arrested in about two weeks by the use of nitric acid and he began to improve very slowly. He was confined to the house about six weeks. The wound healed with a false joint about the 1st of July 1865. In the latter part of June he was sent to New York and fitted with a Hudson's retentive apparatus which he was

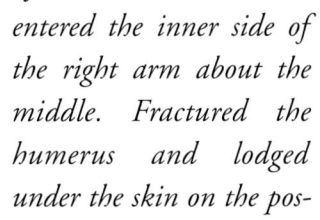

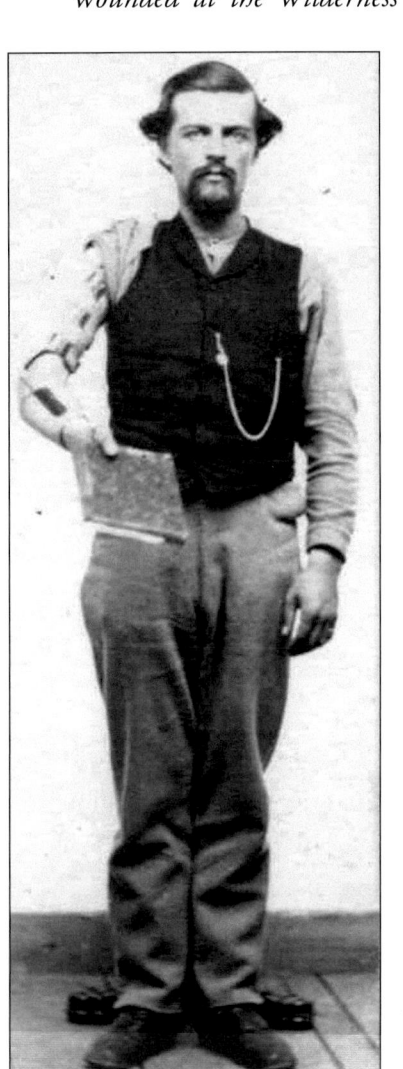

FIGURE 4-8.
A.D.D. with his Palmer leg in 1865.

FIGURE 4-9.
G.T.A. wearing the "retentive apparatus" used to treat his severe upper arm wound.

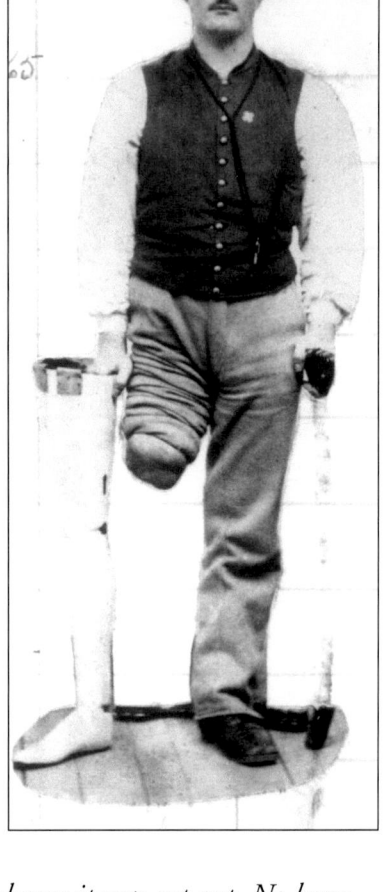

Chapter Four: The College of Medicine Reopens

FIGURE 4-10.
Civil war injury with short leg and obvious foot drop, but preserved limb, in Janes' Casebook.

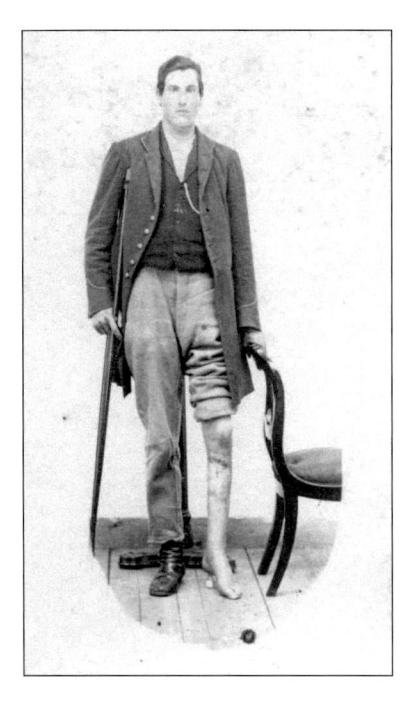

wearing at the time of his discharge from the service Sept. 20th 1865. With this he could write and do almost any kind of light work but without it the arm was nearly useless. He was in good condition and seemed to be doing well up to the time the gangrene commenced. After that the discharge became very profuse; a large abscess formed just above the wound and he became much debilitated. He was in good health when discharged."[51]

Janes returned to private practice in Waterbury following the closure of Sloan Army Hospital in December of 1865. He was the Vermont Medical Society delegate to the UVM medical school in 1868 and became a senior consultant at Burlington's Mary Fletcher Hospital in the 1880s.[52, 53] Janes also taught a course at the College of Medicine entitled "Military Surgery" in 1886.[54] He was an expert extremity and external tumor surgeon, but a failure in the abdomen because of his inability to grasp aseptic technique.[55]

FIGURE 4-11.
Janes' Civil War instruments on display in the museum in his house in Waterbury, VT.

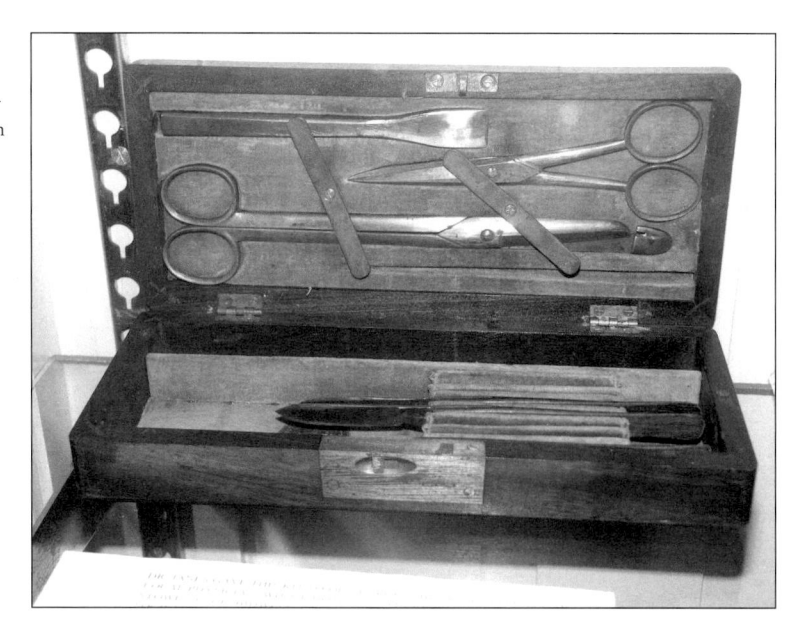

The Professor of Surgery Becomes a Medical Innovator

Benjamin Douglas Howard, the College's professor of disease of the genito-urinary organs since 1866, followed Crosby in 1873 as professor of Surgery. Born in Chesham, England on March 21, 1836, he had made his way to New York City by 1853. He graduated from Columbia's College of Physicians and Surgeons in 1858 and, intending to be a medical missionary, studied at Auburn Theological Seminary. Determined to help end the slave trade, he entered the Army Medical Service in 1861, serving until December of 1864.[56] Among his many innovations were the "Howard" system of artificial respiration, the "Howard" Ambulance Wagon, and an emergency tracheal cannula.[57, 58, 59] Like his predecessors (and successors), he held several other concurrent surgical professorships, including those of the University of the State of New York, the Long Island College Hospital, and the University of Cincinnati.⁶⁰

During the War, Howard pioneered the use of wire to reunite long bones fractured by gunshots.⁶¹ He also successfully removed a minie bullet from a soldier's brain through a small craniotomy.⁶²

His treatment of open chest wounds, on the other hand, was less than satisfactory. He wrote:

"1) Remove foreign material, 2) Control bleeding, 3) Debride wound edges, 4) Close with metallic sutures, and 5) Apply airtight dressings."⁶³ Infections, of course, thrived in the absence of proper drainage, and a high mortality rate ensued before the above practice was abandoned. His failure to appreciate basic physiology became apparent to his students at UVM too, as a member of the class of 1873 later recalled:

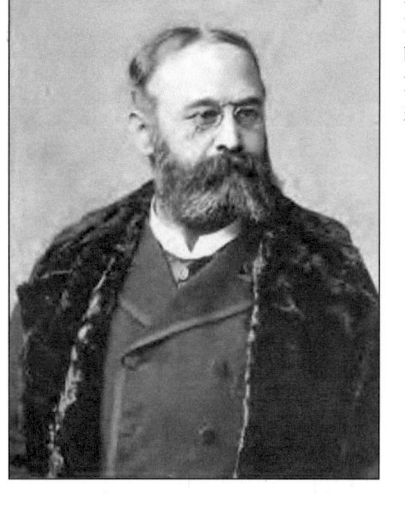

FIGURE 4-12. Benjamin Howard became UVM's Professor of Surgery in 1873.

> "He [Howard] was greatly hampered in his presentation of his subject by the lack of surgical clinics, which prevented him from showing us any operations of major importance. For those of minor importance the patients were never etherized in the lecture room. I remember that once the failure ... to practice what he preached led to a great uproar among the students. A lady came before the class who had what is known as a nævus or tumor of a nerve in the forearm which was very painful. Although it was at a time before hypodermic medication [injectable local anesthesia], and the operation would also be very painful, she consented to removal of the tumor. Before beginning the operation Dr. Howard lectured to the class ... that to avoid hurting her twice, the proximal end of the nerve should be cut off first, and then the distal end. Proceeding with the operation he performed it in a way exactly opposite to that which he had advised in his lecture. His humiliation was evident." ⁶⁴

Howard resigned his academic appointments in 1875 due to worsening "neurasthenia." He traveled the world, convincing authorities in Paris and London to institute "accident-ambulance services" and donated carriages of his own design to both cities. He also worked to reform global prison conditions in the decade before his death from an "affection of the liver" on June 22, 1900.⁶⁵

Howard's career was typical of the medical college's professors at this time. Although individually accomplished, the group probably provided the medical students with an average surgical education at best, compared to other first rate medical colleges such as Harvard. The proficiency of their lectures was significantly reduced in the absence of a teaching hospital. This changed, however, when the school finally obtained the facilities it desperately needed.

CHAPTER 5

New Facilities Breathe Life Into the Program

Acceptance of antisepsis gained momentum as Mary Fletcher's hospital became an integral part of the College of Medicine. Another building, specifically designed for medical teaching, was erected nearby.

The hospital provided sorely needed clinical cases for the school's surgeons. The training program, however, still had largely part-time faculty, lax admission requirements, and offered no in-hospital experience.

The College finally instituted a graded curriculum, along with a practical course in surgery, at the end of the nineteenth century. Academic pursuits, though, were put on hold.

Surgical Techniques Change After the Civil War

The typical Civil War surgeon had treated thousands of wounded soldiers by war's end. Thus, he did not feel that anyone could teach him much about pus, blood poisoning, gangrene, lockjaw or any other postoperative complication. He operated in an old black frock coat that was usually a shabby number long ago discarded from his wardrobe and now after years of use stiff with blood. He took care not to touch the lapels. If he were foolish enough to do so he would certainly get his fingers pricked badly on the porcupine-like field of threaded needles stuck in there so as to be ready, when needed, for sewing up the wound."[1]

"During surgery natural sea sponges are used after some of the sand has been shaken out of them. Afterwards they may be rinsed under the tap and dried for future re-use in surgery. ... dressings were second-hand, soiled, linen rags which the hospital attendants had begged from generous housewives and used on the patient just as they had come in, since no one had bothered to wash them."[2]

John Brooks Wheeler, UVM's future Chief of Surgery, observed the actions of such men first hand as a medical student:

"The old-timers couldn't let their dressings alone. They were accustomed to seeing pus form, collect and make no end of trouble if it was not carefully and skillfully dealt with, so every twenty-four hours they exposed the wound, puttered over it, took out a stitch here and there,

perhaps irrigated it with some solution which happened to have a temporary reputation for the possession of 'healing properties,' put on a fresh dressing and next day went through with the same performance. Of course they almost always found pus sooner or later, as neither their hands nor their instruments were sterile."3

Wheeler watched his professors operate with instruments that had been dropped on the floor and bare hands that had been run through their hair. He recalled that,

"The worst thing of the kind that I ever saw was when a surgeon, operating with knife and forceps, wanted to use his right hand for a moment for something else and instead of laying the knife in the instrument tray or handing it to an assistant, held it in his teeth 'til he had finished his manipulations and then took it in his hand again and went on with his cutting."4

Lister Declares War on Pasteur's Bacteria

French chemist Louis Pasteur had established the link between bacteria and infection as early as 1861. He later demonstrated that these "small corpuscles" could be destroyed through heat sterilization. Upon learning of this breakthrough, English surgeon James Lister took it upon himself to find a substance that would eliminate Pasteur's "germs" from his surgical wounds. After experimenting with zinc chloride and various sulfites, he settled on carbolic acid (the active ingredient in today's Chloraseptic® Sore Throat Spray) as a suitable agent.5

Thinking that bacteria reached wounds through the air, he sprayed the space over the operative field with a 1 to 20 solution of carbolic acid using a steam atomizer. In addition,

"Lister scrubbed his hands with soap and water and a nailbrush and disinfected them, as he thought, by rinsing them in a 1 to 40 carbolic solution. His instruments lay in a tray filled with a 1 to 20 carbolic solution, and he took great care that nothing which had not been thoroughly carbolized should get into the wound or even near it."

"He was particularly careful of his sponges, which were the ordinary sea-sponges, but of fine quality and very carefully cleansed from sand and other foreign substances. They were cleansed first by a thorough beating while the sponge was dry, and then by prolonged washings in tepid water — hot water shrivels a sponge and spoils it — until the water comes clear and free of sand. They were then bleached and disinfected by immersion for forty-eight hours in a solution of hypochlorite of soda, and then kept in a 1 to 20 carbolic solution until they were needed for use."6

Lister wrote in 1867:

"... previously to its introduction [carbolic spray] ... the two large wards in which most of my cases of accident and of operation were treated were among the unhealthiest in the whole surgical division of the Glasgow Royal Infirmary. But since the antiseptic treatment has been brought into full operation, and wounds and abscesses no longer poison the atmosphere with putrid exhalations, my wards, ... have completely changed in character ... so that during the

last nine months not a single instance of pyemia, hospital gangrene, or erysipelas has occurred in them."[7]

Lister's published results were too good for the post-Civil War area practioners to believe. Attempts to replicate his findings met with mixed success, depending on the degree to which each surgeon followed Lister's protocols. It was "No wonder that otherwise excellent surgeons who lacked proper antiseptic training failed to get good results and concluded that Listerism didn't amount to much."[8]

Antisepsis finally came into widespread favor at the end of the 1870/1871 Franco-Prussian War. Wound infections had afflicted over eighty percent of the soldiers injured during that conflict. Upon adopting Lister's methods, German military surgeons reduced that figure to less than five percent in a matter of weeks.[9] Bolstered by their success, Lister came to America in September of 1876 to present similar large-scale results.[10] Many surgeons took his findings to heart, treating their instruments, dressings, and room air with carbolic acid. They continued to operate, however, barehanded and unmasked in their pus-stained coats.

James L. Little, the Big Surgeon

James Lawrence Little, the College's professor of surgery from 1875 to 1885, was a giant in both size and vision. Standing well over six feet tall and weighing at least 250 pounds, he made major contributions to both UVM and the practice of surgery. Born in Brooklyn, New

FIGURE 5-1.
Friedrich von Esmarch performing an amputation, as depicted in John Brooks Wheeler's Memoirs. Wheeler commented: "I suppose the instruments in the little tray are lying in a carbolic solution and that the gentleman who is squirting away with his little hand atomizer thinks he is doing something highly bactericidal."

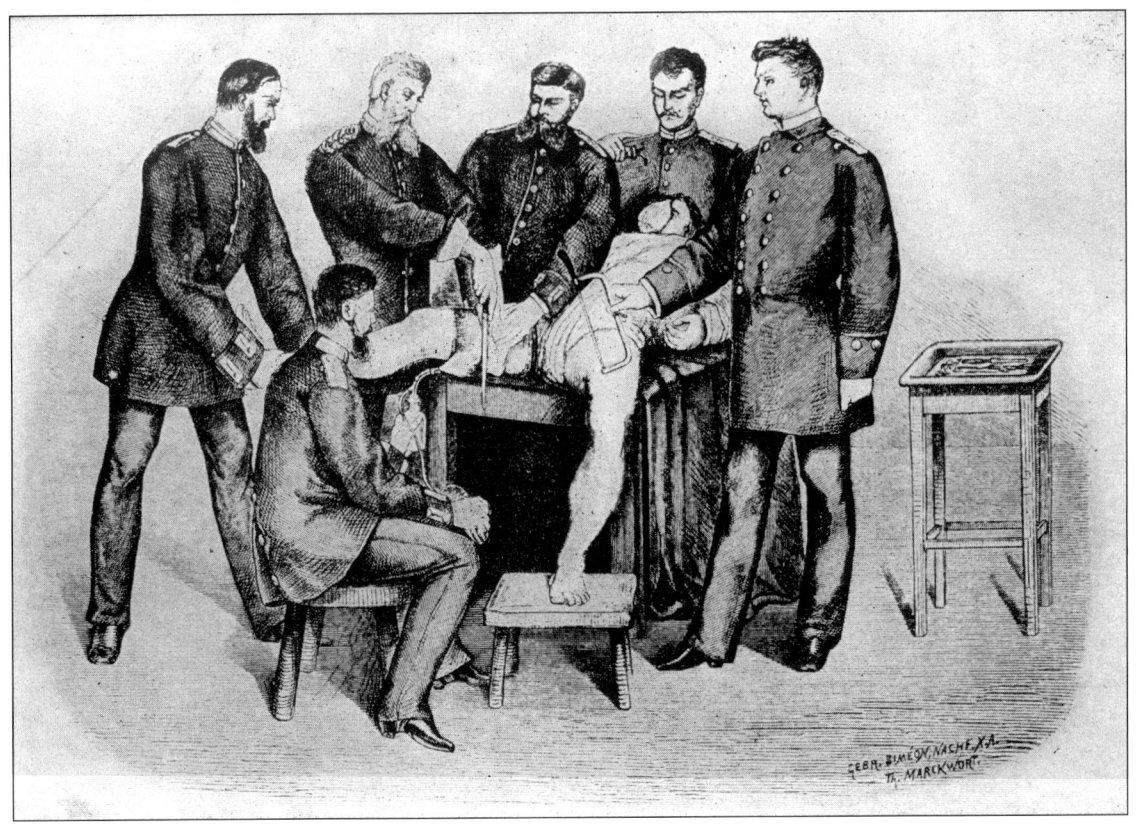

York, on February 19, 1836, he became a bookseller at age twenty, but was fired after spending too much time reading the store's medical books. Interested in learning anatomy, he purchased a pauper's skull from a gravedigger for twenty-five cents. Upon unwrapping the package, however, he found that it contained a decomposing head. Horrified, he threw the entire lot into the East River and chose another course of study.[11]

Little attended the Columbia College of Physicians and Surgeons, graduating in 1860. He became a junior assistant surgeon at the New York Hospital the same year. Little was Surgeon-in-Chief to New York City's 14,000-bed Parks Barracks Hospital during the Civil War, even though he did not serve in the military.[12]

It was during this time that Little came up with his first major breakthrough — the invention of the plaster-of-Paris splint. Beforehand, splints had been made from a troublesome starchy material. Although plaster-of-Paris had been used as a surgical dressing without success, Little was able to adapt the compound to orthopaedic practice. He devised an ingredient mixture and application method that provided an immovable yet porous splint that would conform to any shape desired. His basic technique is still used today.[13]

In 1862, Little began a long association with his alma mater as a clinical assistant. He remained on staff as a lecturer on operative surgery even after becoming UVM's chairman. He eventually left Columbia in 1880 for the professorship of surgery at New York University, but departed after three years when his lecture time was reduced. He held a similar position at the Post-Graduate Medical School in New York from 1883 to 1885.[14]

Like Conant, Crosby, and Howard before him, Little taught in New England during the spring and New York City during the winter. The trip from Manhattan to Burlington was relatively straightforward by that time. A train ran between the city and the far side of Lake Champlain. Passengers then traversed the lake via a ferry service. When the lake froze, a stagecoach line was staked off with cedar bushes. The locals referred to the wintry crossing as "bushing the route." Alternatively, there was a train that ran from Albany through Bennington and Rutland directly to Burlington. Although the journey was long, it was much more pleasant than the arduous overland route from Boston.[15] The train from Boston started soon thereafter and left Boston at 7:30 am, arriving at Burlington at 6:30 pm.[16]

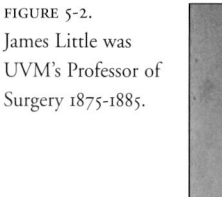

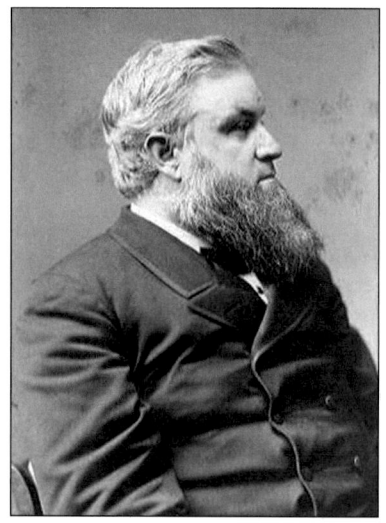

FIGURE 5-2.
James Little was UVM's Professor of Surgery 1875-1885.

Though not as polished as his contemporaries, Little was a popular lecturer nevertheless. One co-worker felt that "He was ungrammatical and incorrect in pronunciation. But in spite of these defects, he was a ready speaker, who knew what he was talking about and could express his ideas clearly and forcefully."[17] Another stated, "His manner was exceedingly simple, in fact, at first distressingly so; but it was earnest, and devoid of mannerisms and self-consciousness."[18]

Little spearheaded the drive to increase the number of UVM lectures delivered by specialists. Using his personal connections, he recruited speakers from New York in the fields of ophthalmology, otolaryngology, and urology, among others. He also convinced his colleagues to give clinical instruction in each of these subjects.[19, 20]

Little was the first surgeon to place a suprapubic catheter for the relief of urinary retention. An early adapter, he was also among the first users of the newly invented laryngoscope and ophthalmoscope during the 1860s.[21] His interests in these instruments led to his next major surgical legacy. In 1879, during the middle of his tenure at UVM, he published the first succinct description of the location in which the majority of all nosebleeds originate.[22] Recognition of this discovery in the United States, ironically, has since fallen to a German laryngologist who reported similar findings in 1884. Thus, the region still known as Little's area in Great Britain is called Kiesselbach's plexus in the United States.[23]

Another field in which Little took the lead, especially at UVM, was "cleanliness," and later, antisepsis. William J. Mayo, an attendee of the Post-Graduate School and founder of the famous Minnesota clinic, remembered that Little was:

> "... a large, handsome man, with a white beard, and hair somewhat scanty on top. He always looked well groomed. At that day tobacco was chewed more than at present, and I have seen some worthy practitioners of years ago whose beards bore evidence of the fact. Professor Little was immaculately clean. His hair and beard fairly shone, and his face was pink rather than congested, as were the faces of so many men in those days from the use of alcoholic beverages.
>
> Little was just beginning to be influenced by the teachings of Lister. His results were excellent, because ... he was clean naturally."[24]

This trait likely had something to do with the presence of "Little's Luck" during his operations. He further improved his results following a visit to London during August of 1881 in which "... he investigated Lister's methods very carefully, and came back to carry out all the details of Listerism in capital operations."[25] The timing was fortuitous, as Burlington had just completed a state-of-the-art facility in which Little's procedures could be performed.

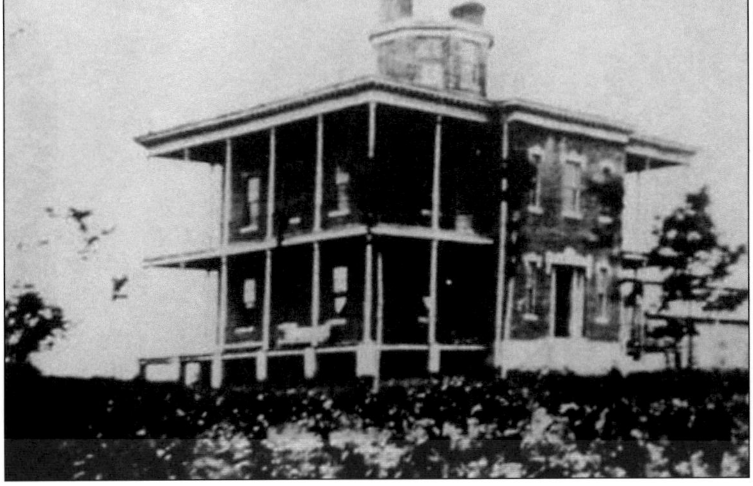

FIGURE 5-3.
The Marine Hospital was Burlington's first. Built in 1858, it stood at the corner of today's I-189 and Route 7.

The College of Medicine's First Hospital

Burlington had been home to a pest house during the 1700s. There had been a "temporary" army hospital at the north end of Battery Street from 1812 to 1815. The city's first permanent infirmary (another military institution) was completed in 1858. Known as the Marine Hospital, it was a two story Italianate-style brick building with a spacious veranda. It was situated on ten acres of land next to Shelburne Road, two miles south of town near the intersection of today's Interstate Route 189. The complex was renamed Baxter U.S. Army Hospital following the addition of nine pavilion-style wards during the Civil War. It treated 2,406 injured soldiers before being decommissioned in 1865.[26] The Sisters of Providence ran a small Catholic hospital at this time as well. Unfortunately, none of these facilities were available to the College for surgical training.[27]

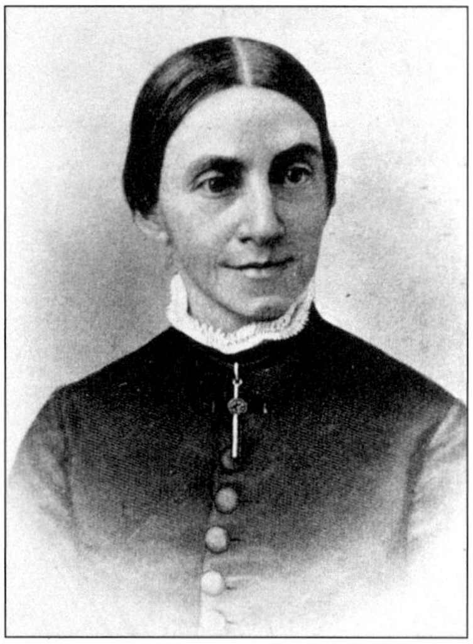

FIGURE 5-4. Mary Martha Fletcher

This was to change following a philanthropic act by Mary Martha Fletcher. Her father, Thaddeus Fletcher, had prudently invested in western real estate during the 1840s, making nearly half a million dollars in the process (although it was rumored that some of his fortune came from the sale of contraband cotton during the Civil War).[28, 29] Thaddeus, his wife Mary Lawrence, and his daughters Ellen and Mary Martha moved to Burlington from rural Jericho, Vermont, in 1853. A single faithful servant, Michael Kelly, saw to all of their needs. Ellen died of "consumption" in 1855 but her sister Mary survived thanks to the care of the family physician, who was incidentally the Dean of the Medical School. Her grateful parents expressed an interest in funding a hospital, but died before a plan could be put into action. Mary, an extremely delicate and exceedingly shy invalid, found the strength to carry out their wishes. In 1876, she donated $25,000 towards the purchase of a site, $50,000 for the construction of a building, and another $100,000 to create a permanent endowment.[30]

The 35-acre Catlin estate was chosen for the new hospital's location. Situated on a hill immediately adjacent to the University, it commanded spectacular views of Lake Champlain to the west and the Green Mountains to the east.[31] Lucinda Allen Catlin, Ethan and Ira's niece, had selected the site after complaining about the view from her Main Street residence. Her husband climbed a tree and remarked "I think Lucinda will think there is enough view from here", and the Catlin estate was built on the present Fletcher House location.[32] The original sixty-year old house and barn were razed, and a new four-story brick building went up in their place. Completed in early 1879, the hospital was named in honor of Mary (Martha) Fletcher's mother, Mary (Lawrence) Fletcher.[33]

A large operating room surrounded by a 200-seat amphitheater occupied an adjacent building, which also contained an anesthetizing room and a recovery room. There was also a pathological room in which autopsies were performed. Little was the first surgeon-in-chief.[34]

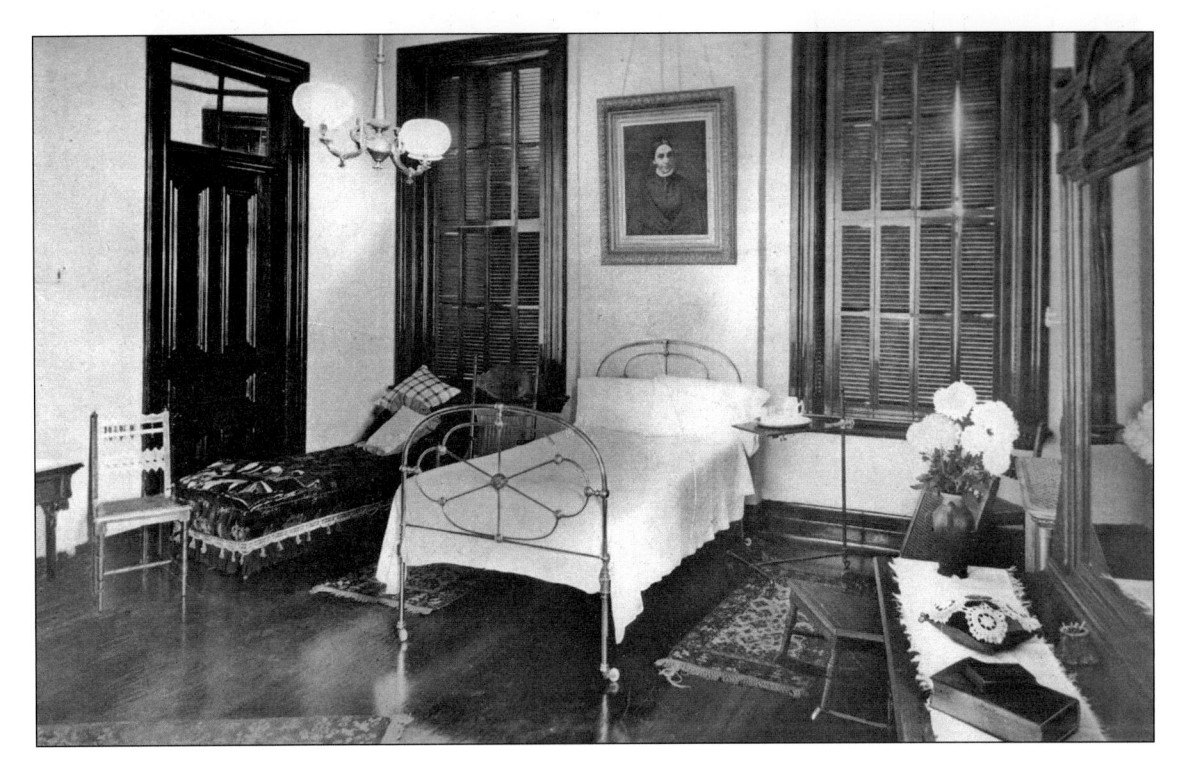

FIGURE 5-5.
Mary Martha Fletcher's private room at her "House". (Fletcher House)

FIGURE 5-6.
The Mary Fletcher Hospital is on the left in this 1882 photograph. The "White Corridor" connects it to the operating amphitheatre on the right.

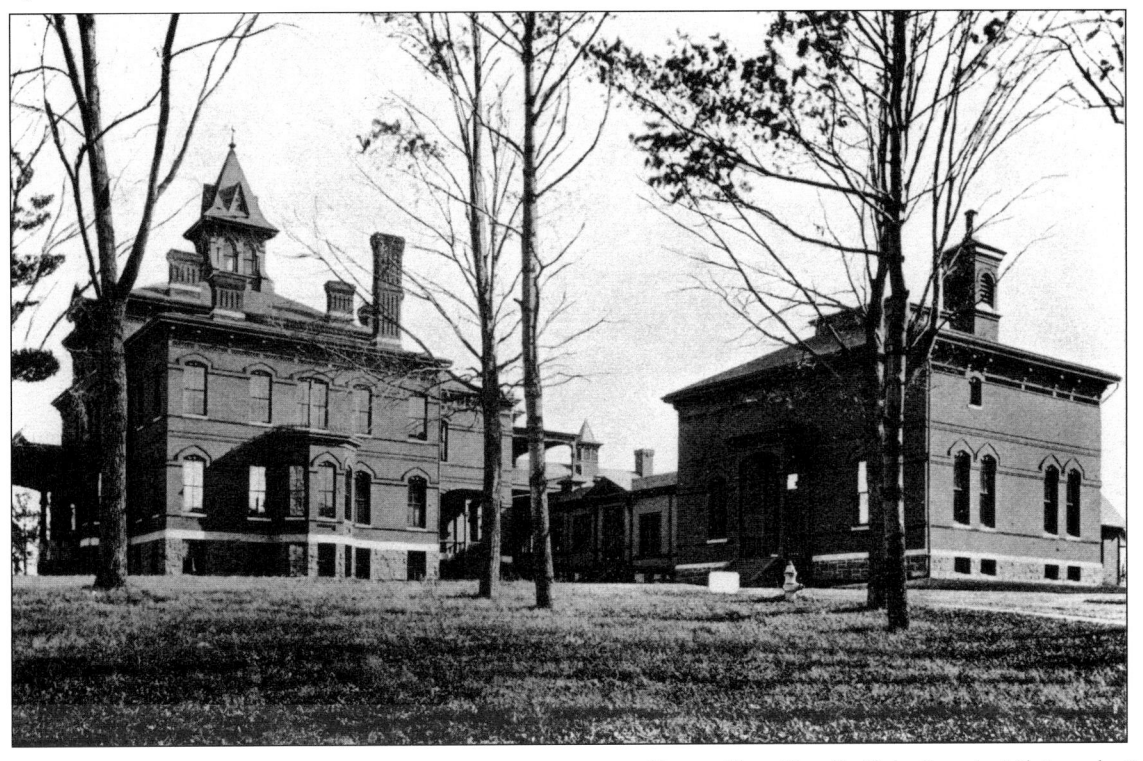

Chapter Five: New Facilities Breathe Life Into the Program 57

FIGURE 5-7.
The Mary Fletcher Hospital as depicted in the 1885 UVM catalog.

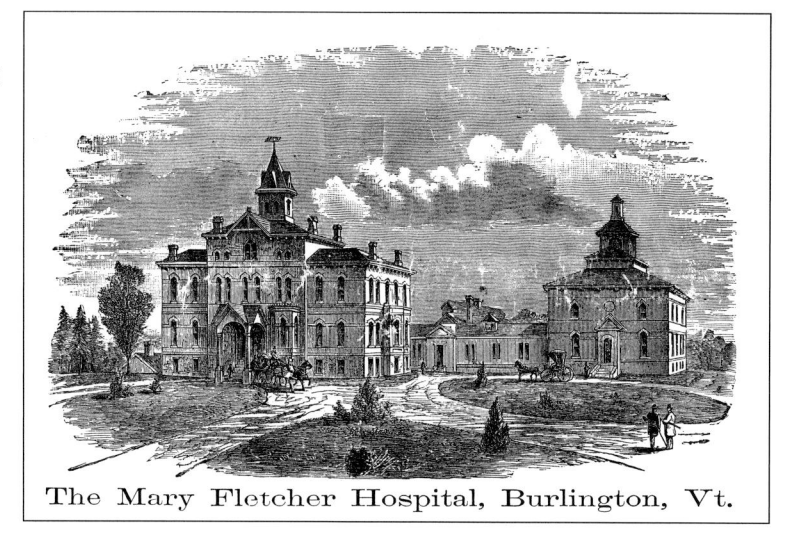

Within a few months,

> "...the streets of the city gave evidence, by the passing through them of numerous people with surgical dressings on some part of the body, and by the great accumulation of the mud-stained buggies of the practitioners of the adjacent towns, as well as by the overfilled wards of the hospital, that a great deal of surgical work was going on."[35]

Surgery occupied a dominant position at the Mary Fletcher Hospital from the beginning. Of the 35 patients admitted during the first six months of 1879, more than two-thirds were surgical in nature. In-patient fees varied from free to $6 per week. The first patient was operated upon by Little on Jan 24, 1879.[36]

Excerpts from the original Mary Fletcher Hospital logbooks give a sense of the operative care provided during that time:[37] The logbooks are written in longhand by the house officer.

> "Mrs. J.J., Charlotte, Vt., Age 32, American.
> Admitted August 11, 1880. Diagnosis: Uterine polypus.
> Patient states that she first noticed her condition 3 years ago ... discharge of blood with considerable pain [and a] weak back. First noticed tumor 6 weeks ago when it began to protrude from the vagina.

FIGURE 5-8.
The original "White Corridor" is still brick-lined and painted white. This well-traveled path connects the Shepardson Building and the Fletcher House.

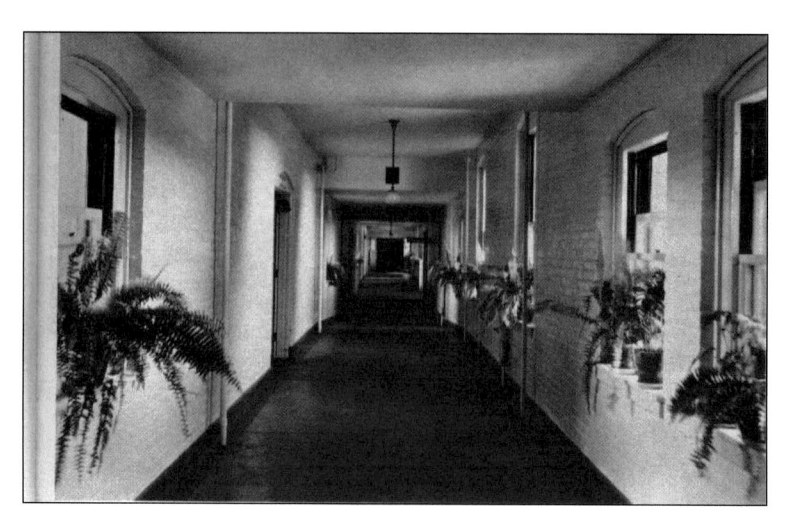

58 CATAMOUNT SURGEONS

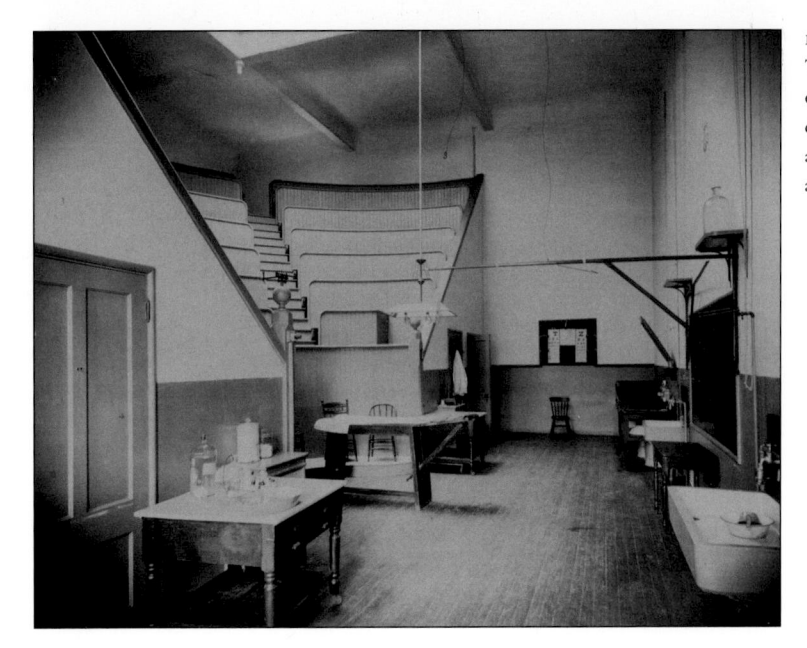

FIGURE 5-9.
The Mary Fletcher operating and demonstration amphitheatre around 1910.

August 14, 1880
Operation for removal by Dr. Kent in the presence of a number of the staff. The ecraseur [wire snare] was used to remove the tumor. No hemorrhage. The tumor was nearly as large as a hen's egg.
August 19, 1880
Discharged. Result: cure.

Mr. J.E.P., Hinesburgh, Vt., Age 21, American.
Admitted September 5, 1880. Diagnosis: Compound fracture of tibia and fibula.
Patient states that he was employed in constructing a dam ... It was nearly completed when it gave way carrying him with it over the rock and down the stream nearly for a quarter of a mile when he chanced to catch hold of a log near the shore. Not knowing that his leg was broken he attempted to get out of the stream and climb ashore. When he stepped on his foot the broken bone came through the flesh. The bone was set by Dr. Fay Miles of Hinesburg with side splints on Friday September 3, 1880 and placed in a fracture box and packed in excelsior [fine curled wood shavings]. Not having any home it was deemed best to send him to the hospital.
Patient was brought to the hospital in a large wagon about noon [and] taken into room No. 60. The bed was protected and made hard by putting in long slats. The dressing was removed and splints taken off by Drs. Kent and Atwater. The odor from the wound was fearful. A few small pieces of bone were removed from the wound and it was syringed out with solution of carbolic acid 1 to 40. There seemed to be considerable swelling and redness.
The leg was placed in the fracture box with small strips of bandage tacked across it to support it and allow free drainage. Oakum [hemp fiber impregnated with tar] packed on each side to prevent its swelling. Extension was made to the lower fragment by means of adhesive strips on each side and a bandage over them with pulley and weights attached. Ordered Quinine Sulfate [and] Aspirin ... One every 6 hours.

Chapter Five: New Facilities Breathe Life Into the Program

September 5, 1880

Wound to be syringed out every hour with 1 to 40 solution of carbolic acid and cloths kept over the wound. Charcoal paste applied. Temperature 102.

September 10, 1880

Patient taken with insomnia; in morning his jaws began to be sore and stiff, and in the afternoon he was unable to open them they were so firmly closed. Patient was ordered five drops of Gelsemium [a weak painkiller] every four hours.

September 11, 1880

Patient remains the same. Bowels were moved freely by the pills. Temperature 99 1/4, pulse 96. There seems to be much swelling and redness of the leg. Decomposition seemed to set in, on removal of the probe it was discolored by the gas showing considerable [chemical] change going on. Wound was opened for more free discharge with knife.

September 11, 1880

A consultation with the staff was called ... large poultices of meal and yeast were applied to the leg and changed often and ... kept hot. Patient drank freely of milk. Spasms of twitching and drawing up of the lower fragment were severe ... toward morning he became more quiet and slept.

September 12, 1880

Patient was etherized, everything removed from limb and redressed and a long side splint applied with extension by Drs. Kent, Lund and Crampton. After coming out of the ether the spasms again returned. Patient made a number of attempts to vomit. Choral was again given.

September 13, 1880

Spasms more intense. Temperature 99, pulse 150. Patient died at 10 minutes past eleven.

Mr. A.W., Port Henry, NY, Age 41, English.

Admitted June 9, 1881. Diagnosis: Perineal abscess and urethral stricture.

About 18 months ago he fell astride a wagon wheel. Had retention of urine for about a week. Became better and was able to urinate with but little difficulty. Became worse in a few weeks. Could not retain water any length of time. Has dribbled away ever since. About a week ago had a chill. Soon noticed a swelling in perineum.

Upon admission: Scrotum enormously distended. Swelling upon perineum half a hen's egg. Considerable pain and tenderness about genitals. Bladder not distended. Urine dribbling constantly. Given cathartic to move bowels and Morphine to relieve pain.

June 10, 1881

External urethrotomy by Dr. Little. A consultation of Drs. Thayer ... and Grinnell decided an operation was necessary and it was performed at once, under ether. A filiform bougie [dilator] was passed down to the stricture. A cut was then made in median line of perineum down upon the bougie. Considerable difficulty was had in finding it. Examination showed that the stricture had been divided about its middle. A knife was passed first up then down upon a director, thus cutting the stricture throughout its entire length. The meatus was slit. A large sound [probe] was passed down to the stricture and then along a grooved staff into the bladder. Lint was placed in the wound and a compression bandage applied around. The incision in the median line had been carried up the scrotum there, leaving a great infiltration of the parts.

Patient slept for some time after the operation. At 4 pm temperature was 101. Given Sulphate of Quinia, 10 grains ... Lint removed at night. Carbolic gauze and compress applied. Very nervous. At 9 pm given Sulphate of Morhine, 1/4 grain. Temperature 101.

June 11, 1881

Catheter removed. Carbolic dressings to wound. Temperature 100 3/4 in am, pulse 79.

June 12, 1881

Better. Urine passes through cut. Bowels move when he strains any. Wound looking well.

June 18, 1881

Number 18 sound passed. Large amount of pus escaped from meatus and incision.

July 6, 1881

Sound passed every 3rd day to date. Patient able to walk about Hospital grounds. Passes most of his urine through penis.

August 26, 1881

Patient passes urine through urethra. Wound completely closed. Number 14 sound passed every three days."[38]

FIGURE 5-10.
The second Medical Building, which opened in 1884, was situated on the corner of Prospect and Pearl Streets — the site of present day Dewey Hall.

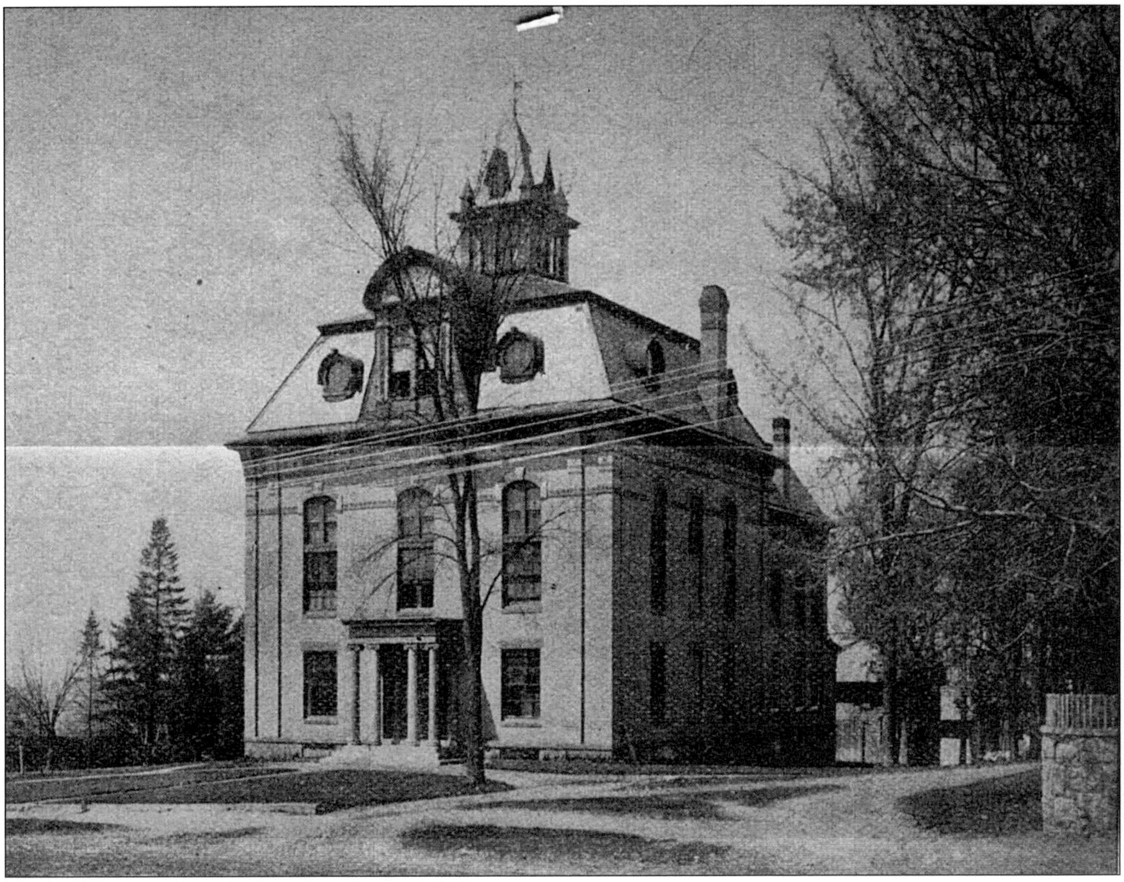

The College Gets a New Medical Building

As Little's reputation spread, enrollment at the College of Medicine steadily increased. By the mid-1880s, the average class size had doubled to around 180 per year. The Medical Building (today's Pomeroy Hall) was updated in 1880 at the faculty's expense, but soon reached the limits of its usefulness. John Purple Howard, another Burlington-based benefactor, came to the rescue in late 1883.[39] He had already used his million dollar fortune to build the Howard Opera House, renovate UVM's "Old Mill" into its current configuration, erect the fountain on the UVM green, and commission the nearby statue of General Lafayette.[40]

Howard purchased a brick mansion on the north side of the campus green (Pearl St), just down the street from the Mary Fletcher Hospital, and had it extensively renovated. When the new medical bulding opened in March of 1884, it held a 350-seat amphitheater in which operative procedures were performed on cadavers.[41] A graduate recalled that,

> *"at the rear of the upper floor was the dissecting room with a well going down to the vault or tank room where the cadavers were kept in a huge tank of fluid. I received 50 cents each for taking care of them, injecting them, and putting them in the tank for preservation. When they were required for dissection, I would draw them to the upper floor by means of a block and tackle through the elevator well."*[42]

FIGURE 5-11.
Floor plan of the second Medical Building. The fire that destroyed the structure in 1903 started in the second floor amphitheatre.

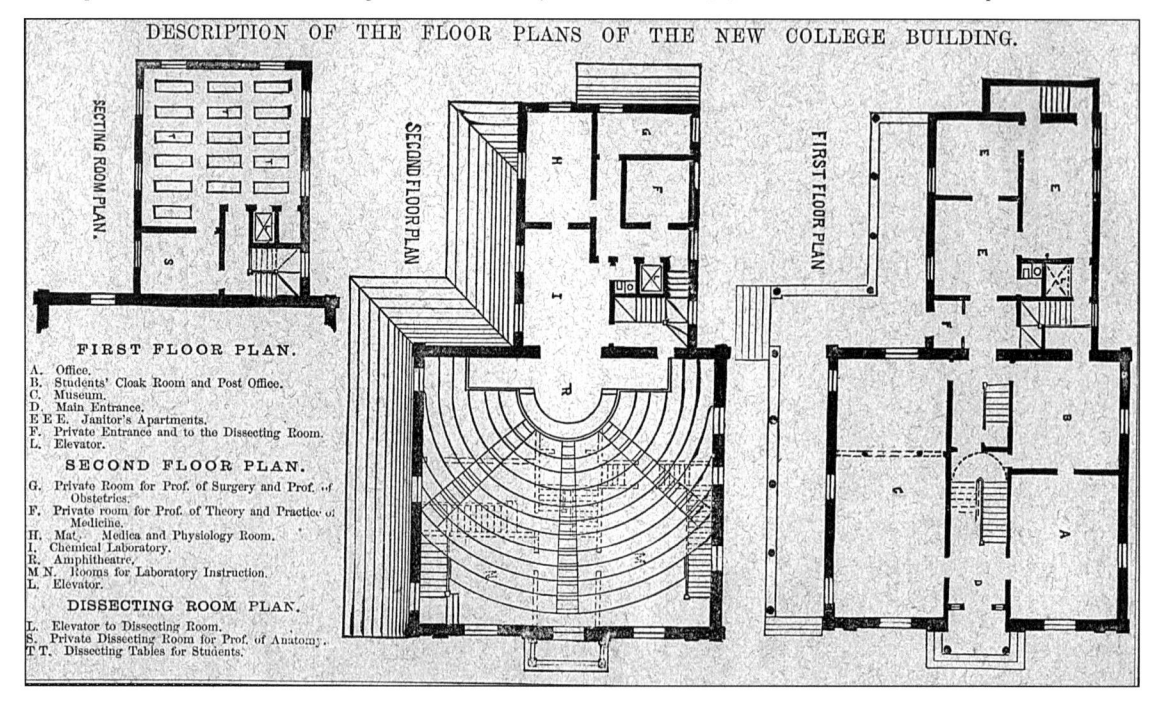

62 CATAMOUNT SURGEONS

UVM's Less Than Advanced Academics

The College's refusal to strengthen its entrance requirements also contributed to its popularity. Harvard's students had to possess a college degree or pass an entrance exam in Latin and Physics prior to admission. UVM was far less stringent, stipulating only that, "the student must register his name with some doctor, who thereby became his so called 'preceptor' and was supposed to give him practical instruction." It didn't matter that some students never went near their preceptors again. "A matriculation examination or any other evidence of educational qualification was unknown."[43]

As of 1871, both Harvard and Northwestern conducted a three year, nine month per year, graded course of instruction. UVM, in contrast, soldiered on with a repetitive two-year program. Students were "required to attend two courses of lectures, each extending over a period of from 4 to 6 months, the last one generally ending at about the same time as his term of registration."[44]

Lectures were a given in Anatomy, Physiology, Chemistry, Materia Medica, Obstetrics, Surgery and Practice. The courses were not graded, so that some students attended lectures in surgery before knowing any anatomy. A small amount of dissection was accompanied by a few amphitheater clinics in Medicine, Surgery, and specialty subjects. True clinical experience still required a preceptorship, which was poorly regulated. "At the end of the second course (the student) was given an oral examination, not unduly severe as to the questions which were asked, nor as to the manner in which the answers were marked. If he weathered this ordeal, he received his diploma, and proceeded to practice upon his fellow creatures with the sanction of his Alma Mater."[45]

The majority of UVM's students "were farmers' sons whose only schooling had been obtained in their native villages." Few had undergraduate degrees, and some were even illiterate. "There were brains enough among the Vermonters, but, as a class, there was less education and though most of them worked hard ... they were not used to studying and it did not come easily to them."[46] The following exchange between William Darling, the school's Scottish professor of anatomy from 1871 to 1884, and an unprepared pupil exemplified the situation:

> "One day at recitation, he [Darling] asked a student what organ passed through the foramen magnum, the large opening at the base of the skull through which the spinal cord goes down into the spine. The student, knowing nothing, but bluffing with the first answer that came into his head, replied, 'The esophagus'. 'Yours does, ye damn fool!' shouted Darling, 'and if God ever gave ye any brains, they've all run down it into your guts!'"[47]

Realizing its curricular shortcomings, the College instituted an optional graded three-year program in 1882. Students could take "examinations in the elementary departments" at the end of their second year, and devote the third to the exclusive study of medicine, obstetrics, and surgery. Additional clinical instruction was offered and the thesis requirement was dropped. Elective practical courses, which included one in minor surgery and bandaging, were added in 1883. Wheeler taught the surgical portion of this course.[48]

A New Chairman and a New Controversy

On April 1, 1885, Little noticed the presence of a dull, steady pain over the right lower portion of his abdomen. His personal physician, having witnessed similar attacks, prescribed cathartics. Little's symptoms, however, continued to worsen. By the next morning, he showed signs of localized inflammation. An operation was considered, but then dismissed upon discovering that Little also suffered from chronic diabetes. He succumbed to the ruptured appendix three days later, at the age of 49.[49] Ironically, pathologist Reginald Fitz of Boston demonstrated the importance of early surgical intervention for appendicitis the very next year.

The faculty chose Joel Williston Wright, Little's successor as professor of surgery at the New York University, to take his place in Burlington for the remainder of the 1885 term.[50] Wright was popular with the students from the start. It was reported that, "his lectures are concise and to the point," and "as an operator he is careful and certain."[51] The faculty agreed with the assessment, and petitioned the trustees for a permanent appointment.[52]

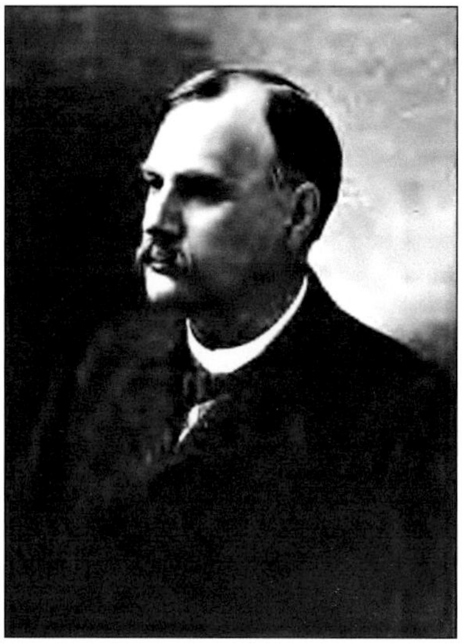

FIGURE 5-12. Leroy M. Bingham was briefly UVM's Professor of Surgery in 1885.

The trustees had previously given the faculty complete control over the school. This time, however, the board decided to end the New Yorker line of succession. They elected "Vermont man" LeRoy Monroe Bingham, Little's assistant at the Mary Fletcher Hospital, to the position instead.[53] Bingham, born in Fletcher, Vermont, on April 10, 1845, had been an infantryman during the Civil War. He graduated from the College of Medicine in 1870, started a practice in Stowe, and then moved to Burlington. He was demonstrator of anatomy at UVM from 1874 to 1880, before being named Vermont's Surgeon General.[54]

Bingham immediately faced several disadvantages. His appointment was unpopular with some faculty as a matter of principle, the students were already fond of Wright, and both groups were familiar with Bingham through his prior work at the hospital. The consensus was that Bingham was a good physician, but "not a successful talker" and certainly not a man of "national ability." Bingham gave his first set of lectures in May of 1886. Within a week, the students called his experience into question after he failed to stress the importance of antiseptic technique. When the faculty and trustees expressed their support for the embattled professor, the student body boycotted classes for the next several weeks. Bingham, realizing the futility of his situation, resigned a month later.[55] He remained on the staff of the Mary Fletcher Hospital until his retirement in 1900, but severed his ties to the College.[56]

The Secret Service Surgeon

Eager to put the entire matter behind them, the trustees named J. Williston Wright to the professorship of surgery in June of 1886, in accordance with the faculty's wishes.[57] Campus politics not withstanding, he proved to be a worthy successor. Born in Sullivan, New

Hampshire on July 30, 1840, Wright was "thin but wiry and muscular, with large hands and a grip that was developed in seven years of life before the mast on sailing vessels, from his sixteenth to his twenty-third year."[58] He served in the 5th Iowa Cavalry from 1863 to 1865, and was rumored to have been a member of the Secret Service.[59, 60] He attended the Geneva Medical College in upstate New York before graduating (like Howard and Little) from the College of Physicians and Surgeons in 1866. He then worked as a demonstrator of anatomy at the New York Infirmary for Women and Children for the next ten years.[61] He succeeded Little as professor of surgery at the New York University in 1879.[62]

"His lectures were clear, methodical talks, pointed and enlivened by stories, generally humorous, drawn from his own variegated experience."[63] He assembled a collection of his most popular talks in the 1884 book, Lectures on Diseases of the Rectum. One of the first works to deal exclusively with anorectal disease, it contained landmark descriptions of procedures for colostomy and extirpation.[64, 65]

Wright's surgical expertise was not limited to the end of the digestive tract. He published accounts of complications following the use of cocaine for local anesthesia, tongue cyst excision, and compound fracture repair.[66, 67, 68] In addition, he lent his name to a rubber-handled "antiseptic" instrument set that came in a "fine Russian leather case, lined with silk velvet."[69] He also assisted Wheeler with the first ovariotomy performed in Burlington. The operation (carried out in the patient's home) was a success, but the patient succumbed to a bladder infection a month later.[70]

The scope of Wright's teaching at the College of Medicine was probably still quite limited, as demonstrated in the 1887 written examination in surgery:

"1. In a stab wound of an artery, at what point would you ligate the injured vessel, and why? How many ligatures would you employ, and what material would you select for a ligature?

2. Give a brief account of Ulceration, Gangrene, Caries and Necrosis.

3. Give the symptoms and treatment of a strangulated inguinal Hernia.

4. What tissues are divided in the lateral operation for Stone in the Bladder?

5. Give the chief points in differential diagnosis between Hydrocele, Hæmatocele and Varicocele.

6. What means are employed for controlling Hemorrhage during surgical operations?

7. What is Dugas' test for dislocation at the shoulder joint?

8. Give the chief varieties of Fistula of the Anus, with treatment.

9. Name the chief varieties of Club Foot, and state what tendons are shortened in each.

10. Describe an excision at the Shoulder Joint, or an amputation at the knee joint."[71]

Of the seventy students taking the exam, only fifty-three passed.

Wright resigned the professorship of surgery at both UVM and New York University in 1889 due to poor health. Within another two years, he retired from the practice of medicine altogether and moved to upstate New York "in broken health." He died on September 2, 1912, in Lake Placid, New York "after a long illness brought about by overwork."[72]

An Orthopod in General Surgeon's Clothing

Wishing to avoid another confrontation, the trustees approved the faculty's recommendation of Abel Mix Phelps as Wright's replacement.[73] Phelps had been Professor of orthopaedic surgery for several years, and was a popular lecturer. Another in the line of New York clinicians, Phelps at least originally hailed from Vermont. A distant cousin of previous surgery professor Edward E. Phelps, he was born in Alburg Springs on January 27, 1851. After attending local preparatory schools, he obtained his M.D. from the University of Michigan in 1873. He spent the next seven years as a company surgeon for the Vermont Central Railroad — a prestigious and profitable position during the age of the iron horse.[74]

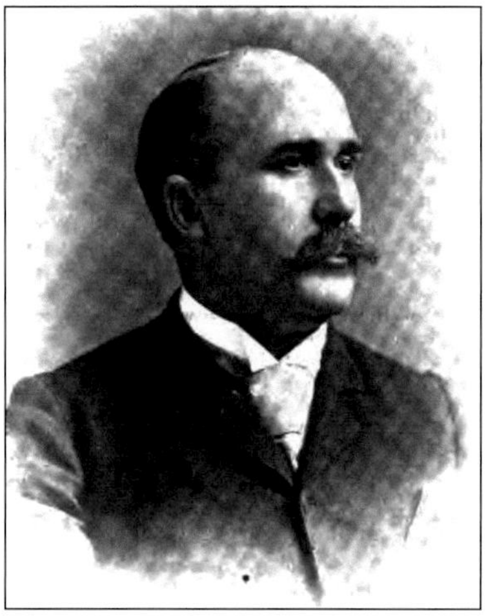

FIGURE 5-13. Abel Phelps, UVM's Professor of Surgery 1890-1900.

Phelps embarked on a grand tour of the European surgical clinics in 1880. He studied with Max Schede, Friedrich von Esmarch, Richard von Volkmann, Theodor Billroth, and Karl Thiersch over the ensuing four years. Already an expert in orthopedic injuries from his railroad days, Phelps ended up introducing new operative techniques to his appreciative hosts. He started a practice in Chateaugay, New York following his return to the United States in 1884.[75] After presenting several novel papers at State Medical Society meetings, he became professor of clinical surgery at New York City's Post-Graduate Medical School in 1887. While there he worked under James Little's successor, Lewis S. Pilcher. Within a few years, he was also named professor of orthopedic surgery at Wright's former institution, New York University.[76]

During his time in upstate New York, Phelps created several inexpensive, practical orthopedic appliances. These included a lateral traction fixation hip-splint for hip joint disease and an aluminum corset for scoliosis and Pott's disease. He had also, out of necessity, devised a number of operative innovations. Among these were improved methods for inguinal hernia repair and cleft lip reconstruction.[77, 78] In November of 1890, shortly after becoming UVM's professor of surgery, Phelps published a paper that outlined a groundbreaking technique for the correction of clubfoot.[79] The procedure became the gold standard of treatment for the next half century and brought worldwide fame to its author.

Progress in Academic Advancement

Phelps's tenure at UVM was also marked by several improvements in the College's standards. In 1890, the school implemented a written entrance exam and a three-year course of study. The preliminary and practical courses were incorporated into the regular teaching schedule the next year, thus creating a graded curriculum. Although advocated by Benjamin Lincoln almost sixty years earlier, the changes were actually made in order to gain acceptance into the Association of American Medical Colleges. Additional laboratory work was added in 1895, and the program was extended to four full years by 1898. The school formally applied for AAMC membership in 1899, a goal it would eventually achieve more than a decade later.[80]

Adjunct professors were appointed in 1892 to help teach the expanded series of lectures.

Phelps promoted Wheeler from instructor in the principles and practice of surgery to adjunct professor of clinical and minor surgery. Two years later, the faculty established a new practical course in surgery that was taught by Wheeler.[81]

The End of the Proprietary Era

The effects of widespread fame had caught up with Phelps by this time. He was a busy doctor and his interests were primarily orthopedic in nature. "His orthopedic work was remarkably good, both as regards operations and appliances. As a general surgeon, his lectures and clinics were not far above mediocrity." It was evident that, "he was not a well-educated or well-nurtured man and his cosmos consisted very largely of ego ... he had an excellent opinion of himself (for which there certainly was some justification) and was never tired of showing off."[82]

A summary of the surgical cases treated at the Mary Fletcher Hospital at that time is provided by Phelps and his House Surgeon, Guy Noyo, as follows:

Patients treated in Phelps' clinic up to Jan 1, 1895.[83]

    370 patients
    299 cutting operations
    84 capital or severe operations

suppuration occurred in	20
Phelps' Club foot operation	18
Phelps' hip splint for hip dislocation	16
Phelps' Hare lip operation	2
Phelps' phymosis operation	4
Excision of the knee	5

Phelps made mention of his dislike for general surgery during his American Orthopedic Association presidential address of 1894: "The orthopaedist was always at war with the general surgeon. There never was a time when they could lie peacefully together in the same bed excepting like the lion and the lamb — one inside the other, and the poor orthopede was always inside. The specialists won the battle in a fair fight upon the field of thought and the profession of medicine awarded them the victory."[84]

Phelps's victory was short-lived. In June of 1898, the faculty staged a coup d'état against the school's Dean. He had been a proponent of the proprietary system and a vocal opponent of change for twenty years; his removal was necessary if the College was to raise its standards. The fallout caused such a commotion among the students and faculty that the University stepped in and assumed complete control of the College. Fed up with the machinations, Phelps resigned at the end of the 1900 term.[85] He returned to New York City, but within two years, required surgery for "an abdominal affection from which he had been suffering for some time." The procedure proved futile and Phelps died of colon cancer with metastases on October 6, 1902.[86]

The resignation of the last of the non-resident professors from New York City, the elevation of standards, and the increase of clinical cases seemed to bode well for the College of Medicine's future. An era of stable surgical leadership and rapid technical advancement was on the horizon. But the school's very existence was about to be challenged again, this time by forces well beyond its control.

PART III

ADVERSITY AND ADAPTATION

1900-1942

CHAPTER 6

Trouble at the Turn of the Century

The tradition of stable surgical leadership began with the appointment of John Brooks Wheeler. His long tenure became characteristic of the position thereafter.

Fire destroyed the Medical Building and the majority of its contents. Within five years, the Flexner Report recommended closing the medical school altogether!

In typical contrarian Vermont fashion, the College ignored the outsiders' advice. The State appropriated funds for a new building, Dean Henry Crain Tinkham reorganized the program, and the Medical College won a temporary reprieve from the American Medical Association (AMA) and the Association of American Medical Colleges (AAMC).

John Brooks Wheeler Becomes Professor of Surgery

UVM's trustees rearranged the College of Medicine's entire faculty in July of 1900. Former assistant John Brooks Wheeler took Abel Mix Phelps' place as professor of surgery.[1] Another native Vermonter, he was born in Stowe on August 13, 1853. He was the son of a prominent lawyer and the grandson of the University's former president. Wheeler made the most of his background by pursuing an extensive education. He graduated from UVM in 1875 then attended medical school at Harvard. After receiving his M.D. in 1878, he completed a one-year internship at the Massachusetts General Hospital — a relatively novel accomplishment at the time.[2]

Wheeler set sail for Europe in July of 1879. Over the next two years, he studied under some of the most important physicians and surgeons of the era. He learned operative surgery from Theodor Billroth and surgical anatomy from Emil Zuckerhandl in Vienna, pathological anatomy from Friedrich von Recklinghausen and microscopic anatomy from Wilhelm von Waldeyer in Strasbourg, and operative surgery from Bernhard von Langenbeck in Berlin. Wheeler studied alongside William S. Halsted while in Vienna, but his most notable brush with fame came during his time in Edinburgh. While there, he not only met Joseph Bell, the real life inspiration for Arthur Conan Doyle's Sherlock Holmes, but also had the opportunity to watch him operate. Bell was the grandson of Scottish surgeon Benjamin Bell whose text was used by John Pomeroy at the start of his Burlington teaching saga.[3]

Wheeler's greatest exposure to Listerism occurred in Austria and Germany (rather than in Lister's home of Scotland) due to widespread European acceptance of antisepsis.[4]

FIGURE 6-1. John Wheeler (center) operating at the Mary Fletcher amphitheatre in 1900. Senior medical student George Sabin (2nd from left in gallery) looks on.

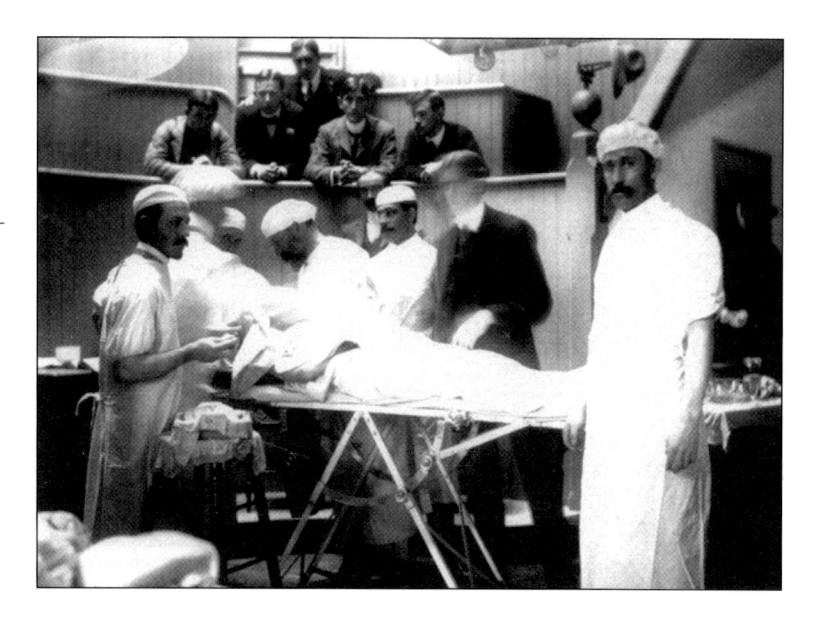

At the completion of his studies, Wheeler was as well trained as any of UVM's previous professors of surgery. Unlike his predecessors, though, he decided to return to Vermont rather than settle in a large metropolitan city. In the fall of 1881, he opened an office on Main Street in Burlington. Within two years, he was an instructor at the College and an attending surgeon at the Mary Fletcher Hospital. Despite lecturing before classes of more than 200 students a year, Wheeler did not enjoy the substantial salary of a full professor. In order to make ends meet, he initially practiced both general medicine and surgery since his patients were poor and surgical cases were few.[5]

Even though Mary Fletcher's hospital had been open for several years, operations were still carried out in patient's homes. Wheeler recalled, "There was a feeling that nobody but paupers were treated at hospitals." The populace was "filled with the idea that hospitals existed for the sole purpose of 'experimenting' on people." As a result of this mindset, Wheeler was often obliged to travel up to thirty miles or more by horseback, carriage, or even sleigh to make a "house" call.[6]

The general public had about as much regard for physicians' advice during this time as they had for hospitals. An incident involving one of Wheeler's first patients (an elderly woman with burns over her lower abdomen and thighs from an overturned lantern) was typical. Wheeler applied gauze soaked with linseed oil and lime water to the burned skin, covered it with a thick layer of cotton, and then changed the entire dressing every day for the next ten days. Just as the surface began to heal, the patient's sister informed him that his services were no longer needed. She felt that the "young doctor" had done his best, but that it was time to switch to a better remedy — a hen manure poultice. Appalled, Wheeler pleaded his case to no avail. "In about a week more this treatment by fertilizer bore the fruit which I had expected, in the shape of a funeral."[7]

Other obstacles to patient care included the conditions under which "outpatient procedures" were conducted. Wheeler operated on boards placed across flour barrels, flap-leaf kitchen tables, and, to his utter dismay, double beds (too wide and too low). He carried a surgical kit, dressings, gowns, and other accessories at all times. Instruments were sterilized on site "by boiling in a milkpan or dishpan, over which another milkpan was inverted, by way of cover."[8]

With experience, Wheeler was able to anticipate problems in the field before they arose. Even so, he was faced with new challenges on a regular basis. One winter's evening, he received a telegram from a country practioner requesting his assistance with a strangulated hernia. Following his arrival at the nearest depot, Wheeler was escorted to his destination by an old man with "a horse apparently about his own age and a sleigh that must have been the first one owned by his grandfather." Undeterred, "we plunged and plowed through the drifts, covering the ten miles between the station and the patient's house in two good long hours."[9]

Upon reaching the "half finished shanty," Wheeler found his 200-pound patient lying on a double bed that nearly filled the room. The doctor who had summoned him sat near the patient's head, ready to give the anesthetic. Another doctor crouched on the opposite side of the bed, prepared to assist. Wheeler unpacked his kit, set up his field, and asked for one of the farmstead's two kerosene lamps. As he later remembered:

> "At first there was no response to my call for a volunteer, but finally a neighbor came valiantly forward, remarking that he had never seen anybody bootchered and he kinder like to know how they done it. So saying, he squeezed into the space at the foot of the bed, lamp in hand, and stood there, radiant. He did nobly for a few minutes, but the sight of blood was too much for him and he made a sudden and peremptory demand that somebody take his place. Somebody did and he made a rush for fresh air, getting outdoors just in time to avoid falling in a faint. Presently he came back, feeling better, and resumed his illuminating function, but before long he again had to make a sudden get-away. He was a good sport though, and came back after the second time, after which there was no fainting.
>
> Everything then went well until I began to divide the constriction, at which point the lamp holder became intensely interested and leaned forward over the bed, holding the light as near to the wound as possible. The anesthetizer had also become deeply interested in watching the operation, so much so that he forgot to keep the patient completely anesthetized, the result being that, just as the lamp holder leaned forward with the lamp, the patient gave a kick and his knee struck the lamp holder's hand. By great good luck the lamp was not knocked out of his hand, but the chimney was knocked off, the lamp went out and we were in the dark, with a knife in the abdomen of a kicking, squirming, half anesthetized patient.
>
> I made a forcible statement to the effect that light was needed and a woman rushed in with the other lamp. By this light the lamp-holder beheld the chimney lying on the bed. He promptly grabbed it, and realizing with equal promptness that its temperature was at least as high as that of boiling water, cast it from him with a yell and pranced into the next room, sucking his fingers, and inquiring at the top of his voice for Helen Blazes. As no response was made, it was evident that the lady must have been at least a half a mile away."[10]

The remainder of the operation was "uneventful." Wheeler spent the rest of the night with his colleagues, and then caught the train back to Burlington early the next morning. With time, the patient made a "good recovery."

Antisepsis Gives Rise to Asepsis

While Wheeler operated on farmhouse tabletops by lamplight, surgical practice underwent another transformation. Although carbolic acid was an effective sterilizing agent, it rapidly dulled knife-edges, irritated intact skin, and inflamed open wounds. It was supplanted by mercuric bichloride (a compound espoused by Nathan Smith!) in the 1880s, which turned out to be just as caustic. Louis Pasteur, whose initial work had inspired Joseph Lister, later discovered that bacteria were as susceptible to heat as they were to noxious chemicals. Franco-Prussian War veteran Ernst von Bergman adapted the principle to the profession of surgery in 1886 when he successfully sterilized his instruments using the recently invented steam autoclave.[11]

Pasteur also found that *everything* that came into contact with a patient contained bacteria — especially the surgeon. Soiled topcoats were traded in for sterile gowns, which were later accompanied by caps and masks. Hands were scrubbed with soap and water, soaked in potassium permanganate until purple, and then rinsed in bleach — at least until William Halsted, Wheeler's fellow student in Vienna, popularized the use of thin rubber gloves.[12] Halsted later admitted, though, that rather than prevent the spread of bacteria from the surgeon to the patient, the original intent was to protect the hands of his favorite nurse (and subsequent wife) from the effects of mercuric bichloride.[13]

By the time Wheeler became the chairman, the practice of antisepsis (destruction and removal of bacteria) had yielded to asepsis (complete elimination of bacteria). Lewis S. Pilcher, James Little's successor at New York's Post-Graduate Hospital and an early advocate of asepsis, summarized the concepts thusly:

> *"The ideal treatment of a wound is that by which a perfectly aseptic condition should be obtained and preserved; where this is impracticable, the object of treatment becomes changed to the application of means to diminish the activity of the septic organisms, to secure the rapid removal of their products, and to increase the resisting power of the wounded tissues."* [14]

"Laudable" pus and its objectionable cousins, "sanious," "puriform," "ichorous," and "curdy" pus were banished. Surgery within the abdomen, chest, and skull — considered murderous at the time of Wheeler's training — became safe and routine.[15]

The Academic Clinician

Wheeler, a widower at age thirty-six, supported his two young daughters, sister, and mother through his busy clinical practice. In spite of the long hours and extensive travel, he managed to contribute to the local medical journals on a regular basis. As an instructor, he published reports on antisepsis and the properties of cocaine.[16, 17] While professor of clinical and minor surgery, he wrote about appendicitis and inguinal hernias.[18, 19] By the time he was full professor, his topics included pelvic organ surgery, prostatic hypertrophy, and medical education.[20, 21, 22]

Wheeler was particularly troubled by tracheotomy failures in diphtheria, especially among youngsters. These emergency operations were done in patients' homes with poor lighting under suboptimal conditions; antibiotics were not yet available. His teacher, master surgeon

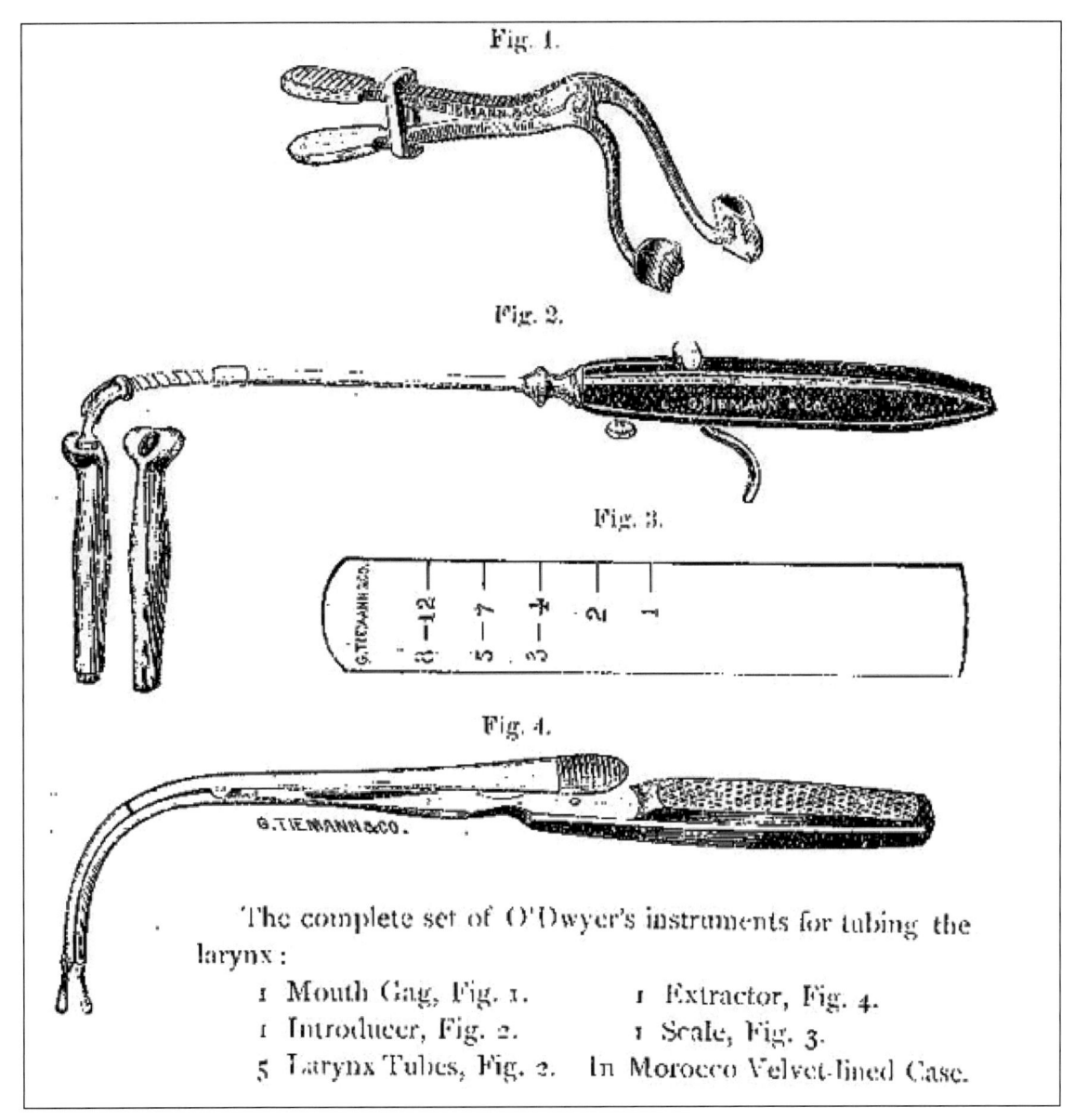

FIGURE 6-2.
Wheeler successfully used the O'Dwyer tube as a substitute for tracheostomy in the treatment of croup. This illustration is from the author's great grandfather's (Lewis S. Pilcher) monograph on tracheostomies.

Theodor Billroth, noted that, "the tracheotomies in children are the most difficult operations I have ever performed."[23] Joseph O'Dwyer of New York devised a tube, which, when introduced into the larynx through the mouth, kept the bronchus open and free of diphtherial membranes. Wheeler went to New York for two months in 1886, learned the new intubation technique, and brought the O'Dwyer tube back to Burlington. Eleven of Wheeler's twenty-five subsequent cases (each under nine years old) made full recoveries. This was felt to be a huge improvement over the results obtained with tracheotomy. Thankfully, the discovery of diphtheria antitoxin in the 1890s spelled the end to this threat.[24, 25]

As professor of surgery, Wheeler gave several didactic lectures and quizzes each week during the term, in addition to a final exam. He conducted an operating clinic in the Mary Fletcher Hospital amphitheater every Saturday followed by bedside instruction in the hospi-

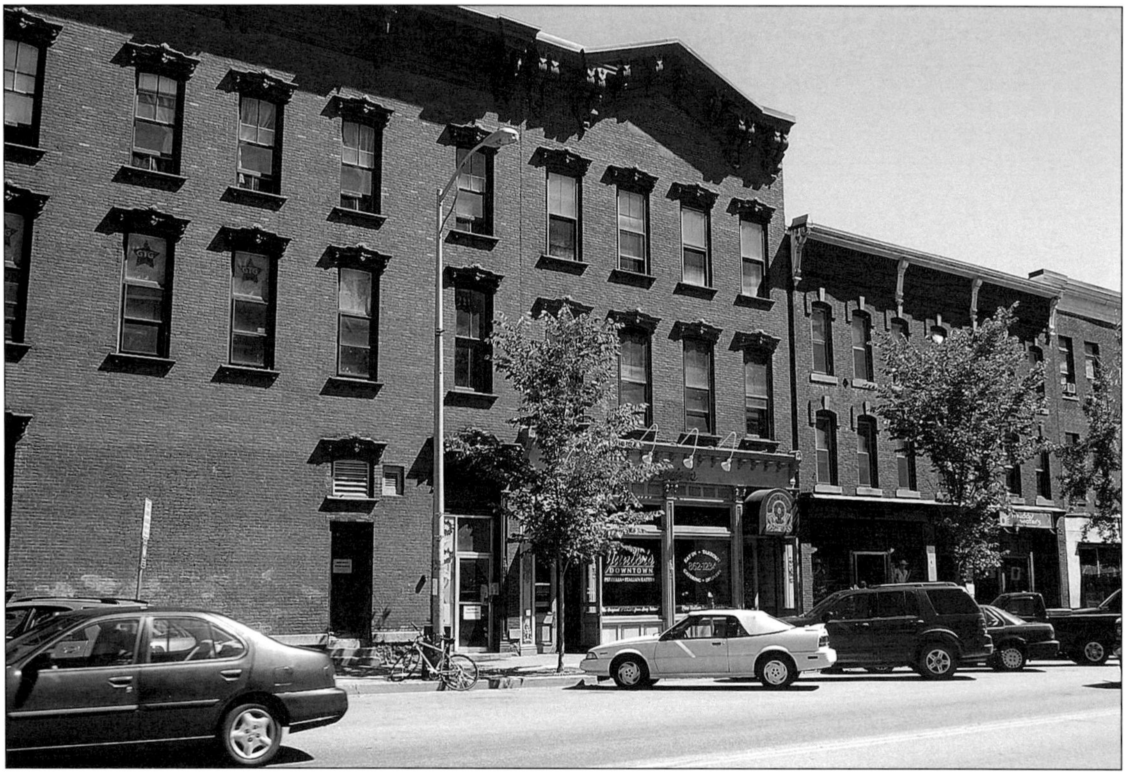

FIGURE 6-3.
John Wheeler's 1900s office was above the present day location of Junior's Pizza on Main Street in downtown Burlington.

tal's wards. In addition, he mentored "office students" who went on house calls, helped with operations, cleaned instruments, and kept his surgical kit in order.[26]

Wheeler taught in the original Medical Building (today's Pomeroy Hall) at the time of his initial appointment. He made the move across campus with the rest of the College when John Howard's "new" facility opened in 1884. Unfortunately, the second Medical Building quickly proved unable to accommodate the additional classrooms and laboratories demanded by the new four-year curriculum.[27]

Fire Destroys the Second Medical Building

Nearly everyone smoked during the ten minutes between lectures. Many "properly raised" students and physicians had taken up the habit, as "it was nearly impossible to endure the odors of the dissecting room unless one smoked."[28] The seats in the second Medical Building's amphitheater were situated on a hastily built wooden incline. Old catalogues, pamphlets, and "the dust and cobwebs of years" occupied the huge open space beneath it. On the morning of December 3, 1903, while the class awaited its next lecture, two visiting physicians got into a playful shoving match. As a member of the class of 1906 recalled:

> *"First one would knock the cigarette out of his friend's mouth, and then he would retaliate by knocking the pipe out of the other's mouth. Unfortunately in the floor below these two seats was a large crack and when the owner of the pipe picked it up he found that the contents were gone — through the crack. After a short while there was a huge puff of smoke in the room."*[29]

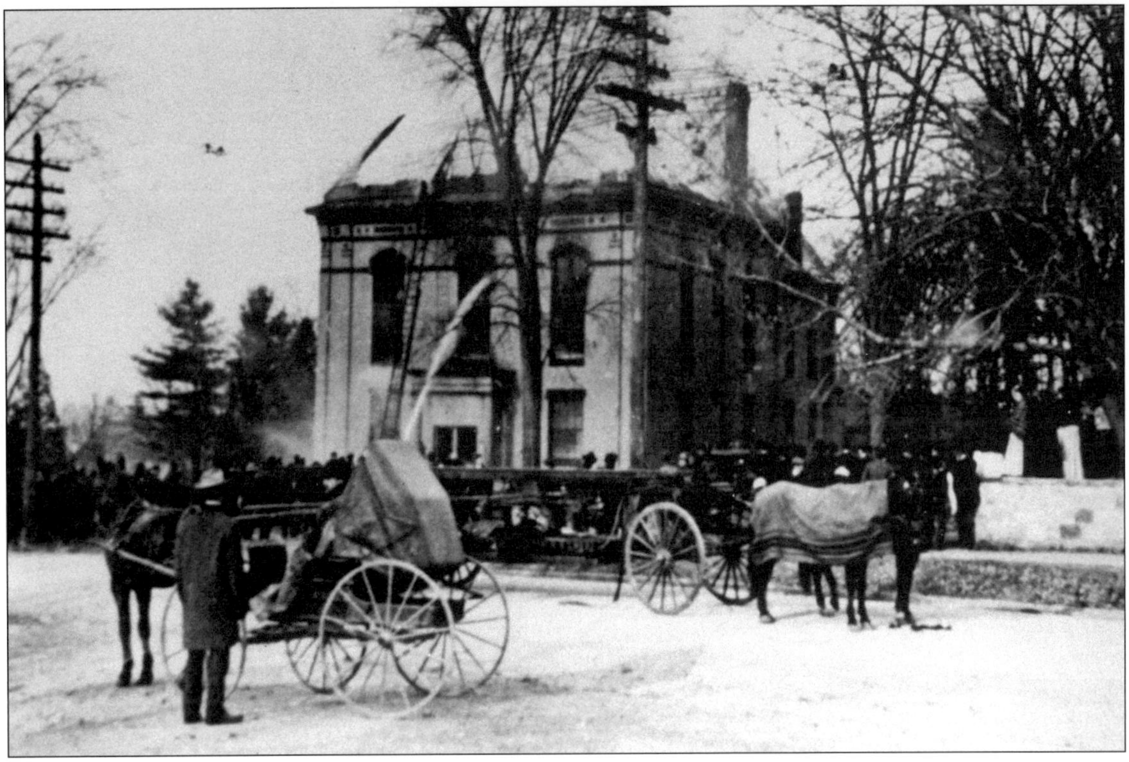

FIGURE 6-4.
The 2nd Medical School Building burned in 1903, ignited by ashes from a pipe smoked during a lecture in the auditorium. Classes were briefly held in UVM's "Old Mill" after the fire.

The conflagration engulfed the chamber within minutes. Its occupants activated the fire alarm and made their way for the exits. The fire department arrived in a timely fashion, but its pumping equipment was not up to the task. Realizing that the building was doomed, the professors and students salvaged what they could. Books from Samuel Thayer's library, museum specimens, and cadavers were spirited through the rear door. Wheeler noted that the dissecting room was:

> "... in the rear of the building, beyond which was an empty barn, which the obliging owner put to our service. In this way the transfer of the cadavers from the college to the barn was effected without observation by the crowd that was watching the fire in front. No doubt the cadavers, though shrouded in old matting, carpeting or anything that would cover them, would have interested the crowd quite as much as the fire did, but we modestly shrunk from the public gaze and felt decidedly easier when the last corpse was under cover. Of course the students, who were assisting in every possible way, were the means of transportation."[30]

Wheeler and the rest of the faculty met with UVM's president that afternoon. The school's close relationship with the University paid immediate dividends, as students were back to work in temporary accommodations within a week. Over the next year and a half, classes were held in the chemical laboratories of the "Old Mill," the amphitheater of the Mary Fletcher Hospital, and a few other University buildings.[31]

The third Medical Building (today's Dewey Hall), an "unpretending and dignified" structure "with abundant room," arose on the site of the old edifice.[32] The $80,000 facility, fund-

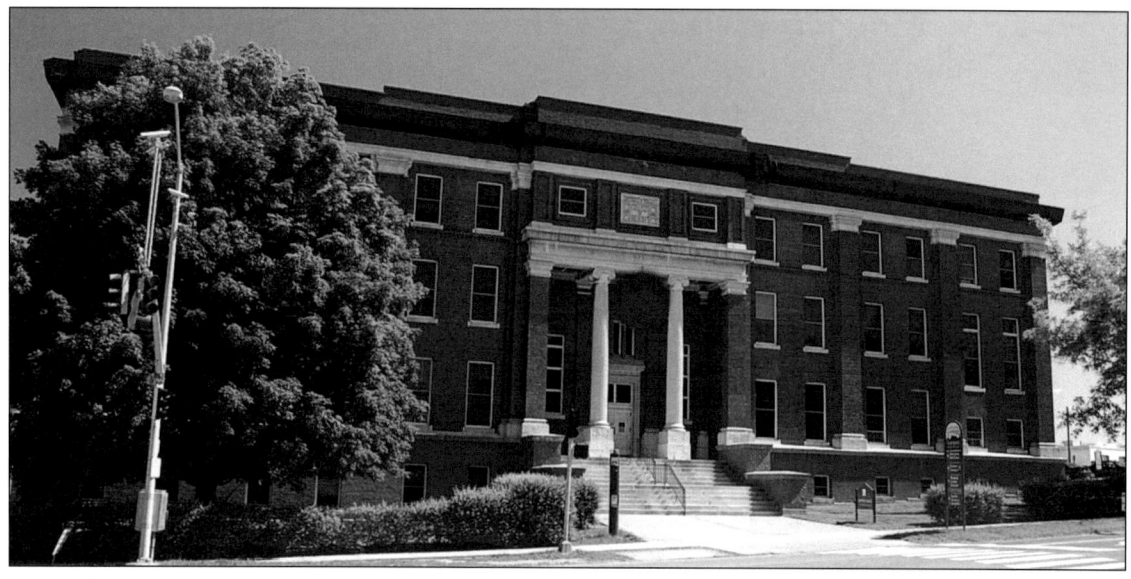

FIGURE 6-5.
The third Medical Building arose from the ashes in 1905, and was hailed as a major improvement. The building was turned over to the Department of Psychology in 1969. (2008 photo)

ed with insurance settlements, alumni donations, and University-backed loans, was formally dedicated on June 27, 1905.³³ A major improvement over the previous building, it was appreciated by students and professors alike. Patrick E. McSweeney, the adjunct professor of obstetrics, and a busy general surgeon, expressed a prevailing sentiment at the following year's commencement when he said:

> *"I wish to extend on behalf of myself and the faculty, the thanks to the medical class of 1906 for burning down the old school, thereby attaining a long-wished want for a new one."*³⁴

FIGURE 6-6.
The Mary Fletcher Hospital operating room in 1900. Note the electric overhead lights. Frank Norris MD operating.

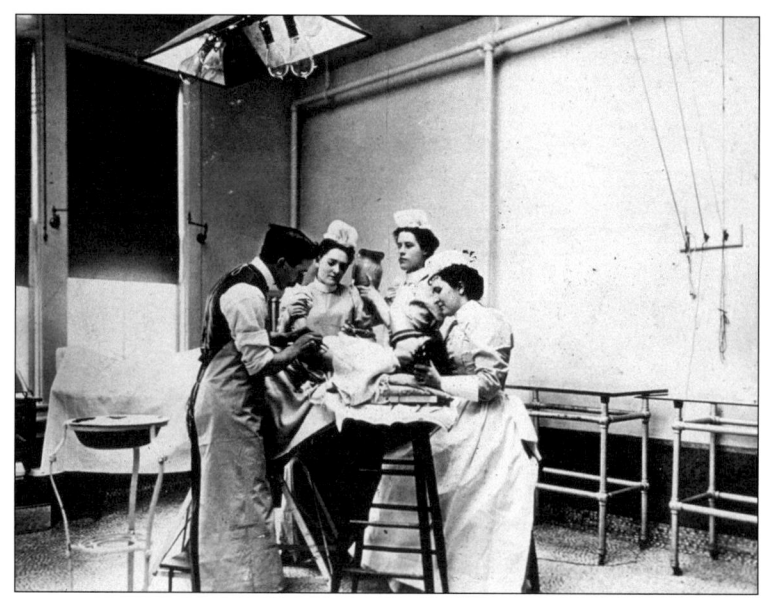

78 CATAMOUNT SURGEONS

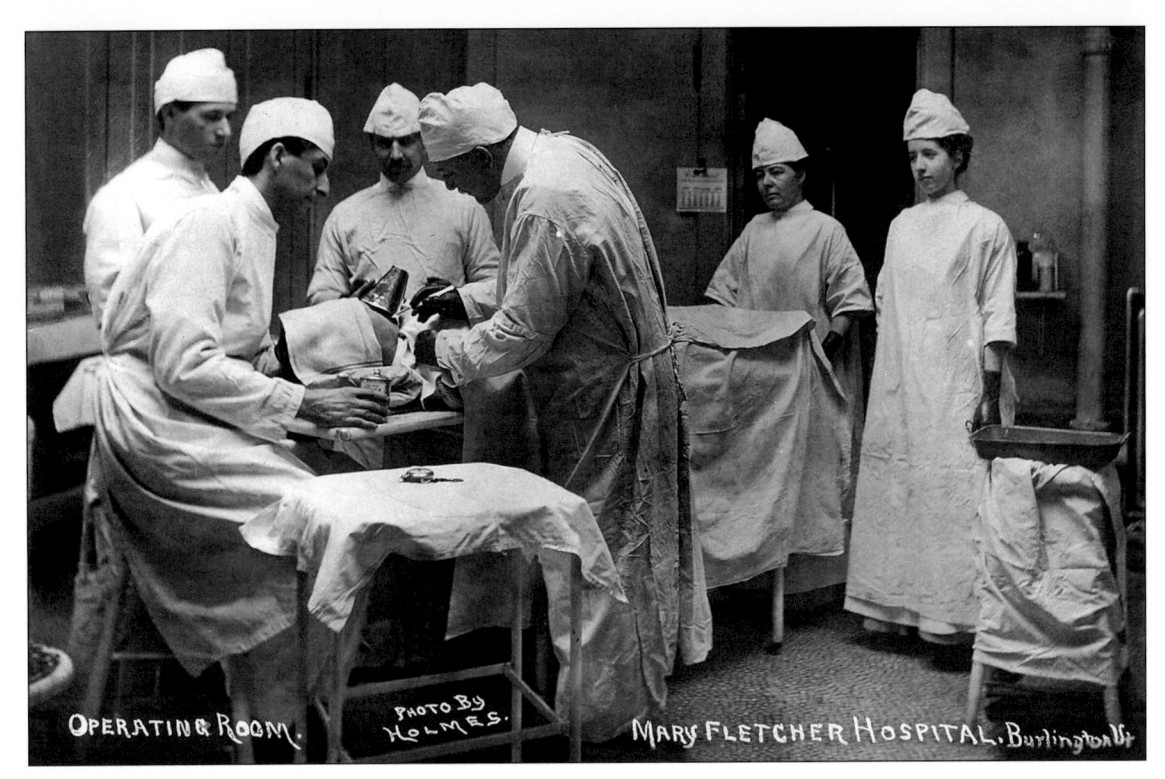

FIGURE 6-7.
Henry Tinkham operating in 1910. The gown and gloves seem modern for this period.

The "Other" Professor of Surgery

The successful completion of the College's new building was due largely to the efforts of the School's new Dean, Henry Crain Tinkham, who was also a surgeon. Wheeler noted that, "his clear and forcible demonstrations to the University Trustees, of the absolute necessity of a first-class, up-to-date building, if the College was to continue to exist, resulted in the erection of the present building."[35]

Born in Brownington, Vermont, on December 7, 1856, Tinkham's great-grandfather Seth was yet another Bunker Hill veteran. Tinkham received a local preparatory education, and then attended the College of Medicine, where he studied under Wheeler. After graduating in 1883, he started a Burlington-based surgical practice and took a job as demonstrator of anatomy with his alma mater. Over the course of the next ten years he advanced to instructor, adjunct professor, and then full professor of the same department. His fellow professors elected him Dean in 1898.[36]

At the time of the 1900 reorganization, the trustees created a new professorship in clinical surgery, which was filled by Tinkham. Like Wheeler, he held a weekly surgical clinic at the Mary Fletcher Hospital and taught at the bedside. "His clinical talks were admirable. He was not a highly educated man, but he was a ready fluent speaker who knew what he was talking about and expressed himself clearly and convincingly." His operative technique was honed by years spent in the dissection room, which "increased the natural deftness with which he was endowed."[37]

Tinkham wrote several surgical papers in spite of the demands of a busy practice and two full professorships. Among the topics covered were uterine cancer, care of the surgical patient, surgical management of the biliary tract, right-sided abdominal pathology, and superior mesenteric artery syndrome.[38, 39, 40, 41, 42]

The requirements of the Deanship, however, occupied the majority of Tinkham's time over the rest of his long career. Spearheading the recovery from the fire turned out to be one of his easier tasks. By 1905, the College's curriculum had fallen 860 hours short of the number recommended by the Association of American Medical Colleges. Adjustments were made, but at an increased expense to the school. At the same time, enrollment began to decline. Faced with dwindling student fees and salaries, the faculty grudgingly let the University take complete financial control of the College in 1908. Unfortunately for Tinkham, however, conditions only got worse.[43]

The Flexner Report Suggests Closing the Medical College (1910)

The American Medical Association had unsuccessfully tried to reform medical education throughout its entire history. In 1904, the AMA established the Council on Medical Education to promote systematic instruction nationwide.[44] The following year, the National Confederation of Examining and Licensing Boards adopted the educational criteria set forth by the AAMC.[45] Medical schools were suddenly forced to comply with standards that had been merely "recommended" in the past.

Members of the Council inspected each of the country's 160 medical schools during 1906. Every institution received a grade based on its entrance requirements, course offerings, facilities (classrooms, laboratories, dispensaries, and hospitals), faculty, and board certification rate. Eighty-two schools, including the UVM College of Medicine, were deemed "acceptable" and granted Class A status.[46]

Although the results were not publicized, the perceived intrusion on the part of the Council was resented by many of the medical colleges, especially those in the "doubtful" and "unacceptable" categories of Classes B and C. Seeking to minimize resistance to reform, the AMA approached and urged the Carnegie Foundation for the Advancement of Teaching to conduct another study. The Foundation was in the process of funding a similar project under the direction of noted educational innovator Abraham Flexner. In the winter of 1908, the two agencies agreed to join forces.[47]

Flexner started by calculating the ratio of physicians to occupants in each state, thereby determining whether a region was over- or under-served. He personally assessed every school's entrance requirements, attendance, teaching staff, resources available for maintenance, laboratory facilities, and clinical activities. He then compared individual institutions to Halsted's idealized European system at Johns Hopkins University.[48] The Report was thoroughly researched, logically constructed, and intelligently written. Its impact was groundbreaking.

Released in 1910, the work came to the same conclusion that Benjamin Lincoln had reached seventy years earlier — that the training of properly qualified physicians was in the public's best interest and that incompetent institutions should be identified and eliminated. Of the 155 colleges surveyed, only a handful met with Flexner's approval. Others (such as Yale), needed work, but were salvageable. The remainder, however, were condemned in no uncertain terms. The words "filthy," "disgusting," "rudimentary," and "foul" appeared throughout his descriptions of the more questionable facilities. Several summations contained the phrase "The school is a disgrace to the state whose laws permit its existence."[49] The UVM College of Medicine escaped such vitriol, but just barely.

During his visit to Burlington in May of 1909, Flexner found that students were still admitted without a high school education, that there was only one full-time faculty member, that thirteen of the thirty-three teachers were from out-of-state, and that the faculty *never* met as a group. In addition, he noticed that the school lacked a library, museum, and teaching accessories. There were 200 beds available in a limited way, but they were primarily surgical (Flexner believed that there should be more medical and obstetrical cases). There were no signs of active research at either the laboratory or animal level.[50]

He noted that Burlington, a town of 22,690 people, was home to 60 physicians, and thus over-served. He also pointed out that the College did not utilize the University's "intelligent advice" when it came to checking the credentials of its students. On the plus side, Flexner applauded the fact that the school was "now an organic part of the university," and that the state had "lately appropriated $10,000." In addition, he wrote that, "The school has an attractive new laboratory building adequate to routine teaching of anatomy, pathology, histology, bacteriology, physiology, and chemistry."[51] In the end, however, he felt that New England should only support Harvard and Yale:

> "...it is unnecessary to prolong the life of the clinical departments of Dartmouth, Bowdoin, and Vermont. They are not likely soon to possess the financial resources needed to develop adequate clinics in their present location; and the time has passed when even excellent didactic instruction can be regarded as compensating for defective opportunities in obstetrics, contagious diseases, and general medicine. The historic position of the schools in question counts little as against changed ideals. Dartmouth and Vermont can, however, offer the work of the first two years with the clinical coloring made feasible by the proximity of a hospital."[52]

The College of Medicine Fights Back

Tinkham was furious. His school had improved several of its practices following Flexner's evaluation, yet was not credited with doing so in the final Report. The College had started requiring a year of collegiate study prior to admission and was in the process of hiring more full-time instructors.[53] Tinkham declared that, "Mr. Flexner has been unjust in many instances. The whole trend of his work seems to be an attempt to forcibly crush out the small colleges and build up the great institutions." The Dean felt that it would be "impossible to argue the small school into oblivion by the results of any such pedagogic investigation as this."[54]

Wheeler and the rest of the staff, naturally, came to Tinkham's defense:

> We of the Vermont Medical Faculty thought that at least one smaller school was necessary in order to supply well trained medical practitioners for the smaller rural communities. We thought it was very unlikely that men who were able to make the necessary financial invest-

ment for attendance at a school in one of the large centers, and who had experience of life in such a place, would be willing to settle down for life in some small country village. Yet such places had a right to the best medical service ... and there is now no question of the need of training schools to fill this want. [55]

Using this argument, Tinkham applied for AAMC membership again in 1911. The findings from the Association's follow-up investigation, however, mirrored those of the Flexner Report. There still were not enough full-time staff members, teaching accessories, or clinical facilities. Acting on the AAMC's suggestions, Tinkham embarked on another wide-scale faculty reorganization. By the time it was done, there were five full-time basic science professors, another five full-time instructors, and only one non-resident professor. The school was admitted to the AAMC in 1912, with the understanding that it would improve its clinical situation.[56]

Tinkham drummed up public support for the College with the help of the president and local businessmen. He called the Carnegie Foundation "vicious" and "unfair," implying that a "conspiracy" was underway to squeeze the smaller medical schools out of existence. As the legislature debated the school's financial future, Tinkham convinced the AMA's Council on Medical Education to refrain from changing the College's rating until the upcoming 1915 inspection.[57]

The Mary Fletcher Hospital, in the meantime, was unwilling to underwrite a maternity ward or a free dispensary for the College's benefit. Tinkham appealed to UVM's president, who in turn obtained another appropriation from the state legislature. Money in hand, the hospital provided rooms for a dispensary and opened a twelve-bed obstetric ward.[58] A "large percentage" of the patients were "practically turned over to the College of Medicine," under the "direct supervision" of the clinical professors.[59] As Wheeler later put it:

"Vermont's reaction to the announcement was characteristic. Vermonters are not in the habit of letting outsiders manage their affairs for them. They thought they were capable of deciding for themselves whether they needed a medical college or not, and when they realized a Class A institution would cost money, the Legislature, which contains a representative for every town in the State, voted an annual appropriation of a sum of money to enable the University of Vermont to teach medicine in accordance with modern ideas of medical education. Thus did the State of Vermont assist her College of Medicine to carry on and to meet the requirements of a Class A institution, without calling on outsiders for help." [60]

The Dean's next job was to address the chronic shortage of clinical cases. A second dispensary, staffed by the city physician, was established on Pearl Street. The directors of the Mary Fletcher Hospital, in turn, generously granted access to all patients except those in the private ward. Despite these measures, though, the number of available beds still fell short of the number recommended by the AAMC.[61] The College's attention soon turned to the little hospital four and a half miles north of town.

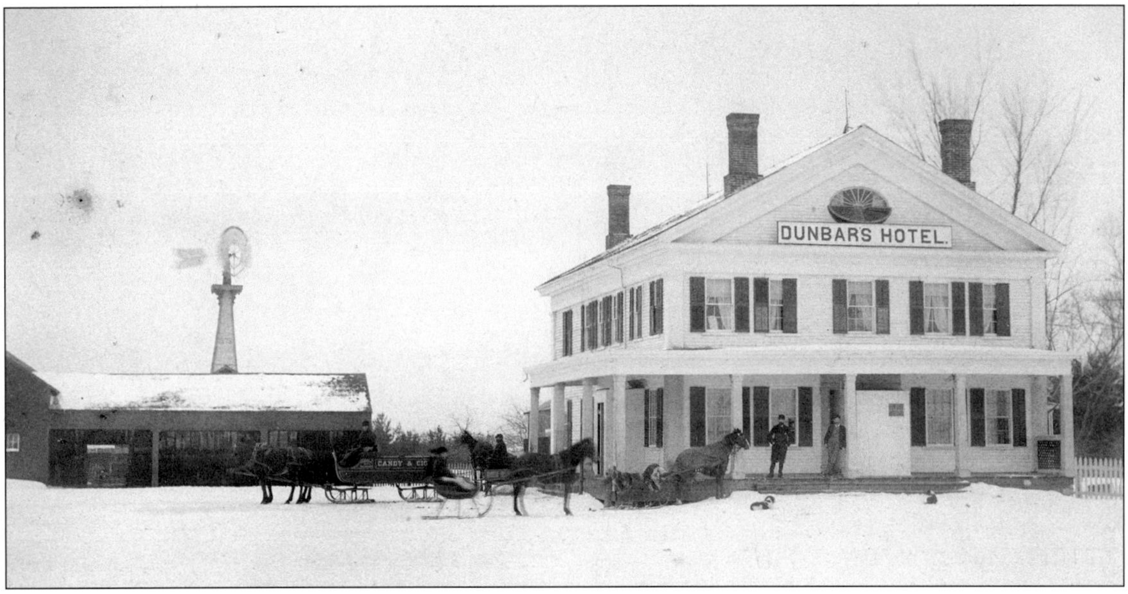

FIGURE 6-8.
Colchester's Dunbar Hotel prior to its conversion into the Fanny Allen Hospital.

Frances Margaret Allen and Her Hôtel-Dieu

Twenty years earlier, in May of 1894, a group of nuns belonging to Montreal's Religious Hospitallers of St. Joseph (RHSJ) arrived in neighboring Colchester. Summoned at the behest of Burlington's visionary bishop, Louis DeGoesbriand, they worked in concert with his successor John S. Michaud to create a caring retirement home for his priests and a hospital for the poor. The sisters (who were also professionally trained nurses) took charge of a dilapidated old tavern donated for that purpose. Within five months, the structure formerly known as Dunbar's Hotel was re-christened as the Fanny Allen Hôtel-Dieu.[62]

The new hospital's namesake was the youngest daughter of Green Mountain Boy Ethan Allen. Born on November 11, 1784 to the Vermont hero's second wife, she was raised by her stepfather, Dr. Jabez Penniman, following Ethan's demise. Penniman, a colleague of John Pomeroy, provided young Frances Margaret with a first-rate education. In 1807, while studying French in Montreal, she underwent a religious transformation. She converted to Catholicism and, in 1810, made history as the first woman of New England birth to become a nun.[63]

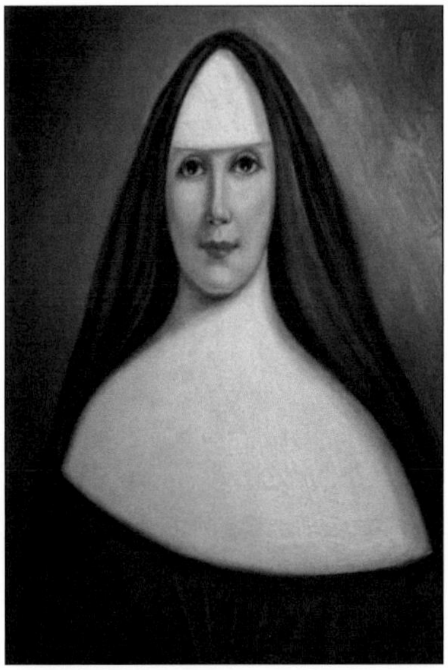

Fanny Allen joined the Congregation of the RHSJ and went to work at Montreal's Hôtel-Dieu. Founded in 1642 by Jeanne Mance and staffed by the RHSJ since 1659, the hospital treated indigent patients from across the region. The "lovely American nun" ran the apothecary as the facility's chemist. Her kindness and compassion were remembered by many, long after her death from "a lung ailment" on December 10, 1819.[64]

FIGURE 6-9. Ethan Allen's daughter Frances Margaret Allen converted to Catholicism in 1810. Her order, the Royal Hospitallers of St. Joseph, staffed and administrated her namesake hospital.

Chapter Six: Trouble at the Turn of the Century 83

FIGURE 6-10. Mary Fletcher's servant and companion Michael Kelly donated the land on which the Fanny Allen Hospital was built.

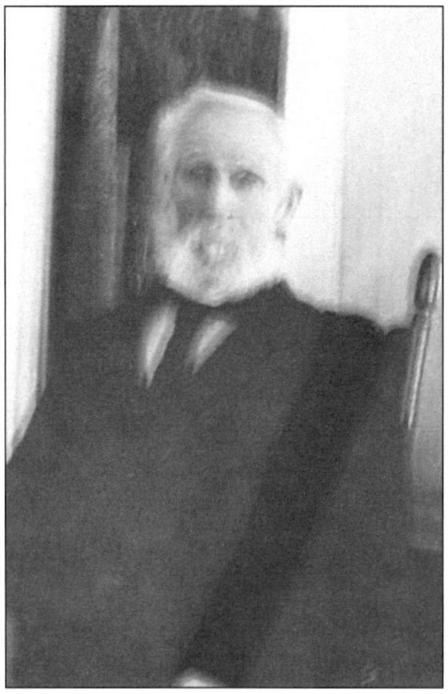

Penniman, meanwhile, bought a large tract of land from Ira Allen in 1809. He subdivided the Colchester property in 1830, and sold a portion of it to Arad Merrill, who then proceeded to erect a tavern on the site. Frank Dunbar purchased the tavern in 1877, whereupon he converted it into a hotel. Dunbar ran into financial difficulty and, in May of 1889, mortgaged his assets to Michael F. Kelly of Burlington.[65]

Kelly, the devoted servant and "man-of-all-work" to Miss Mary Margaret Fletcher, had inherited a substantial amount of money from his former employer. Using skills he had learned from Mary Fletcher's father, he parlayed his newfound wealth into sizable real estate holdings. Dunbar died in 1892, and Kelly foreclosed on the property a short time later. He then deeded the entire 25-acre lot to Bishop Michaud for the establishment of a hospital.[66]

The fifty-bed institution catered to unwed mothers, people with contagious diseases, and those with mental illness. The first two floors contained separate wards for the men and women, and an operating suite that doubled as a waiting room for visitors when not in use. The sisters reserved the use of the attic for themselves.[67] The old bar of the Dunbar Hotel was used to dispense drugs and medicines, instead of beer and whiskey.[68]

Only four years later (1898) a new operating room was constructed that remained until the 1973 renovation. The roof was of glass to admit light, and there was a huge plate glass window on the east wall facing the hospital farm, the site of a former race track.[69]

The "new" hospital remained independent of UVM for many years due to religious differences and physical distance, although a trolley did run between Burlington and Essex Junction. The region's French Canadian population remained loyal to the Fanny Allen Hospital over the ensuing decades despite the proximity of the better-equipped, but Protestant based, Mary Fletcher Hospital.

Several surgeons, including Wheeler and Tinkham, held appointments at both hospitals. This was not a two way street, however. Physicians with appointments at the Mary Fletcher

FIGURE 6-11. The trolley shelter at the base of Mary Fletcher's "Hospital Hill".

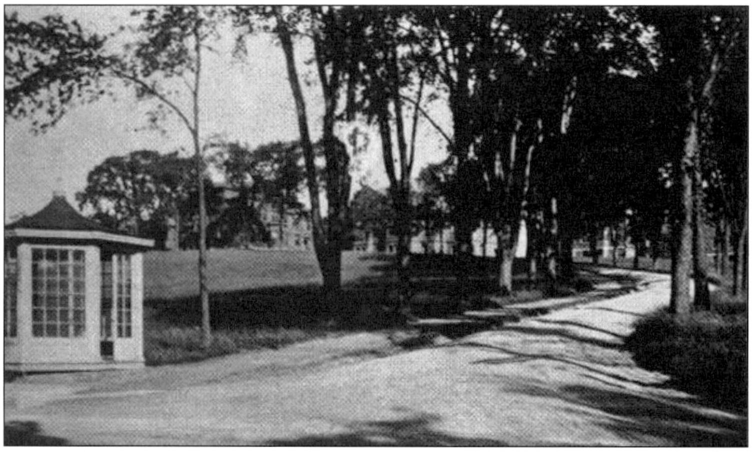

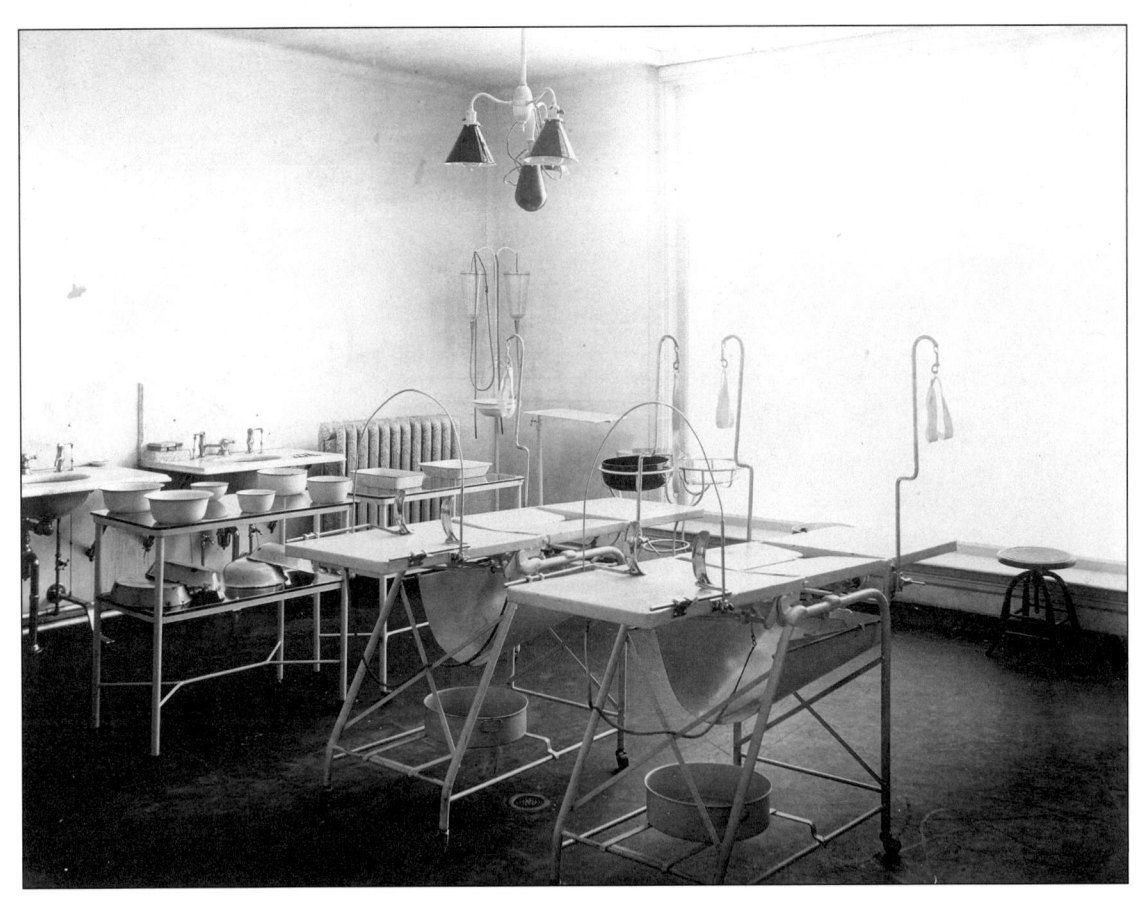

FIGURE 6-12.
The Fanny Allen Hospital's operating suite following an 1898 renovation. The huge glass windows provided light.

Hospital held UVM appointments as well, and usually had privileges at the Fanny Allen Hospital. Most of those with primary privileges at the Fanny Allen Hospital, on the other hand, did not receive a UVM or Mary Fletcher appointment.

Patrick McSweeney, a surgeon and an adjunct professor of obstetrics at UVM, was the first president of the Fanny Allen medical staff. In 1905, he performed the first cesarean section in Vermont at that hospital.[70]

A case from the 1906 hospital casebook is interesting in the apparent requirement for multiple opinions prior to surgery. The entire record for one patient follows:

"Mrs. J.B.P., Burlington, Vt.
Admitted July 7, 1906.
Age 42 years, Nat'y. French, Married, Housewife.
Family History: Negative.
Previous diseases; Measles and Scarlet fever in childhood.
Present Disease: Two years ago patient experienced a sharp and sudden pain in the abdomen which in a few hours became localized in the right iliac fossa and was accompanied by tenderness over McBurney's point. This attack lasted nine days. Three weeks later she had another similar attack which lasted four days. One month ago she had another attack which lasted but one day. On July 6, 1906, patient was taken suddenly ill with pain in the

Chapter Six: Trouble at the Turn of the Century

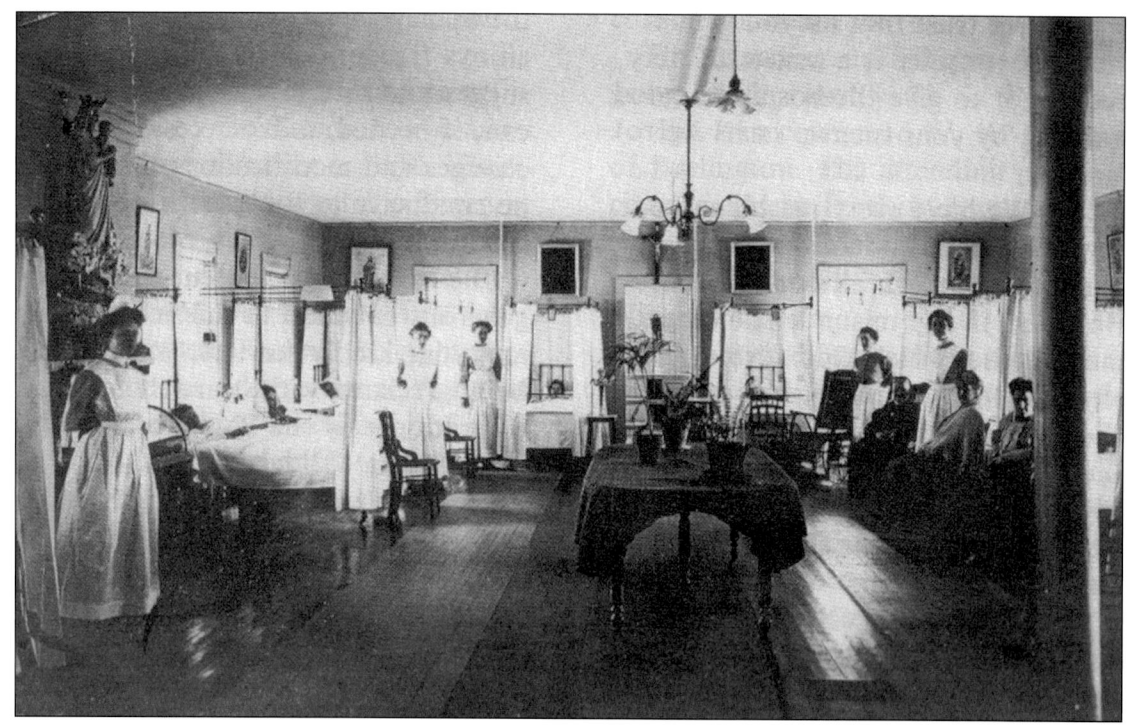

FIGURE 6-13.
Fanny Allen wards had electric lights and nurses wearing starched uniforms by 1910.

FIGURE 6-14.
Balanced traction applied for a fractured femur at the FAH in 1918.

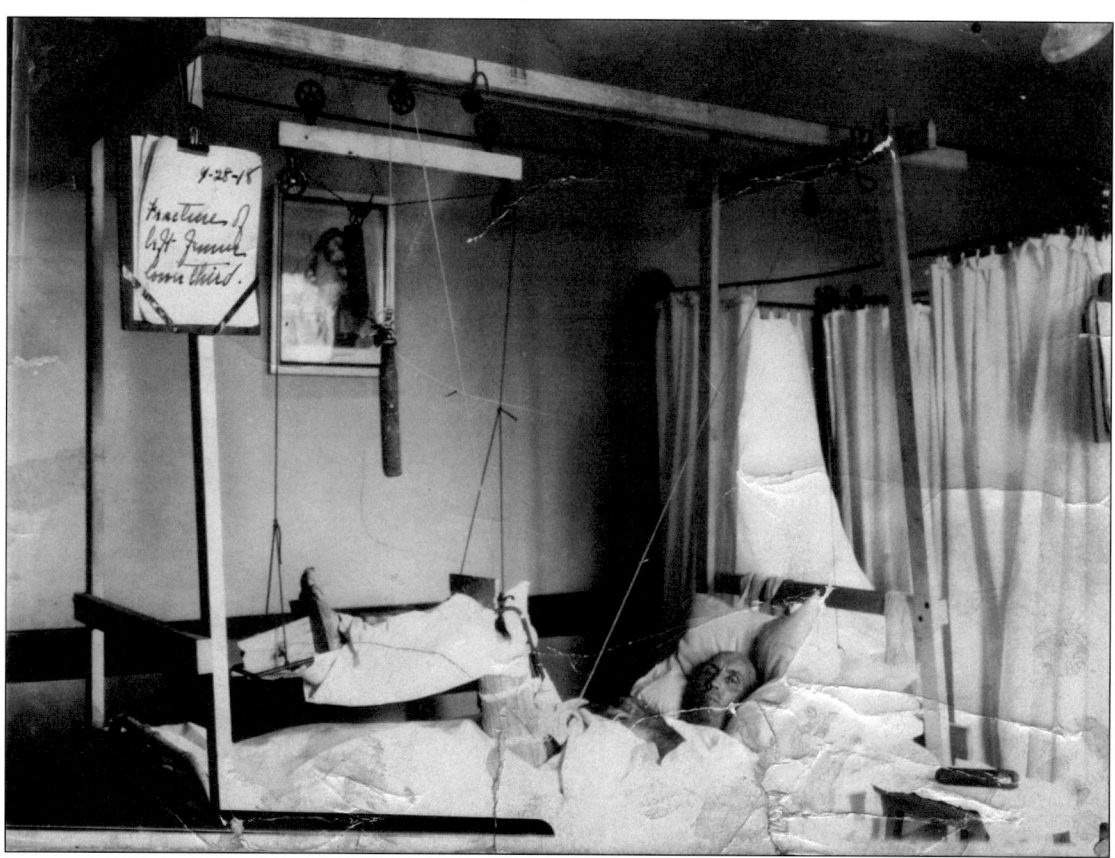

epigastrium which later became localized over McBurney's point and was associated with tenderness. Patient had some fever, but did not vomit.

Diagnosis: Dr. McSweeney – Appendicitis; Dr. Allen – Appendicitis; Dr. Thabault – Appendicitis; Dr. Wheeler – Appendicitis

Treatment: Operative.

Patient was prepared for operation in the usual way. Ether administered by Dr. Johnson. Operation performed by Dr. McSweeney. Incision made over McBurney's point, appendix was found inflamed and bound down with adhesions. Appendix ligated and removed. Wound closed, dressings applied and patient taken to her room in good condition.

After treatment: Strychnine gr.1/60 t.i.d. for five days, Calomel and salts.

Stitches removed from the wound on July 15, 1906.

Patient made a rapid recovery.

Discharged July 21, 1906. Cured."[71]

The College of Medicine Retains Its Class A Status

In 1914, Tinkham and McSweeney asked Bishop Michaud's successor, Bishop Joseph J. Rice, to provide more beds for teaching cases at the Fanny Allen. Rice, eager to "come into the city," saw this as an opportunity to also build a new Catholic hospital near the UVM campus.[72] Within a few months, the Legislature finally committed its financial support for the College of Medicine and its needed new hospital. Although the College continued to have deficiencies, the AMA was impressed enough to maintain its Class A status.[73]

Nathan Smith's other rural schools indicted by the Flexner report, Dartmouth and Bowdoin, did not fare as well. Dartmouth, unable to meet clinical case requirements, became a two-year medical college in 1913. It would not offer a four year M.D. program again until 1968. Bowdoin, in contrast, lacked financial resources. In 1920, it dropped its medical school altogether (although the State of Maine later developed a formal relationship with UVM to provide training for its medical students).[74]

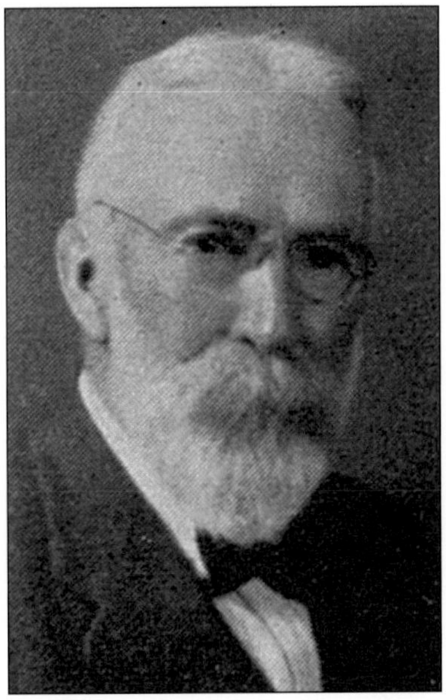

Further reforms were forestalled by the outbreak of World War I. Wheeler, hoping to retire in 1917 at age 65, was instead commissioned for military duty. He became a first lieutenant in the Medical Officer's Reserve Corps and was appointed Medical Aide to the Governor. "The job was by no means a sinecure. In addition to the visits to the Governor, it involved reports to him and correspondence with medical examiners all over the State and with recruits who were dissatisfied with the result of their medical examination. The Governor's Medical Aide was the court of appeal in all cases of the kind, and there were enough of them to take up a good deal of such spare time as I had in those days."[75]

Tinkham, however, was looking ahead. He kept up with

FIGURE 6-15. John Brooks Wheeler, Chief of Surgery 1900-1924.

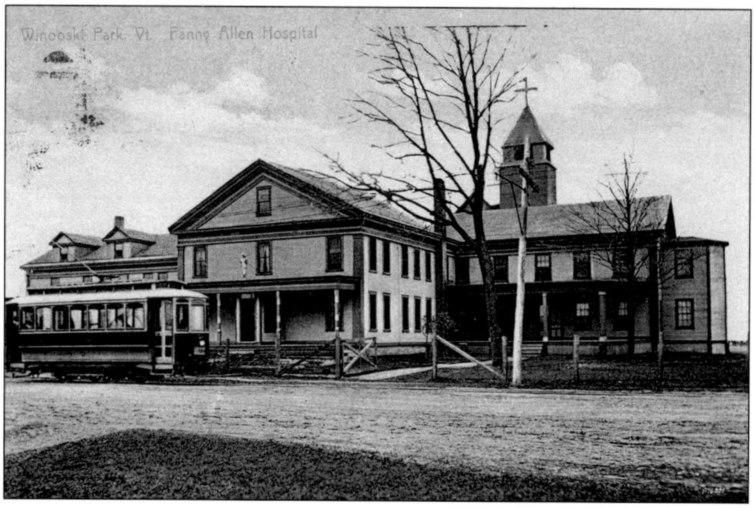

FIGURE 6-16. The trolley in the lower left corner connected the Fanny Allen to Burlington and Essex Junction.

the latest educational advances and implemented them whenever feasible. Faculty meetings included efforts to integrate scientific and clinical teaching. By 1924, he was prepared to introduce clinical training during the first and second years. It would have been a revolutionary move had he succeeded. Unfortunately, he developed a chronic illness that took his life within a year. In his last act of service, he left his extensive library to the College and donated his operating instruments to the Mary Fletcher Hospital.[76, 77]

With Tinkham gone, and Wheeler about to turn 72, surgical training at UVM again found itself at a crossroads.

CHAPTER 7

New Leaders and New Hospitals Fail to Solve Old Problems

Hometown surgeon Lyman Allen succeeded John Brooks Wheeler as chairman. Excellent clinical teaching continued in the absence of academic research.

Another Catholic hospital arose within sight of the Medical Building. The staff, however, was not fully accepted at the University or at the protestant hospital on the hill.

The College of Medicine, unprepared to meet the demands of an academic medical center, was placed back on probation in 1935 by both the AMA and the AAMC, and took five years to emerge from this state.

Wheeler Relinquishes the Chair of Surgery After 25 Years

Wheeler, professor of surgery for an unprecedented twenty-five years, finally stepped down in 1924. He had treated Samuel Thayer's gangrenous foot, accepted referrals from Henry Janes, and operated alongside James Little, Leroy Bingham, J. Williston Wright, and Abel Phelps during his illustrious career. He had taught dozens of young surgeons and had mentored several more who become leaders in their own right. Foremost among that group were his colleagues Henry Tinkham and Lyman Allen.

Homegrown Chairman

Allen, a distant relative of Ethan, Ira, and Fanny, spent all but one year of his life in the shadow of the UVM campus. Born on May 21, 1872 to a prosperous family, Allen grew up in the former home of John Johnson, the builder of the "Old Mill" and the original Medical Building. The house, located on the corner of Main Street and University Place, occupied the site of today's Morrill Hall. As Allen later recalled:

"Our land ran back to the top of the hill ... we owned about half the grove, the college the other half. It was really a rural sort of community. Everyone farmed more or less, and the college boys helped themselves to the grapes and apples ... before I can remember the College Green was covered with pine trees. They were cut down to make the first college building ... that building burned down. You see there was no running water. The reservoir was just where it is now. The water would trickle into the basements of the houses, but they couldn't

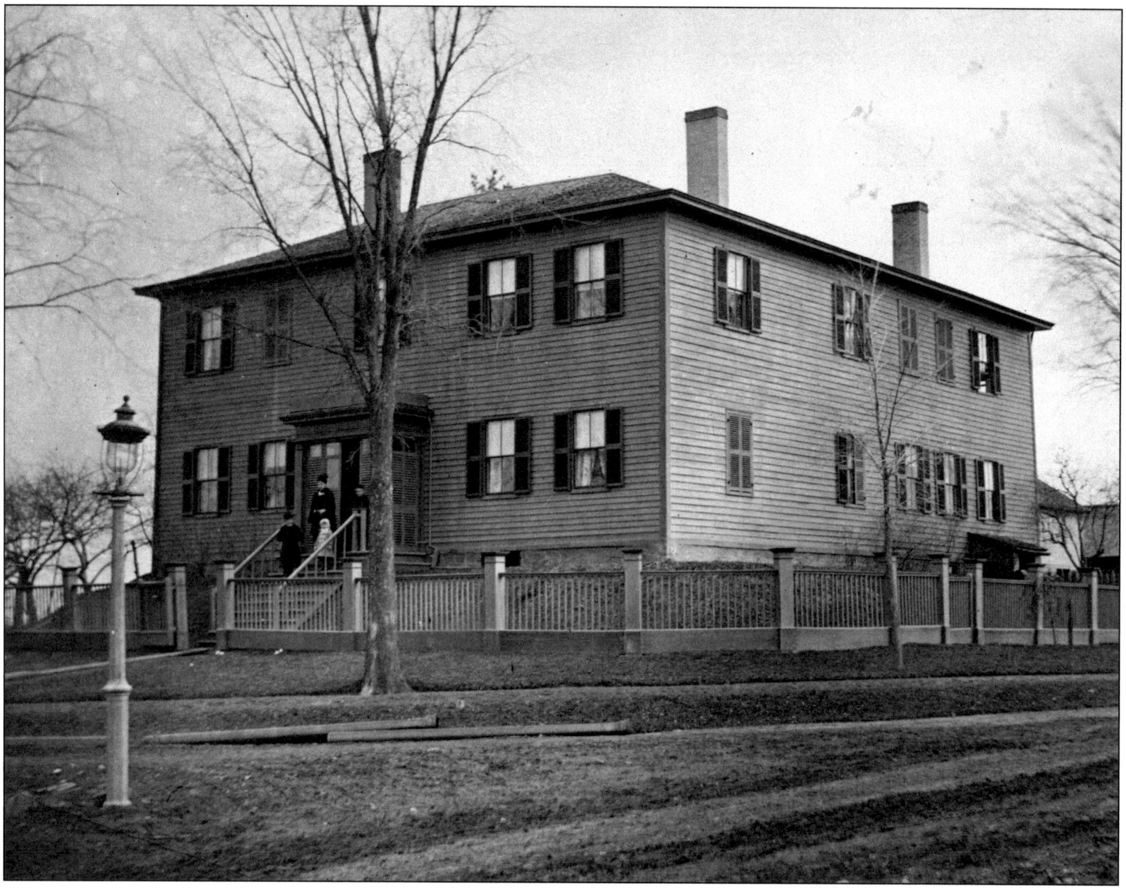

FIGURE 7-1.
Lyman Allen's boyhood home stood next to the UVM Green, diagonally across from Pomeroy Hall.

get it up to the kitchen floor. There was no water in the college buildings. The reservoir was not high enough. Water had to be carried around in pails. ... there were ... gas lights all around the green ... after they got the pine trees off the Green they decided to plant elm trees ..." [1]

Following an appropriate preliminary education, Allen obtained his Bachelor's degree from UVM in 1893. An accomplished student, he was elected to Phi Beta Kappa at the time of his graduation. He was also a standout football and track star, and was the captain of the school's championship baseball team for four straight years.[2] He continued to play baseball while attending the College of Medicine, and even convinced the faculty to underwrite part of the team's tuition. This generous offer was extended with the understanding that the students "shall not be called upon to sacrifice their medical studies to the interests of baseball by absenting themselves from lectures."[3]

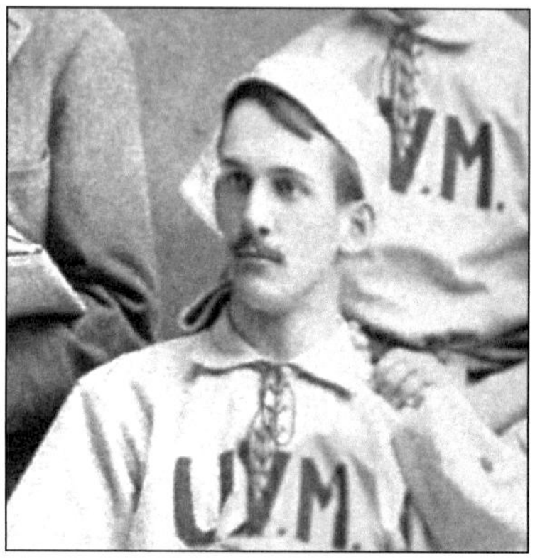

FIGURE 7-2.
Future Chief Lyman Allen was the star of the 1891 UVM baseball team.

As one of Wheeler's "office students," Allen accompanied his preceptor on several epic journeys. During the winter of 1895/1896, the two traveled over one hundred miles to northern New Hampshire. By the time the duo

90 CATAMOUNT SURGEONS

reached their destination, the temperature had dropped to twenty-five degrees below zero. Their patient, a Dartmouth football player, had been suffering from diffuse abdominal pain for ten days. Wheeler remarked:

> "He was in very bad condition when I saw him, very septic, temperature 101.5, pulse 120, feeble, mind cloudy, face duskily flushed, abdomen tensely distended. He had been vomiting fecal matter since morning. Death seemed certain, but there was a faint chance that it might be avoided by operation. An operation was accordingly done and an abscess was found which occupied a third of the abdominal cavity. There was a gangrenous, ruptured appendix. The appendix was removed and the abscess cavity disinfected and drained."[4]

After surviving the near-derailment of their rail car on the return trip, Allen was back in class the next morning. The patient, unfortunately, did not do as well. He "made something of a rally after the operation," but succumbed the following day "in spite of internal and hypodermic stimulation and external heat."[5] Such outcomes were common in the days before antibiotics, especially with delays in obtaining treatment.

After receiving his M.D. in 1896, Allen (like Wheeler) augmented his medical education with a one-year internship. Upon completing his training at Boston City Hospital, he returned to Burlington and established a practice. In 1899, he secured a position at the College of Medicine as adjunct professor of physiology. He became the assistant to the chair of surgery under Wheeler in 1900, and succeeded Horatio Nelson Jackson as instructor in surgery the following year.[6] Jackson, in turn, went on to achieve more lasting fame in 1903 as the first person to drive an automobile cross-country.[7]

Appointed adjunct professor of surgery in 1907, Allen was named assistant professor following Tinkham's 1911 faculty reorganization, and then associate professor in the early 1920s.[8,9] During this time, he produced articles on the relationship between temperature and infection, the use of Bismuth in wounds, and the favorable results of early mobilization after knee injury.[10,11,12] Later, as full professor, he authored papers on blood tests for appendicitis, omental torsion, and arterial injury following knee dislocation.[13,14,15]

One of Allen's more pertinent publications reflected his interest in the burgeoning field of Neurosurgery. In it, he discussed the mechanism, diagnosis, and treatment of traumatic brain injury, correctly concluding that,

> "Increased intracranial pressure, no matter how produced, causes brain injury [by interfering with the circulation of the blood or of the cerebrospinal fluid] and must be relieved. There are several methods of doing this, so choose the one most applicable to the given case. The absence of "localizing symptoms" must not be allowed to affect at all the diagnosis of possible brain injury. The stage of cerebral exhaustion is too late for successful operative measures. Operate in the stage of cerebral stimulation as soon as it becomes obvious that the symptoms are not improving. Keep the patient under close and constant observation from the very start. No case of head injury is so trivial as to be ignored or so severe as to be despaired of."[16]

Allen was also committed to professional development. He held several executive positions within the Vermont State Medical Society between 1904 and 1932.[17,18] As a faculty member

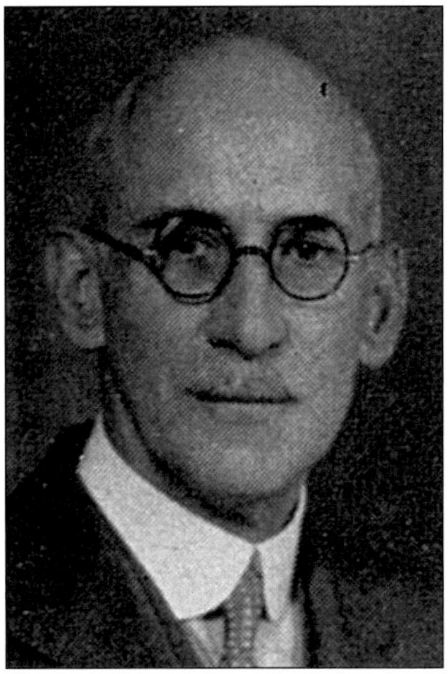

FIGURE 7-3.
Lyman Allen,
Chief of Surgery
1924-1942.

at a school of medicine, he was invited to be one of the several hundred "Founders" of the American College of Surgeons (ACS) in 1912. The group, an outgrowth of educational clinics sponsored by the publishers of *Surgery, Gynecology & Obstetrics*, a prominent surgical journal, quickly gained widespread acclaim for upholding ethical and professional standards in practice.[19] Four years later, Allen helped Wheeler, Tinkham, and fifteen other surgeons from across the region establish the New England Surgical Society. Similar in philosophy to the ACS, it provided a forum in which the surgical leaders of the Northeast could present papers, attend clinics at major hospitals, and socialize with fellow practitioners.[20]

Back in Trouble

By 1924, almost all of the school's chairmen were graduates of the College of Medicine. This was in keeping with the Association of American Medical Colleges' recommendation that local physicians administer specialty subjects. UVM's relative isolation (despite the presence of the railroad) and the lack of other rural New England medical schools, however, led to a diminished pool from which to choose its instructors. An unintended consequence was that accomplished itinerant professors were often replaced with inexperienced inbred teachers.

Wheeler was in the process of turning over the professorship to Allen, though he continued to operate and teach during his emeritus status. Mackay describes him around 1930 with a long white beard which in the operating room flowed down the front of his gown. "He never wore a mask, saying that he thought any surgeon who was, in fact, able to or apt to spit in the wound should not be in the operating room."[21]

The American Medical Association's Council on Medical Education inspected the College in late 1926. Within months, UVM faced another downgrade to Class B status. The AMA felt that there still weren't enough full-time pre-clinical teachers. In addition, it thought that students ought to start their clinical training earlier and should have better access to dispensary and hospital patients. And, as before, it determined that the number of available inpatient beds was inadequate for the school's clinical needs.[22]

Obstetrical training in Burlington was non-existent, so students were assigned to spend three weeks in New York City at the Lying-In Hospital. One student related that he was in the home for a delivery and announced to the father that there were to be twins. The father insisted there be only one baby, and sat down with a sawed off shotgun outside the door to enforce this concept. The UVM student was upset, but soon had an idea. The Lying-In hospital had a routine of sending out a team to the home if no report was received within two hours. So he gave the patient 15 mg of intravenous morphine which stopped her labor "He said nothing to the father and carefully observed her and then returned to the kitchen, read and smoked and passed the time, all the while the old man sitting in front of the only exit with the sawed off shotgun. A second dose of medicine was necessary to maintain the patient who was having no difficulty and the fetal heart rate was satisfactory. After the two hourly period had passed, a resident, two interns and two medical students came downtown to see what was going on, broke into the apartment and overpowered the old man with no difficulty."[23]

UVM applied to the Legislature for additional appropriations, which it used to hire more teachers. It also reduced the amount of didactic teaching, thereby bringing its hours in line with the national average.[24] Additional clinical cases, though, were harder to come by. The city's dispensaries and the Mary Fletcher Hospital ran at near capacity. The Fanny Allen Hospital was available theoretically, but it was too far away for daily student visits. Fortunately, the College found a solution right across the street.

The Bishop DeGoesbriand Hospital Opens

Even though the Fanny Allen Hospital had been brought into the College of Medicine's fold back in 1914, it was not an integral part of the school. Physical distance aside, it failed to fit in for a number of other reasons. The first problem, as alluded to earlier, was its overt religious affiliation. The second difficulty involved the native tongue of its patients, the majority of whom were French Canadian. The last, most glaring problem was that the facility (originally opened in 1894) was not suited for "modern" medical practice. Patrick McSweeney's grandson (E.D. McSweeney Jr.) recalled that, "Even in 1924 ... the facilities were woefully antiquated. Only a few could believe what the operating room at the old Fanny Allen was like. There was a skylight, and that's where the light came from — that was it." [25]

The College, for its part, remained distant. The majority of the Fanny Allen's surgeons were not given appointments at either the university or the Mary Fletcher Hospital. In addition, greater Burlington's Catholics were culturally divided. The French were centered in Winooski, whereas the Irish lived in Burlington. It became apparent that erecting a new facility near the city's existing medical campus might address many of these issues.

Burlington's third Bishop, Joseph J. Rice, agreed that the city needed another hospital as well. In fact, he had intended to build an up-to-date infirmary on church property as early as 1916. The Great War precluded his plans, as both building materials and manual labor were in short supply. The Bishop gathered support for the scheme while he waited for the economy to improve. Finally, in March of 1922, the project was formally announced. Ground was broken the ensuing year, and by June 10, 1924, the brand-new hospital was ready to admit its first patient.[26]

The building was erected as a memorial to Louis DeGoesbriand, the first Bishop of Burlington. DeGoesbriand, the son of a French nobleman, had emigrated from Brittany in 1840 following his ordination. He then ministered in Cincinnati and Cleveland before coming to Vermont in 1853. Over the next forty years, he recruited priests and nuns, built churches, and established schools and charitable institutions throughout the state.[27] In 1885, he presided over the marriage of Michael Kelly — Mary Fletcher's longtime servant — to Miss Fletcher's seamstress. Within weeks of the ceremony, Kelly (at the Bishop's suggestion) purchased the land on which the Fanny Allen Hospital was to be erected.[28]

DeGoesbriand made several real estate transactions of his own. In 1854, he bought the former "Pearl Street House" with funds he had inherited from his family in Brittany. Located on the corner of Pearl and Prospect streets, the tavern had originally been built by Eli Barnard, an associate of Ira Allen and Moses Catlin. The building served as an orphanage

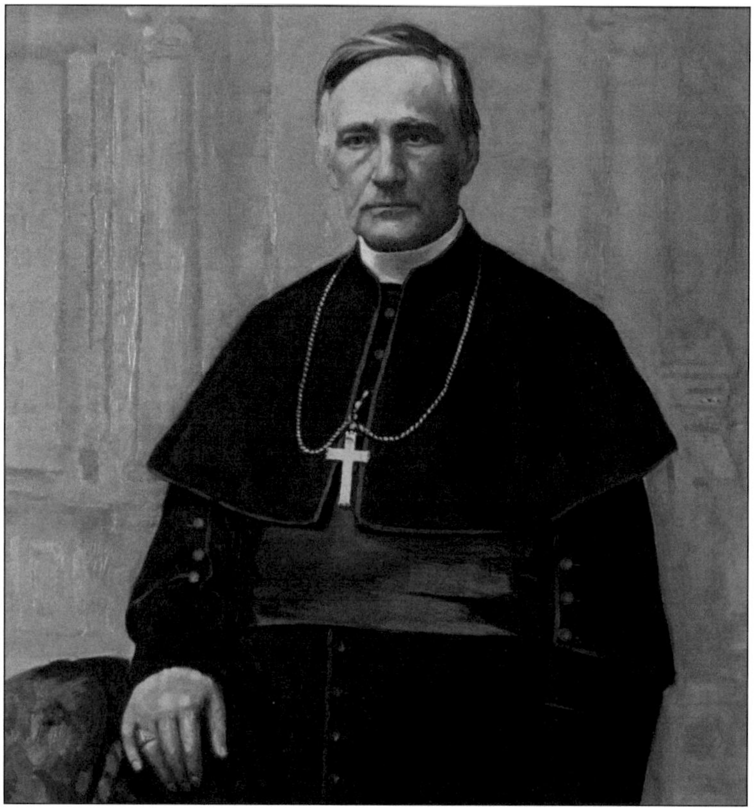

FIGURE 7-4.
Louis DeGoesbriand, the first Bishop of Burlington, was instrumental in the founding of the Fanny Allen and DeGoesbriand Hospitals.

until 1884, whereupon it was converted into St. Joseph's College for Boys and Young Men. The college closed in 1900 and the dilapidated structure was torn down shortly thereafter. Fittingly enough, the Bishop's property then became the site of his namesake hospital.[29]

Patrick McSweeney, gynecologist and surgeon, with his Irish roots, was a dominant figure during and after the building of the new facility. He performed the DeGoesbriand's first operation (insertion of radium needles into a cancerous growth), and was president of the medical staff from the time the hospital opened until his death in 1938.

As with the Fanny Allen Hospital, the Sisters of the Religious Hospitallers of St. Joseph provided the staffing. McSweeney personally recruited several of the hospital's senior nurses for the new venture. Years later, one of the Fanny Allen Hospital's elderly nuns mistook his grandson, Douglas McSweeney Jr., for the old obstetrician. Cornering him, she snapped, "Pat McSweeney, I will never forgive you for taking all the nuns to Burlington!" McSweeney Jr., always quick with a comeback, replied that he only took "the Irish sisters and left the French sisters at the Fanny."[30]

Patrick McSweeney was also out front when it came to innovation — in one case a little too far.

> *"A former student remembered watching McSweeney use an unproven sine-wave machine on a patient with general peritonitis. The device would, by electrical stimulus, cause a massive contraction every 30 seconds to all muscles of the patient's abdominal wall in an attempt to correct the patient's ileus. He later realized, of course that nothing was calculated to make the peritonitis spread faster or to prevent the patient from localizing his own infection."*[31]

The idea was abandoned.

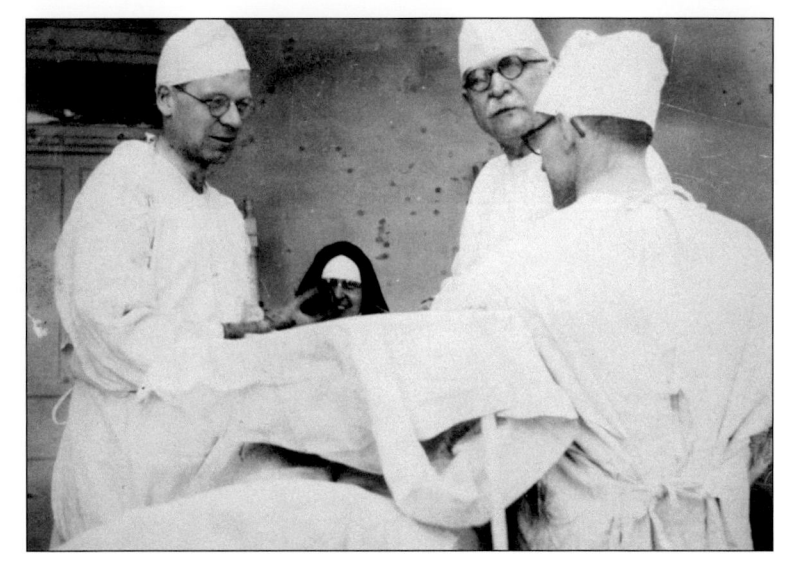

FIGURE 7-5. Patrick McSweeney, (center) operating at the FAH, was the driving physician force behind the DeGoesbriand Hospital.

Surgery Becomes an In-hospital Specialty

Technical innovation notwithstanding, surgery and hospitals soon became synonymous. Wheeler, reflecting on some of his earlier "house calls" at the time of his retirement, noted that,

> "Experiences of this kind are not nearly as common as they used to be, for two reasons: First, because the people realize much better than they used to, the great advantage of treat-

FIGURE 7-6.
The DeGoesbriand Hospital opened in 1924. The main entrance was on Prospect Streeet. (1949 photo)

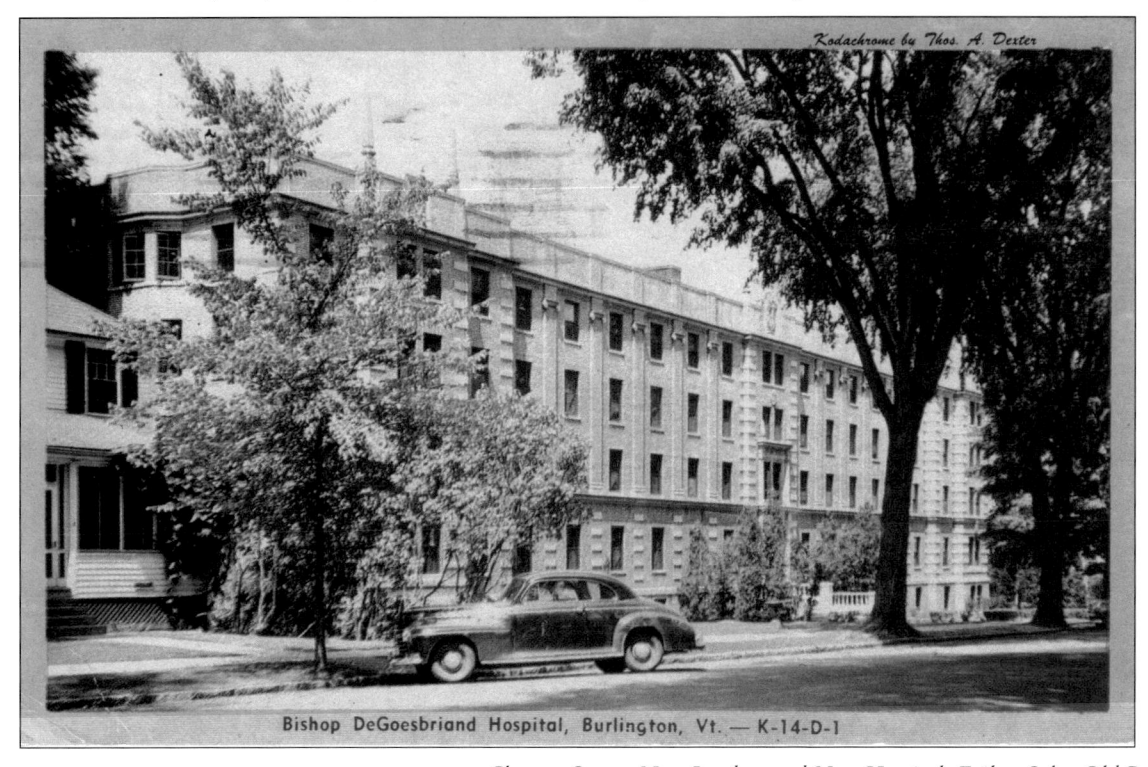

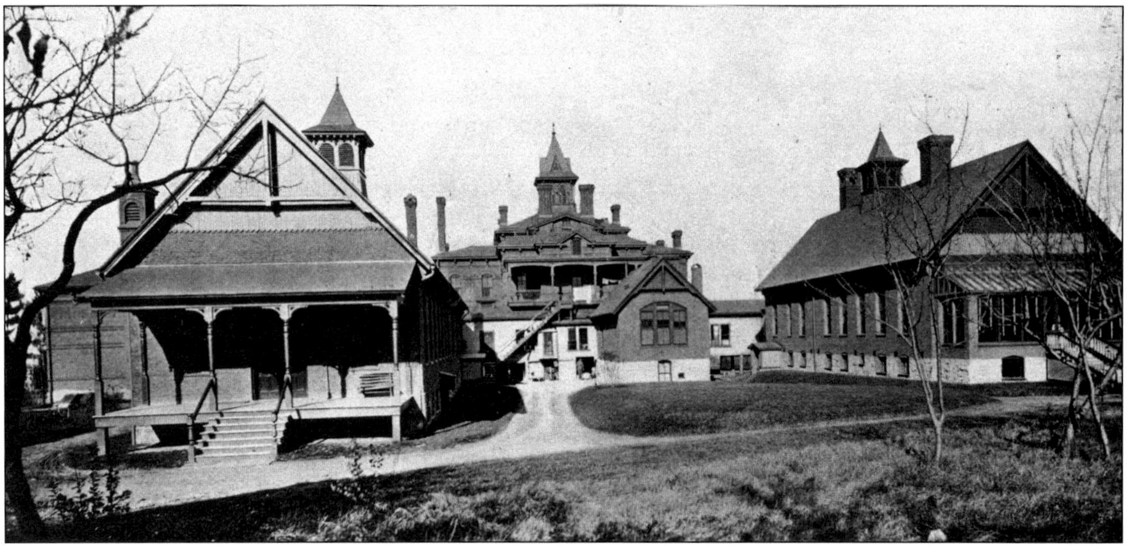

FIGURE 7-7.
Rear View of the Fletcher House in 1902. The Men's Pavilion is on the left, and the Children's ward (pavilion) is on the right.

ment in a well appointed hospital, and second, because the automobile has solved the question of transportation to the hospital. Comparatively few people with any serious ailment, especially if it is surgical, are unwilling to go to a hospital, and the cases are few that cannot be easily and safely transported in an automobile."[32]

The Mary Fletcher Hospital kept pace. Individual pavilions (the legacy of Florence Nightingale and UVM chief of surgery Crosby) were built between 1887 and 1907 for female, male, children, and private patients. An entire surgical building containing operating rooms and improved teaching facilities replaced the original amphitheater. A children's ward arrived several years later, along with other physical plant improvements. Electricity supplanted gaslight as gowns, masks, and rubber gloves became a regular part of the operating room scene.

Although the world's first x-rays were taken in 1895, several years elapsed before their medical potential was realized. The Mary Fletcher Hospital obtained its first Roentgen device in 1905. By 1919, there was an entire X-Ray Department with its own wing. The Fanny Allen Hospital, working with a smaller budget, had to wait until 1914 before it could afford a machine. This equipment, so long in coming to the Fanny Allen Hospital, was "donated" to the Bishop DeGoesbriand Hospital when it opened in 1924. The Fanny Allen replaced it with a portable unit made by the Wappler Electric Company. This contraption, distinctly inferior to the equipment at either of the Burlington hospitals, was not replaced until 1943.[33]

Other scientific advances were in store in the early twentieth century. During World War I, English chemist Henry Dakin, working in concert with French surgeon Alexis Carrel, devised a solution of sodium hypochlorite buffered with sodium bicarbonate that destroyed superficial infection without harming underlying tissue. In 1922, Canadian orthopedic surgeon Frederick Banting isolated pancreatic extracts that lowered blood sugar levels. Within months, insulin was in widespread use. And in 1928, Alexander Flemming, a Scottish surgical student, turned bacteriologist, discovered the antibacterial properties of the penicillium fungus (although a clinically useful version was not available until 1945.) All three "surgeons" were eventually awarded the Nobel Prize.[34]

The Nascent Department Grows

The Department of Surgery was also starting to take shape. Technically in place since the 1880s, it had never amounted to more than a professor and an assistant until Wheeler became chairman. There were other surgeons in Burlington, but they were not to be found on the UVM faculty lists. Staff members were progressively added throughout Wheeler's tenure as encouraged by educational reform. By the time Allen became chief, there were multiple assistant professors and clinical instructors under his supervision. As before, though, the faculty consisted mainly of UVM graduates with little to no experience outside of Burlington.

Clifford Atherton Pease (1874-1931) was one of the Department's first instructors. A member of the medical class of 1899, he spent a year as a "house surgeon" at the Mary Fletcher. After additional training in Vienna, he became instructor in neurology and clinical assistant to Henry Tinkham.[35] Active in public affairs, he was appointed State Director of the Bureau of Medical Service during World War I.[36] He was an attending surgeon at the three local hospitals and wrote a number of medical articles. Among these were works on traumatic Fourth of July injuries, applications of local anesthesia, and an overview of Dakin and Carrel's breakthroughs in wound care.[37,38,39] Pease was promoted to assistant professor of clinical surgery following Tinkham's death in 1925 — a position he held until his own demise.[40]

Another assistant from this era was George Millar Sabin (1873-1958.) Sabin studied alongside Pease and graduated a year later. After practicing in his native town of Malone, New York, he returned to Burlington in 1903. That same year, he was hired as instructor in gynecology and clinical surgery — an unusual combination now, but typical in the days before specialization.[41] He authored a few papers, including a case report of a double ectopic pregnancy, however he was not as prolific as his colleagues.[42] Leaving gynecology behind, he advanced to assistant professor of clinical surgery in 1926, and then full professor of clinical surgery within ten years.[43,44] Sabin is credited with introducing spinal anesthesia to Burlington.[45]

Allen's successor, Albert G Mackay, operating with Sabin during the 1940s, recalled that, "he had only one good eye. Therefore, he had no depth perception, and in my years of assisting him, when he put a scissors down to cut a suture or tissue, he would rely on me to push the scissors ... to the proper depth."[46] Sabin compensated somehow, as he managed to keep working until he was 81 years old.[47]

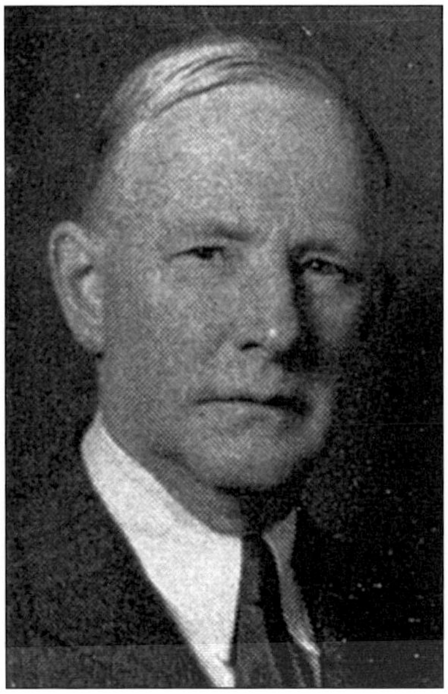

Sabin was also known for his willingness to review unfavorable outcomes. "Clinically honest" to a fault, he discussed fractures that "all had a failure of union or some kind of complication" during teaching conferences. Even though "He was told that it might not be a good idea to advertise his mistakes," Sabin "was thinking only of telling

FIGURE 7-8. George Sabin was an active faculty member for a record 51 years. He retired in 1954 at age 81.

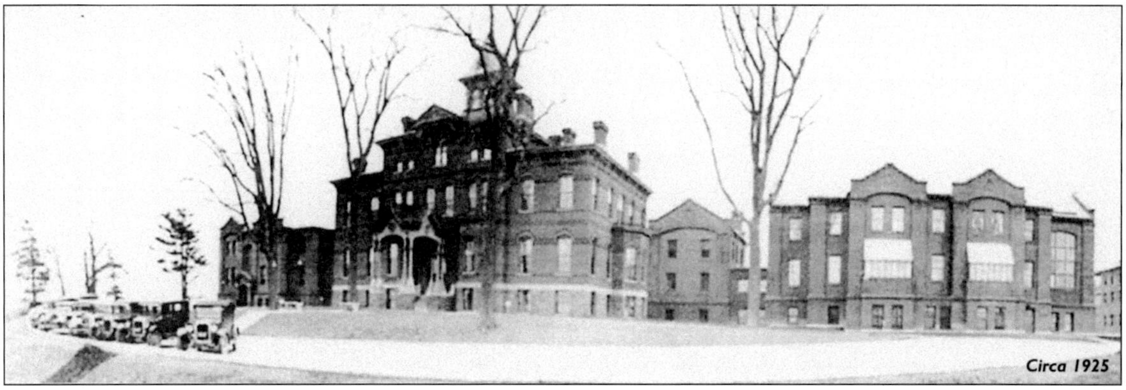

FIGURE 7-9.
Mary Fletcher Hospital in 1925 with private pavilion on left, Fletcher House, and the operating suite on far right.

people what not to do as well as what to do in the practice of surgery."[48] This philosophy was certainly ahead of its time. It foreshadowed the rise of the Department's morbidity and mortality conferences in the 1960s.

Vermont's First Colo-Rectal Specialist

Benjamin Dyer Adams (1878-1961) almost matched Sabin's longevity. Upon completing his medical studies at UVM in 1908, he too became an instructor in surgery.[49] A stint in the Army during the First World War gave him a taste of conditions beyond his home state.[50] He returned to Burlington, resumed his position at the College, and became director of the free dispensary shortly thereafter. He continued in these roles until the mid-1930s when he was named assistant professor.[51, 52] A fixture at the Mary Fletcher Hospital, he eventually retired in 1956 at the age of 78.[53]

Adams, like his fellow faculty members, performed a wide range of operations. Ultimately, however, he became a self-taught specialist in proctology. Although "he was not fond of teaching nor very good at it," he was a popular instructor.[54] This was in spite of the fact that he also possessed a bit of a temper, according to a former student:

> "I recall one day when Dr. Benjamin Adams, a very reputable Burlington surgeon, had scheduled an appendectomy at the Mary Fletcher Hospital. Just before "scrubbing" for surgery he was reminded that he could not proceed until the "second opinion" was obtained. With no one else available, he asked Dr. "Mickey" McMahon, a nose and throat specialist to contribute.
>
> Dr. McMahon was a personable, humorous physician, highly skilled in his own field. To oblige Dr. Adams he visited the patient, touched his abdomen, explained the "second opinion" rule, and scribbled, "I concur" on his chart. Then, looking for a little mischief, he came down to the O.R. dressing room and spoke loudly to Dr. Adams, who was answering a call of nature.
>
> "I can't sign the chart," he declared. "I see no signs of appendicitis." Out of the restroom emerged Dr. Adams, holding his pants in one hand and angrily shouting, "Where in hell did you go to medical school?" Dr. McMahon began to laugh — and all was well."[55]

One of his younger colleagues noted that "One was never sure how radical or minor an operative procedure would be when Ben Adams got started." The colleague was, "in the uncomfortable position of being a younger chief over these older men." At one point, "I had to warn [Adams] that unless he was willing to allow a patient to be transfused who had lost enough blood to go into shock, he would have to stand the consequences." In the end, "the patient who had suffered the massive hemorrhage made an uncomplicated recovery and Ben, with a wide smile said to me: you see, I was right all the time."[56]

Another staff member recalled a similar encounter with the proctologist:

"There was a patient coughing post-operatively following a gastrectomy. I said, 'If she keeps coughing she's going to open up her wound. We've got to stop this cough.' Ben looked at me and said, 'Codeine, codeine is what she needs.' I said, 'How much?' Adams replied, 'One-half grain [30 mg — a substantial dose] whenever she coughs.' I said, 'Dr. Ben, you'll kill her!' He said, 'Nonsense, she'll stop coughing first.' So I wrote in the orders, 'One-half grain codeine every time she coughs.' Sure enough, she was alive the next morning."[57]

Adams did have a softer side, though, and often came back to the hospital late at night to visit his patients. He told his students, "Make rounds after dark. Your patients will appreciate it, they'll love you." A lifelong bachelor, he eventually amassed a substantial fortune. It was said that, "for his time, he was very well to do."[58] In fact, before he retired, he had already made a sizable contribution to the recently organized Shelburne Museum.[59] His last charitable act was to make a similar donation to the hospital, which was used to build a dormitory for the house-staff.[60]

Adams, characteristically, was parsimonious to the end. Stooped over a table, his shoulders wrapped in a blanket, he was about to sign the transaction papers when "he suddenly dropped the pen and said, 'I don't think I'll go through with this.' His sister Helen, sitting right behind him, said, 'Now brother Ben — you've got all these nice people here, of course you're going to go through with it.' She put the fountain pen in his hand and he signed his name 'B.D. Adams,' and drew $250,000 out of his estate for the hospital."[61]

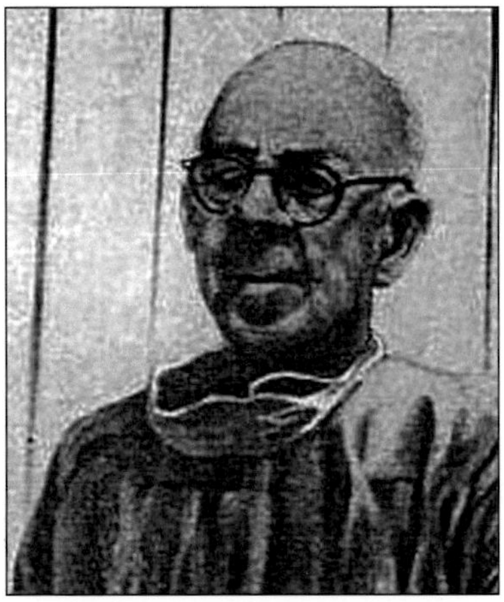

The "Benjamin D. Adams Residential House," completed in 1961, contained multiple bedrooms, a lounge, a library, and a squash court. Connected to the back of the original hospital, it provided an overnight home for generations of interns and residents. Unfortunately, it was deemed out-of-date within forty years. Having outlived its usefulness, it was torn down in 2003 to make room for further hospital expansion.[62]

FIGURE 7-10. Benjamin Adams, benefactor of the "Adams Residential House", which was razed in 2003.

The AMA Returns

Although the College of Medicine was able to maintain its Class A rating in 1926, it did not fare as well following the AMA inspection of 1935. The school's enrollment, funding, and endowment had dramatically declined during the Great Depression. As a result, it was unable to keep up with the Council on Medical Education's expectations. Inspectors found that there were only a dozen or so full-time faculty members. Several pre-clinical professors were not fully trained in their fields of expertise. Junior medical students continued to attend too many lectures. And, as always, students did not spend enough time in the hospitals. The medical class had "no actual contact with patients except in connection with amphitheatre clinics in medicine and surgery."[63]

Most damning of all, the curriculum had not significantly changed since Tinkham's death. His successor had created an extramural service in which students shadowed rural practioners for a month and then staffed State institutions for another three months. The preceptor rotation was intended to provide further clinical experience, but it was unregulated and unsupervised, and thus of dubious value.[64] The inspectors concluded that despite the "fine spirit of idealism and a desire to serve on the part of the faculty, there would seem to be little reason for the attempt to carry on medical education under the (present) conditions."[65]

In light of its "manifest deficiencies," the College was placed on probation in December of 1935. "If UVM is not in compliance by June of 1939, the Council will at that time review the standing of your school and take appropriate action."[66]

A month later, the Association of American Medical Colleges reached a similar conclusion. Citing the poor credentials of incoming students, the diminished number of pre-clinical instructors, and the continued reliance on non-resident clinical professors, it too placed the College on probation. The secretary of the AAMC recommended that the staff, the didactics, and the clinics needed to be completely revamped "if the school is to proceed along the lines of an acceptable medical school."[67]

The faculty bypassed the Dean and took matters into their own hands, just as they had done when Tinkham's predecessor (Dean A.P. Grinnell) was ousted in 1898. A reorganization committee was established and funds were appropriated from the university. The committee then set to work fulfilling the AMA and AAMC's requirements. The anatomy, chemistry, and physiology departments were substantially overhauled. The Department of Obstetrics and Gynecology was divided into two sections following Patrick McSweeney's retirement. Several new departments were created, including ones in Ophthalmology, and Otolaryngology/Rhinology.[68]

Didactic teaching, which had been "overemphasized, and not always well done," was restructured.[69] Clinical utilization of the Fanny Allen and Bishop DeGoesbriand Hospitals was increased. In addition, students and faculty were given access to Fort Ethan Allen's 158-bed military hospital in Colchester, just down the road from the Fanny Allen.[70]

Mackay described patients checking in to the Mary Fletcher for the winter where they had a warm bed and good food for $2.50/day. They gave material for the medical students and kept their residence as patients, by constantly having an elevated temperature. This they achieved by warming their thermometers on the radiator when not observed.[71]

In accordance with AMA guidelines, the school also obtained control of the medical staff at its primary teaching hospital. After a series of tense negotiations, the chairmen of the College's clinical departments became chiefs of service at the Mary Fletcher Hospital.[72] The Department of Surgery (which had not had a full professor of *clinical* surgery since 1924) named long-time assistant professor George Sabin to the position.[73]

The school's Committee on Reorganization made sure that all future faculty were adequately trained and credentialed. In 1937, it declared that, "No person shall be appointed as professor or as head of a department in any subject until he shall have ... received certification by the American Board of that subject."[74] It was a timely move, as the American Surgical Association, in cooperation with the A.M.A., the A.C.S., and the New England Surgical Society (among others) had formed the American Board of Surgery earlier the same year. Every surgeon already belonging to one of the aforementioned societies became a member of the founders' group, along with all full, associate, and assistant professors of surgery at each Class A medical school.[75] Allen, Sabin, and Adams were automatically admitted, despite UVM's probationary status.

The Department's junior faculty, however, were not professors and had not practiced the minimum fifteen years required for exemption from board examination. Each of the instructors had finished a one-year internship, which had included some surgical training. A few had spent an extra year in pathology or anatomy, but none had completed a formal surgical residency. This meant they did not automatically become board certified. As a result, UVM provided several staff members with leaves of absence and financial aid to undergo proper postgraduate training at metropolitan medical centers.[76] In surgery this included Mackay and Gladstone. The investment paid off for within a decade both former "residents" became full professors and chiefs of service at UVM's hospitals.

The reorganization committee kept the AMA and AAMC fully informed of its activities. Upon reinspection by the AAMC in December of 1938, it was noted that the school had "done a splendid piece of work" and had "gone far to rehabilitate the college."[77] Hardy A. Kemp was hired as Dean, specific teaching appointments were made at the Catholic hospitals, and additional clinical opportunities were created for upperclassmen over the next few years.[78]

The AAMC finally rescinded UVM's probationary status in November of 1940 following yet another evaluation. The AMA, however, did not follow suit, as "conditions made it uncertain when such inspection would be made."[79] With war looming on the horizon, the Association had decided to overlook the College's few remaining discrepancies — at least for the time being. It was a short-lived reprieve for the members of the Department of Surgery, who soon found themselves facing new challenges at home and on the front.

PART IV

WAR AND ITS AFTERMATH

1942-1969

CHAPTER 8

World War II Brings Dramatic Changes to Surgery at UVM

A number of new surgical instructors were appointed at UVM's teaching hospitals. Several of them went on to receive additional specialized training.

World War II led to an acceleration of the training program in order to produce more doctors, but the effort was negatively impacted by the faculty's enlistment into the military service.

Albert G. Mackay assumed the chair of surgery and occupied it for the next 27 years. The AMA removed the school from its list of institutions placed on probation just as the troops returned home.

The Mary Fletcher Hospital Sits Proudly on the Hill

The Mary Fletcher Hospital treated 5,708 inpatients during 1940. An observer noted that its surgeons wore white gowns, caps, and aprons while they worked in the hospital's "modern operating rooms." Their attire was "folded up and baked for half an hour by live steam in special ovens." It came out "terribly wrinkled," but sterile, as "the entire process of sterilization would be robbed of its one aim were clothes ironed." Instruments were treated in a similar fashion, and the "old-fashioned sea sponges" gave way to sterilized disposable gauze pads. Surgeons scrubbed their hands "with brush, soap and water for ten or fifteen minutes, and then soaked them in a special disinfecting solution and then pulled on sterile rubber gloves."[1]

The observer added that, in contrast to Mary Fletcher's day, "Surgery is also now a matter of highly trained teamwork in which some six to eight persons take part. There is the head surgeon, first and second assistant surgeons, the anesthetist, and three or four nurses: one to keep the instruments in order and readiness, another to handle the sponges and account for every one, and the supervising nurse to stand by and see that every co-ordinated movement is technically and aseptically correct."[2]

Some of this surgery was performed in the hospital's latest addition, today's Shepardson South building. The four-story structure — connected to the old Surgical Wing by means of a service corridor and an ambulance entrance — contained the X-Ray division, the Diagnostic Clinic, a minor surgery room, and post-surgical wards. It also featured such long-discarded amenities as patient solariums and open rooftop decks. Upon its completion in 1942, the overall number of beds and bassinets at the Mary Fletcher increased from 150 to 230.³

The Department Continues to Grow

Advances in surgical technology, improvements in hospital care, and demands of ever-increasing educational standards prompted further expansion of the Department as well. Over time, Lyman Allen, George Sabin, and Ben Adams were joined by another batch of attending surgeons. Prominent among them were Vermonters Walford Rees, Keith Truax, and A.G. Mackay.

Walford Tupper Rees (1900-1965) graduated from the College of the Medicine in 1925 and became an instructor in anatomy the following year. Although he was named assistant professor of surgery at the young age of 28, Rees never compromised his surgical integrity and

FIGURE 8-1. (L to R) A.G. Mackay, E.L. Amidon, and Keith Truax in 1932.

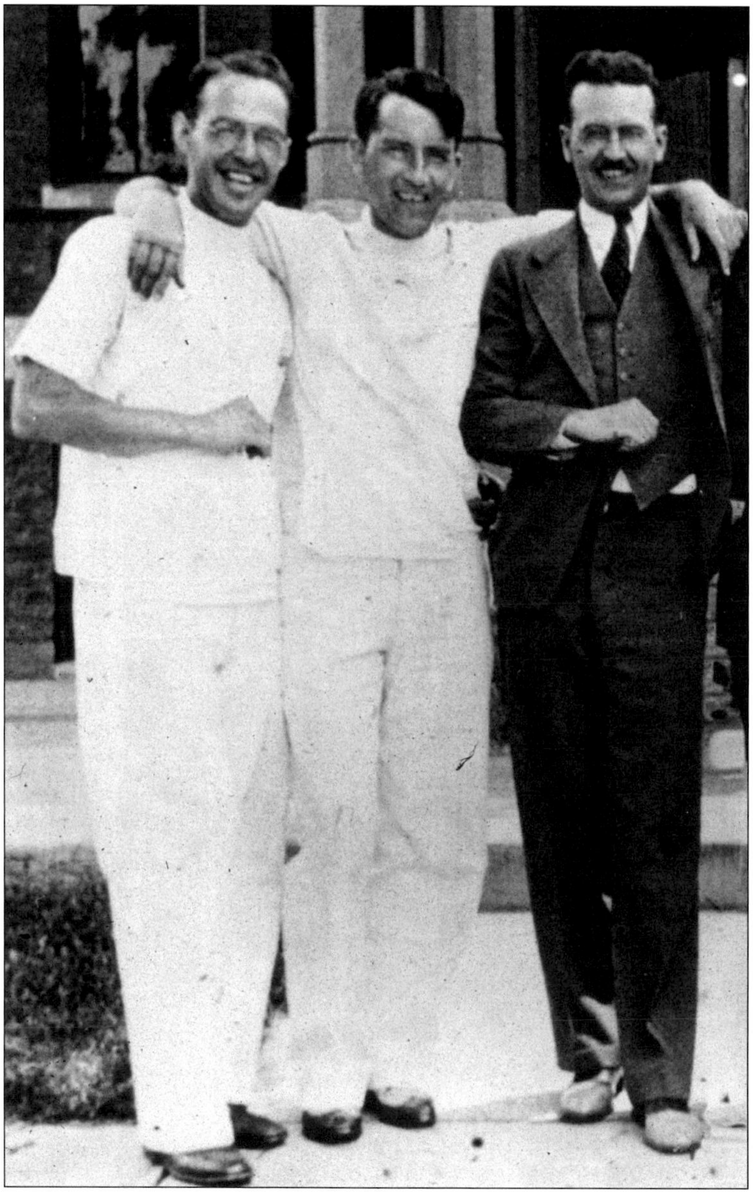

principles.[4] He was ready to criticize poor management or incorrect treatment even if it meant others would not refer him cases. An author of papers on cutaneous anthrax and goiter treatment, he was later "remembered for his undying effort to maintain surgical excellence in the community and on the faculty."[5, 6, 7]

Keith F. Truax (1904-1974), a member of the UVM medical class of 1932, joined the staff after his graduation as an instructor in anatomy, then pathology, and finally surgery. He also studied in Vienna in 1936. This wasn't satisfactory so he returned to take a course in NYC.[8] He was promoted to assistant professor of surgery in 1938, and soon succeeded Ben Adams as director of the free dispensary. Ten years later, he advanced to the position of associate professor of surgery.[9] Like his contemporaries, his interest was not primarily in academia, but he did write an article on burn treatment.[10] He also reported a rare case of prepubertal malignant melanoma, which is still cited in reviews of the subject.[11]

From 1948-1965, Truax and his hunting partners, Raymond Towne (a general practitioner from Cambridge) and Robert Hunziker (a UVM Radiologist), had a wonderful annual party in May at their West Bolton hunting camp, "Buckfever Lodge." All of the surgical house-staff and attendings were invited, and huge amounts of steak and beer were served. The event was held on a Saturday night. Since half of the house-staff were on-call, the party was repeated for their benefit the following Saturday when they were off duty. This also accommodated the attendings' call schedule.

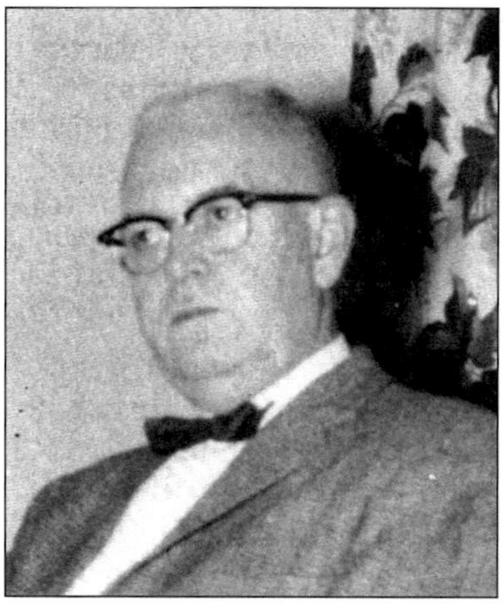

FIGURE 8-2. Keith Truax shortly before undergoing aortic aneurysm repair in Texas by Michael DeBakey.

Truax was an otherwise unpretentious and enigmatic surgeon. He rarely said anything in the Operating Room or the Doctor's Lounge, either before or after surgery. He was an avid photographer, and for years took the official house-staff photographs for the hospital.

UVM's Future Chief of Surgery Grows Up in Peacham, Vermont

Albert George Mackay (1907-1978), the youngest member of this group, ended up playing the largest role. "A.G." was born in Peacham, Vermont, the hometown of former chairman Edward Elisha Phelps. His father, Albert James Mackay, was an accomplished physician and politician.[12] The elder Mackay died from a ruptured appendix, having delayed his own hospitalization to care for another patient. The event — which occurred when A.G. was only nine years old — undoubtedly influenced the youngster's subsequent choice of career.[13, 14]

The family was left in financial straits, but A.G. and his siblings managed to support each other through school. Mackay earned a B.S. in 1928 and an MD in 1932 through UVM's seven-year combined course program. He served in the R.O.T.C. and spent several of his summers in Carlisle, Pennsylvania on active Army duty. Mackay felt that his fellow medical students set an example for the rest of the University since they were the only group on campus that wore jackets and dressed professionally.[15]

During his junior year, Mackay took an eight-week "internship" at northeastern Massachusetts' Beverly Hospital under UVM alumnus (and founder of the New England

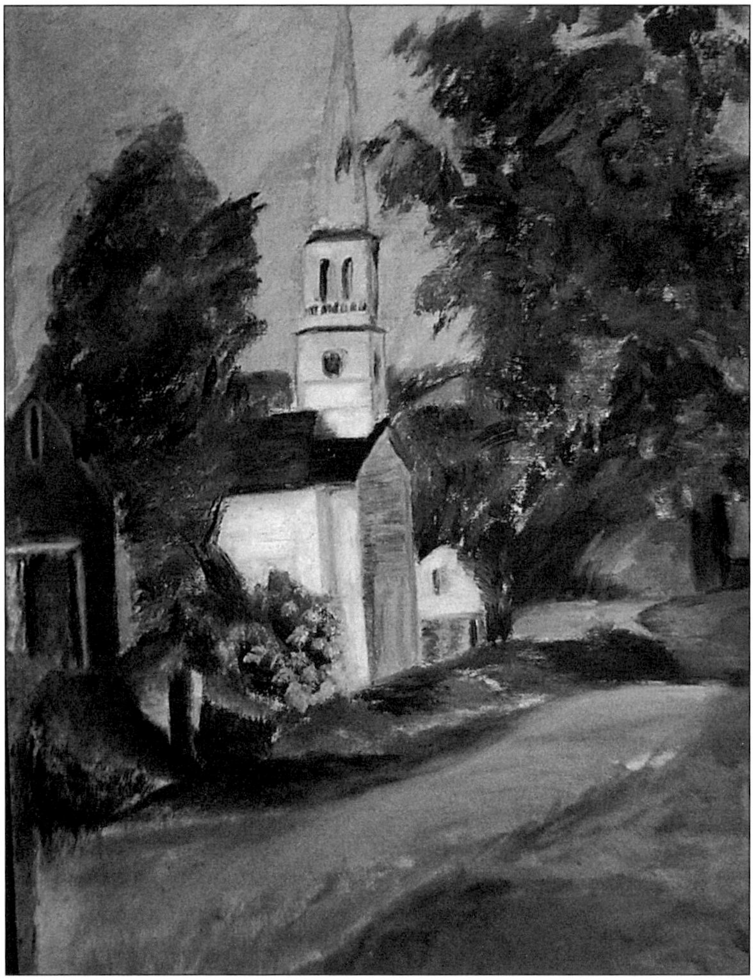

FIGURE 8-3. Main Street and the Congregational Church in Peacham, VT as depicted by the author's (DBP) grandmother, Stella Bogart. Peacham was the childhood home of Edward Phelps and A.G. Mackay, and the retirement home of neurosurgeon Henry Schmidek.

Surgical Society) Peer P. Johnson. After graduating, Mackay stayed on at the Mary Fletcher Hospital for his formal internship. He followed this with another year of training alongside the hospital's sole medical resident, E.L. Amidon. Thus, Mackay's claim to be the "first surgical resident at the Mary Fletcher" was true, even though the hospital didn't actually have a surgical residency.[16]

E. Hiram Buttles, UVM's legendary professor of pathology, kept a close eye on the hospital's "first surgical resident." Buttles berated A.G. during his internship for omitting to do a history and physical on a patient with diphtheria (the attending physician had ordered him to avoid the contagious case.) Later, after Mackay had become an instructor in anatomy, pathology, and anesthesia at the College of Medicine, Buttles scolded him again for being seven minutes late to work (the home delivery of his son had delayed him.) When Mackay complained to fellow instructor Brad Soule about the tongue-lashings, he was told, "Al, I think you've got it made! If Hi Buttles thinks enough of any intern or student to spend twenty minutes giving you the devil, he certainly thinks you have the potential for something great in the future, and I think you are to be complimented."[17]

Mackay was sent to Boston City Hospital in 1937 for a "two-year house officership in surgery."[18, 19] While there, he fulfilled his board certification requirements and furthered his anesthesiology training. He also spent time at Temple University in Philadelphia with Chevalier L. Jackson, the country's foremost endoscopist, and at the University of

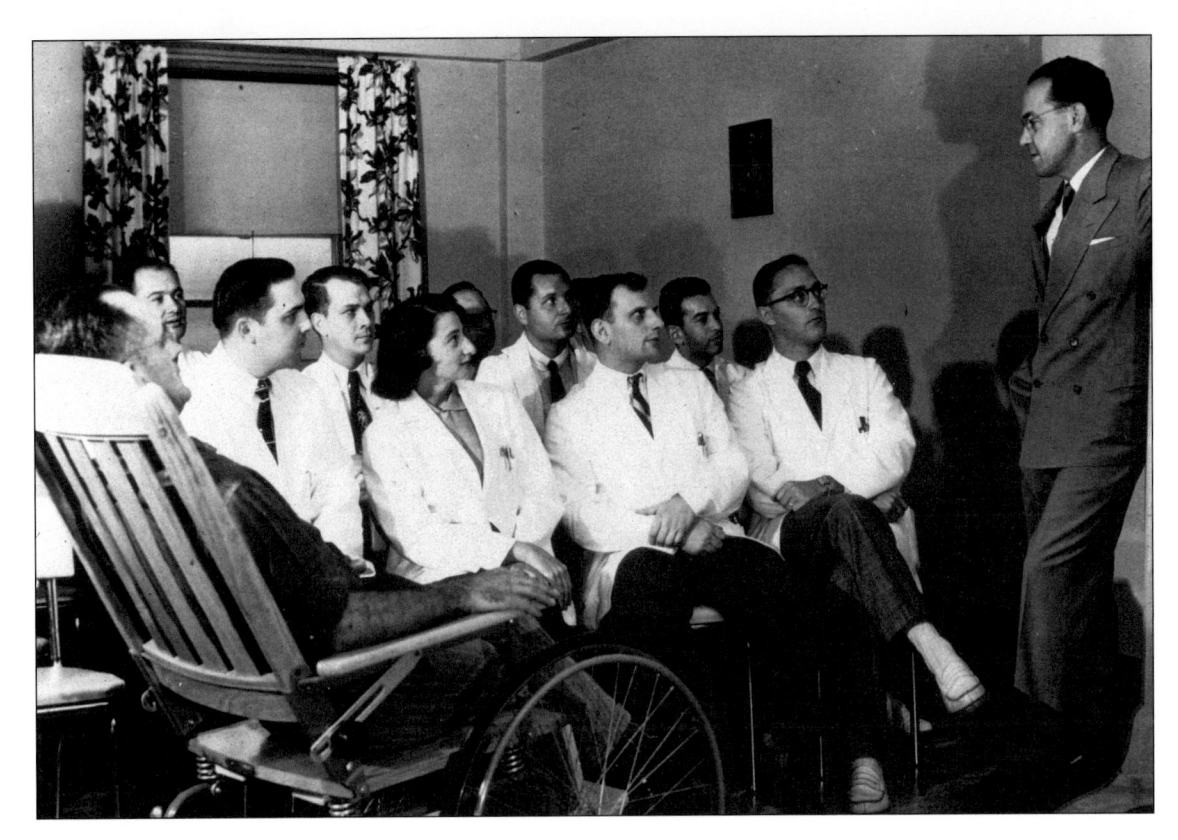

FIGURE 8-4.
A.G. Mackay teaching clean-cut medical students around 1940.

Chicago.[20, 21] Upon his return to Burlington, Mackay accepted an instructorship in surgery. He was rapidly promoted to assistant professor, and then associate professor over the next several years.[22]

Mackay later recalled treating a patient with an unusual problem during his early days as a surgical instructor:

> "She was admitted for consultation and the nurses on the floor called me to say that they had given Martha an enema, and when she went to return it in the bathroom, she collapsed on the floor because both legs were too weak to hold her body. That afternoon Dr. Amidon and I went to work on her and made an exotic diagnosis of a perispinal epidural abscess. We could not sell this diagnosis to anyone else, although she had a history of having had a pustule on the face when she was at Johnson Teachers College, which had been squeezed by her roommate about seven to ten days previously. We could not get [radiologist] Brad Soule to undertake the process of doing a myelogram and so, in the evening, we took the patient down to x-ray and did a myelogram on our own. In the course of doing this we did not encounter any pus, but we did show a deformity of the spinal column. I reported to Dr. Rees that I thought we needed to invade the spine and explore for a possible abscess, which would be fatal if not drained that night. Dr. Rees differed with me and felt that I was wrong in the diagnosis, but he refused to take the position that I could not operate. I called on Dr. Sabin and one other man, possibly Dr. Allen, and got no further help. We decided to take the bull by the horns and go ahead with the exploration.

The stage was set, and the old small amphitheatre that held only ten students on a stand-up rack was in place, and just as I was ready to make the incision, Dr. Rees walked in to watch this procedure. We went down through skin and deep fascia and approached the spinal column, and everything was quiet. There was not a word said in the room. Dr. Amidon stood off on one side, our medical visitor, waiting to see the outcome. About five minutes later, as I approached the epidural space, to my great relief, thick creamy pus welled up into the wound and we established drainage. There was a sigh of relief from the nurses. Dr. Rees got down from the stand and went out, and from that point on he and I never discussed the case again — nor did I ever understand how he felt about the procedure. At any rate, I grew several years older in one night at that time." [23]

The Catholic Hospitals' First Surgical Instructors

A number of teaching appointments were also made at the Catholic hospitals during this era. Among the most notable newcomers were surgeons Louis Thabault, Albert Crandall, and Arthur Gladstone. Their longevity at their respective institutions (each practiced well into the 1970s) was only matched by their service to the greater Burlington community. The trio, born within two years and twenty miles of one another, followed somewhat divergent paths before settling into their roles at the University.

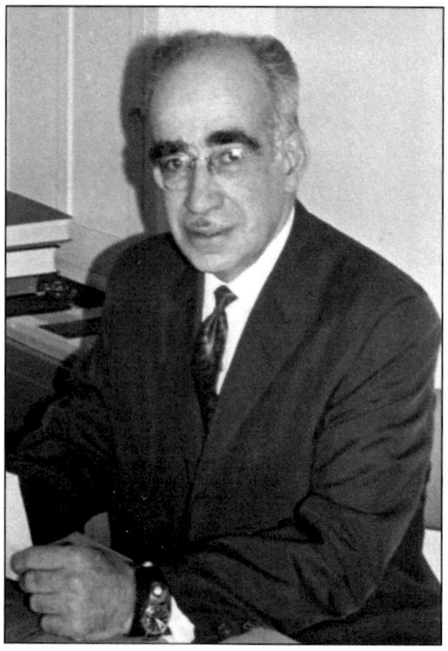

FIGURE 8-5.
Louis Thabault held reign at the Fanny Allen Hospital until his 1974 death.

Louis George Thabault (1907-1974), like the majority of Winooski's residents, was of French Canadian descent. He followed in the footsteps of his father, George J. Thabault, one of the first general practioners at the Fanny Allen Hospital and a beloved physician in his own right. Dr. "Louie" graduated from UVM in 1927 and the College of Medicine in 1930. He interned at St. Mary's Hospital in Philadelphia before moving across the city for a surgical residency at Frankford Hospital. Despite the uncertain political climate overseas, he was able to study in Vienna, Austria from 1936 to 1937. Initially a family physician, he later specialized in general surgery.[24]

In addition to being an instructor in surgery, Thabault was also asked to chair the Fanny Allen's new surgical student program. This proved to be an excellent choice, as "he was an avid reader of surgical books and journals." Thabault was a stickler for proper procedure. His widow recalled that, "Certain cases that he had, he would worry about them and be up at four in the morning reading surgical books. Then he would come back and say the operation went fine and he did exactly what he learned."[25]

Albert James Crandall (1909-1982) joined Thabault at the Fanny Allen in 1939. A native of nearby Huntington, he had also attended UVM for both his undergraduate and medical education. After obtaining his MD in 1933, he completed an internship at St. Francis Hospital in Hartford, Connecticut, and then became an assistant to Burlington community surgeon B.J.A. Bombard. He later completed post-graduate courses at the New York

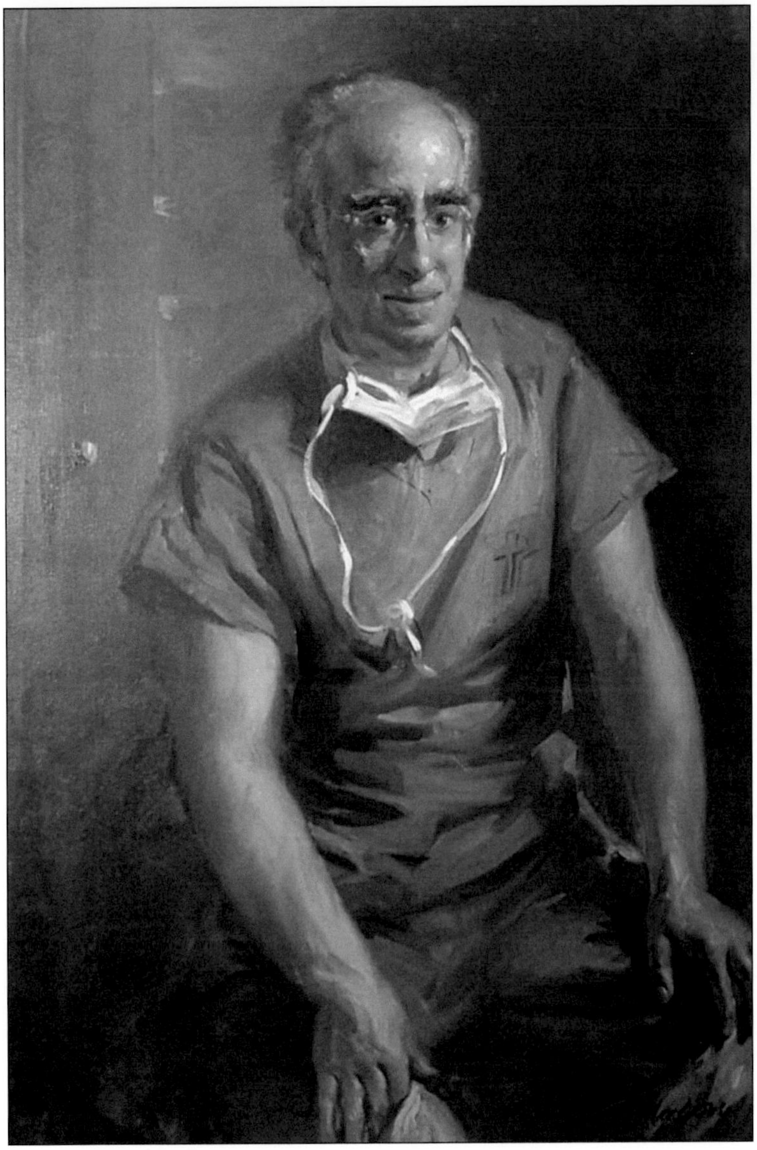

FIGURE 8-6. Louis Thabault benevolently watches over all who enter the FAH operating suite. This portrait was commissioned by Dr. Louis' staff and friends under the organization of surgical resident F.S. Cramer and painted by Frank Mason of NYC. Thabault, for some reason, never cared for the picture.

Polyclinic Hospital and Medical School and, with Thabault, studied at the University of Vienna in Austria.[26, 27]

Crandall became an instructor in clinical surgery upon his arrival at the Fanny. He was "a gentleman and highly competent surgeon; an outstanding physician who frequently remained day and night at the bedside of his patients who were seriously ill; a surgeon who had many appealing offers at prestigious medical centers; held in high esteem by all, for he was an unassuming individual."[28]

A Jewish Surgical Leader for the Catholic Hospital in Town

Arthur A. Gladstone (1907-1980) occupied the position of Chief of Surgery across town at the Bishop DeGoesbriand Hospital. A denizen of Burlington's small Jewish community, he too had obtained Bachelor's and Medical degrees from UVM, ending his studies in 1931. He finished an internship at the Maine General Hospital, but had to put his career on hold after developing a severe corneal inflammation. His sight was restored a few months later after tak-

Chapter Eight: World War II Brings Dramatic Changes to Surgery at UVM ing a self-prescribed course of the newly invented sulfa drugs. Following an extended recovery, he returned to Burlington in 1933. He became associated with Ben Adams, and a short time later, decided to pursue additional training in proctology.[29]

Gladstone spent some time at the Massachusetts General Hospital's Outpatient Department with noted proctologist Parker Hayden. This experience led to a surgical residency at the University of Pennsylvania, followed by another year of residency at Mt. Sinai Hospital. Gladstone later wrote that:

> *"When I returned to Burlington in 1939, I knew more about diseases of these areas than anyone else on the scene. I had worked long and intensively at Mt. Sinai with Dr. Burrill Crohn who first described ileitis, an inflammatory process involving bowel segments, which became known as Crohn's disease. Dr. Crohn was a medical doctor, but the surgery developed for the management and cure of this disease was due to the efforts of Drs. Garlock, Ginzberg, and Oppenheimer. Because of my experience with these men, I was assigned this subject for teaching at the University of Vermont's College of Medicine."*[30]

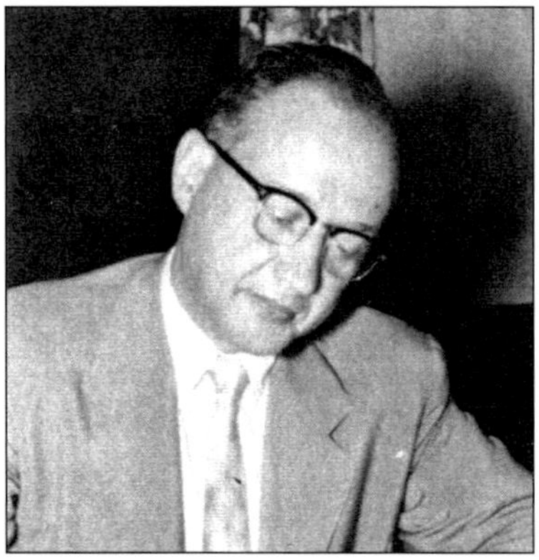

FIGURE 8-7. Arthur Gladstone, Burlington's first trained colorectal specialist, in 1939.

Gladstone although Chief at the DeGoesbriand, only held the postion of an assistant surgeon at the Mary Fletcher Hospital. Thabault and Crandall, on the other hand, had appointments and operating privileges at the Bishop DeGoesbriand but not at the Mary Fletcher. Although cooperation between the hospitals remained difficult for the next twenty years, the College and its students benefited from exposure to these three well-trained individuals. In fact, surgery at the Fanny Allen was a popular rotation for the senior medical students, since the hospital did not have interns.

Medical Education is Accelerated as a Part of the War Effort

The Department's expansion efforts, unfortunately, had to be reformulated because of the outbreak of World War II. Once American involvement became a foregone conclusion, the College of Medicine took action. Recognizing the pressing need for military physicians, it received permission from the Board of Trustees to increase its annual class size from 32 to 36. The academic program was accelerated (at the expense of vacations) so that four years of academic work were completed in just three. At the same time, every able-bodied class member was inducted into the short-lived Army Specialized Training Program (ASTP).[31, 32]

The ASTP served to generate a steady supply of military engineers, diplomats, and eventually, physicians. The program proved mutually beneficial to all involved over its two-year existence. The military ended up with a stream of well-trained personnel, the College of Medicine had full classes throughout its nine-month academic "year", the University's administrators avoided dealing with local draft boards, and the students got to be in the Service without having to immediately ship off to war.[33]

ASTP participants were assigned the rank of private, first class. The designation was accompanied by a stipend of $80 a month — a sum that greatly improved the status of many a medical student. The privates attended surgical lectures, learned practical surgery, and observed clinical cases as before. War-specific topics, such as tropical medicine and military science, were also covered. Students continued their education as long as they maintained their grades. Those who failed to do so were reclassified and ordered into other duties as enlisted men.[34]

The young doctors-in-training were enlisted for the duration of the war plus six months. Upon graduation, they were technically discharged from the military into an internship, but were then reactivated as first lieutenants six months later. A few forestalled the inevitable assignment as general medical officers by completing a residency, but within another nine months they too were in uniform and overseas.[35]

Mackay Mans the Home Front Virtually Alone

Although medical school instructors were exempted from military service, twenty-five members of the College of Medicine's faculty went to war. Of those, eight were from the Department of Surgery.[36] Rees, a commander in the Navy, was sent to the Philadelphia Naval Hospital.[37] Anesthesiologist John Abajian, Jr. was named Consultant Anesthetist to Patton's Third Army where he made history through his innovative use of regional anesthesia.[38] Urologist Winthrop Flagg, orthopaedist Maurice Bellerose, and clinical surgeon Ralph Cudlipp also entered the Army's Medical Corp.[39]

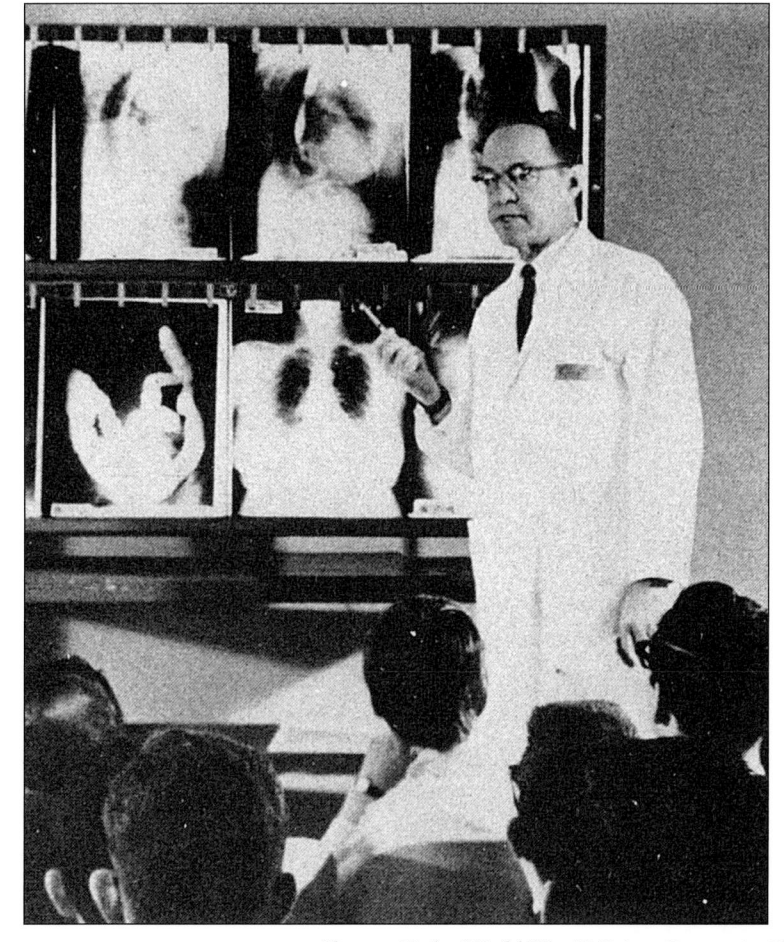

FIGURE 8-8.
A.G. Mackay holds forth at a 1965 conference.

Mackay, left alone in Burlington, recalled that, "Our staff was decimated. Our anesthetists were all gone. Our urologists were all gone. Our orthopedic surgeons were all gone. It was difficult to tell where one could serve best." Mackay eventually concluded that, despite his own Reserve Officers Training Corps (ROTC) background, he "could probably serve better here than there" by training as many additional medical officers as possible.[40]

"We were turning out forty-eight to fifty new first lieutenants every nine months, teaching around the clock, and having one graduation in June, the next one in March, and the next one in December. We found many of the students in those years were more interested in not getting sent overseas than they were in getting a real medical education. It was a question of whether we had real draft dodgers or real enthusiastic undergraduate medical students." Mackay had to evaluate his charges carefully, as *"it was an unpatriotic thing to flunk a medical student who could serve his country as a medical officer in those years."*[41]

Mobilization for the war effort led to a shortage of surgeons throughout Vermont. Mackay pitched in where he could. "I remember living in my straight-eight cylinder Oldsmobile, with a windshield wiper on the back and on the front, and lecturing in Burlington then operating in St. Johnsbury, nailing a hip on the X-Ray table in Barre, and then going to Porter Hospital that night for two more cases, and sleeping in different towns. All the while we were trying to keep a semblance of an active teaching curriculum going, and help the outlying hospitals."[42]

Gladstone's eyesight kept him out of the military and, initially, it looked as though a chronic condition might disqualify Thabault for service too. Dr. "Louie" had sustained a lower extremity fracture as a child that was subsequently treated with a long leg cast. The injury healed satisfactorily, but left him with a foreshortened limb and a limp. The Army, however, conveniently overlooked this problem. Thabault was commissioned as a major in due course, and was eventually stationed at military hospitals in England, Wales, and France.[43]

Crandall's Unit was the Forerunner of the MASH

Crandall joined the Army in June of 1942, and became the leader of the first airborne surgical team to land by gliders in France behind enemy lines the night before the European invasion of France in 1944. The team again saw action at Operation Market Garden in Holland. Crandall was taken prisoner during the earliest days of the Battle of the Bulge, and was marched 80 kilometers through the snow into western Germany. Crandall, eventually escaped, and, fifty pounds lighter and suffering from beriberi, was sent back to Washington, D.C. for interrogation and rehabilitation.[44, 45] A detailed description of these events is contained in Crandall's report to the Surgeon General.[46] (see Chapter 29)

Deemed too valuable to discharge, but too fragile to send back to the front, Crandall was reassigned stateside. He reviewed airborne medical operations and developed units for future use in Washington, and then worked at Missouri's O'Reilly General Hospital until the war's end. He completed a general surgery refresher course at the New York Academy of Medicine in early 1946, before finally returning to the Fanny Allen.[47] By that time though, Thabault — a loved, respected, and powerful leader — had acquired the major portion of the surgical practice.

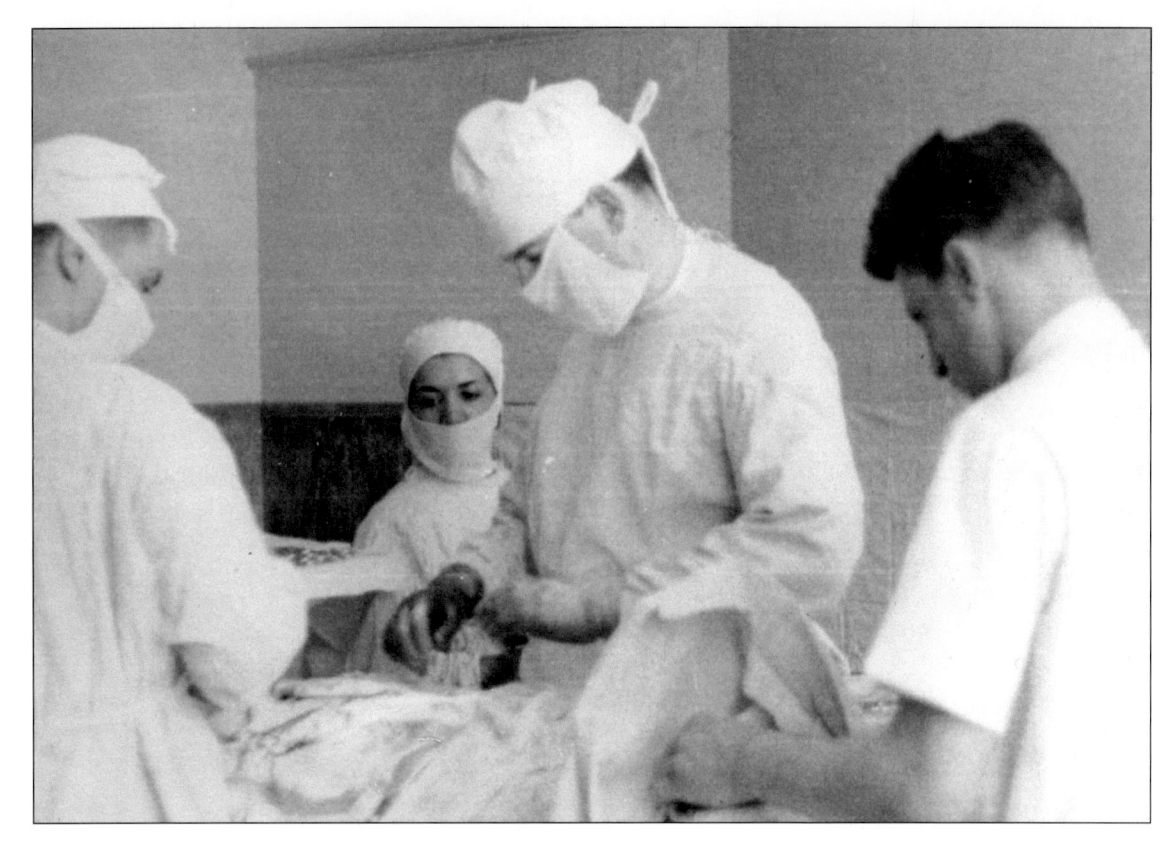

FIGURE 8-9.
Albert Crandall operating at the FAH around 1939.

A private and humble man, Crandall resumed his low-key role as a surgical instructor. Few people beyond his immediate family ever knew the details of his war experiences.

A.G. Mackay is Appointed Chief of Surgery

Wartime faculty shortages, larger class sizes, and accelerated training programs took their toll on the Department of Surgery. Salaries, supplies, and morale steadily declined. John Brooks Wheeler, the Department's patriarch, died in May of 1942 at the age of 89. That fall, in the midst of the turmoil, 70 year-old Lyman Allen stepped down as chair in favor of a surgeon from the next generation. It was thus under these less than ideal circumstances that A.G. Mackay — still five years removed from his 40th birthday — became the next chairman of surgery.[48] Remarkably, he was able to overcome these difficulties and remain chief for the next twenty-seven years.

Although Mackay's training and skills were impeccable, his relative youth worked against him. "I had come back from Boston, in '39, as full time instructor in surgery, but soon found that I had little cooperation from the other older surgeons on the faculty." As a result, "Dean Jenne and I agreed within a year's time that I should, in fact, be part time — and would have better cooperation from the other men." The war, however, postponed this plan. Interestingly, "On Rees' return (from the Navy) I asked him if he would care to take over the Department of Surgery as administrative officer, which he graciously declined, but he did enthusiastically accept my suggestion of a professorship of clinical surgery."[49]

Mackay then turned to other problems. The College of Medicine, on probation since 1935, was long overdue for a re-evaluation. The AAMC had lifted its probation of UVM in 1939, but the AMA had temporarily avoided the issue. The AMA finally conducted its inspection in mid-1944. Although a few deficiencies remained, the inspectors recognized that the overall clinical situation had, "appreciably strengthened since the last survey."[50] The College's probationary status was lifted, with the understanding that the school hire more full-time clinical instructors, improve its leadership, and engage in meaningful research.[51]

An executive committee was established to advise the Dean and act as an intermediary with the faculty. Among those appointed were Amidon, Buttles, and Mackay. The group's role was never properly clarified, and it was often left out of major policy making discussions. After Mackay successfully lobbied to increase the College's budget by $40,000, he resigned from the committee (which disbanded shortly thereafter) realizing that the school's management was changing.[52]

Although successful at campus politics, Mackay's real forté was in the area of clinical practice. Born left-handed, he skillfully developed his right hand in order to perform surgery, becoming notably ambidextrous in the process. Even today, when people are asked about Mackay, the first thing they mention is that he was ambidextrous. Perhaps his colleagues were jealous of this ability. Or perhaps he made a point of emphasizing this trait himself. Either way, Mackay was a technically excellent surgeon. He was also an adept endoscopist, and was called upon throughout his career to use his skills with rigid bronchoscopy and esophagoscopy.

Mackay performed large numbers of hiatal hernia repairs, partial gastrectomies, bile duct reconstructions, and thyroidectomies. He was often asked to bail out fellow surgeons during complicated biliary procedures. At one point, he presented a personal series of 63 subtotal gastrectomies. This was the standard operative treatment for peptic ulcer disease during the 1940s and '50s before being replaced by vagotomy and pyloroplasty.[53] Given the effectiveness of current anti-ulcer medications, it is unlikely that any surgeon will ever perform as many gastrectomies for ulcers again.

The Chairman closed his post-thyoidectomy incisions with "Michelle" clips, which resulted in cosmetically excellent scars. The clips everted the skin edges in a manner similar to today's staples. This was long before disposable skin closure devices came into vogue. Residents were uniformly skeptical that acceptable cosmesis would result, but Mackay proudly showed them his late results. The dressing consisted of a folded green operating room towel, which was held to adhesive tape on the chest wall by towel clips. This set-up allowed quick access to the neck wound in case of airway obstruction. Mackay insisted upon keeping scalpels ready at the bedside for emergency tracheotomies. No one ever remembers having to do one, but a co-worker does recall having to reopen such an incision in an elevator once.[54]

Mackay's influence was felt beyond the hospital as well. He always drove a slightly older than current model Oldsmobile. When asked why he didn't have a Cadillac (which he could obviously afford), he replied that his patients might think he was becoming affluent by overcharging them! Following his example, none of the Department's surgeons ever drove a Cadillac or other luxury car during Mackay's tenure.[55] Of course, more than a few attending surgeons have clandestinely owned high end and vintage vehicles (including a DeLorean) since then.

Mackay remembered that before the war, "A usual operating day was probably from 8:30 to 12:30 with doctor's offices from 1:00 to 3:00, and those like Dr. Rees and Townsend (urologist) that used to enjoy playing golf, or Dr. Pike (internist), would be on the golf course by 3:00 p.m., doing their full day's work and yet being free to enjoy sports on almost every afternoon aside from having an emergency." The tempo of practice increased markedly, however, as former medical officers returned home. "We have never returned to the lackadaisical, easygoing, low key days of practice such as Drs. Sabin, Townsend, and Rees used to enjoy in surgery as a matter of habit at the time of our internship."[56]

Part of the reason for this lay in the increased efficiency and demands for speed learned in military service. But the faster pace of surgical life was also due to a number of other factors. The war, for all its destruction, had led to several medical breakthroughs. As more effective antibiotics and less noxious anesthetics found their way into hospitals across the country, patient confidence increased, and more people sought medical care. At the same time, the population steadily grew as soldiers returned home. Increased demand once again led to openings for more surgeons.

Jay Keller is the First to Return From the War

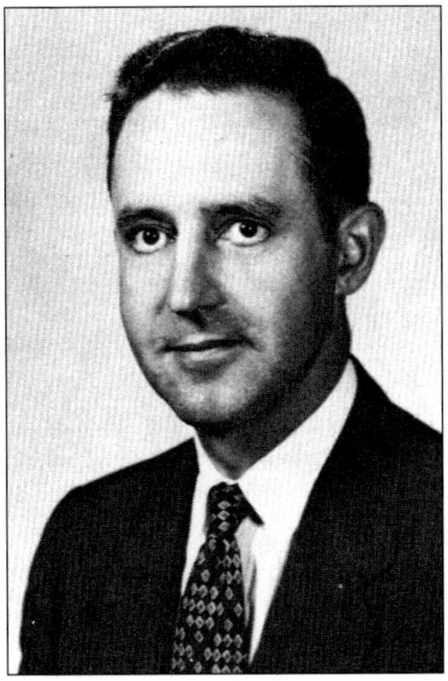

Jay Edgar Keller (1914-) had graduated from the College of Medicine in 1940. As a senior medical student, he had been freed from his clinical responsibilities at five o'clock each afternoon. Keller made the most of this situation by going to the Fanny Allen Hospital every night where, in return for room and board, he assisted with surgery. He took a one-year rotating internship in Newark, New Jersey following graduation, and then established a general practice in Essex Junction. Keller credits his medical experiences at Vermont, and his surgical rotations during internship with preparing him well for his military experience. He was able to perform surgical procedures, such as appendectomies and cholecystectomies when he started practice in the army, based on his experiences and training.[57]

FIGURE 8-10. Jay Keller returned to Burlington from WWII prematurely because of a severe asthmatic attack. He was still going strong at age 95 in 2009.

Keller joined the army in 1942 (as did most of his peers), but was discharged less than two years later after suffering a severe asthmatic attack. Upon his return to Vermont, he found that gasoline rationing had severely curtailed civilian travel. Many patients, in fact, were unable to make routine office visits. Keller though, as a physician, had unlimited access to fuel. As a result, he ended up making a considerable number of wartime house calls.[58] He recalls that he would drive his car as far as road conditions would allow in the winter, and be met by a sleigh, pulled by horses, to take him the rest of the way to the patient's house. He also remembers renting a frozen food locker in Essex, because in those days some patients would pay their bills by bringing in "chickens or strawberries or other such foods."[59]

By the late 1940s, Burlington's hospitals had begun to grant privileges based on board certification. Knowing that he could not meet the new requirements (despite having performed a significant amount of surgery in just three years), Keller saved up for a surgical residency at New York University's Bellevue Hospital. In order to cut costs, his family remained behind in Vermont. His wife worked for the Vermont Transit Company, so was able to hop a free bus ride to NYC when he was able to get away from his busy schedule. Although the GI Bill helped some, Keller didn't have enough money for his chief year. Short on cash, he came back to Burlington and started a surgical practice. Mackay acted as his preceptor for a year, which satisfied the American Board of Surgery's eligibility requirements at that time.[60]

Most surgical practices were concentrated at the Mary Fletcher Hospital. Nevertheless, the Bishop DeGoesbriand Hospital's Emergency Department was nearly as busy as its neighbor on the hill. Shortly after joining the DeGoesbriand's staff, Keller was assigned responsibility for surgical emergencies. He took call every night for three years, until three new surgeons signed on allowing for the creation of a rotating schedule.[61]

When George Sabin and Benjamin Adams joined Lyman Allen as emeriti professors (although both practiced to some degree into the 1950s), the Department once again needed to recruit and expand. This time around, however, growth mandated the incorporation of subspecialties and the conduction of scientific research if UVM was to remain competitive with New England's other medical centers. Mackay assessed the situation accordingly, and called in the troops.

CHAPTER 9

The Need for Growth

Military-trained surgeons returned to Vermont at the end of World War II and subdivided into areas of practice based upon areas of special competence or interest. UVM established a broad-based surgical residency program suited to the needs of its rural population.

The Department of Surgery started a remarkably successful research division thanks to the inventiveness and determination of one man, Julius H. Jacobson, II. UVM became the world leader in microvascular surgery shortly thereafter.

The Department's quest for academic recognition stalled after Jacobson's departure. His successors tried, but were unable to maintain UVM's former status. That step was left for a new chairman to take.

Sub-Specialization Follows World War II

Consumer goods and services were in great demand at the end of the Second World War, and health care was no exception. In response, the Mary Fletcher Hospital expanded again, doubling its footprint through the construction of the Medical Center Building in 1952. The

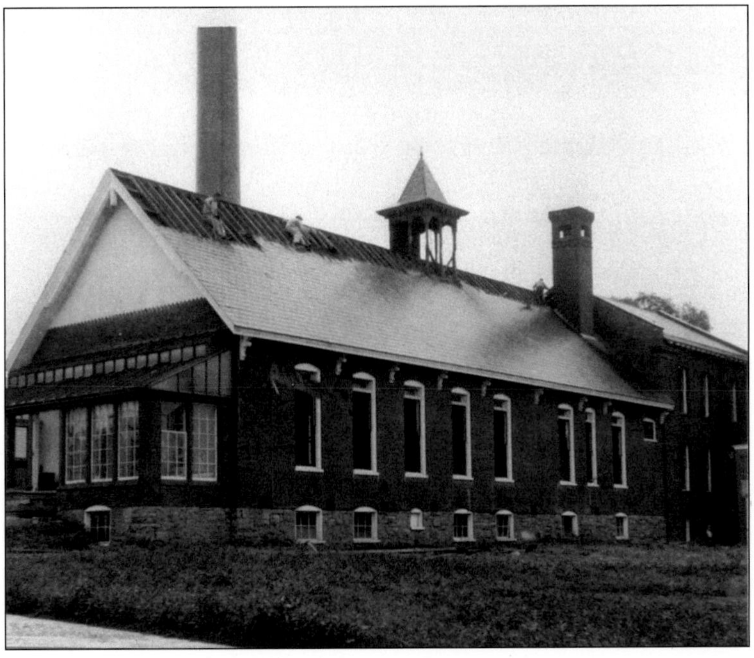

FIGURE 9-1.
The Men's Pavilion was demolished in 1958 to make way for the Adams House.

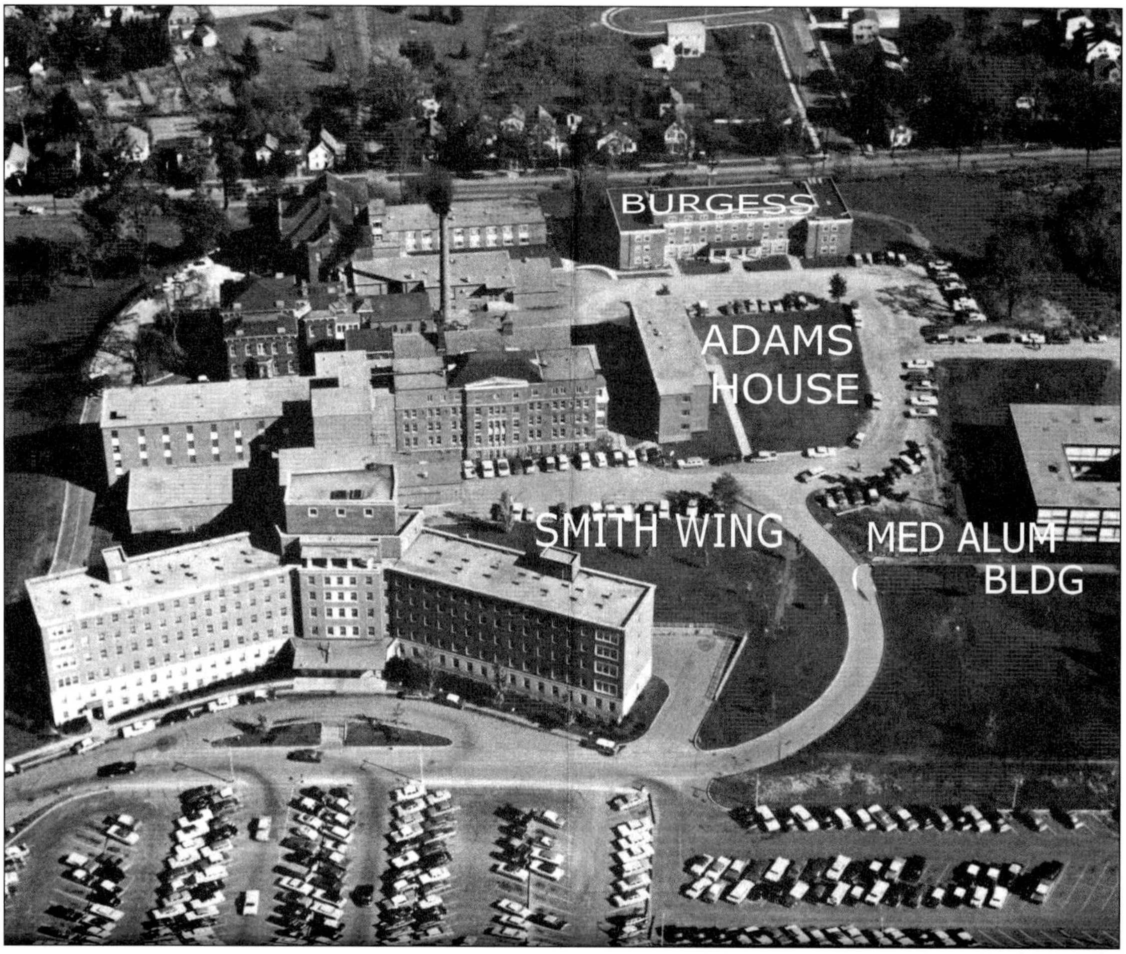

FIGURE 9-2.
The Mary Fletcher Hospital in 1962. The lower 2 stories of the front of the Smith (right) and Patrick (left) Buildings were painted white to resemble angel's wings according to John Mazuzan. The Durfee surgical clinic was in the lower level of Patrick and had its own entrance. The operating rooms were on Smith 2. The ICU was on the second floor of the center section. The Adams Residential House was adjacent to the Burgess Nursing residence. The Medical Alumni Building housed Surgical Research, Pathology, and Psychiatry.

main Operating Rooms (housed in the old Surgical Pavilion since 1908) were relocated to the second floor of the new building's Smith wing, one flight up from the facility's state-of-the-art Emergency Room, and adjacent to the laboratory and blood bank.[1]

The Urology Department had had one professor of Urology since the early 1900's. The only change seen was the succession of "Tod" Townsend by Winthrop Maillot Flagg, and his designation as Chief of Urology. In 1945 Urology was designated as a division of the Department of Surgery. The Department of Ophthalmology, Otology, and Rhinology had a part time chief E.G. Twitchell who was appointed in 1937 supplanting his "special lecturer status."[2] By 1945 this was formally listed as a Department with John Cunningham as chief. Otology (renamed Otolaryngology) and Rhinology was a division of that department with Rufus Morrow as division chief.[3] John Abajian had been hired in December, 1939 as Chief of Anesthesia, so perhaps that was the first designated division of the Department of Surgery. Orthopaedics comprised of professors, and visiting and special professors, formally became a division of the Department of Surgery in 1946 with the appointment of John Bell as chief.

Other specialties overseen by visiting professors now required more formal designation. Thus, Raymond Madiford Peardon Donaghy, a combat-tested alumnus of the College of

Medicine, was hired to launch the Division of Neurosurgery. Donald Barker Miller came on board to start a Cardiothoracic Surgery Division, Bernard B. Barney began an "unofficial" Division of Plastic Surgery. Later, R. W. Paul Mellish initiated the Division of Pediatric Surgery.[4]

The Department had established a surgical residency in 1946 keeping in step with the increasing subspecialization of surgery. (There were two residents in 1942, then none until 1946.) Interns and residents worked hard, but gained a huge amount of experience in the process. UVM's program trained one or two residents at a time for one to three years in an apprentice-style manner.

UVM's First Residents Stay On as Attending Surgeons

Most of the school's post-war surgical staff had served in the military. Several returned to town afterwards and became the nucleus of the Department's expanding staff. Arnold Caccavo joined Jay Keller, and former students Nolan Cain and Bill Shea, to practice mainly at the Bishop DeGoesbriand under chief Arthur Gladstone. Carleton Haines, Bishop McGill, and Gordon Page went into practice at the Mary Fletcher alongside A.G. Mackay, Walford Rees, and Keith Truax.

F. Arnold Caccavo (1917-) obtained his MD from UVM in 1943. He finished an internship at Salem Hospital the following year, and then fulfilled his Army obligation. Although initially successful at parlaying his military experience into an operative practice, he eventually succumbed to the necessity of Board certification. After completing his residency in 1954, he went into partnership with Gladstone. Caccavo worked part-time for General Electric in Burlington and, years later, he left his clinical duties for a full time position with General Electric.[5, 6]

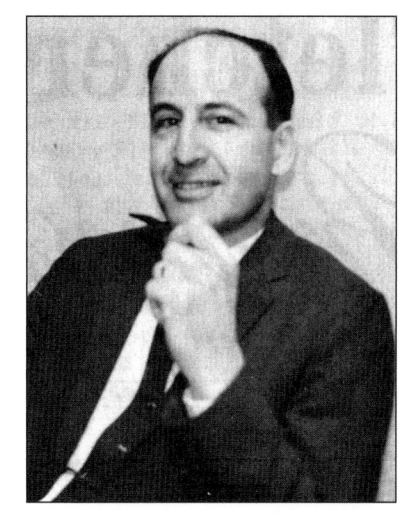

FIGURE 9-3. Arnold Caccavo in 1960. He had partnered with Gladstone before leaving to be General Electric's Burlington company physician.

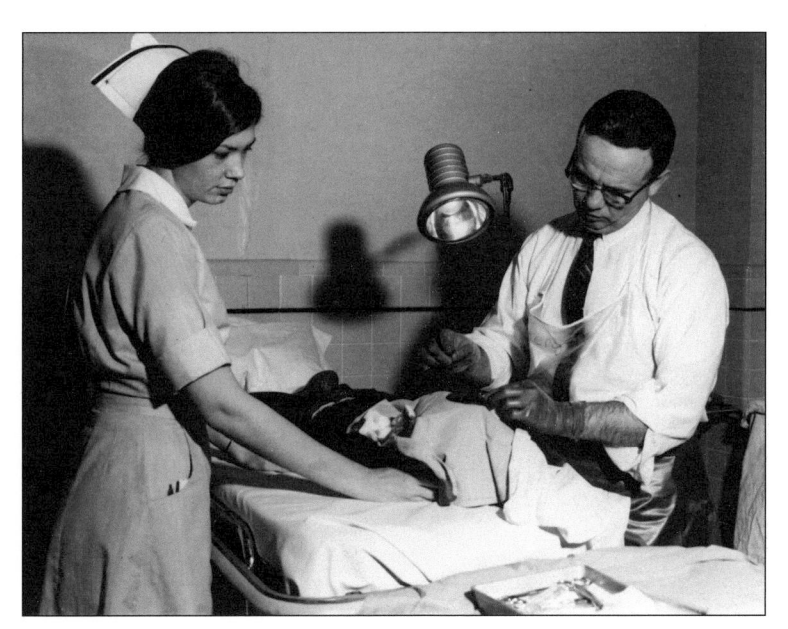

FIGURE 9-4. Nolan Cain performing minor surgery at the DeGoesbriand in 1967.

R. Nolan Cain (1921-1997), a student in the accelerated program, graduated from the College of Medicine in 1945, three calendar years after matriculating. Assigned to a Veteran's Hospital in Maine, he underwent two years of surgical training, which were then supplemented by a rotating internship in New York City. Cain completed fellowships in Pathology and Anesthesiology at UVM before spending another two years in surgical residency at a Boston Veteran's Affairs Hospital. He eventually started his Burlington practice in 1953.[7]

FIGURE 9-5.
William Shea, Cain and Keller's partner, in 1964.

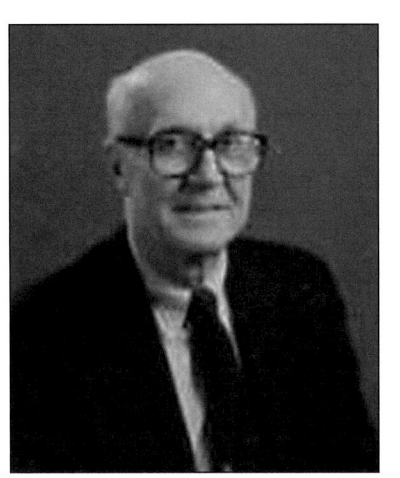

William Ireland Shea's (1914-1989) adoptive mother told him that he was going to attend Holy Cross College, that he was going to be a doctor, and that he was going to UVM for medical school. Shea did as he was told, ultimately graduating from the College of Medicine alongside Jay Keller in 1940. He completed a rotating internship at the DeGoesbriand at a time when the Hospital's non-surgical house staff were segregated from their counterparts at the Mary Fletcher — even though both programs were affiliated with UVM. This was followed by a combined Internal Medicine and Anesthesiology residency at St. Vincent's Hospital in Manhattan. Shea then joined the Army, where he worked as a surgeon in the South Pacific for three years.[8, 9]

Returning to Burlington, Shea found that despite his military experience, more training was necessary if he were to remain a practicing surgeon. He spent a year as a resident at UVM. Louis Thabault then came to his rescue, financing a three-year residency at Boston City Hospital in General Surgery, Orthopedics, and Hand Surgery. This was followed by an additional year in Vascular Surgery at Columbia-Presbyterian Hospital. Shea finally joined forces with Keller and Cain at the DeGoesbriand in 1953. The trio practiced together for twenty years before becoming members of Surgical Associates in 1973.[10]

Shea conducted a noteworthy outreach program in Ticonderoga, New York. Although the town's small hospital had an ample surgical population, it did not have a trained surgeon. Shea made the hour-and-a-half drive almost every week to operate. He often took a resident with him, which not only added to the house staff's surgical caseload, but also gave them a sample of life at a rural community hospital.[11]

FIGURE 9-6.
Carleton Haines in 1954 after becoming director of the Division of Cancer Control for the Vermont Department of Health.

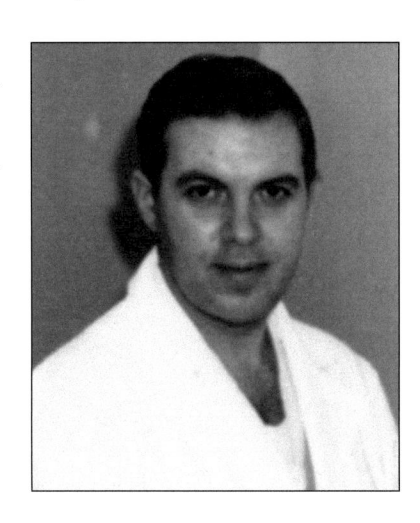

Carleton R. Haines (1919-), a member of the first group of accelerated training program students, received his MD in 1943 — just two years after obtaining his UVM undergraduate degree. Once he had completed his nine-month internship, the Army sent him to the Philippines, and then to Japan. Haines returned to UVM at the end of the war, where he finished his surgical residency in 1950. He then spent two years as a fellow at the Massachusetts General Hospital, followed by another year at the nearby Pondville State Cancer Hospital.[12, 13]

Haines became an instructor in the Department of Surgery, advancing to the level of Associate Professor by the time of his 1989 retirement. Building on his fellowship training, he became the school's first Tumor Clinic and Registry director. He was also the Director of the Division of Cancer Control for the Vermont Department of Health from 1954-1974 (a position that originally paid all of $3000 a year). Haines was an adept, reliable surgeon and teacher who, in addition to running a number of clinical trials, trained the surgical residents in cancer surgery of the head and neck. His patience in this endeavor was legendary.[14]

J. Bishop McGill (1922-2007), of the College of Medicine's class of 1946, came to practice solo at the end of his UVM surgical residency and after a stint with the Air Force in Spokane, Washington, in a community where others had formed alliances. Originally from St. Johnsbury, Vermont, he lived one block from the Mary Fletcher, when not on the lake, or at his home in Stowe. He championed two innovations that have since become standards-of-care: outpatient surgery and the repair of inguinal hernias under local anesthesia. McGill also brought the Shouldice herniorrhaphy to Burlington at a time when the town's surgeons were still doing either Bassini or McVay repairs. His fervent use of infection-resistant wire sutures was before his time, and his compulsive attention to detail was a model for the residents. Despite their dislike for tying knots with wire, the residents learned the technique.[15, 16]

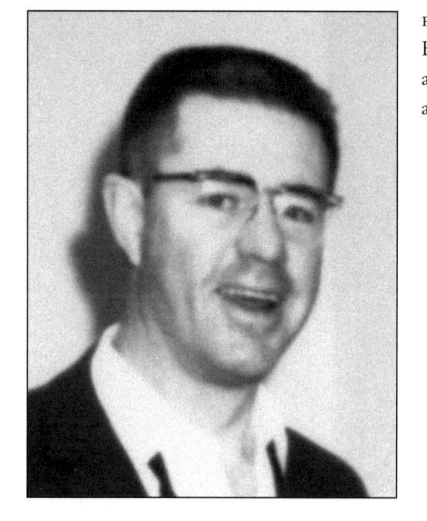

FIGURE 9-7. Bishop McGill was always a fitness advocate.

McGill devoted a great deal of time to community service and physical fitness. He was a past-president of the Vermont Medical Society, the medical director of the Mount Mansfield Ski Patrol, and a co-founder of the sports-oriented Northeast Medical Association. McGill, like nationally known thoracic surgeon Richard H. Overholt, tried to convince those around him that smoking was bad for their health. McGill stood alone when he preached this though, as his fellow UVM surgeons were usually the worst offenders. He always found a resident or an attending to pick on; sometimes he actually grabbed packs of cigarettes, crushed them, and threw them away.[17]

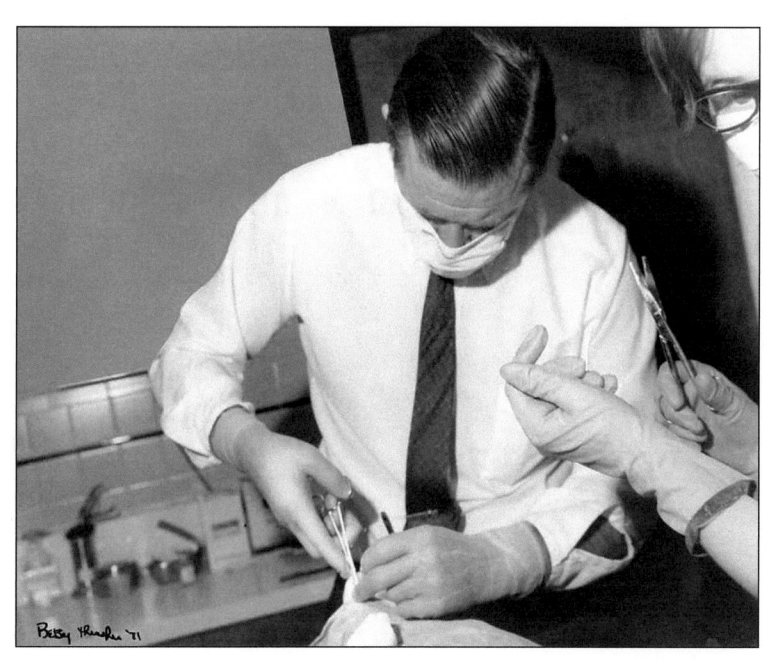

FIGURE 9-8. McGill was a meticulous surgeon with a delicate technique. No one wore gowns in the 1950s for minor surgery.

Chapter Nine: The Need for Growth 123

Page Becomes the Second-Busiest Surgeon in Burlington

H. Gordon Page (1918-) was born and raised on a farm in Groton, Vermont. He enrolled at the Vermont Agricultural College (a technically distinct, but intimately connected entity within UVM), "thinking I was signing up for premed. I got in with a bunch of Ag Boys — and went right along with the agricultural class."[18]

Page remained interested in medicine as an undergraduate, however, and applied for a job as a surgical orderly. Ushered into Dean Brown's office (Room 311 of the original Mary Fletcher Hospital), he patiently waited for his interview. Brown entered the room and, without saying a word, sat down behind his desk and proceeded to open a large pile of mail. When he had finished, he glanced over at Page and said, "So, you are looking for a job as an orderly?" Page replied, "Yes sir." Brown, without any further comment, responded, "We don't have any openings."[19] And so ended the interview.

After graduation, Page spent the summer studying organic chemistry and physics in order to meet the College of Medicine's entrance requirements. He also took a job as an Agricultural Agent for Chittenden County. Although it was a good position, it came back to haunt him on his first day of medical school. As soon as Page walked into Hall A, one of his classmates hollered, "Be quiet, here comes that little barn boy. He's probably still got cow's ... on his boots." "Well," remembers Page, "that didn't make opening day any better."[20]

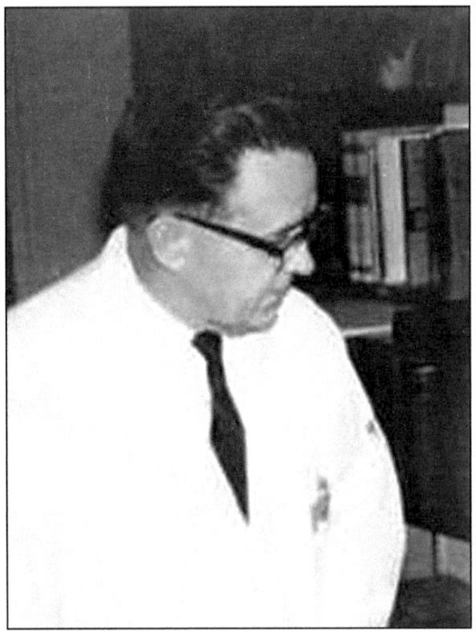

FIGURE 9-9. Page in 1967 when he had a corner on vascular surgery in Vermont.

World War II broke out during the middle of Page's first year of medical school. He was inducted into the "Army Specialized Training Program" as a private, along with the rest of his classmates. Although a sizeable number of faculty members went to war, a few old-timers stayed behind and taught. Page recalls an episode with one of the remaining senior surgeons:

"I scrubbed with this surgeon one Saturday afternoon on a twelve year-old girl with appendicitis. The abdomen was entered and there was this little tiny appendix, which looked perfectly benign and warm. The old doctor would pinch it, scrub it, put a clamp on it, go and look around somewhere else, and come back to it. Finally he took it out. He took this appendix and walked right into the bathroom and flushed it down the toilet. He said, "[pathologist] Hi Buttles will never see this one."[21]

Page graduated from the College of Medicine in 1945. He technically left the Army at this point to take a rotating internship at the Mary Fletcher Hospital. After a few months, he requested a meeting with Mackay's old colleague E.L. Amidon, who had since been promoted to Chief of Medicine and was now in charge of the interns. Page wanted to know why the interns only received $25 a month while the janitor received $25 a week. Amidon answered that "house staff were easy to come by, but a good janitor was hard to find. He looked up and said, 'Page, are you learning anything?' I said, 'Yes, of course. I'm learning every day.' 'Then,'

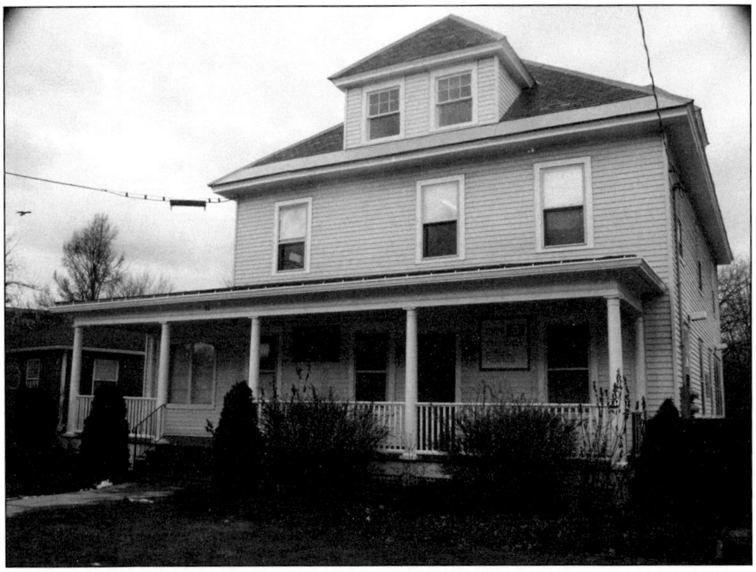

FIGURE 9-10. Mackay and Page turned their Fletcher House faculty offices over to the thoracic surgeons after they purchased this building at 96 Colchester Avenue.

he said, 'if you're learning, you ought to be paying tuition.'"[22]

During this time, Page assisted a gynecologist with a hysterectomy. All was fine until, without warning, the peritoneal cavity began to fill with urine. Page said, "I think the ureter is cut in half!" The attending looked and said, "I believe you are right. I don't remember ever seeing that before — and I'll forget about this soon." The gynecologist then proceeded to put a stent in the bladder, thread the ureter over it, and attach it to the bladder with four sutures. The patient did well, and was never told of the misadventure.[23] Surgical disclosure has certainly changed since then!

Upon finishing his internship, Page was re-inducted into the Army as a first lieutenant to serve at Walter Reed and then in Germany as an orthopedist! While in Germany, he had the opportunity to visit several innovative European surgeons. He was back home by 1948, at which time he started his "official" surgical training at UVM.

Two years later, near the end of his residency, Page received a phone call in the Operating Room. He remembers Jackie Roberts, head O.R. nurse, coming in with the telephone: "Captain Page, 057936?" "Yes" ... "In 24 hours be in Texas. And be prepared to ship to Korea!" Page was one of many doctors mobilized in this manner as the Korean War erupted. After three days of "officer training," he was sent to Japan with a group of doctors. The new arrivals were told that a list would be posted the following day; half of them were going to Korea, the other half were staying in Japan.[24]

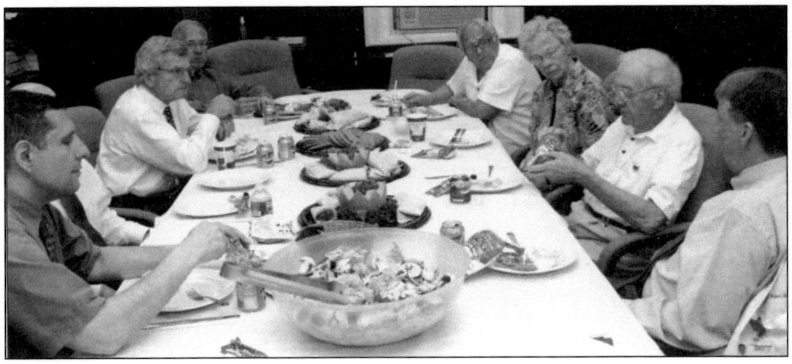

FIGURE 9-11. Surgical Associates' Friday noon luncheons were held in the Given Building, then the UHC conference room, and then the Abrams Library. This later-day luncheon is enjoyed by (left to right): Ricci, Shackford, Vane, Page, Mrs. H. Howe, Harry Howe, and Hebert.

Chapter Nine: The Need for Growth

Page was stationed in Osaka, Japan at a busy 2000 bed hospital where he often operated non-stop for two days at a time:

"We would sometimes get 300 patients and have to triage them into different wards. It was nothing to operate twelve hours on and twelve hours off around the clock for five or six days until we got the rush over. At the time of the Choisin Battle, casualties were arriving with intraperitoneal wounds having their clothes still on and not having been treated for three days. The ability of these young soldiers to withstand such delayed treatment was testimony to their youth and vigor." [25]

He eventually returned to Burlington in 1951, finished his residency, and then went to Massachusetts' Fort Devens for additional Army "pay back time." He attended Thursday afternoon Vascular Surgery rounds at the Massachusetts General Hospital when Robert Linton was Chief Surgeon, and Stanley Crawford was Chief Resident. This later stood Page in good stead when he went to Houston to watch Crawford and his associate Michael DeBakey perform vascular surgery. Resident (and later attending surgeon) Martin Koplewitz joined Page for the Texas one-week mini sabbatical.[26] In the 1950s, apparently all that was required to conduct such surgery (and even title oneself a "vascular surgeon") was to watch another physician operate.

Finally done with the Army, Page partnered with Mackay. UVM's chairman was the busiest surgeon in town by far, having developed a broad referral base by war's end. Amidon, in particular, sent all of his surgical patients to Mackay. This was not a trivial matter, as the Chief of Medicine held a monopoly on the Mary Fletcher's patients. Amidon reluctantly accepted Page's services on the rare occasions when Mackay was unavailable according to Page. Since Page was always around, he rapidly developed his own huge practice.[27]

Patients entered the pairs' office at 96 Colchester Avenue through a narrow hallway. If they turned left, they found a very small waiting room that contained the secretary's desk. Beyond this was Page's cramped office, through which everyone passed to get to the examining room. If patients turned right, they entered Mackay's much larger waiting room, followed by his office and his adjacent two examining rooms. Secretary Doris Bell took care of Mackay, and

FIGURE 9-12. Mackay (2nd from L) operating with resident Martin Koplewitz (2nd from R) in 1958. Gino Dente (far R) is giving anesthesia.

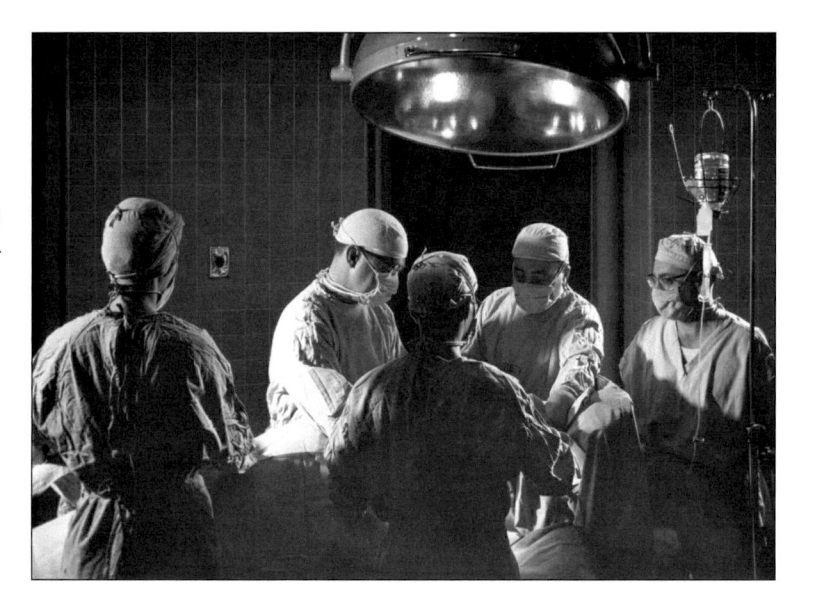

for several years, Page as well. She did the scheduling and billing, and sent academic information to the students and residents.

The upper floor was rented to John W. (Jack) Heisse, an otolaryngologist. The basement housed the group's medical supplies alongside Burlington's first tanning parlor containing Mackay's sunlamp. Thinking that he looked more wholesome and appealing to his patients with a slight tan (rather than a Vermonter's sallow pallor), Mackay maintained a lightly bronzed complexion throughout the winter months.

Patients were often admitted for diagnostic workups during this era. Those needing barium enemas, for instance, were brought into the hospital the night before for castor oil purgatives and tap water enemas. Page had a patient from Corinth, Vermont, who had made a fortune in West Texas oil. The old prospector called Page whenever he wasn't feeling up to snuff; Page then arranged for a full workup, putting his patient and his wife in adjacent private rooms. The couple typically stayed one to two weeks, paying out-of-pocket upon their discharge.

At one such check-up, the gentleman's wife was found to have a colon cancer by barium enema and sigmoidoscopy. Page re-admitted her and got the husband into the room next door so that he could visit whenever it was convenient. In the course of the woman's colectomy, the spleen was inadvertently torn. Page repaired the injury with carefully placed mattress sutures and bolstered it with a piece of omentum, performing in the process perhaps the first splenic repair at the Mary Fletcher Hospital. Page always followed his postoperative patients carefully, but this time he went overboard. He clucked around like a mother hen for the first eight hours, worried that his VIP patient might bleed. Her recovery, to the relief of all, was uneventful.

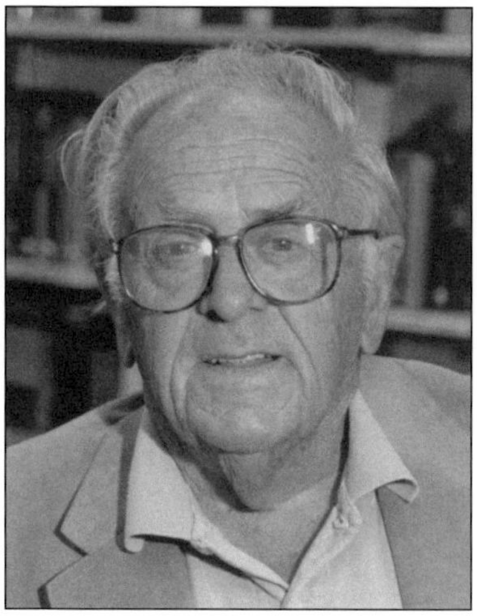

FIGURE 9-13. H. Gordon Page had a long career at UVM as an astute clinician and busy surgeon.

Page was also the surgical consultant to the Vermont State Psychiatric Hospital in Waterbury, a sprawling turn-of-the-century facility that held over 200 beds. The setup was much like that in the movie "One Flew Over the Cuckoo's Nest," except that the staff respected and cared for the patients. Elsie, an experienced O.R. nurse, staffed the hospital's lone Operating Room. She was present for every surgery, usually assisted by nurses from various other disciplines. Supplies were extremely limited. For example, Sears Roebuck catalogs substituted for surgical step stools. When asked for a 2-0 silk, Elsie often responded with a 3-0 cotton suture — the only type she had available.

The resident medical director notified Page whenever a patient was in need of an emergent surgery. Elective cases, on the other hand, were saved for routine visits. Page didn't mind the thirty five-mile travel distance (even though he was one of Burlington's busiest surgeons) since he still owned the family farm in nearby Groton. Every trip to the State Hospital was thus accompanied by a stopover at his beloved homestead.

During the late '60s, Page took a Surgery resident (myself, DBP) and an Anesthesiology resident (Rodrigue Charles, who had never been to the State Hospital before) to help with an operation. Our patient turned out to be a chubby 50 year-old with a large ovarian cyst. While we prepared for surgery, Charles turned the patient onto her side and placed the spinal needle. As he reached for the syringe that contained the anesthetic, the patient leapt off the table. She sprinted for the door with an open gown, a disconnected intravenous line, and a half-buried spinal needle still in her back.

Charles lunged for the needle, Page and I tackled the patient, and the three of us wrestled her back onto the operating table. Charles decided to use general anesthesia instead and turned on the Halothane®. Within a few minutes, the room started to smell of Halothane. The patient, meanwhile, stayed awake. It turned out that the ancient anesthesia machine's rubber bellows bag had deteriorated and sprung a large leak.

Page told Charles to prepare another spinal tray and then disappeared into a back room. As Charles gathered his supplies, Page injected the woman with Pentothal®. The spinal anesthetic was calmly given in due course, with Charles none the wiser. The Pentothal wore off just as paralysis from the spinal set in. The operation proceeded smoothly from then on, and the patient recovered without incident. Page later bought us ice cream cones before retiring to his Groton farm for the night. Shortly thereafter, such surgical resident experience at the Vermont State Hospital ceased due to new policies and alignment with other hospitals.[28]

Surgical Residency During the 1950s and '60s

UVM's surgical residency became a four-year program in 1957, continuously graduating one or two residents per year from that point onward. The residents usually operated at the Mary Fletcher, as the bigger cases tended to be done there. They also had the option of scrubbing at the Bishop DeGoesbriand if a major procedure (such as an aortic aneurysm graft) was on the schedule. The residents rarely visited the Fanny Allen Hospital during this period, as there were more than enough clinical opportunities for them in Burlington. Cardiac surgeon Donald Miller was in charge of the house staff and their schedules.

The Fletcher and DeGoesbriand both had active Emergency Rooms. Call was an every other night, in-hospital affair during this time (1963-1966). The Chief Resident was allowed to go home if all was quiet, but was required to return immediately when summoned. Those on call "in-house" slept (whenever possible) at Benjamin Adams' Residential House. During their time off, they exercised in the building's squash court or took the aluminum rowboat, donated to the house staff by the medical staff, out for a cruise on Lake Champlain.

Just before I (DBP) started my residency in Vermont, one of the senior residents took further advantage of this rowboat. He was required to complete dictations and sign off on all of his medical records in order to advance. He rowed the records out into Shelburne Bay one dark night, and weighted them down to sink into the mud bottom. They, however, floated ashore, and needless to say as a result we had one fewer resident in the program.

David B. Pilcher Prepares to Become a Resident Under Mackay at UVM

I (DBP) had no option but to go to medical school and become a surgeon. My father, Lewis Stephen Pilcher II, had trained with UVM's first thoracic consultant, Richard Overholt, at the Lahey Clinic in Boston.[31] My father had approached Lyman Allen in 1935 about practicing at UVM, but was told there was no room for him in Burlington. He went

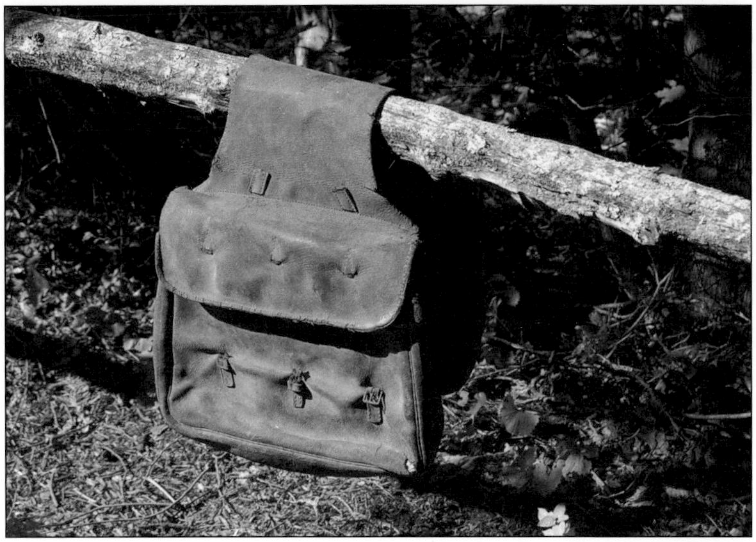

FIGURE 9-14. Saddlebags used by the first of the six generations of Pilcher physicians as he visited patients by horseback in Michigan during the mid-19th century.

on to have a long, successful community surgery practice in Newton, Massachusetts.[32] My grandfather, Paul Monroe Pilcher, had been an expert in the diseases of the urinary tract and was considered one of Brooklyn's foremost surgeons at the time of his death.[33] My great-grandfather, Lewis Stephen Pilcher, had written a number of surgical texts, had founded the *Annals of Surgery*, and had succeeded UVM's James Lawrence Little as Professor of Surgery at New York's Post-Graduate Medical School.[34] Even my great-great grandfather, Elijah Holmes Pilcher, had been a physician. He had received his MD degree in 1859 at the age of 49, which had made him the oldest University of Michigan medical school graduate up to that point in time.[35]

Gaining Acceptance to Medical School in the 1950s

Achieving academic excellence at Amherst College was necessary in order to gain acceptance to medical school. But how could I overcome a "D" in freshman German and calculus? I ended up telling the admissions committees that I hadn't applied myself before deciding on a medical career, and that my performance over the last three years represented my real potential when motivated.

There was a lot of truth in this explanation. At Amherst, the physics professor had set himself up as the gatekeeper for future medical practitioners by eliminating students who were not true scientists. He set high standards for the physics course required for medical school admission. This course was also a prerequisite for physics majors, and there was no compromise for potential medical students. My pre-med roommate struggled with physics, working much harder in this class than in any other. He subsequently received a "D".

I spent time in Boston during the summer, so I took the pre-med oriented physics course at Harvard's summer school and easily received an "A". At the same time, I worked as an orderly in the community hospital, thus enhancing my chances to become a medical student. Along these same lines, I rowed on the crew team and joined the Drama Club. This certainly made me appear well rounded, even though my Drama Club role was to play a "rock" in Oedipus Rex!

I was accepted at the University of Rochester under the early admission program. My roommate from Amherst with the "D" in physics, who had also been a "rock" in the Drama Club, finally eked into Long Island medical school via the waiting list. His later surgical career was nevertheless a huge success. He ended up using his physics expertise to develop a widely used prosthesis for total hip replacement procedures.

The Demands of Medical School (1956-1961)

Medical school tuition was $5,000 per year in 1956. My fellow students and I worked during medical school and the summers to cover living expenses and pocket money. My parents footed the tuition bills. Today's government-sponsored medical education loan programs were not yet in full swing.

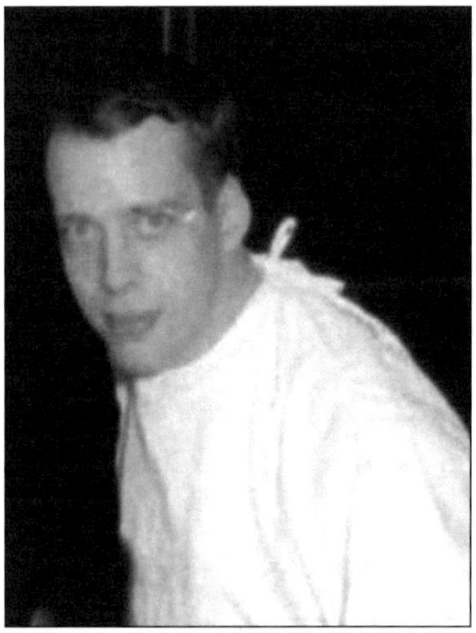

FIGURE 9-15. The author (DBP) as a medical student at Rochester, NY in 1957.

Graduate students in other disciplines got help with their expenses through work/study programs or by becoming research assistants. Medical students, in general, had limited free time to work gainfully, except in part-time jobs. I was able to work four hours a day in the cafeteria, washing trays. This job had the bonus of free meals attached to it. I rented a single room in a house with a family with two small children — which ended up being a place to sleep, rather than a place to study. Anatomy and microscopic work required that I be at the medical school anyway. I worked evenings and some weekends at a community hospital, doing lab work and drawing blood samples.

I remember one night in 1958 when I was called to the emergency room to draw a blood sample. There was a nine-year-old girl with croup noisily gasping for air. Her skin had a bluish tinge in spite of the presence of an oxygen mask over her mouth. The Emergency Room resident and an Ear, Nose and Throat physician were laboring to insert a tube through her nose past her swollen upper airway and into her trachea. Unfortunately, they were unsuccessful despite multiple attempts. As I watched in awe, one of them grabbed a scalpel and incised her neck to perform a tracheotomy. The wound immediately filled with dark blood. Direct pressure was applied and the operation was abandoned. The doctors then tried to place the tube through her mouth. As they continued to struggle, the patient arrested and died. I had never seen anyone die from a failed technical procedure before and the event became deeply etched into my mind.

My great-grandfather had kept track of the tracheostomies that he had performed in a diary. The experience reminded me of a handwritten quote that I had once seen in his little notebook from Theodor Billroth, dated 1881: "I think that the tracheotomies in children are the most difficult operations I have ever performed."[36]

During my second year of medical school, I was married to Jean Rogers. We then moved to a two-room apartment. She worked summers, as did I, and then taught school to cover our subsistence. Studies became slightly less demanding. I grew a garden, and we attended cultural events around town such as the symphony. We were frugal and stuck to the straight and narrow path. A $10 washing machine and $15 second hand TV were our big expenses. Hamburger and spaghetti were the order of the day, rather than the choice meats of my youth. Imaginative cooking paid off.

As I entered clinical studies, the evening hours away from home increased, but the intensity of academic work dropped a level. We actually had more free time at home when we were awake, and not dog-tired or sleeping. I do remember that Jean went to the family doctor one day complaining of nausea. Neither she nor I, the great medical student, realized that she was pregnant with Jonathan, our first *in utero* doctor-to-be.

I may not have shown much promise as a diagnostician, but at least I did better as a third year student when it came to surgery. The patient was our cat, who had gone into heat one too many times, and the assistant was my brother-in-law, first year medical student John Frymoyer. The successful hysterectomy was performed in the morgue, which certainly lacked sterility, but otherwise served us well. Unfortunately, we used non-absorbable sutures, so our pet required a second anesthetic for their removal.

Fifty percent of Rochester's medical students took an additional research year. This helped with family relations as well as family finances. I spent my year in pathology doing research on drug toxicity using rats as the animal model.

Surgical House Officer Years in Boston (1961-1963)

After graduating from the University of Rochester School of Medicine and Dentistry in 1961, I returned to the Boston area for a surgical residency at Tufts-New England Medical Center. My first rotation was on Neurosurgery. Within three weeks I had developed a huge carbuncle on the back of my neck. The neurosurgeons did not want my infection on their wards, and told me to come back when and only when the infection was totally gone. I thought that soaking my neck in the salt water of my family's Cape Cod beach home was an ideal addition to the prescribed antibiotic therapy. Luckily, it was summer time, and it didn't even count against my vacation!

Once this serendipitous sabbatical was over, surgical internship proved to be strenuous and demanding. I remember one afternoon when we uncharacteristically had a break in the action. I asked my chief resident if I could sneak out to get a haircut. I was immediately told: "You are off this coming Saturday afternoon aren't you?" The responsibility and the clinical experiences were unbelievably exciting, and confirmed that surgery was the correct career choice for me.

It was lucky for my family that our parents were around, because a tired intern doesn't do much else except sleep once he or she gets home. Vacations were very restricted, and income was inadequate to support a wife and two children. Luckily, a student loan program came along. The Benjamin Franklin Fund had been created many years ago out of Benjamin Franklin's fortune in order to provide loans for apprentices in Boston and Philadelphia. Eligible candidates were hard to find, so the Fund's board decided that medical house officers met the definition of an apprentice. A very low interest loan was offered to me, and I gladly accepted it.

Vermont Beckons (1963-1966)

During my second year of residency, I learned that there was an opening in UVM's residency program at the third-year level. Remembering the summer research fellowship I had taken in Burlington as a medical student with UVM pioneer Jacobson, I took the spot and moved to Vermont with my wife Jean and children Jonathan and Susan.

In the era of the Vietnam Conflict, physicians were not allowed to complete their residencies unless they committed themselves to military service upon graduation. Other options were to join the National Guard or Reserves (both of which provided deferments) or to receive a physical exemption. Surgical residents who had not made such arrangements were often called-up during the middle of their residencies to function as general medical officers, rather than as surgeons. Residency programs, therefore, were reluctant to accept and retain non-committed residents whose departure might leave them short-handed. This requirement led to my subsequent service in the Army upon completion of my surgical residency.

I arrived from Boston in July of 1963, and was warmly welcomed into the residency along with one other resident at my level, Robert Dewitt. Coming from an every other night in-house call system, which resulted in my getting home at eight pm on my nights off, Vermont was far more humane. There were still a lot of every other night rotations, but I got home early on my nights off. The teaching seemed equivalent to that which I had experienced in Boston. Supervision by attending surgeons was ever present and constructive. Didactic lectures were not frequent, but there was a lot of one-on-one teaching. We were also expected to be up-to-date with the surgical literature. Candid, responsible morbidity and mortality conferences supplemented constructive criticism.

Journal club was held monthly in one of the attendings' homes. This led to a great camaraderie and esprit d'corps, and we got to know staff families well and to appreciate that better days were coming for us in terms of lifestyle. We also got to see the attendings' houses. McGill always had the July journal club at his house, and all enjoyed his pool and backyard view of Mt. Mansfield. In addition, on Sundays there was free noontime dinner for all house staff and their families in the Mary Fletcher Hospital cafeteria. We certainly always took advantage of that.

As surgery residents we rotated through anesthesia, obstetrics/gynecology, and orthopaedics. I remember being on Obstetrics when my youngest son Chris, who later became a doctor, was born. I decided that the best place for me was to be having breakfast in the cafeteria, although today it would be more politically correct for me to have been in the delivery suite with my wife. Allowing families in the delivery suite was not the rule in those days, the argument being that if something went wrong, the family being present might inhibit proper medical practice.

I remember giving anesthesia for a delivery using nitrous oxide 20%/oxygen 80% by mask. My patient was turning blue, and there was fetal distress. The problem was luckily remedied and patient and fetus were unharmed. We discovered that the wall oxygen outlet and air outlets were interchangeable, and that I had been giving 80% room air/20% nitrous — a guarantee for hypoxia! The system was changed to make the process fail safe with dedicated unique attachments for each of the gases.

Attending surgeons were expected to be present at every admission, although sometimes a case admitted during the early hours was not seen until morning rounds. The attendings supervised whenever a patient was taken to the operating room. It is my recollection that the Department inadvertently took a unique approach when it came to surgical billing, listing surgical residents as assistants at the time of surgery around 1965-66. Our insurance carriers accepted this practice for a time, although it later was disallowed.

Chief Residents ran their own service through the Fletcher Hospital's Durfee Memorial Clinic, a dispensary that provided services based on a patient's ability to pay.[37] Cases were presented to an attending, but the chief resident made the clinical decisions and scheduled surgery. An attending was always in the Operating Room during "service cases," and scrubbed for anything more complex than an appendectomy. This was in sharp contrast to some metropolitan teaching centers where an attending may not even have been in the hospital when such cases were performed.[38]

The Mary Fletcher did not have a Recovery Room until the early 1970s. This was because John Abajian, the head of the Division of Anesthesiology, advocated the use of either halothane, a rapidly excreted inhalation anesthetic, or regional anesthesia for most cases. Patients were kept in the Operating Room until they were awake enough to be cared for on the surgical ward. This demanded a high level of skilled nursing care on the wards, but also biased the choice of anesthetic technique. Abajian claimed that he could numb a thyroidectomy with a spinal. In fact, many major abdominal operations (including cholecystectomies) were done under spinal anesthesia. On occasion, patient comfort dictated additional sedation — sometimes to the extent of a general anesthetic!

Harry Elwin Howe, a General Surgery resident from 1953 to 1957, recalled the free-wheeling nature of those days. Howe felt that he needed more sub-specialty exposure in order to meet the broad requirements of a rural surgical practice. He approached Miller and asked for a four-month rotation on gynecology, orthopedics and urology. Miller, to Howe's gratification, granted the request.[39]

Howe learned most of his orthopaedics from Charles Rust, a notably rapid surgeon. He knew he had arrived when Rust told him, "Slow down, you shouldn't try to operate as fast as I do!" On another occasion, Rust let Howe take over during the repair of a fractured hip. As Rust gave Howe the knife, he commented, "You are the first resident I have ever let do a hip nailing." Unfortunately, the hardware eroded through the sub-cutaneous tissues the following year. With the fracture healed, Howe removed the Smith-Peterson nail in the Emergency Room under local anesthesia.[40]

Abdominal surgery was in its heyday. Laparoscopy was the sole domain of the gynecologists. The few general surgeons who did attempt the technique decided that they could do better with open procedures. Physicians were trained to insert orotracheal or nasotracheal tubes in the Operating Room for anesthesia. These tubes were soon readily available on "Code Carts" throughout the hospital. Respirators were used for post-operative recovery, and volume resuscitation with Ringer's lactate became prevalent. Patients in shock were rescued through prolonged Intensive Care Unit stays. Blood component therapy was on hand, as was renal dialysis.

Closed chest compression replaced open heart massage for patients in cardiac arrest. Prior to 1960, it was generally believed that chest compressions were inadequate to circulate blood.

Thus, many a physician opened the chest cavity and squeezed the heart directly during a "code" situation. Test tubes containing sterile scalpels were kept taped to the walls for just this purpose. Gloves were not worn, and sterile conditions were not observed in such a crisis. That a chest opened in this manner could heal without infection was amazing.

Howe was present for such a case during his 1956 rotation with John Maeck, the Chief of Obstetrics & Gynecology. Their patient, an otherwise healthy woman, suffered a cardiac arrest after her spinal anesthetic went too high. Howe stood by with the scalpel, awaiting Maeck's command. When Maeck nodded, he opened the chest through the left fifth interspace. Just as Howe was about to massage the flaccid heart, Maeck pushed him aside and took over. Howe was left to close the wound and explain to the patient why she had an incision in her chest, rather than her lower abdomen. Surprisingly, the woman was spared any brain or cardiac damage. The understanding and grateful lady went on to have her hysterectomy a month later under general anesthesia.[41]

UVM surgery residents rotated on Obstetrics and Gynecology until Davis took over the Department of Surgery in 1969. John Van Sicklen Maeck was Chief of Ob/Gyn during these years (starting in 1948) and was greatly appreciated by the surgical residents. He was a demanding but fair teacher, and a superb technician. He taught me (DBP) the concept of knowing the surgical anatomy involved completely, and then staying away from the danger areas (such as the ureters in hysterectomy), and ligating the vascular pedicle at its origin going to the uterus, rather than multiple times close to the uterus, because one didn't understand the anatomy. He taught us: either stay away from the area of the trouble, or identify the endangered structure so you can avoid damaging it.

Mackay was a tough but fair mentor to the residents. "For Dr. Mackay, a rite of surgical passage was successfully closing a patient's abdominal wound with less than industrial strength silk. ... senior residents initially broke sutures and then mastered the subtle technique ..."[42]

I (DBP) personally recall closing a patient with "new and improved" Davis and Geck® 3-0 silk suture that had been coated with silicone so that bacteria couldn't get into the thread's interstices. The fact that the silicone also made the surgical knots less secure was never conveyed to the surgeons. As our patient was being extubated, he gave a prodigious heave and popped all of his sutures because the knots slipped. Mackay found out about the change to slippery sutures, and he banished all Davis and Geck products from the Operating Room. The Mary Fletcher Hospital (and its successor, the Medical Center Hospital of Vermont) thus became an exclusive Ethicon® customer for the next fifteen years!

Mackay Tries to Embrace Academia

Pressure mounted on Mackay to improve his department's academic standing. This also applied to himself as chief. Mackay was a superb surgeon, blessed with excellent judgment and technical skill. For some reason though, he was not inclined to conduct research or contribute to the surgical literature. In fact, of the eleven papers that carried his name, Mackay was the primary author on only four.[43] He had to be more than just a role model interested in teaching if he were to meet the criteria for a chairman of an academic surgery department.

Mackay began receiving a salary from the College of Medicine in the 1950s, thereby becoming the Department's only full-time faculty member. The rest of the attending staff remained part-time and received fee-for-service reimbursement directly from their patients. Most of the faculty were home bred and educated. Few of them engaged in research, although Haines and Page each wrote a few articles.[44] The Department's members went to New England Surgical Society and American College of Surgeons' meetings, but did not usually present papers.

Although he rarely vacationed, Mackay did attend regional and national surgical meetings in order to bolster his scholastic credentials. The New England Surgical Society named Mackay president in 1964, but this was in recognition of his leadership as UVM chair rather than his academic or scientific contributions. His failure to be elected to the more prestigious American Surgical Society was a major disappointment to him, according to the recollections of Page.

It came as no surprise then that the Residency Review Board criticized the UVM program for its lack of full-time faculty and commitment to research. One solution would have been to hire a more academically-oriented chairman, but Mackay held on to the power base. He chose to bring in outside talent to remedy the situation — an approach he continued until he stepped down in 1969. It was under these circumstances that up-and-coming surgeon Julius Jacobson started the school's first surgical research laboratory.

Julius Jacobson Brings Surgical Research to UVM (1959)

Julius H. Jacobson, II, another World War II veteran, started his surgical journey with a detour. He had graduated from high school at age 15, but did not have enough money to go to college and "pursue my goal of becoming a physician."[45] According to Jacobson:

> *"I worked as a photographer taking pictures of school children and peddling them to their parents in the evenings. On turning 16, there was still no money for college. I hitchhiked to Toledo, which had a University I could attend tuition-free. Beginning there in 1943, credit could be obtained for a course if a student passed the final exam. By age 17, I had 3 years of credits but the war in the Pacific was heating up and patriotic fervor intervened to have me enlist in the Navy. I was made a Pharmacist's Mate and placed on independent duty aboard a small ship with a 200-man crew, a frightening memory when I think of how little I knew. While doing this I received orders to report for Fleet Marine Force training, which was almost tantamount to a death sentence, since the Fleet Marines set up aid stations on the beaches as the Marines stormed in. I've always felt my life was saved by the atomic bomb. It was dropped — and I was discharged."*[46]

After completing his last year at Toledo, Jacobson applied to 23 medical schools amidst a glut of postwar candidates — and was promptly rejected by all of them. Undeterred, he took a job in a research laboratory at the University of Pennsylvania studying *paramecia* under a microscope. He spent "all day every day" in the lab. Jacobson believes to this day that had he "not been rejected from medical school and spent the year in the laboratory, microvascular surgery would have arisen elsewhere."

FIGURE 9-16. Julius Jacobson operating with the binocular single scope in the basement of the Medical Alumni Building's surgical research laboratory. Note the "Bird Respirator®" on the left.

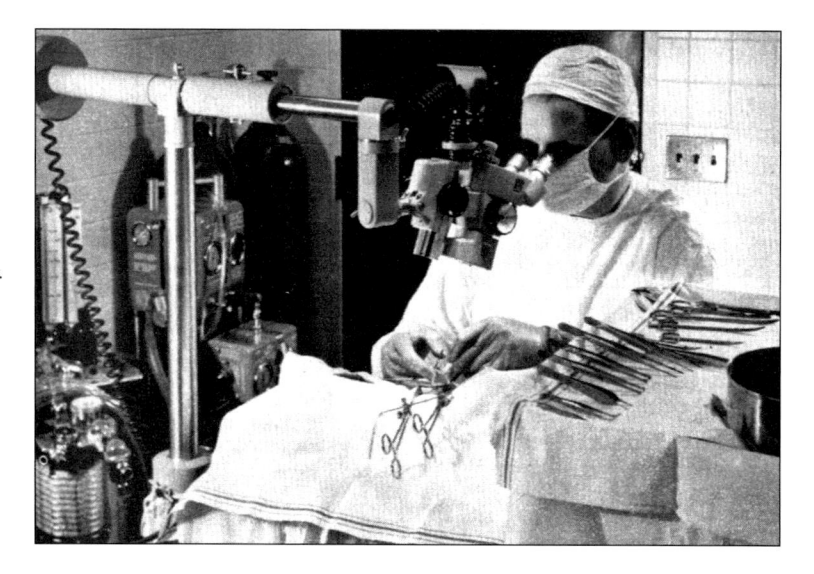

With recommendations from Penn's nationally prominent cell physiologists, Jacobson reapplied to the medical schools that had rejected him the year before. This time around, he was accepted at every one. He graduated from Johns Hopkins, and then completed a seven-year general surgery residency and a thoracic surgery fellowship at New York City's Columbia-Presbyterian Hospital.

During his internship year, he worked with Arthur Blakemore treating aortic aneurysms. Blakemore "was applying constricting bands to the aorta just proximal to the aneurysm with the aim of decreasing pressure within the aneurysmal sac." Jacobson, typically, "would spend my evenings observing these patients and in the majority, calling and telling him either there was still a strong pulse in the aneurysm, or, that the patient's legs were ischemic." As Jacobson noted, "this productivity eventually accounted for the appointment that led to the microsurgical development."[47]

Upon completing his fellowship in 1959, Jacobson was recruited by Mackay to start a research program at UVM. He accepted the offer, and was soon appointed Associate Professor of surgery and Director of Surgical Research. Not bad for someone only a few months out of training! He was generously funded by the College of Medicine, the Department of Surgery's clinicians, and the United States Public Health Service, which "was pouring money in to upgrade the smaller schools."[48]

Jacobson drew upon his interest in thoracic surgery and his prior experience with the operating microscope. The Department of Pharmacology asked him to help with a study that involved denervation of the canine carotid artery. "It became clear that the only sure way to achieve this was to divide and reanastamose the artery." After working on the 3 mm arteries, however, "It became obvious, that the problem was the eye not being able to see well enough to guide the hand properly." Experimentation with magnifying loupes was undertaken in short order. "Suddenly the epiphany occurred. I remembered wandering into an ear, nose, and throat operating room at Presbyterian Hospital and peering through the microscope during a stapes mobilization."[49] The rest unfolded as follows:

"I immediately went to the Mary Fletcher Hospital to borrow an operating microscope. The resistance to moving an expensive piece of equipment and contaminating it in the ani-

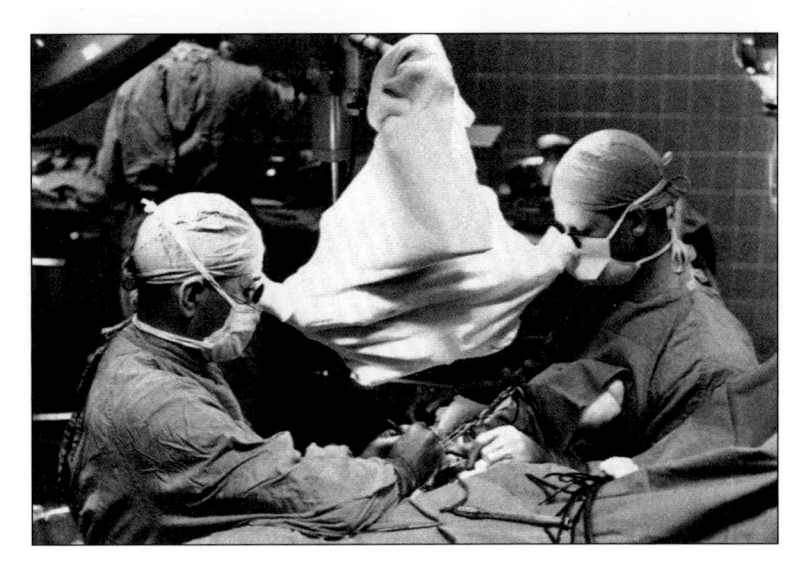

FIGURE 9-17. Jacobson (left) operating with the original "Diploscope" which now resides at the Smithsonian Institute in Washington, DC.

mal laboratory was monumental, even as it might be today. However, that same day we did the first canine carotid anastomosis with the microscope. I shall never forget how appalled I was by all the loose fibers sticking out of the surgical sponges. From then on the anastomoses were successful, but the instruments were crude, the sutures and the needles were too large, the operating field was neither stable nor controllable, all of us had some degree of tremor, and the first assistant could not see to be of help."[50]

"The local jewelry store solved the forceps problem. Spring-handled instruments had been developed for use in eye and ear surgery and simply had to be modified for our deeper operations. The instability of vessel clamps was easily resolved by placing them in holding clamps attached to the operating table and providing a screw attachment to control the position of the vessel ends. The problem of the tremor resulting from the party the night before was resolved when I remembered the use of the lathe rest in a machine shop course I had once taken. We all soon learned to rest the instruments on a stable part of the operative field."[51]

"Another immediate need was suture and needle miniaturization. The finest sutures then available were #6-0. The Ethicon suture people were extraordinarily helpful. They developed a needle that was 0.0005 inches in diameter and found a machinist capable of drilling a 0.0001 inch hole into the stock which would accommodate the 0.0001 inch suture that was then swaged in place."[52]

"The final major difficulty was securing a microscope that would allow the surgeon and the assistant to see the operative field simultaneously, at the same or at different levels of magnification. The Carl Zeiss Company was different [from other manufacturers] and sent over the engineer who had devised the original single binocular operating microscope. He observed what we were able to do, and without further consultation, agreed to build one (and only one) of the desired double binocular microscopes, later named the Diploscope."[53]

Jacobson was given a wing in the basement of the new Medical Alumni Building. It contained an office for himself, an office for a fellow, an office with several divided carousels for students, and three rooms that could function as animal laboratory operating rooms. There was enough cage space for 160 dogs, a luxury unheard of today.

Jacobson hired Clement Comeau, a Mary Fletcher O.R. assistant, and Rodney Larrow, who had been working for a local veterinarian, as his laboratory technicians. He recruited Ernesto L. Suarez, a gifted young physician from Argentina, to be a research associate. Suarez, like Jacobson before him, eventually developed superb skills operating under the microscope.[54]

During the summer months, medical students were paid $300 apiece to work in the new lab. The 1960 crew included two students from UVM, Robert Guiduli (who later became a South Burlington-based ophthalmologist) and Charles Pitman; and one from the University of Rochester, myself (DBP) thanks to my family's summer connections in the greater Burlington area. Guiduli and I worked with the operating microscope under Jacobson and Suarez's tutelage.

UVM's Early Attempts at Cardiac Revascularization

Coronary revascularization (in the form of endarterectomy) was just coming into vogue at this time, although "it was obvious that better technical performance was needed."[55] Jacobson thought that the operating microscope could be useful in this regard. He started removing the inner layers of coronary arteries using the Diploscope to determine "If endarterectomies are done in young animals, will the repaired arteries grow appropriately as the animals mature?"[56]

Coronary angiograms were quietly performed on Jacobson's bovine patients at the Mary Fletcher Hospital. The calves were coaxed through the back door of the X-Ray suite under the cover of darkness to avoid detection or even worse, publicity! Jacobson's group also tried their experiments on pigs, but found that cows were more amenable to the surgical approach (and more in keeping with Vermont's image.)

Anesthesiologist John Abajian zealously believed that halothane, with its high percentage of oxygen delivery and rapid excretion, was the safest inhalation anesthetic available. During his tenure, UVM probably used more halothane than anywhere else in the world. Halothane, therefore, became the natural choice of anesthetic for the calves' coronary endarterectomies. Comeau acted as both the perfusionist under Jacobson's direction, and the anesthetist under Abajian's instruction.

When the calves were a year old, they were re-angiogramed and then sacrificed. Those of us working in the lab thought that it would be appropriate to harvest the prime cuts, rather than discard them — a concept that would certainly appall today's Institutional Review Boards. As it turned out, science settled the issue for us as the halothane rendered the meat inedible.

Donald B. Effler, the Chief of Thoracic Surgery at the Cleveland Clinic, came to Burlington to observe the new developments in microsurgery firsthand. Effler stayed for a week learning to do small artery anastomoses. Jacobson, "fully realizing the potential, sent Suarez back to Cleveland to aid in training their surgical staff." Suarez subsequently completed a cardiothoracic fellowship under Effler.[57] The Cleveland group, in turn, "put coronary bypass on the clinical map."[58]

Jacobson and Donaghy Join Forces

UVM neurosurgeon R.M.P. Donaghy started using the operating microscope in Jacobson's lab, hoping that the device might open new avenues in the surgical treatment of blood vessels both within and leading to the brain. He and Jacobson took their first subject to the Mary Fletcher Hospital's Operating Room on August 4, 1960. Using the surgical research lab's Diploscope, the two performed the first-ever middle cerebral artery endarterectomy on an individual who had suffered a stroke. The patient, however, didn't miraculously recover. Jacobson reported the case (along with later work) before the Harvey Cushing Society in 1961 and published it in the Journal of Neurosurgery in 1962.[59]

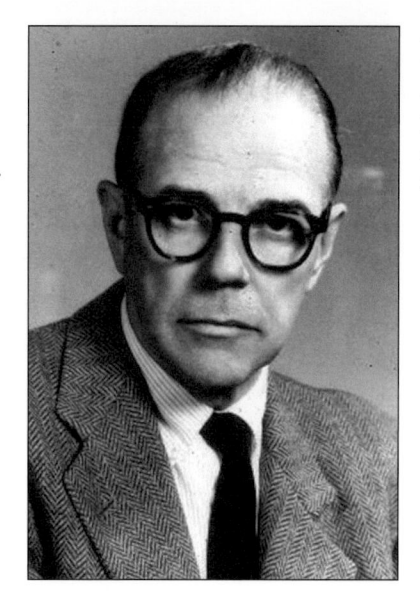

FIGURE 9-18. "Pete" Donaghy collaborated with Jacobson in the original surgical research laboratory.

Donaghy persisted in his faith in the operating microscope. A fellow from Switzerland, Mahmut Gazi Yasargil, came to work with him in the lab at Jacobson's suggestion. Together, the pair developed the extra-cranial to intra-cranial (EC/IC) bypass procedure for occlusive cerebral arterial disease. Using Jacobson's microsurgical methods, they anastomosed the superficial temporal artery to a cortical branch of the middle cerebral artery beyond the occlusion, thereby restoring blood flow.[60] (see Chapter 21)

Jacobson utilized the Diploscope in many other inventive ways. He reversed vasectomies in experimental animals and in patients by creating vaso-vasostomies — a procedure that has become commonplace among Urologists. He also restored the patency of scarred Fallopian tubes, a technique now rendered obsolete by the success of *in vitro* fertilization. Veins, lymphatics, nerves, and ureters were approached in a similar fashion. Limbs and digits were replanted and rat kidneys and hearts were transplanted.[61]

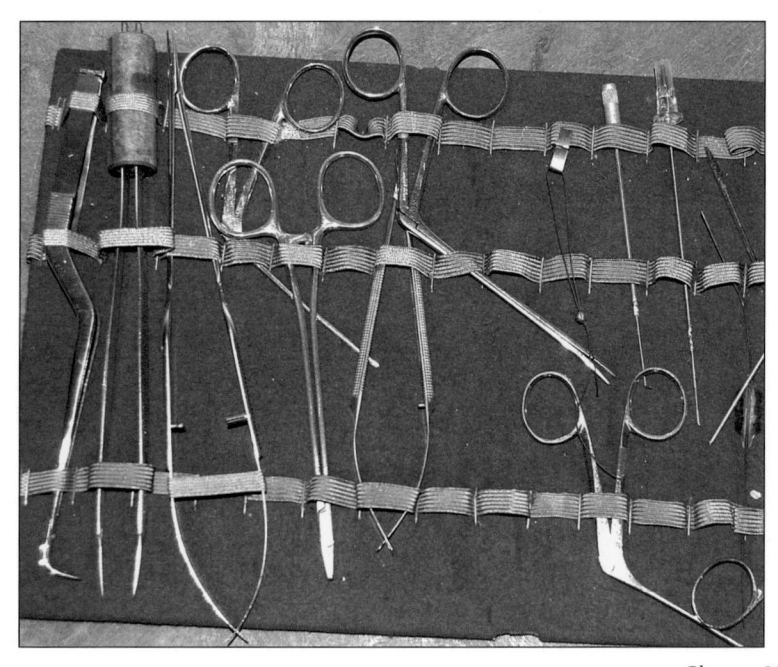

FIGURE 9-19. Donaghy's micro-neurosurgical instruments currently reside in the Given Building's surgical research corridor museum.

Jacobson was a trailblazer when it came to instrumentation too. He promoted the use of operating loupes (which have, ironically, now replaced microscopes in most microsurgical applications) in lieu of cumbersome magnifying spectacles. Moreover, many of the forceps and needle holders used today for vascular and neurosurgical procedures are the offspring of equipment Jacobson either modified or invented.[62]

The manner in which Jacobson handled blood vessels proved to have value in other types of vascular surgery. By carefully stripping the adventitia from the ends of tiny arteries prior to an anastomosis, Jacobson prevented even the smallest amount of collagen from becoming a thrombogenic focus within the artery. Small vessel replantation procedures and low-flow vascular operations such as distal bypasses and in-situ vein grafting have greatly benefited from the application of this technique.[63]

Having secured his reputation, Jacobson returned to New York City at the end of 1962 to pursue a wonderfully successful career. He is presently Director Emeritus of the Vascular Surgical Service and Professor of Surgery at The Mount Sinai Hospital. Since his retirement, he and his wife have generously funded vascular surgical professorships at three separate institutions. They have also established the "Jacobson Innovation Award" and more recently, "The American College of Surgeons Joan L. and Julius H. Jacobson Promising Investigator Award" through the American College of Surgeons.[64] In 2002 his interactive audio book entitled "The Classical Music Experience" was published.[65]

Surgical Research Decelerates After Jacobson Leaves

Mackay's next research lab director was William M. Stahl, Jr. Stahl had trained at New York University and then returned to his hometown of Danbury, Connecticut to practice surgery alongside his father. While in private practice, he wrote articles and even a textbook on the surgical aspects of renal failure.[66] Stahl eventually returned to academia after seven years of private practice — one of only a few doctors to successfully make such a transition. He focused on renal hemodynamics and lymphocyte physiology during his time at UVM, eventually publishing close to a dozen papers.[67] Stahl's lab also had an active microsurgical component, although Donaghy was now the school's dominant force in microvascular surgery.

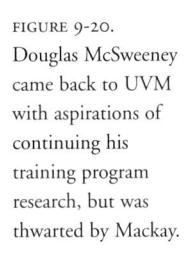

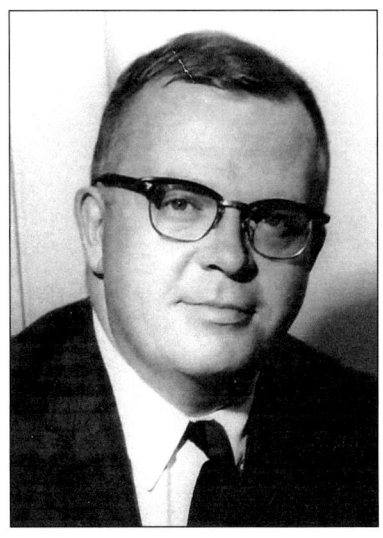

FIGURE 9-20. Douglas McSweeney came back to UVM with aspirations of continuing his training program research, but was thwarted by Mackay.

E. Douglas McSweeney, Jr. (1928-2002) — the grandson of Patrick McSweeney, the legendary gynecologist, surgeon, and co-founder of the Bishop DeGoesbriand Hospital — arrived on the scene within a year of Stahl. Although "Doug" (as the son of a Burlington gynecologist) had grown up within a few blocks of UVM, he was the only member of his extensive family of physicians that did not attend the UVM College of Medicine. He instead obtained an MD from the University of Ottawa in 1958, finished a surgical residency at Montreal's McGill University in 1964, and then completed additional studies in Oregon and California.[68]

McSweeney had done significant research at each of these locations. He joined UVM as a full-time surgeon thinking that he would do research here as well. Mackay, though, had already brought Stahl on board to fill the "research" slot. Mackay told McSweeney, "There's only room for one of you — there's only one that's going to be doing research."[69] Discouraged by the turn of events, McSweeney left the Department, set up a private practice on Pearl Street, and became a part-time faculty member. In addition to practicing full time, he also served two terms in the Vermont Senate, from 1978-1982.[70]

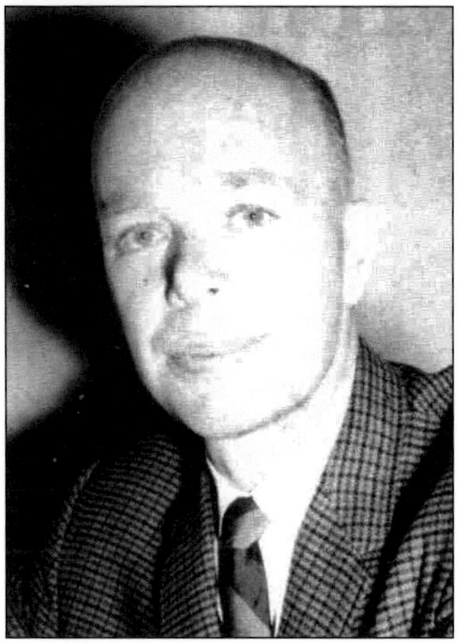

Stahl was a dedicated teacher and an obvious choice to be the chairman of an academic surgery department had there been an opening. Mackay made it clear, however, that he was staying on as chief. Stahl apparently knew that he had to leave in order to advance his career. His subsequent vice-chairmanship of the New York Medical College Department of Surgery from 1980 to 1999, and position as Chief of Surgery at the Lincoln Medical and Mental Health Center, were testimony to his leadership abilities.[71]

When Stahl left in 1967, Mackay turned to Emil Blair (1922-1998), a thoracic surgeon from the University of Maryland, to not only perform research but also rejuvenate the stalled cardiac surgery program.[72] Having spent the previous ten years working on hypothermic, hypovolemic, and septic shock, Blair decided to study blunt thoracic trauma.[73] Whereas others had recreated chest injuries by impacting anesthetized monkeys with moving objects, Blair implemented an intricate model in which the animals were slung down rails at high speeds into stationary objects.[74] In the end, his research methods produced few promising results. Blair worked hard, but failed to lead UVM to academic prominence, and to revive the cardiac surgical clinical program.

FIGURE 9-21. William Stahl made the successful transition from private practice to academia at UVM and directed the research laboratory.

Formation of a Full Time Group Fails to Revitalize Surgery

Rees and Truax, meanwhile, had both stopped operating. Mackay was unable to convince any of the remaining part-time surgeons to join the faculty on a full-time basis. Page had signed on briefly, but soon returned to private practice. Mackay finally brought pediatric surgeon Paul Mellish in from Philadelphia.[75] Recently graduated residents Gerald Howe and Cemalettin Topuzlu, and Canadian James MacKenzie, eventually supplemented Mellish as general surgeons. These new surgeons formed into a group practice called "Surgical Associates". This was a non-profit group, and the majority of its income came from Mackay's huge practice. The practice group was to endure, although the participating surgeons (except for Mellish) had short tenures.

Howe (1934-2006) was a gifted surgeon and a devoted teacher who was loved by the students. He left Vermont for private practice in Colorado.[76] Topuzlu (whose surgeon-grandfather was a pioneer in the development of open chest cardiac massage) was both a superb surgeon and researcher.[77] He ultimately went back to his homeland of Turkey where he pursued a productive academic career. MacKenzie relocated to Hamilton, Ontario's McMaster University. While there, he helped revolutionize medical school teaching through the creation of an innovative Problem-Based Learning curriculum.[78]

Mackay also tried to extend the Department's influence across town. Maine native Clarence Bunker had graduated from the College of Medicine in 1962. He went to Stanford for his surgical residency, but by 1968 he and his wife (an alumna of UVM's nursing school) longed to return to Vermont. Their timing was propitious since the Fanny Allen Hospital's Crandall had just retired. Bunker was hired by Surgical Associates, given a salary of $16,000, and positioned at the Fanny Allen. Thabault still dominated the Fanny Allen area's practice of surgery, however. Bunker's UVM full time affiliation didn't pose much of a threat but his nascent practice lagged. Bunker wondered if this was partly due to a town/gown attitude of referring doctors.[79]

Mackay Seeks a New Leader for Surgery

Mackay admitted that his attempts to solve the school's academic problems had failed. "Inasmuch as I have found that, at sixty-one years of age, I am unable with my background to recruit the type of scientific personnel with immunology training, etc., to complete the picture for the development of this new phase of surgery, I am willing to relinquish my chair and go on with my professorial duties, allowing my successor to have the responsibility for recruiting these new men."[80] Mackay's 27-year reign as chairman ended. His contemporary loyal troops soldiered on, however, ready to help a visionary new leader revitalize the Department.

PART V

MATURATION INTO ACADEMIA: THE DAVIS YEARS

1969-1989

CHAPTER 10

Resurrection of the Department of Surgery

A.G. Mackay stepped down as Chief and was replaced by John Davis of Cleveland. Davis brought new faculty members and nationally recognized research to town.

At a time when others were leaving academia to pursue lucrative jobs, Davis convinced the community's surgeons to form a single, dedicated practice. Davis also helped develop UVM's broad-based specialty practice group.

Davis became president of the American Association for the Surgery of Trauma and editor-in-chief of the Journal of Trauma. Just as he reached the height of his success, disaster struck.

Mackay Steps Down After 27 Years as Chief of Surgery

The inability to maintain a full-time staff and establish a permanent research program wasn't the only problem facing Mackay before he stepped down. The Department's teaching and

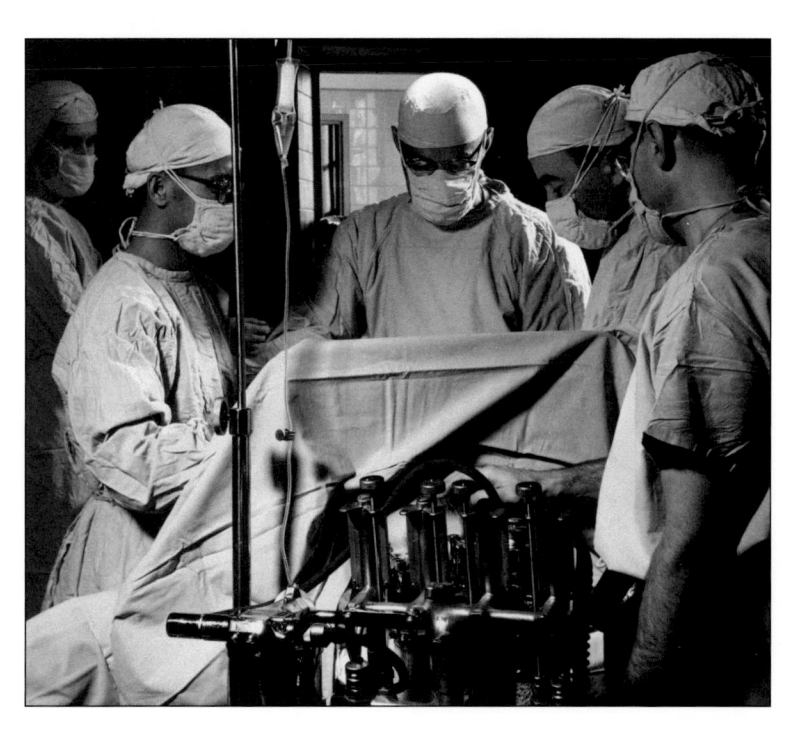

FIGURE 10-1.
A.G. Mackay performing an abdominal-perineal resection at the Mary Fletcher with resident Martin Koplewitz (2nd from R) in 1958.

145

FIGURE 10-2.
The Arnold Wing at the DeGoesbriand Hospital, housed the surgical service on the 6th floor. The operating rooms were on the top floor of the adjacent St. Joseph's Pavilion (the older building on the right in this photo).

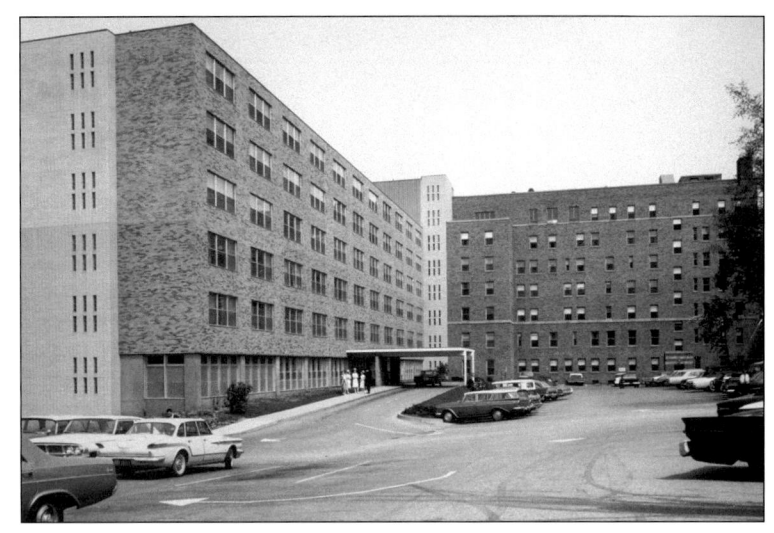

FIGURE 10-3.
The Shepardson North wing was built in 1958. The Women's Pavilion to the south was later converted into Shepardson South.

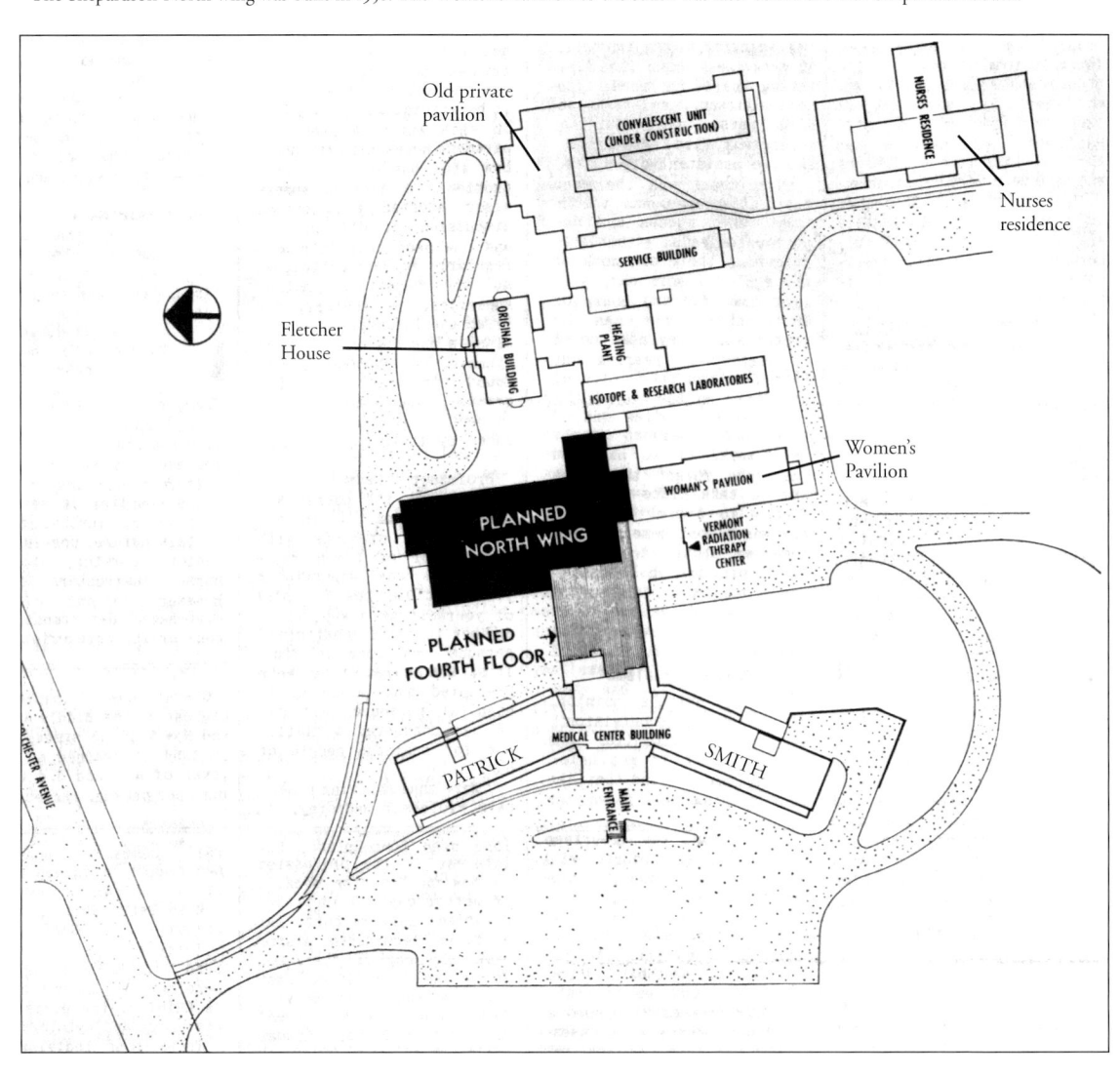

146 CATAMOUNT SURGEONS

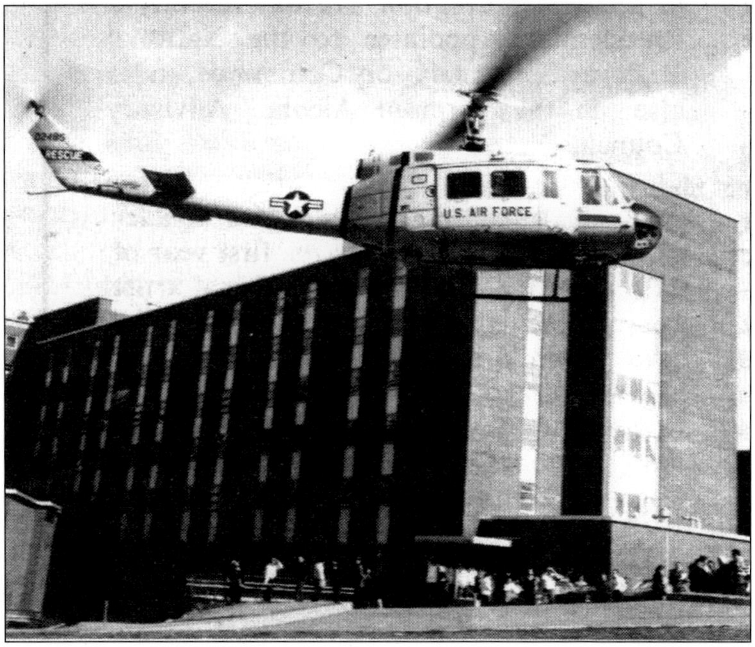

FIGURE 10-4. The Baird Wing dominates this 1974 view of the Mary Fletcher. Surgical patients were located on Baird 3 at the time, one floor up from the ICU on Patrick 2 and the operating rooms on Smith 2.

operating costs were escalating. At the same time, a shift from fee-for-service to third party payers was reducing reimbursement. The creation of Medicare and Medicaid foreshadowed further decreases in hospital stays and charges.

The Formation of the Medical Center Hospital of Vermont (MCHV)

Burlington's two hospitals, though, were in the midst of a major building spree. The city's Catholic institution (renamed the DeGoesbriand Memorial Hospital in 1956) embarked on a disastrous course in which it tried to keep pace with improvements at the Mary Fletcher. By the early 1960s, the construction of the Rehabilitation and Research Center, the Arnold Pavilion, and a Cobalt radiation facility had drained its coffers.[1] The Mary Fletcher, meanwhile, had torn down the old Surgical Pavilion to make way for the Shepardson North building, and was in the process of erecting the Baird wing.[2]

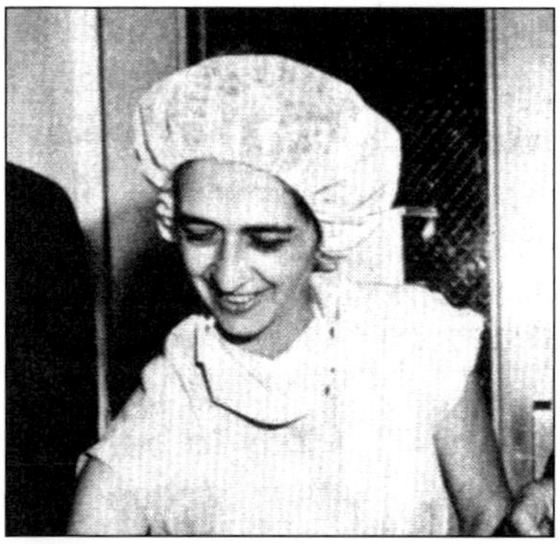

By 1965, the two hospitals had a total bed capacity of 584. Realizing that further expansion and duplication of services were doomed to economic failure, the directors of both institutions entered into an affiliation agreement. This (as well as work done by intra-hospital liaison Arthur Gladstone during the 1950s) paved the way for the 1967 merger into a single entity called the Medical Center Hospital of Vermont.[3]

FIGURE 10-5. Mary Fletcher operating room head nurse Beverly O'Neill (seen here in 1972) always had a smile for everyone.

The hospitals were re-christened the Mary Fletcher Unit (MFU) and the DeGoesbriand Memorial Unit (DMU). Mackay became the Chief of Surgery for MCHV, while Gladstone relinquished his title as chief at the DeGoesbriand. Most of the community surgeons continued to base their practices with their old hospital affiliations. In the end, both Units functioned as before, with the merger initially existing in name only.

The DMU's emergency room remained full-service, although most of the serious cases

FIGURE 10-6. The DeGoesbriand's operating rooms were filled with light from large windows. Windows were abandoned in later O.R.s to allegedly minimize surgeon distraction.

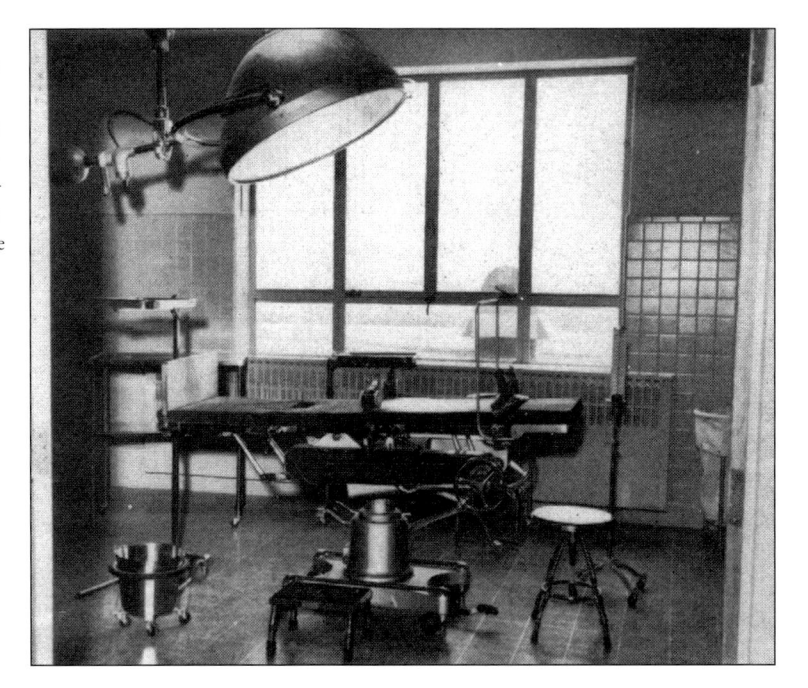

went straight to the Mary Fletcher. The surgical residents already served both hospitals, so their roles did not change. A second or third-year resident staffed the facility overnight, and the two chief residents went to the DMU to operate whenever a desirable case presented itself.

The DeGoesbriand's operating rooms were located on the sixth floor of its 1948 addition, St. Joseph's Pavilion. Each room had a large picture window from which one could view the lake in the distance and the pigeons in the foreground. O.R. #1 had a separate glass panel through which students and nurses observed surgery. The six operating rooms emptied into a single corridor. The nurses sat at one end of the hallway between cases and drank coffee. The surgeons relaxed at the opposite end, which overlooked the UVM green and the Ira Allen Chapel. The floor's only dressing room was reserved for the male doctors; the nurses and other females had to change on the maternity ward, one flight down.

Once the economies of scale became evident, the DMU's emergency room and operating rooms were closed. Inpatient admissions and educational opportunities dwindled following the loss of acute care and operative capability. As a result, the AMA and the AAMC

FIGURE 10-7. Sister Monica Rock was the DeGoesbriand's head operating room nurse for many years. Here, William Paganelli talks with a pediatric patient before inducing anesthesia.

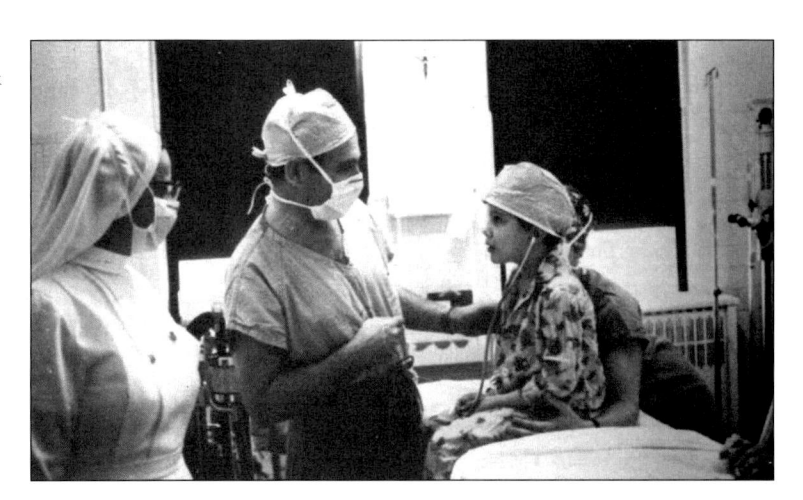

criticized the newly formed MCHV for its insufficient number of housestaff cases. Mackay's replacement was going to have his hands full from the start.

John Herschel Davis, Chairman for Rebirth

John Davis always wanted to be a surgeon. It was an interesting choice for a young man without any direct medical contacts (aside from a close friendship with the family physician's son) to make. Nevertheless, the southwestern Pennsylvania native liked to work with his hands, and he enjoyed cabinet making. After scoring well on a statewide high school merit examination, Davis received a full scholarship to Allegheny College, which he accepted without hesitation. His timing was fortuitous, as accelerated degrees were all the rage following the United States' entry into World War II. In fact, one of Davis' first professors at Allegheny recommended that he apply to medical school immediately. Davis took his advice, and was accepted by the School of Medicine at Western Reserve University "with the stipulation that he continue research in college."[4]

A year later, after learning that another friend had died while in the service, Davis left college and enlisted in the Army. Starting out as a private, he advanced rapidly, eventually becoming a drill sergeant in charge of training engineers. When the Army learned that Davis had already been accepted to medical school, it transferred him to a military hospital near Cleveland, and then discharged him a few months later. Davis thus started at Western Reserve in 1944, after attending only one year of college. He married his high school sweetheart, Peg, in 1946 and received his MD in 1948.[5]

Davis remained at Cleveland's University Hospital for his internship and surgery residency. While there, he studied under arterial injury and shock expert Fiorindo Simeone. Davis spent a year in the research lab sponsored by a grant from the U.S. Army Surgical Research Unit evaluating the role of antibiotics in wound infections. At the end of 1950, he was "asked" to go to the unit's headquarters, Brooke Army Medical Center at Fort Sam Houston, Texas, to pursue further investigations. Davis complied, rejoining the Army as a captain in the process. Following his arrival, he went to work in the Burns Study Program with future military surgeon Curtis P. Artz as his resident.[6]

The Korean War was in full swing at the time and casualties were mounting. Davis was sent to Korea with a research team to evaluate surgical care, and ended up with a Mobile Army Surgical Hospital (MASH). He treated renal failure caused by inappropriate volume resuscitation via the first war zone use of hemodialysis.

Davis was re-assigned to the Brooke Army Medical Center upon the completion of his Korean tour of duty. Curtis Artz, who had been his resident at Brooke, replaced him in Korea.[7] Later he reunited with Artz at Brooke. They quickly resumed burn care studies — a continued military concern in the era of the atomic bomb. Building on the principles of Davis' fluid resuscitation work in Korea, the group sought to improve the survival of the severely burned.[8] Their efforts led to the development of the Brooke Burn Formula (and its successor, the Modified Brooke Formula), which helped surgeons calculate the massive volumes of Ringer's lactate and plasma required for resuscitation after large burns.[9] This innovative formula has since stood the test of time.

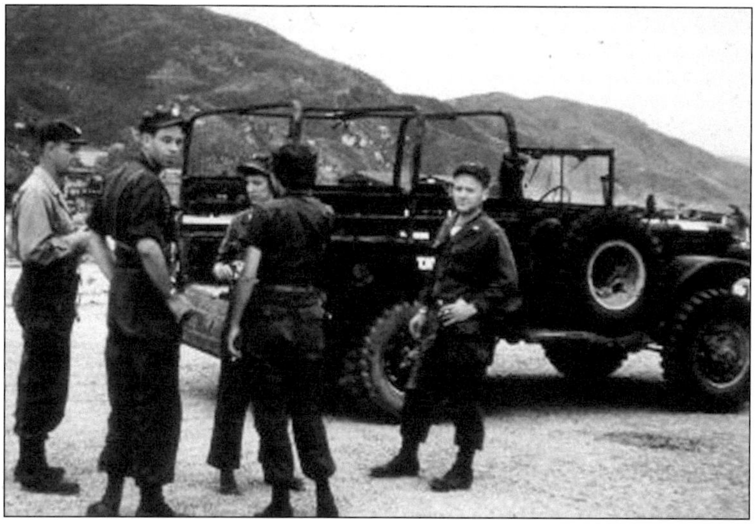

FIGURE 10-8.
A slim and trim John Davis (2nd from left) assigned to a MASH in Korea.

Davis returned to civilian life in Cleveland, finished his surgical residency, and in 1956, became an instructor at Western Reserve's medical school. He was rapidly promoted, and was eventually named Chief of Surgery at Cleveland Metropolitan General Hospital. Davis conducted research while engaging in his clinical duties, continuing to pursue his interests in metabolism, red blood cell physiology in disease, infection, trauma, vascular surgery, and burns.[10]

A Full-time Chief of Surgery Arrives From Out of State

The College of Medicine's Dean, Edward Andrews, approached Davis in 1968 to interview for UVM's Chief of Surgery position. Davis was not looking for a new job, but he was in need of a vacation, so he agreed to come to Vermont for an interview. Davis, his wife, and their three young daughters left for Burlington in mid-August. John Abajian, the Chief of Anesthesiology, picked them up at the airport and drove them down Spear Street "at 90 miles an hour" for a view of Lake Champlain. Upon checking into the Sheraton, the family found that the showers didn't work, so they improvised with a couple of pitchers of "ice water."

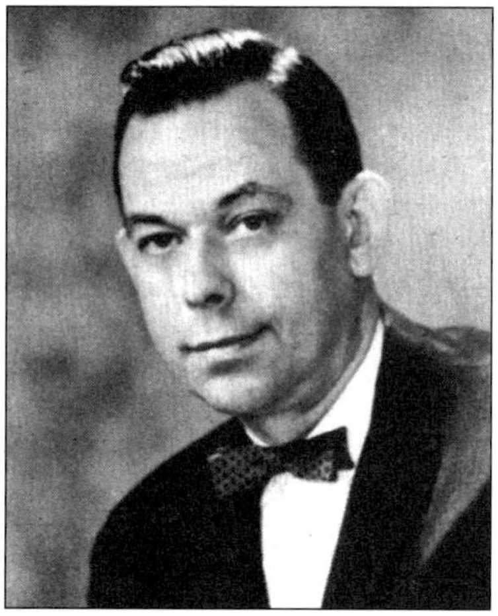

FIGURE 10-9.
Davis on the verge of making the move to UVM in 1968.

Matters didn't improve much at the restaurant. After everyone ordered lobster, the waitress informed the five of them that, "there are only two lobsters left." An hour went by without any further attention.[11]

In spite of the inauspicious start, the rest of the trip went well. Interviews were conducted over two days. Davis liked the faculty and the fact that they were trying new things. He came back (alone this time) for a second interview, feeling that he was the school's first choice for the chairmanship. Mackay told him, "I don't want to step down, but go ahead and I will support you to the fullest. If you'll take the job, I'll be happy."[12]

Davis became the Chief of Surgery on January 5, 1969. Although the surgical offices had been on the third floor of the old Fletcher House, Davis was given space in the College's brand-new Given Medical Building. The Department's research facilities were also moved — in this case from the basement of the Medical Alumni Building to the Given Building. In a more troubling move, Mackay's remaining full-time staff (with the exception of pediatric surgeon Paul Mellish) left for greener pastures.

Jerome Sanford Abrams, Vice Chair Complementary to Davis

Davis shored up the Department as quickly as possible. He called Jerry Abrams (who had been his vice-chairman at Cleveland) and offered him a similar position at UVM. Davis had known Abrams since 1958, first as a resident at University Hospitals of Cleveland, and then as a fellow instructor at Western Reserve. Abrams came for a visit, saw what UVM had to offer, and signed on. He arrived in June of 1969, and was placed in an office adjacent to Davis.[13]

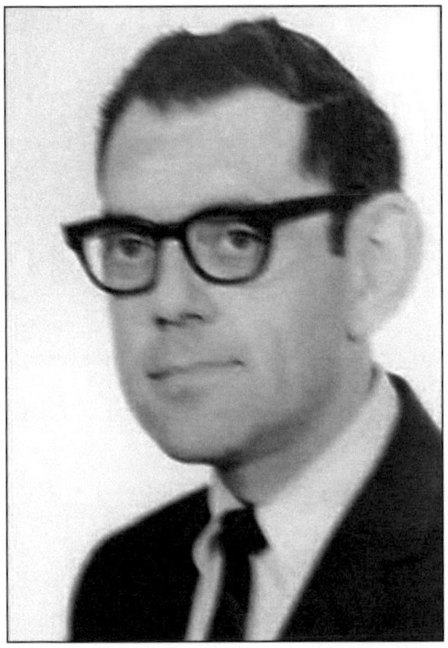

FIGURE 10-10. Jerome Abrams accompanied Davis from Cleveland as his right hand man and Vice Chair of surgery.

Abrams, a very diligent worker with a classic "Type A" personality, ran the academic and research functions of the Department. He was a firm taskmaster with high standards, and a fair and supportive boss overall. As such, everyone respected him. Davis positioned him as the Department's hard bargainer and expediter, while Davis himself maintained a more fatherly image.

Abrams channeled his clinical and research interests into improving the diagnosis and treatment of gastrointestinal disease.[14, 15] He recognized the need for improved colorectal surgery, especially with respect to inflammatory bowel disease.[16] Abrams also worked with the Vermont Chapter of the American College of Surgeons (ACS), and the Cancer Committee of the ACS to deliver better colon cancer care statewide.[17, 18, 19]

Ironically, years later, the hard working Abrams' own rectal bleeding was diagnosed too late. Davis resected the advanced rectal cancer and the piece of bladder it had invaded with considerable difficulty. Abrams' postoperative recovery was complicated by severe back pain. Initially felt to represent metastatic disease, it turned out to be the result of a paraspinal infection. Just when things started to look up, Abrams (a heavy smoker) suddenly succumbed from a ruptured ventricle, the after-effect of a heart attack suffered at the time of his operation.

Abrams' family and friends made contributions to the Department's library, which is still located in the old Fletcher House, and had it named in his honor. At first, a picture of a grinning, tuxedo-clad Abrams graced the room, keeping watch over those attending conferences and luncheons. A more refined portrait, placed during a 2005 remodeling, currently adorns the walls of the "Abrams Library."

Roger Sherman Foster, Oncologic Surgeon

Davis continued to expand the Department's core staff through his Cleveland connections. Roger Foster, a fellow alumnus of the Western Reserve Medical School, was the next to be

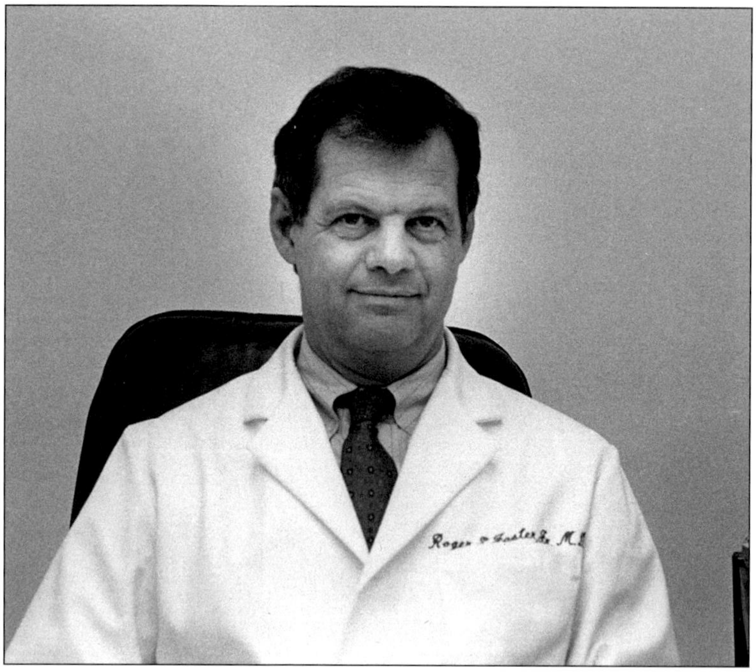

FIGURE 10-11. Roger Foster, UVM's first oncology-trained surgeon, was one of the initial members of the Davis team.

hired. Foster, like Abrams, had been a surgical resident at University Hospitals of Cleveland, and had considered Davis his most inspirational teacher at that program.[20] Foster went to Buffalo's Roswell Park Memorial Institute (today's Roswell Park Cancer Institute) in 1966 for a two-year surgical oncology fellowship. While there, he performed basic laboratory research on mouse bone marrow tissue cultures, which eventually led to the development of the white blood cell boosting compound Granulocyte Colony Stimulating Factor (GCSF).[21, 22]

Foster, like many other young doctors during the days of the Vietnam War, went into the Army. He ended up at Fort Irwin, a training and deployment base in the Mohave Desert. The Fort's light surgical schedule and remote location provided Foster with a chance to finish his research papers and gradually gain clinical confidence.[23]

As he neared the end of his time in the Service, Foster started to search for an academic surgical position. His options eventually came down to either Yale or UVM. Foster's ties to Davis ultimately drew him to Vermont, despite his wife's reservations about raising a family "on the frontier." The couple rented a lakeside camp during their first summer, which they shared with their giant Newfoundland dogs. The quantity and quality of dogs continued to

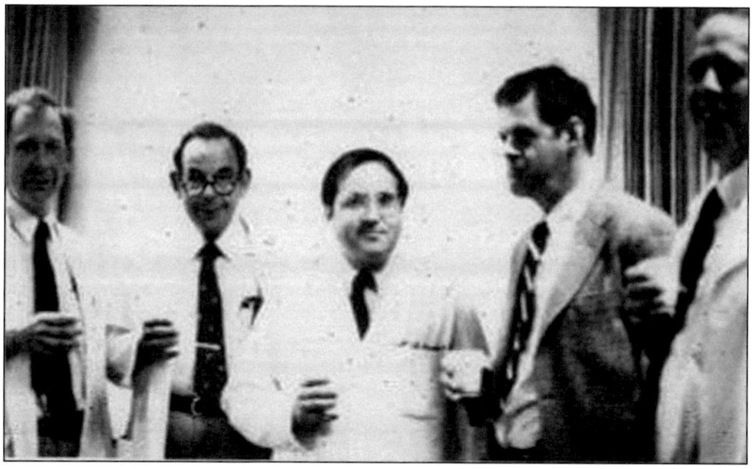

FIGURE 10-12. A few of the Surgical Associates in 1983 (left to right): Allen Browne, Davis, Gamelli, Foster, Pilcher.

152 CATAMOUNT SURGEONS

grow after the construction of a house and professional kennel deep in the woods of nearby Shelburne.[24] The family's subsequent Christmas cards seemed to show more dogs and more children each year.

Foster's overwhelming interest in cancer surgery had been influenced by his relationship with the Cleveland Clinic's George W. Crile, Jr., whose daughter Foster had married during medical school, and whose own father had co-founded the Clinic.[25] Crile, controversially, felt that certain cancers were systemic in nature, and that radical surgery alone was not the solution. Although Foster performed extensive cancer operations with great skill, he too believed that disease prevention and adjuvant therapy were important components of cancer treatment.[26]

Foster's research was centered on the early detection of cancer. He participated in the generation of randomized prospective data by enthusiastically contributing to the efforts of the National Surgical Adjuvant Breast Project.[27] Foster, in conjunction with Carleton Haines, also conducted a five-year study on Breast Self Examination (BSE) that showed a higher survival rate in women who performed BSE. Convinced beforehand that BSE was of no benefit, Foster became a convert when the data showed the opposite to be true.[28]

Foster continued his original bone marrow studies as well, timing chemotherapy doses to maximize toxicity against tumors while minimizing harm to normal cells.[29] He started UVM's kidney transplant program in 1971, partly because of the similarities he observed between the side effects of chemotherapy and rejection. In 1976, Foster became the director of the Vermont Regional Cancer Center, a clinic "without walls" that was one of the multidisciplinary approaches to the disease. It turned out to be a very time consuming position, one that subsequently led to a reduction of his basic research duties.[30]

David B. Pilcher, Vascular and Trauma Surgeon, Returns to Vermont

I (DBP) had often thought about practice opportunities during my UVM surgical residency, military service, and UCLA vascular fellowship. Commuting to Boston from suburbia didn't seem like a good idea. The final decision rested between practicing in an academic setting, UVM or Dartmouth; or working in a smaller community, such as Gloucester or Plymouth, Massachusetts. My father's example of being a city bachelor while the family summered on Cape Cod or in Vermont helped me make my choice. In Vermont the workplace

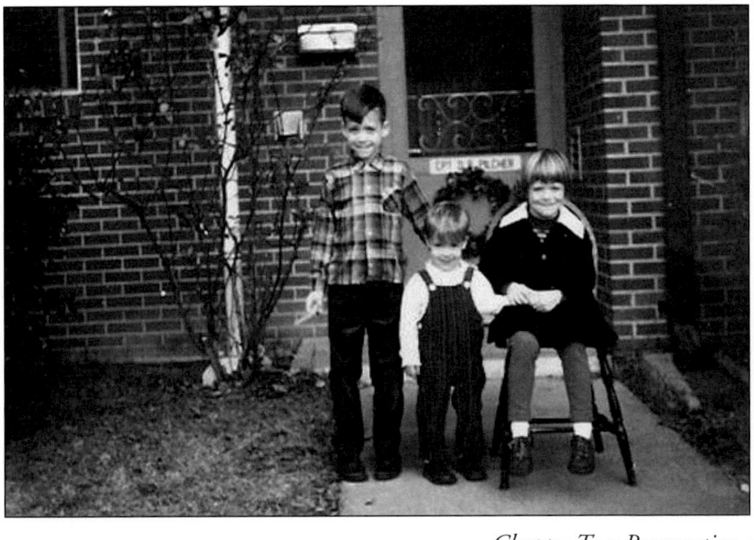

FIGURE 10-13. The author's children in Virginia in 1967 while I ponder options.

and the vacation spot could be the same.

Davis became UVM's chairman while I was finishing at UCLA. I interviewed with him in Cleveland, just before he made the move. I was hired soon thereafter at a salary of $18,000 a year. The deal included a leased car, which for my growing family turned out to be an Oldsmobile station wagon. I was provided with an office in the Given Building for research and academic pursuits, and separate clinical space to see patients. My military background led to my appointment as director of the emergency room, as well as practicing trauma, vascular, and general surgery.

Amalgamation Into a Full-time Group

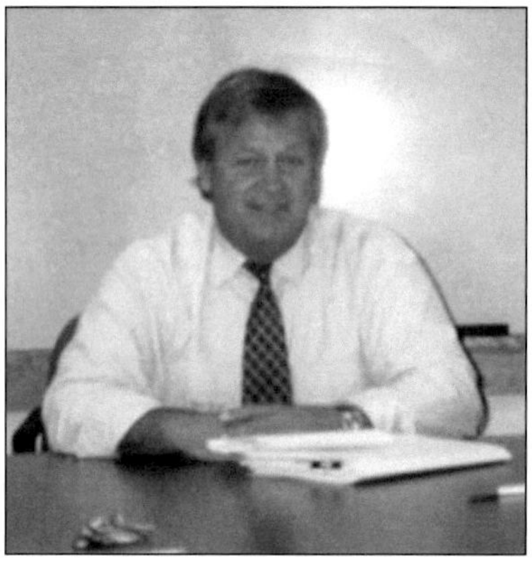

FIGURE 10-14. James Reuschel served as the Department of Surgery's administrator under both Mackay and Davis.

Davis realized that the best way to extend the Department's reach was to bring the rest of the region's surgeons into the fold. This would give the Department the means to control both its day-to-day management and its future expansion. Davis' business manager, Jim Reuschel, obtained tax returns from each of the city's surgeons. He and Davis made counter-offers that matched prior private practice incomes, added academic credentials, and provided fringe benefits. Individual's salaries were to remain stable as their productivity decreased with age. Under this plan, for senior members, the number of nights on-call was to diminish, allowing the quality of life to improve. Davis noted that, "Most of the surgeons, to my surprise, accepted the offer and we had a full time staff to provide clinical care, teaching and research."[31, 32]

By the end of 1970, almost every surgeon in Burlington had decided to join the venture. The ensuing group, "Surgical Associates Foundation," was organized as a tax-exempt corporation. Sacrifices were made for the sake of unity. Newcomers kept their accounts receivable and collected a salary from day one, even though some didn't live up to their end of the practice agreement. In the beginning, there was little evidence that the previous part-time faculty, who were now "full-time" faculty, changed their practice patterns, teaching, or research efforts. The bulk of teaching and research was left to the Department's original full-time staff.

Those of us without private practices set up shop at 96 Colchester Avenue. Mackay maintained his office and examining room at the front, along with his secretary Doris Bell. Gordon Page kept his tiny examining room across the hall. Mackay's back exam room was turned over to the rest of us. Patients were occasionally seen in Mackay's front examining room if he wasn't busy. A single secretary, sitting in a makeshift hallway office, assisted Davis, Abrams, Foster, Mellish, and me. I later had a small basement room renovated into my dedicated office with its own waiting area, desk, and examining room. It still amazes me that we tolerated such cramped conditions!

All professional fees were billed through Surgical Associates. Each surgeon received a clinical salary from the corporation, and a teaching salary from UVM. Surgical Associates essentially reimbursed the University for the University's portion of the surgeons' salaries. The University, for its part, provided the group with health care benefits and a tax-deferred savings account. The business plan provided everyone with a leased car, which at that time was still a legitimate expense. Oldsmobiles were the order of the day due to Mackay and Reuschel's longtime dealership connections. Mackay himself never wanted to drive anything that could be considered ostentatious by Vermont's standards.

When it came to salaries, the whole group put its faith in Davis. No one, to my knowledge, ever had a written contract. We got a letter from the Dean and Davis each year that outlined our annual remuneration — and that was it! There were allowances for books and travel. The travel budget was limited, but Davis liberalized it for those of us presenting papers at meetings or teaching postgraduate courses. The entire Department went to the ACS meetings. This was academically advantageous, but it left little surgical support in town. I remember flying out of Burlington one year at the crack of dawn, arriving in San Francisco just in time to give my presentation, and then immediately taking the red-eye back to Vermont in order to provide vascular and trauma coverage!

Our cramped, tight quarters were alleviated once the group moved to the DMU. Davis, Abrams, Foster, and I had academic space in the Given Building and clinical space at the DeGoesbriand. We were each entitled to one secretary, equal to the staffing that Gordon Page, Bishop McGill, Douglas McSweeney, Jay Keller, Nolan Cain, and William Shea kept in their old private practice offices. For example, I shared an academic secretary with one partner and a practice secretary with another. I later had a single secretary who spent half of her time at the Given Building and the other half at the DMU during office hours. Pamela Bizzozero and Marilyn Driscoll were the constants in our lives, as office locales and academic spaces varied.

FIGURE 10-15.

The Department of Surgery grew under John Davis through the formation of new divisions and the addition of community surgeons to the full-time group.

Top row (left to right): Howard Yeaton, James Hebert, Allen Browne, Henry Schmidek, Howard DeLozier, Alan Irwin, David Pilcher, Donald Miller, William Shea, Philip Aitken.

Bottom row (left to right): Roger Foster, Gordon Page, Kathleen McGuire, Richard Gamelli, Jay Keller, Martin Flanagan, John Davis, Jerome Abrams, Steven Wald, Nolan Cain, Bernard Barney, Martin Koplewitz.

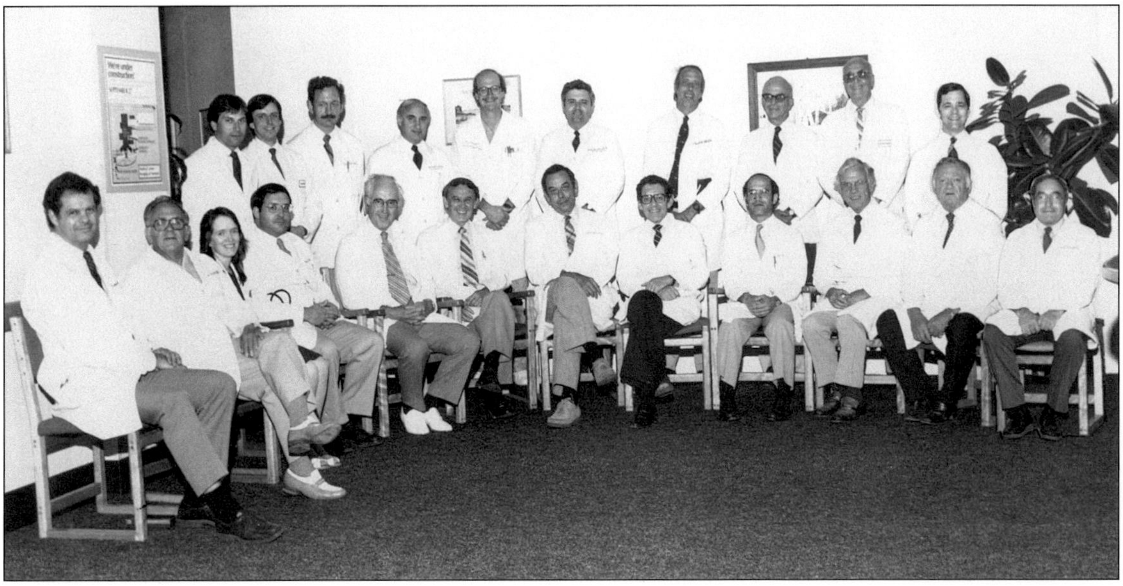

A group lunch was served every Friday in the Surgical Associates' conference room at the DeGoesbriand. The weekly meal — which always featured the same New England clam chowder — was later offered at the Given Building. Davis' successors have continued the tradition at the Abrams Library.

Davis ran Surgical Associates as a virtual monarchy, with input from Abrams and Reuschel. Most policies were decided in his Given Building office. The rest of the group gathered at the Shelburne Inn once a month after hours. Cocktails and a large shrimp bowl were usually presented beforehand. These business meetings, at which the predetermined policies were discussed and voted upon, followed the main meal. New ideas and suggestions were volunteered, but the policies themselves were rarely altered.

Davis' group brought in significant revenue, and because of this, contributed a large amount to the University and to research. In return, the Department of Surgery received about $300,000 from the medical school, which it used to support the faculty's base salaries. During the same time frame (early 1970s), the Department of Orthopaedic Surgery's budget was only around $60,000.[33]

The University Health Center

MCHV had also come under fire from the AMA and AAMC for its lack of adequate outpatient facilities. The College of Medicine needed to teach ambulatory care in a coordinated manner and have access to a sufficient number of clinical patients. Dean Andrews' successor, William Luginbuhl, asked Davis to tackle the issue. Drawing on the Surgical Associates business model, Davis convinced nine other specialty practice groups to join forces. The University Health Center (UHC) was launched in 1971, with Davis serving as CEO.[34]

By 1977, the DeGoesbriand was virtually empty, and the UHC practice group needed space. Davis recommended turning the DMU into an ambulatory facility, similar in concept to the Mayo Clinic. Davis and Dean Luginbuhl pitched the idea to MCHV Board of Trustees president Stuart "Red" Martin, and the board approved it. MCHV donated the building to UVM, but the University "wouldn't put a cent into it." UHC paid for the $12 million renovation with a $1.2 million grant from the Given Foundation and six different twenty-year loans. The UHC physicians were to pay the loans back with "rental" income generated from each specialty.[35] The University would then own the building when the loans were finally paid off twenty years later.[36]

Davis's original proposal included an adjacent parking garage with a motel on the top to attract and accommodate out-of-town patients and their families. The Airport Parking Corporation of America agreed to build the complex and a connecting skyway at no cost to MCHV if it could collect and keep all parking fees. UVM allegedly "put the squash on it as competing with downtown parking." UHC was subsequently hampered by a lack of adequate parking space for the next twenty-five years.[37]

The New Fanny Allen Hospital

Even though the Diocese of Burlington owned it, the Fanny Allen (FAH) did not enter into the affiliation between Burlington's hospitals. The Diocese did not want to bring the ancient facility, which was still run under the auspices of the Religious Hospitallers of St. Joseph (RHSJ) up to code. The RHSJ pointed out that the Diocese had to invest something, as it owed them seventy years' of compensation for their services. Realizing that the Sisters had made a valid point, the Diocese agreed to transfer the hospital to the nuns.[38]

The RHSJ quickly raised over a million dollars in private funds for a new building. Former Burlington mayor C. Douglas Cairns, who had once received life-saving care from Albert Crandall for a bleeding esophagus, greatly assisted in this endeavor. A modern, two-story structure containing Intensive and Cardiac Care Units opened in 1968. An Emergency Room and surgical wing followed suit five years later.[39] It seemed as if the DeGoesbriand had moved across town to the site of the Fanny Allen!

Surgical conditions improved in another major way. Louis Thabault, as Chief of Surgery at the Fanny Allen Hospital, had always had strained relations with Mackay. Thabault's brother recalled that:

"When Davis came on the scene in the late sixties as Chairman of the Department of Surgery at the University of Vermont as well as Chief of Surgery at the Medical Center, it was a great source of aid to Louie to be able to dialogue with a person along the lines of caring for the sick and leaving politics behind. From that day on for the rest of his remaining years as Chief of Surgery [at the Fanny Allen Hospital], the relationship between what was now referred to as the Medical Center, and not the Mary Fletcher, was a most amiable one." [40]

Davis expanded the residency program, placing an intern and a third year resident at the hospital. David Browdie, whom Davis had brought from Cleveland, became the Fanny Allen's first such trainee. Since there were no orthopedic or gynecologic residents at the hospital, the surgical resident experience in these two disciplines was substantial. The senior surgical resident assigned to the Fanny Allen Hospital was always on call, but could go home if things were quiet.

In 1973, former College of Medicine student and MCHV surgical resident Donald Majercik started a private practice in Essex Junction. Davis tried to dissuade him, but Thabault, Bunker, and McSweeney encouraged the move. Their advice proved sound, as Majercik soon became the Fanny Allen's busiest surgeon.

Thabault died unexpectedly in 1974. A life-size portrait was hung in the hallway leading to the Operating Rooms to remind the surgeons and staff of his accomplishments as they entered the surgical stage. In order to avoid a conflict of interest, Clarence Bunker left Surgical Associates and supplanted Thabault as the Fanny Allen's chief.[41] His resignation from the full time group helped smooth the way, and make him more acceptable to the Fanny Allen staff, some of whom still perceived a strained relationship with the Burlington hospitals.

In 1984, chief resident Tom Schwarcz was helping Majercik with a presumptive bowel obstruction. Upon opening the peritoneum, their charge was found to have a ruptured retroperitoneal abdominal aortic aneurysm. Being the on-call vascular surgeon, I was summoned to the scene. Closing the abdomen and transferring the patient was impossible, so we repaired the aneurysm using the few vascular instruments on hand. The Fanny Allen didn't have an adequate surgical ICU, so we sent the intubated individual to MCHV for his post-op care. The MCHV resident thus inherited the patient without having done the case. This made for some loud complaining about itinerant surgery.

Pagers and the Answering Service

The Mary Fletcher Hospital's switchboard was located in the front lobby during the 1960s. Doctors checked in as they came and went. The operators knew the physicians by sight, and how to reach them. Loudspeakers throughout the hospital loudly "paged" doctors on a frequent basis. The chief operator, Mary Crowley, was a fountain of knowledge about all that went on in the medical community. When mobile pagers came into being, the telephone switchboard was banished to the basement of the Smith wing. The paging station, meanwhile, moved to the basement of Gladstone's South Willard Street office. Mary left the hospital to become Gladstone's lead paging operator.

Two-way pagers were available, but they were as large as a carton of cigarettes and weighed over five pounds. Messages came through a speaker that broadcast the emergency to all within earshot. McGill, McSweeney, and orthopedist Philip Davis bought a transmitter for their own use in 1964, and had it placed atop the Mary Fletcher's roof. They identified each other as Blue Mobile (McGill doing general surgery), Red Mobile (McSweeney, who did some vascular surgery), and White Mobile (P. Davis, who did hand surgery.) McGill turned his radio pager over to the ski patrol whenever he hit the slopes at Stowe, thus leaving his fellow patrolmen to find him in the event of a Burlington emergency.

Gladstone's paging service grew and prospered as advances in technology led to smaller, more confidential units (although the afore-mentioned color mobiles maintained their independence.) In an unwritten rule that continues to the present, residents were not bothered at home if they were not on call. Not so for the attendings. During the early years of the service, the attending of record was called for any patient problem. The actual on-call surgeon was contacted only if the attending of record was unreachable.

Koplewitz Emigrates From St. Albans to Burlington

Martin J. Koplewitz took a tortuous route in order to join UVM's faculty. The Far Rockaway, New York native and child of the Depression was accepted to the College of Medicine in 1948. He graduated planning on a career in anything but surgery. He changed his mind during his internship, however, after rotating on the surgical service at Boston's Beth Israel Hospital. Koplewitz started a surgical residency at Brooklyn's Maimonides Hospital, but was drafted during the Korean conflict. After spending 1954-56 in Spokane as an Air Force surgeon, he finally finished his residency at UVM in 1959.

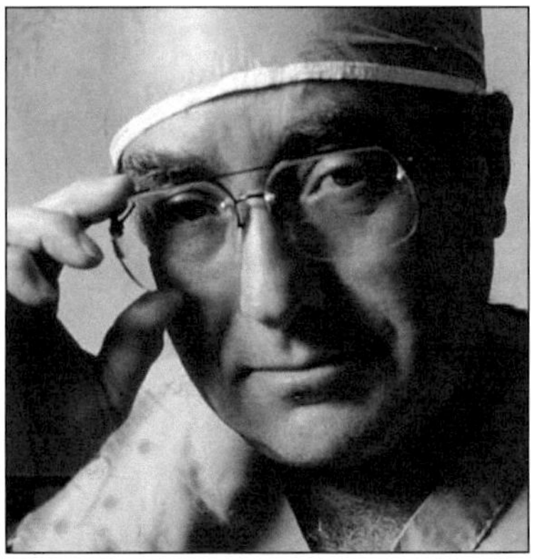

FIGURE 10-16. Martin Koplewitz, in 1983.

Koplewitz wanted to stay in Burlington, but Mackay told him there was no room, as he felt there were already too many surgeons in town. Koplewitz tried practicing in Long Island, but was disillusioned by the medical environment there. Koplewitz looked at Middlebury, where early UVM resident Ray Collins had a surgical monopoly, but determined that there wasn't enough room for both of them. Mackay suggested St. Albans, where Koplewitz was welcomed with open arms. Within two years, he was the busiest surgeon in that town.

By 1970, Koplewitz decided that he had to come to Burlington for the sake of his children's education and his wife's graduate classes. Davis had supplanted Mackay as Chief, but still told Koplewitz that he wasn't needed. Gladstone offered Koplewitz a partnership, and before long the "unneeded" surgeon had a huge practice. Koplewitz opened an office in South Burlington's Aesculapius medical center the next year, which was surrounded by referring internists. Davis offered him a Surgical Associates partnership in 1973, and Koplewitz was fully accepted.[42]

Moonlight(ing) in Vermont and Other Tales of Residency

Surgical residents supplemented their income during the Mackay and early Davis years by moonlighting at neighboring emergency rooms. This was most prevalent at Ticonderoga's Moses-Ludington Hospital on account of Shea's outreach program there. Unfortunately, a sleep-deprived resident got into a bad automobile accident on his way back from Ticonderoga in 1970 and ended up with a serious head injury. While recuperating, the resident was visited by one of the attendings. He asked the attending (in all seriousness) to taste his apple juice — which was really a cup of urine. Needless to say, the resident underwent further recuperation before resuming his patient care duties and the practice of moonlighting was put to an end.

Residents were still given a certain degree of latitude as their training came to a close. Former resident Monica Morrow told the following story about Davis:

"I was awakened as a surgical Chief Resident one day by the sun streaming into my face. Now everyone knows something is dreadfully wrong if a surgical resident is still in bed when the sun is up. I looked at my clock to see with horror it was 8:30. I was supposed to be in a case with Dr. Davis, and feared my junior resident might have seized the opportunity to replace me doing the case. I called in to the O.R. to find that no one was helping Dr. Davis, who had started the case alone. So for the first time I could remember, I jumped out of bed and hurried to the O.R. without a shower or makeup, most uncharacteristic for me. Dr. Davis said "good morning" and "overslept did you?" and we proceeded to do the case as if nothing was unusual. That night at 9 pm, I received a call from Dr. Davis at home. He said I should turn my clock around and pull out the little white button in back to turn ON the alarm. The episode was never again mentioned."[43]

Residents received attending support on other fronts. Frank Ittleman remembers a DeGoesbriand-based patient Koplewitz had who went into shock following a colon resection. Koplewitz, meanwhile, was busy operating up the road at the Mary Fletcher:

"When [Koplewitz] was informed of this unexpected turn of events, he suggested we contact Dr. Page for assistance. Dr. Page was at home soaking a sore knee in the bathtub.

Though physically indisposed he rose, dressed, and was in the Operating Room in the blink of an eye. With Dr. Moore and me assisting as residents, Dr. Page instructed the scrub nurse (whom he affectionately called "nursey") to keep the needle holders loaded with heavy catgut and the instrument table piled high with sponges. With Gordie maintaining a steady stream of encouragement, the sponges flew in and out of the abdomen with lightning speed. Many settled like parachutes on the floor of the Operating Room. Before I had time to take a deep breath, the middle colic artery was ligated with heavy catgut and Gordie was back to his lukewarm bathtub. My only comment to Dr. Moore was, "Who was that masked man?" [44]

During the Davis years, I (DBP) invited the entire surgical housestaff and a few of the attendings to lakeside picnics at my summer camp. Sailing, water skiing, and power surfing (standing on a sailboard while being towed behind a motor boat) were popular pastimes. We usually finished the day with hand-churned ice cream topped with homemade maple syrup. The gatherings were thrown on consecutive Saturdays so that those on call the first weekend could attend the following weekend. One year, resident Gene Moore held an overnight pig roast on the wooded part of my property. Attendings, including myself, were NOT invited. The pig roasters obtained their privacy — along with several cases of poison ivy.

The residents often conducted a different kind of "roast" at their formal graduation celebration, usually taking the opportunity to lampoon the faculty. In 1976, Moore and his fellow Chief Residents, Jim Linta and David Coletti, instituted the Teacher of the Year Award in recognition of an outstanding surgical mentor. As the first recipient of this award I (DBP), as well as subsequent faculty so honored, were extremely gratified.

The Journal of Trauma and Additional Research Come to UVM

Davis, with his interest in burns and infections, had joined the American Association for the Surgery of Trauma (AAST) in 1960. Following in the footsteps of his friend and former resident Curtis Artz, he was named the Association's president for 1975. Davis also became editor-in-chief of the AAST's official publication, the Journal of Trauma, the same year.[45] For 25 years, the journal was edited from the corner office — UVM's version of the U.S. President's Oval Office. The AAST gave Davis a small stipend for his efforts, which he applied toward the salary of his editorial assistant, Joan Young. Davis used his own UVM salary and office space for all other Journal business. The Journal was prepared to pay him an editorial salary, but for some reason Davis never took it.

Abrams and I were appointed associate editors. The three of us reviewed submitted manuscripts until Abrams' death in 1985. Davis and I then divided the manuscripts fifty-fifty, before sending them on to the final reviewers. Many manuscripts didn't pass our initial screening and were summarily rejected without further consideration. The Journal of Trauma flourished with Davis as its editor, and he maintained its national prominence in the field during his stewardship.

Unfortunately, Davis' prior laboratory studies did not continue to receive funding after he came to Burlington. A well-financed research project was, however, developed in 1977 by new recruit James Coil, one of Davis' last Cleveland residents. For years, splenic rupture was treated with splenectomy to prevent exsanguinating hemorrhage. It was thought to be without consequence to the future health of the patient. But in the 1970s, increasing episodes of late death from overwhelming pneumococcal sepsis were observed.

Coil, teaming with UVM pediatrician Joseph Dickerman, investigated the effects of pneumococcal pneumonia on splenectomized mice.[46] The duo's grant money was used to purchase an enormous centrifuge capable of infecting hundreds of mice at a time. The machine (which still lurks in the bowels of the Given Building) provided the Department with a unique, rapidly employable model that was the envy of other investigators. The post-splenectomy pneumococcal sepsis project proved to be more durable than Coil's presence at UVM. Coil left for Marshall University in 1980, became Vice Chairman at SUNY Brooklyn in the late '90s, and eventually settled down in Phoenix.[47]

Richard L. Gamelli Joins the UVM Surgery Staff

The newly united Department of Surgery underwrote a modest amount of research with its own meager clinical funds. Residents did some of this work in conjunction with the established attendings. One such resident was Richard L. Gamelli. The Agawam, Massachusetts native had graduated from the College of Medicine in 1974, and then finished his MCHV internship and residency in 1979. Upon joining the staff, he quickly became a major force in the Davis inner circle.[48]

Gamelli assumed a great deal of administrative responsibility, and spearheaded efforts to study the infectious and nutritional aspects of burn care, the role of granulocyte colony-stimulating factor (GCSF) in burns, chemotherapy, pneumococcal sepsis, and the utility of bariatric surgery.[49] He became the leader of the unofficial, but functional Trauma Division in the early 1980s. This division became a model for clinical teaching at UVM. Gamelli was named Vice Chairman of the Department in the wake of Abrams' illness and fatal heart attack.

James C. Hebert Continues Research and Becomes the Surgeon for All Jobs

Another research resident turned attending was James C. Hebert. The Waterville, Maine native had become interested in medicine at the age of ten when, during a hospitalization following an accident, he was cared for by a doctor that happened to be the father of one his friends. Hebert attended Holy Cross College, and then matriculated at the College of Medicine with the class of 1977. He paid in-state tuition as a Maine contract student, and received a need-based scholarship due to his family's limited financial resources. The two provisions significantly reduced his education costs.

Davis had initiated a Senior Major Project for each medical student. Hebert worked on his senior major project in Coil's lab. He demonstrated, for the first time in the pneumococcal pneumonia model, that diabetic mice had an increased susceptibility to pneumococcal infection. The work was published in the Journal of Surgical Research.[50] Hebert stayed at UVM for his surgical residency, and then joined the faculty in 1982. He has since carried out additional post-splenectomy studies over the ensuing decades.[51, 52]

Hebert and Gamelli were among the second generation of "new" faculty under Davis. Hebert was a jack-of-all-trades, and a master of many. He never refused an assignment. He was a stalwart for colorectal surgery, trauma surgery, and laparoscopic surgery, and a ready fill-in for pediatric surgery when needed. In order to allow time for research, Abrams initially let Hebert only take pediatric surgery call. This didn't work out well, so Hebert soon found himself on the general surgery coverage schedule. His string of legendary, bad on-call experiences started his very first day — the day of the Vermont Amtrak disaster.

Hebert, having been trained by Abrams, became the go-to colonoscopist in the 1980s. He became a skillful upper endoscopist after a mini-sabbatical at the MGH. His interest in the upper GI tract led to expertise with complicated biliary and pancreatic surgery. Hebert was the region's Whipple expert for many years. He stayed on during the Shackford years, succeeding Gamelli as Director of the Surgical Residency Training Program. He subsequently served as the Associate Dean for Graduate Medical Education for eight years, and the Chairman of the Division of General Surgery for six years. Under Hebert's watch, each general surgeon gained special competency in specific realms of procedures.

Hebert was UVM's representative to the Accreditation Council for Graduate Medical Education, the Residency Review Committee, the National Board of Medical Examiners, and the American Board of Surgery. In 2000, the New England Surgical Society decided that a surgical history of each member state should be presented at the annual fall meeting. The request came just four months before the event. In typical fashion, Hebert accepted the challenge, and prepared an excellent history of surgery in the State of Vermont. This was presented at the NESS meeting, published in the Archives of Surgery, and later placed on the UVM surgery Web site.[53]

A Resident's View of Training in the 1980s at UVM

Stephen Payne, now practicing in St. Albans, recalled his days as a resident at UVM under Davis and his staff:

"Resident training in the 80s was filled with clinical and operative experience. We usually took call every third night and averaged about 110 hours a week in the hospital including

FIGURE 10-17. G-4 surgery resident Stephen Payne, nephew of UVM surgeon Bishop McGill. Payne practices in St. Albans, and is the author of an extensive number of short stories.

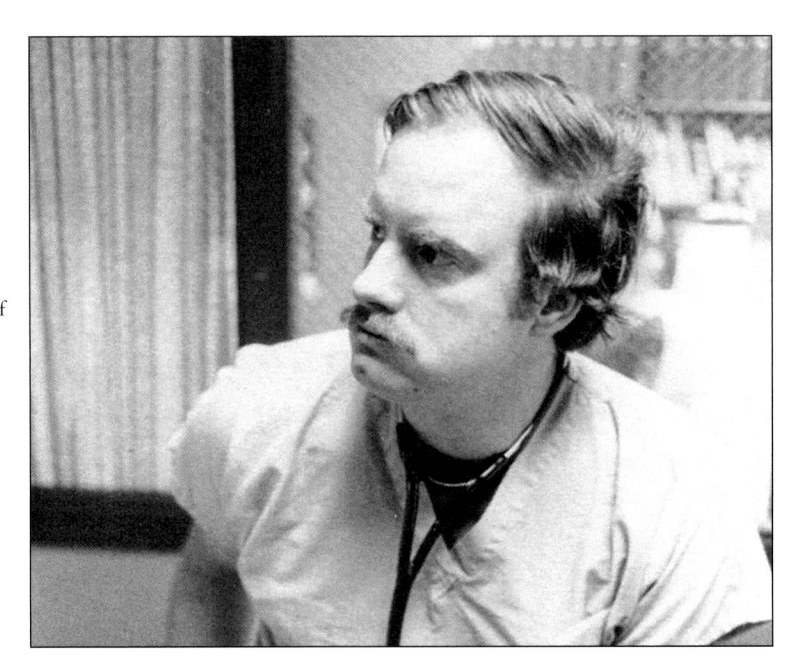

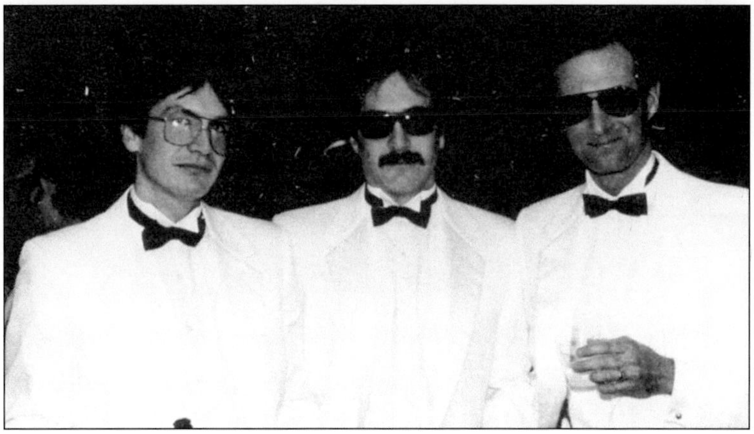

FIGURE 10-18. Ittleman was reported to hold Miami Vice parties with the residents. Here he is joined by William Cioffi (left), and Jeff Kaplan (middle).

call. When I graduated in 1988 I had over 1200 cases in my logbook. This tremendous hands-on experience prepared us for a comfortable transition into practice as attendings. Spending that much time "in the Zoo", as we often said, fostered a close relationship between many residents and attendings who, remarkably, attended every single surgery that we did. There was a great balance to the faculty from the revered father figure/master surgeon Davis to the tremendous in-the-trenches-with-us teaching of Gamelli, Hebert, Koplewitz, Page, Pilcher and many others. Abrams pushed us especially hard academically, smiling and looking sternly at us seemingly all at the same time. We were cajoled and comforted by DeMeules, and Haines, while Coffin tried, usually without success, to teach us about classical music which filled the room while opening the chest with him on a CABG. McSweeney also did a lot of teaching then, holding Saturday morning teaching rounds at the blackboard in the Fanny Allen locker room.

One of the kindest and hardest working attendings was Frank Ittleman. He would sidle up to you around dinner time when your eyes were starting to get blurry and gently ask you if you'd do yet another heart with him, which was often his third and sometimes the fourth of the day! He would often have hot pizza delivered to the ICU and we would enthusiastically watch episodes of Miami Vice together on some intubated patient's TV. One of my favorite memories was a Miami Vice party Frank held at his new house in Shelburne. He and Bill Cioffi put it together and we all dressed up like Sonny Crockett, ate a great dinner, drank lots of beer and then watched the show together.

Journal Club rotated from one attending's house to another on a monthly basis. The much-anticipated July meeting always being held at McGill's house on East Avenue. The literary part of the evening always seemed to be cut short as we soon found ourselves abandoning the discussion for a little R & R in his pool.

Sometimes we got to know attendings in unexpected ways. When I was an intern at the DeGoesbriand with Bill Cioffi as my G-2, we were doing a case with Page very early one morning when he suddenly became ill, fell back from the table and had to be taken to the ER at the Mary Fletcher. Bill and I started an IV and attended to him and to the patient. The only thing Page said as they wheeled him out was: "You boys finish up, now, won't you?" We finished the case, Page fully recovered, and then one day he called Cioffi and me and said he'd cleared us for an afternoon off with Davis, to thank us for taking care of him. With excitement and a bit of trepidation, as we never "took an afternoon off," Page picked us up

FIGURE 10-19. Richard Gamelli essentially became the Department's Vice Chair after Jerry Abrams' untimely death, while still pursuing his significant research initiatives.

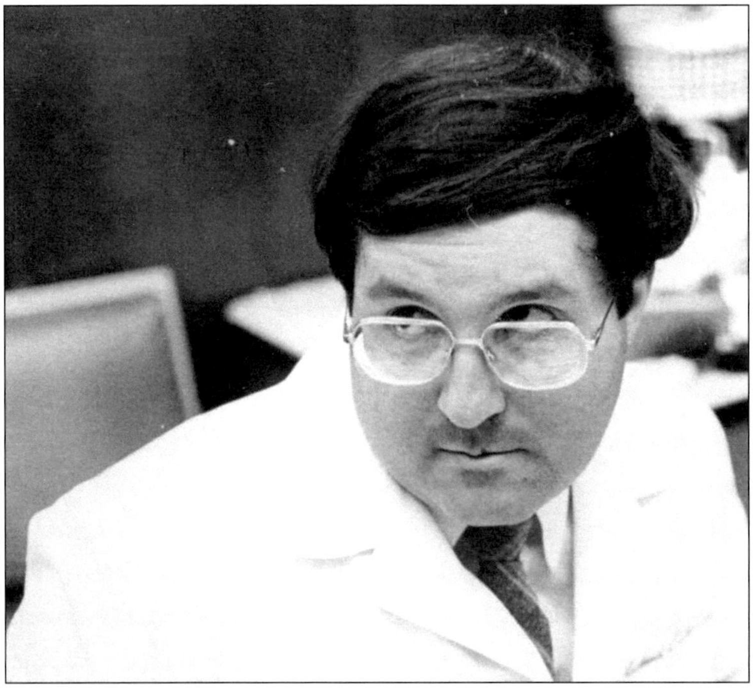

in front of the hospital in his 1968 Oldsmobile Cutlass Supreme four barrel convertible, and actually let us drive his dream machine around town, on our way to an elegant lunch at the exclusive Ethan Allen Club. It was very thoughtful and a lot of fun and I assure you none of us returned to duty till the next day!

Research was largely done on your own time though we were afforded four months in the laboratory in our G-4 year during which we were off service, but took call at night for pediatric surgery, and covered vacations.

Finally, I have to say a few words about the author of this book, mentor and friend. Dr. Pilcher, now retired after nearly four decades with the department, who not only taught us vascular and trauma surgery, but also was a constant source of encouragement and camaraderie. We crewed for him at the Thursday night J-24 races on Mallett's Bay. We watched him cheer up patients by bringing them fresh orchids from his own greenhouse. We learned from his wonderful humanity and humor as evidenced by the little Geo Metro convertible he drove to work, onto which he had glued Jaguar nameplates. I still laugh thinking of the team doing an aortic aneurysm case and Pilcher asking nurse Eunice Pasho for some stitch he'd never used before. To her frustrated expression he would usually reply: "Eunice, we always do it the same way ... except when we don't!" I've borrowed that line many times over the years." [54]

Paralysis Strikes the Chief of Surgery

The AAST held its 1986 meeting in Hawaii. Davis rarely took an out of town vacation, so he used the opportunity to spend some time with his family. He was in peak form during the meeting, both as the Association's past president and the Journal of Trauma's respected editor. His staff, residents, and past residents presented many of the meeting's most important papers. One evening, Davis wowed everyone by hitting the dance floor and dancing a

Jitterbug with his wife Peg. He chaired the Journal's editorial board meeting the following day, vacationed in Maui, and then flew back home to Vermont.

Two weeks after returning to Vermont, he performed what was to be his last surgery, a carotid endarterectomy. He noticed that his right great toe was a little numb. He couldn't figure out why this should be. As he walked down the hill to his office, he noticed his right leg was acting funny. "It didn't act like it recognized me." He called his internist, Henry Tufo, who examined him and announced that Davis was coming down with Guillian-Barré syndrome, and sent him home. A neurologist then examined him at home and concurred with the diagnosis of Guillian-Barré, adding that Davis would be well in eight to ten days.

The following morning, Davis had breakfast. Planning to go to the hospital, he stood up at the kitchen table and promptly fell flat on his face. "I lost both legs." He managed to crawl back to bed and call an ambulance. He was admitted to MCHV thinking that his condition was still temporary. He became discouraged when there was no improvement after seven days, and feared that his paralysis was permanent. "But you can't hope but think maybe with me it'll reverse and I'll be all right."[55]

FIGURE 10-20.
Davis came to his office on a regular basis despite being confined to a wheelchair with T-6 paraplegia. Secretary Ruth Gilbert helped him carry on as Chief.

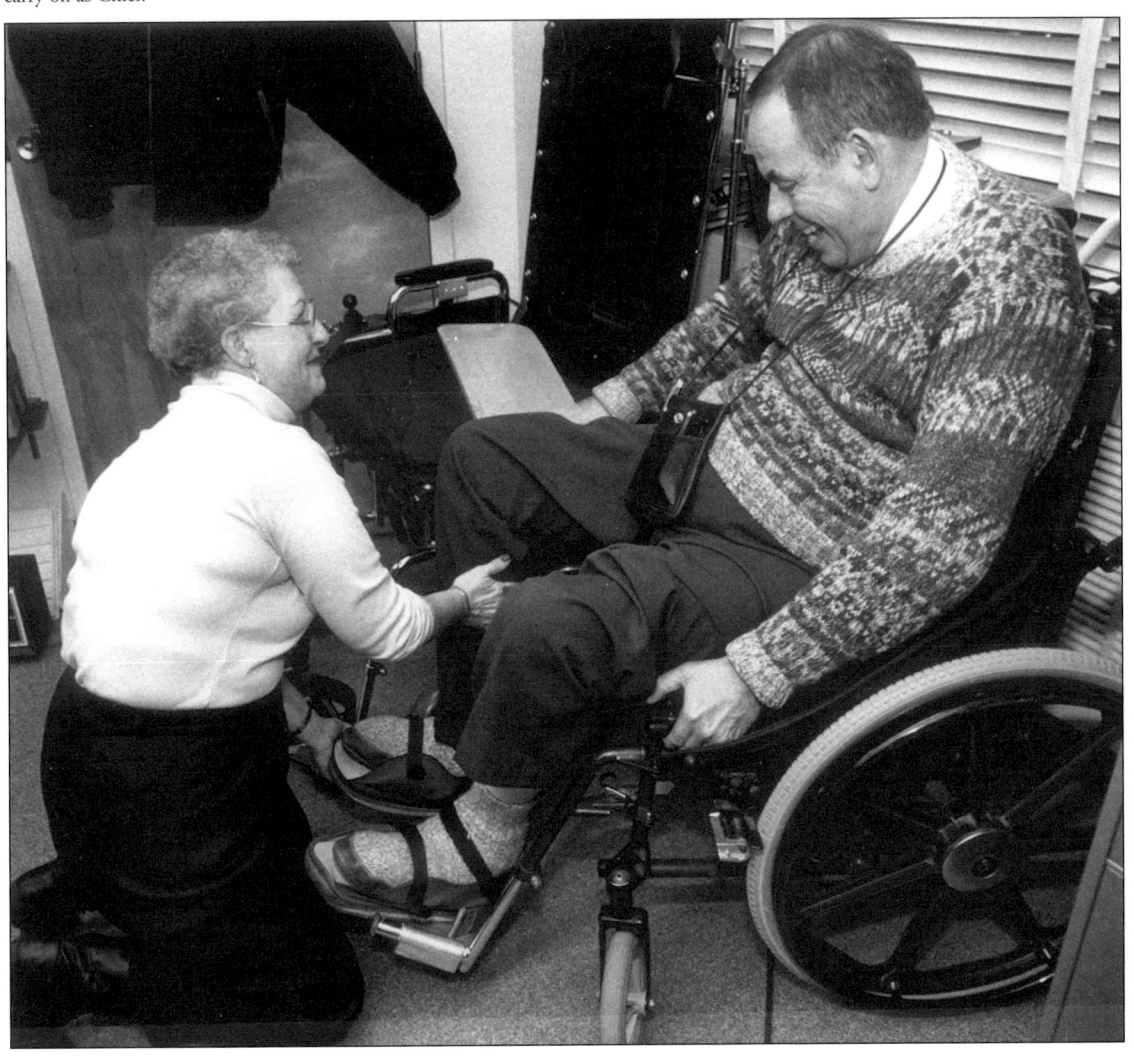

His symptoms were also suggestive of encephalitis, since he was easily fatigued and unable to think clearly. Later, as that component cleared, Davis' belief that his paralysis might eventually improve delayed his rehabilitation efforts. He subsequently developed bilateral heel ulcers and sacral decubiti. Being over 60 didn't help.

Davis eventually left the acute rehab unit and returned home. His wife and youngest daughter provided much of his daily care. His basement office was moved to the first floor. A stair-lift was installed that provided access to the greenhouse and woodshop, but it was rarely used. The family's van was equipped so that Davis could drive it from his wheelchair, but this was not utilized either. A ramp with raised flowerbeds was built outdoors by the Department's residents and attendings so that he could at least enjoy his passion for gardening.

Although these endeavors failed, Davis' outpatient rehabilitation proceeded as scheduled. He remained ensconced as the Department's Chairman, MCHV's Chief of Surgery, and UHC's Chief Executive Officer. Gamelli (who had succeeded Abrams as Vice Chairman) became MCHV's acting Chief of Surgery in all but title. Foster filled the gaps as needed. James Reuschel, the Department's longstanding business manager and treasurer, continued as UHC's administrator and treasurer, and took up additional slack. Editorial assistant Joan Young kept the Journal of Trauma running smoothly, just as she always had, and I temporarily assumed the role of de-facto editor-in-chief.

At the time of his illness, Davis was in the final stages of assembling his magnum opus — a comprehensive new surgical textbook that utilized the Problem-Based Learning approach to medicine. The book was eventually published through the efforts of Foster, his wife Joan, and Gamelli.[56] Davis' out of town associate editors helped, but Foster and Gamelli did the lion's share of the work. The two spent many an evening editing and rewriting material.

Davis continued to travel to national meetings, accompanied by an entourage of family and associates to help him navigate the mazes of less than accessible airports and hotel rooms. Even with all of this help, air travel was a chore that put stress on Davis' decubiti and interrupted his carefully orchestrated routines. Eventually, septic episodes and a fractured femur

FIGURE 10-21. Davis still conducted teaching rounds with the students after his paralysis. The sessions were extremely popular, and were at one point conducted from his home bed after he developed a decubitus ulcer.

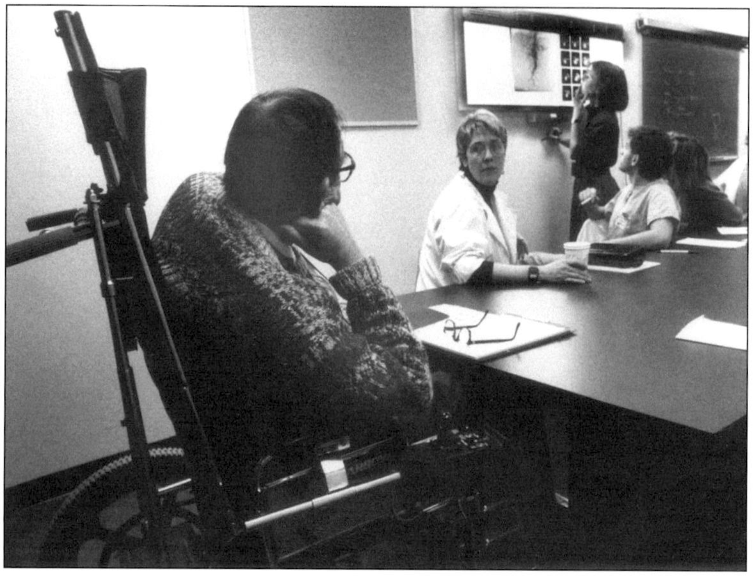

incurred during a lift by trained ambulance personnel put an end to out of town travel. Davis successfully used his own van to attend the annual lectureship endowed in his honor. These were held in the Davis Auditorium, which adjoined the new ambulatory care facility and had been generously named in his honor by the medical staff and his surgical colleagues.

It became obvious after two years that Davis, now unable to operate or even provide patient care, could not continue as an effective Chief of Surgery. And, despite all of the help, he was equally overextended as Department Chairman and UHC CEO. The Department shifted its Thursday Grand Rounds from 7:30 in the morning to 4:00 in the afternoon so that Davis could be present. Unfortunately, attendance was abysmal, since many surgeons were otherwise occupied with cases or clinics at that time of day. Even worse, the residents and attendings that did show up frequently dozed off. Yet another good idea that ultimately failed!

Davis' ability to effectively manage the UHC practice group was also called into question. The issue simmered for a while until Dean Luginbuhl abruptly announced that he was going to replace Davis. It fell to Page to go over to Davis' house and tell him that he had been removed from the position.

While Davis — relieved of his duties at MCHV and UHC — continued as the Department's Chairman, the search for his successor as Chief of Surgery at UVM and MCHV got underway. A number of surgeons from UVM's staff and greater New England's academic medical centers were seriously considered. It appeared that an experienced candidate with Davis' educational, clinical, managerial, and interpersonal skills was going to be hard to find.

PART VI

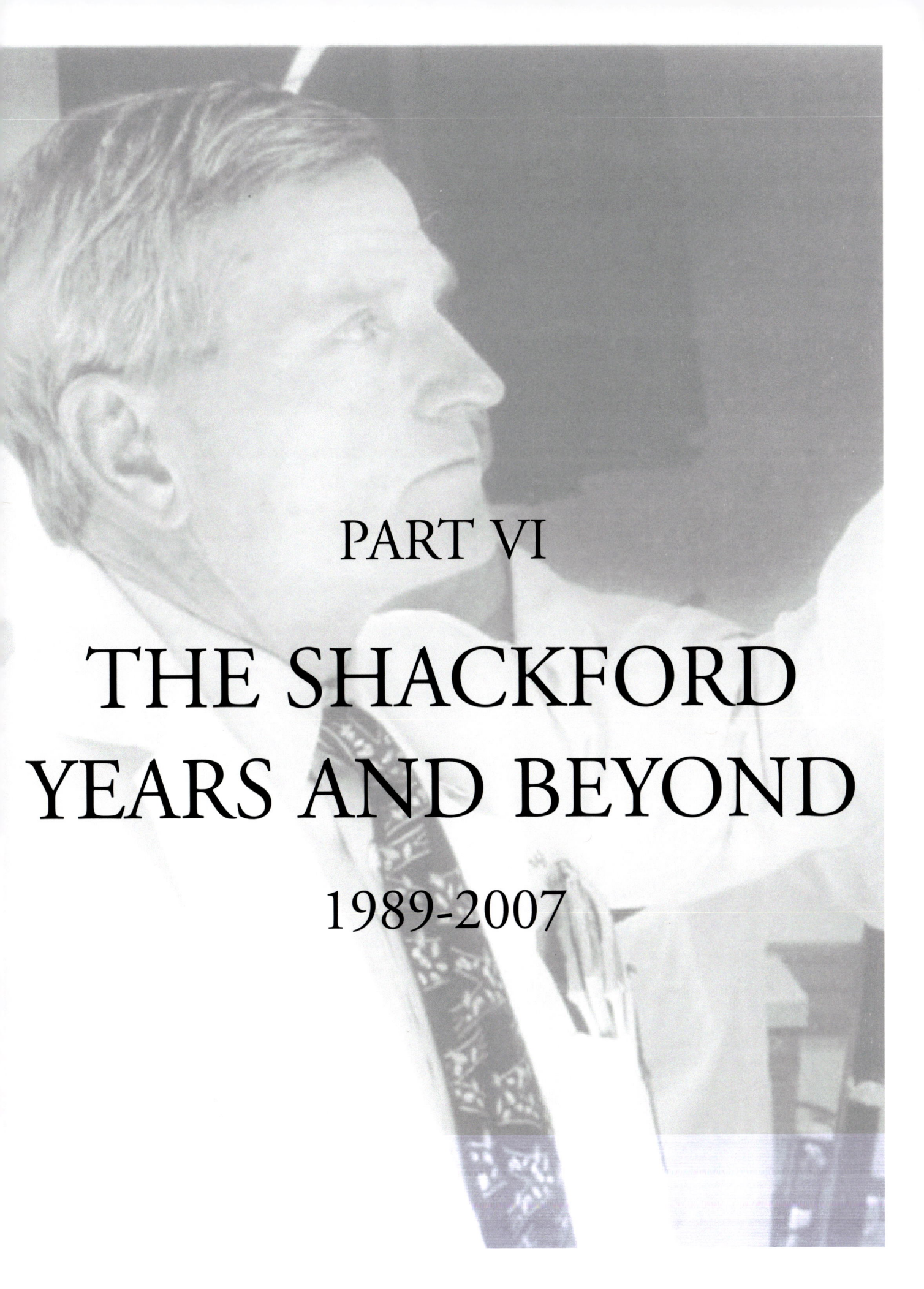

THE SHACKFORD YEARS AND BEYOND

1989-2007

CHAPTER 11

Tragedy and Transition: Rebirth of the Department

Steven Shackford replaced John Davis as Chief, attracting a dynamic new staff in the process. Divisional structure was reorganized, the residents started a mandatory research year, and teaching received renewed emphasis.

A new era was launched with regard to compiling outcomes data. A charitable "giving back" sabbatical was formalized. A surgical newsletter was instituted, along with other collegial activities.

Although a residency program oversight led to ACGME probation, the Department continued to grow. Shackford, having steered UVM into the 21st century, voluntarily stepped down at the top of his form.

The Search for a New Chair Proceeds

Although the Department of Surgery had made do during John Davis' illness, it could not function indefinitely without an actively practicing chairman. Dean Luginbuhl's search committee interviewed many excellent candidates for the chair, including the department's own Roger Foster and Richard Gamelli. It was no secret that the Dean did not favor internal candidates. UVM also interviewed many nationally prominent candidates. I (DBP) approached a fellow Orange County trauma conference attendee and urged him to consider the UVM position.

I knew that Shackford was already happily employed as the Chief of the Division of Trauma at the University of California at San Diego. I also knew, however, that he had written extensively in two areas of interest to UVM: quality trauma care and preventable deaths. He had a military background (like Davis) and was board certified in vascular, trauma, and critical care surgery. Acknowledged to be an excellent speaker and teacher, Steven R. Shackford seemed destined for success.

Influenced by the example his family physician set, Shackford had decided to pursue a career in medicine at the age of seven. He attended the University of Southern California where, like prior UVM Chairman Lyman Allen, he played collegiate baseball. Lockers were assigned alphabetically. Shackford's was next to a fellow who went on to achieve a bit of notoriety of his own — O.J. Simpson.

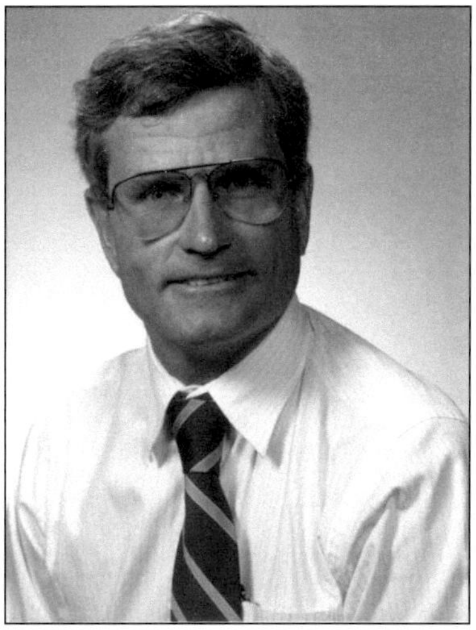

FIGURE II-I.
Steven Shackford, ready to start rebuilding the UVM department, in 1989.

Upon graduating, Shackford applied to St. Louis University Medical School. Placed on the waiting list, he opted to follow in his father's footsteps and enlist in the Navy. As he stood in line, ready to sign up, his father called him at the recruiting station. "Have you raised your hand and sworn in yet?" "Not yet." "Well don't — your acceptance letter just arrived from St. Louis." Shackford stepped out of line, went home, and started making plans for medical school.[1]

Money was a problem, so he looked for another way to finance his education. He went back to the Navy, applied for a scholarship, and got it. That commitment, together with a general surgery residency and a vascular surgery fellowship at San Diego's Naval Medical Center, led to a fourteen-year military career.

During his residency, Shackford cared for an engaging young nurse who had sustained a pelvic fracture after falling off a cliff. Ethics dictated that doctors not have personal relationships with patients under their care. Shackford therefore waited (and waited) until she was declared well enough and discharged from the trauma clinic. As soon as she left the building, he called and arranged a date for the following evening. His patience was rewarded, and marriage to Ellen was imminent.[2]

The Chairman of Surgery at the University of California, San Diego, Abdool Rahim Moosa, recruited Shackford to be the director of the newly created Division of Trauma. The position also included a busy vascular practice at the local Veterans Administration hospital. Shackford, working without much precedent, developed a trauma system that focused on the care of seriously injured patients. He studied preventable deaths both before and after the implementation of the system, and published landmark papers on the results.[3, 4] His group also established triage guidelines for trauma center patient selection.

Aware of UVM's national prominence through Davis' involvement with the American Association of the Surgery of Trauma and the Editorship of the Journal of Trauma, Shackford applied for the chairmanship position. The search committee was impressed with his credentials and his conduct during a face-to-face interview. Shackford was inspired by the opportunities UVM offered. He was also, oddly enough, fascinated by the following local headline: "Burlington resident stabbed in arm during candy store break-in." He realized that if this was considered front-page news, Vermont was going to be a much better environment in which to raise a family than crime-ridden San Diego![5]

Shackford was offered (and accepted) the chairmanship in the spring of 1989. When he arrived at UVM, he found himself with a dilemma — how to find an appropriate place for Davis in the department, while still having his own space? Shackford admired his predecessor, stating that, "my desire for the Department is to maintain John's high standards for patient care, research and education."[6] He could not, however, share an office with Davis, or evict him from his existing territory. He promised Davis that he could have a desk and a secretary as long as he wished. As with every promise that he made, Shackford kept his word. Davis's office eventually moved from the original location in the Given Building to the DeGoesbriand Unit, but he always had his own space. For years Davis continued to conduct popular teaching rounds with surgery students, initially at his DeGoesbriand office, and later at his home.

In an excellent decision, Shackford moved his own new "oval office" into the original Mary Fletcher hospital, leaving Davis in his space. The Department of Medicine objected to the reassignment, having used the building's choice areas during the Davis years (they obviously forgot that the surgeons had occupied this so-called "new" space for most of the preceding century!) Shackford hired Page's longtime secretary, M.J. Cahill, as his administrative assistant, and started reorganizing the Department.

The Surgery Staff Turns Over

A great deal of turnover occurred during this period. Mackay's remaining recruits had either retired (Keller and Shea) or were ready to step down (Page, Haines, Cain, and McGill). Davis' inner circle and subspecialists were also on the move. Chief neurosurgeon Schmidek had gone to Boston's Deaconess Hospital. Gamelli became Professor of Trauma Surgery (and later, Chair of the Department of Surgery) at Loyola University. Pediatric surgeon Browne went to the Maine Medical Center, transplant surgeon Haisch ended up at East Carolina's Brody School of Medicine, and Foster was appointed Professor of Surgery at Emory University and Chief of Surgical Services at Crawford Long Hospital in Atlanta. The ensuing gaps were problematic, but gave the new Chief opportunities to attract new innovative talent.

A Vascular Surgeon Embraces Change

Davis' remaining staff, including myself (DBP), strongly supported the new chief. My surgery workload intensified, but was offset after a while by having more partners with which to share call as new hires appeared. UVM's on-call policy did not change as one became more senior, so I took vascular call until the night before my retirement. I did, however decrease my nighttime stress level by electing to forego trauma call when the trauma service was reorganized. I assumed the official titles of Chief of the Division of Vascular Surgery and Director of the Non-invasive Vascular Laboratory, legitimizing the duties that I had been fulfilling on a de-facto basis for years. Teaching became a priority, and was a truly rewarding part of my affiliation with an academic institution.

I married Suzanne Wulff around the same time that Shackford arrived, and this rejuvenated my life. Suzanne provided the loving support that I needed to succeed. It has been unbelievably wonderful to live with someone whose love is unconditional and unwavering. I hope that most surgeons in relationships share this sentiment.

Suzanne's daughter Wendie inspired me in many ways, and helped with my post-retirement writing career. Suzanne's son Warren, having changed course from engineering to medicine, subsequently attended the College of Medicine and became an orthopaedic surgeon. I was understandably gratified to have the opportunity to teach my sons Warren Wulff and Jonathan Pilcher during their UVM surgical clerkships. I also accepted the fact that Christopher Pilcher, my other son, took his UVM surgery rotation at the Maine Medical Center. Chris and I had been a close team when we raced our J-24 sailboat, Doctor's Orders, so perhaps that stress led to his decision to pursue his surgical rotation elsewhere!

It was nevertheless extremely satisfying to place the graduation hoods on all three sons when they received their UVM medical degrees. Only parents who are on the faculty are allowed this privilege. Stanford Law School didn't give me any recognition when my daughter Susan Pilcher obtained her JD, nor did Carnegie Mellon when my daughter Wendie Wulff accepted her PhD, but I am equally proud of their accomplishments.

Shackford Recruits New Troops

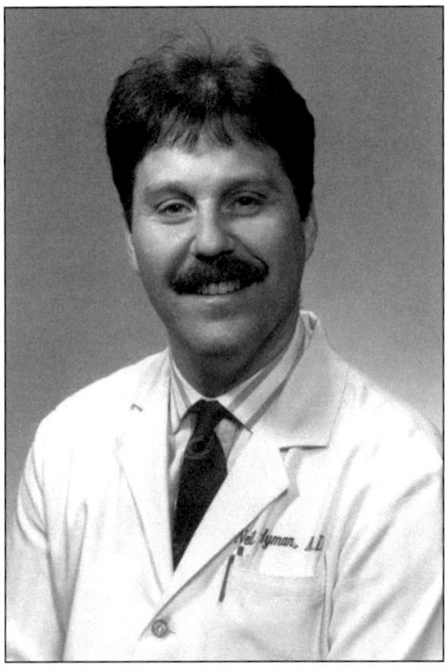

FIGURE 11-2. Neil Hyman was Shackford's first new recruit.

Shackford's first new faculty appointment, Neil Hyman, was a city boy. When it came time to choose a medical school though, he decided to come to UVM and see what it was like to "live in a log cabin." He returned to NYC for a general surgery residency at Mount Sinai, followed by a colorectal fellowship at the Cleveland Clinic. The plan was to finish training, return to New York, and take a position at Mount Sinai. Hyman's only remaining obligation was to chair a symposium on ethics and residency during an upcoming American College of Surgeons' meeting.[7]

Shackford and Hebert attended Hyman's presentation. Shackford was taken with his performance, especially after Hebert mentioned that Hyman was a UVM graduate. Shackford called Hyman shortly thereafter and offered him an interview. Hyman "was flattered that anyone would ask me." Shackford, as he did for all future applicants, conducted the final interview session. He outlined the job's specifics, and then asked Hyman if he was interested. Hyman was taken aback since "I didn't know you were supposed to come to an interview ready to accept!"[8]

Hyman tactfully replied that he'd have to go back to the Sheraton and discuss it with his wife, Jennifer (who was, incidentally, eight months pregnant). Shackford went to the hotel lobby and rang Hyman's room. He clarified the offer and expressed his willingness to wait while Hyman thought things over. The couple discussed the pros and cons of each institution during the drive back to Cleveland. Hyman contacted the Chief of Surgery at Mount Sinai, Arthur H. Aufses, Jr., and asked his advice. After considering their options, they decided on Vermont.

Hyman started work on July 15, 1990, relieving Hebert and Koplewitz from months of holding down the general surgery fort. According to Hyman, the pair promptly announced that they were taking the next six weeks off upon his arrival as compensation for their efforts. Ricci (Davis's last official hire) was on board in vascular, but he wasn't operating or taking call yet. As a result, Hyman was on call six of his first eight days in town — right in the middle of new intern and resident season.

Hyman was followed over the next four years by pediatric surgeons Dennis Vane and Andrew Hong, trauma surgeons Fred Rogers and Krista Kaups, surgical oncologists David Krag and Seth Harlow, transplant surgeon Jeffrey Reese, and colorectal surgeon Peter Cataldo. The new Shackford team's individual histories are in part detailed within their respective divisional chapters.

Financial and Administrative Reorganization

Cordell Gross, the new Chief of Neurosurgery, was named Vice Chairman and Director of Research. He filled both roles admirably until his untimely illness and demise from cancer in April of 2000. Business and administrative duties were briefly handled by pediatric neurosurgeon Steven Wald. After a short stint in private practice, Wald returned to the UVM full time fold. The Department, at that point, was woefully behind in computer literacy. Wald was given the task of bringing everyone into the digital age. Computers were purchased and distributed to each of the attendings and their secretaries. Wald unpacked the machines, set them up, and even mentored some of the less skilled users before leaving for another academic center.

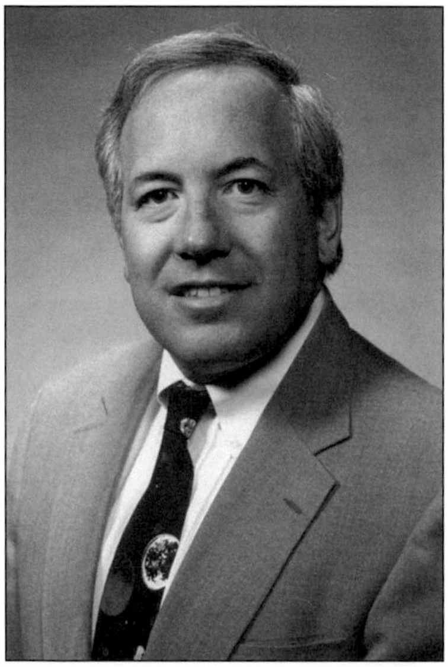

Administrative management was eventually turned over to Dennis Vane who, as Vice Chairman for Clinical Affairs, sorted out the Department's finances in concert with the MCHV managerial expert, Lisa Goodrich. After seeing the complexities of the task before him, Vane enrolled in UVM's business school. He subsequently earned an MBA while still leading the Division of Pediatric Surgery (with considerable help from junior member Kenneth Sartorelli). One of Vane's biggest administrative contributions was to tie compensation to productivity.

FIGURE 11-3. Dennis Vane was both a pediatric surgeon and an administrator capable of running the business side of the Department.

The Department's 32 surgeons had billed roughly fourteen million dollars a year during Davis's tenure, ninety percent of which was ultimately collected. Individual salaries, however, were only eighteen cents for every dollar billed. Thus, each surgeon on average generated $437,500 in revenue, but received less than 1/5th of that in salary.[9] Overages were used for research activities, Journal of Trauma operations, and services (like a photography studio) some of which were duplicated by the College of Medicine. Funds also supported non-surgical UHC providers, the College, and the Dean. Where all the money was allocated is unclear to this historian.

There had been functional divisions in the past, but they had been loosely defined and managed. The divisional structure was now formalized and expanded. An executive advisory committee (consisting of the vice-chairmen and the division chiefs) was created that contributed to the department's decision-making process. Individual divisions were soon responsible for their own budgets. The respective division chiefs decided compensation distribution with Shackford's input.

Rejuvenating Research

Shackford stressed the importance of surgical research and critical thinking throughout his career. He believed that:

> *"...close scrutiny of a problem leads to creativity in constructing a means to solve the problem. That creativity has broad application, not only in the science and art of surgery, but*

also in the process of living. Research ... teaches patience and humility — two traits highly desired in the operating arena. Production of scholarly work improves both analytic and communicative skills — attributes ... surgeons lack." [10]

As a condition of his appointment, Shackford stipulated that UVM provide salaries and benefits for three research fellows each year. Although the first few residents entered the laboratory on a voluntary basis, twelve months of continuous research between the second and third years of training eventually became a mandatory commitment. The research fellows participated in conferences, journal clubs, and all other academic activities. There were no clinical responsibilities assigned to them and NO moonlighting was allowed. The program's impact was evidenced by the large proportion of UVM graduates that later pursued fellowships and academic careers.

The National Institutes of Health had awarded Shackford a research project grant just before he left San Diego. After a considerable amount of effort, he was allowed to conduct his investigations at UVM. Shackford reviewed the curricula vitae of his newly inherited residents, seeking one with a scientific background. He subsequently chose Joseph Schmoker to "volunteer" for the first research year (which was followed by another, and then another.) Shackford and Schmoker's work was the first to show that hypertonic saline improved head injury resuscitation, a finding that dispelled the longstanding prohibition against its use.[11, 12, 13]

Shackford also performed funded research on secondary brain injury for many years.[14] This work carries on under the present Chief of Trauma, Bruce Crookes. The Division of Neurosurgery followed similar paths. Gross' successor, Bruce Tranmer focused on cerebral smooth muscle cells and vasospasm.[15] His associate, Paul Penar, evaluated the mechanisms and modulation of malignant brain tumor invasion.[16]

Select research activities below were part of a wider effort not entirely included here.

Hebert continued his work with the Davis-era aerosolization chamber and splenectomized mice. His pneumococcal infection studies helped promote the splenic preservation movement of the 1980s.[17]

Ricci's lab examined arteriovenous reversal, a technique in which ischemic limbs without suitable bypass targets were revascularized by arterializing a vein and its outflow bed.[18] When this didn't pan out, he started studying the effects of beta-blockers and other agents on the growth of experimental rat aneurysms.[19, 20] Ricci was also involved with telemedicine's application in remote radiological assessment, follow-up patient care, and continuing education.[21] Later, Fred Rogers, as the Director of Research, examined the use of telemedicine in trauma.[22]

Laboratory research was complemented by case reports, population studies, and clinical trials. David Krag's landmark investigations occupied a significant amount of the department's energies.[23] All told, hundreds of papers were published under Shackford's watch by various students, residents, and faculty members. As always, the emphasis remained on improving the delivery of quality care to patients in a rural setting.

Reforming Curricula and Recognizing Academia

The College of Medicine instituted a new three-part curriculum at the start of the Davis era. One-and-a-half years of basic science classes were followed by a year of clinical core clerkships in Surgery, Medicine, Pediatrics, Psychiatry, and Obstetrics. After a basic science review, students embarked on a "senior major" program tailored to their individual choice of specialty.[24] The three-month surgical clinical core provided one-to-one mentoring through a successful preceptor system. The corresponding senior major included engaging in a scholarly project that was presented at a year-end conference. These studies were frequently published in nationally known journals.

The senior major program was faced with elimination in the early 1980s. When the Department caught wind of this, it held an emergency meeting in the DeGoesbriand's cafeteria. It was unanimously agreed that if the senior major program were discontinued, the surgeons would leave the full-time group and start their own private practice. The surgical protest was so strong that the College rescinded its decision. The other senior majors were disbanded in favor of a senior selective program (with less rotation requirements and no scholarly projects), but the surgical senior major program was allowed to continue.

The College, bowing to healthcare reforms calling for more generalists and fewer specialists, reduced the surgery and medicine clinical clerkships by a month apiece to create a new family practice rotation. Hebert, the department's faculty representative, agreed to the changes with the provision that the rest of the school's courses undergo a similar reassessment and update. He headed a curriculum task force that gave rise to 2003's Vermont Integrated Curriculum (VIC), while also serving as the Associate Dean for Graduate Medical Education from 1999 to 2007.

The VIC resembles the senior major in surgery without the scholarly project. The curriculum integrates more clinical subjects earlier, and includes additional basic sciences later. An online component — College of Medicine Educational Tools (COMET) — was initiated with the arrival of the Class of 2007 (whose members were each given a laptop computer and a PDA to facilitate participation!) COMET is a completely web-based teaching system that supports course materials with contact information, PowerPoint presentations, interactive documents, case studies, animations, virtual reality models, and other advanced multimedia features. Developed with the help of the Blackboard Learning System™, it has put UVM at the forefront of hybrid educational technology.[25]

Hebert replaced Gamelli as Residency Program Director. The apprentice-like training of the Mackay days had evolved into an intern/junior/senior resident team approach under Davis. This system was codified and applied across the major surgical divisions (general/colorectal, surgical oncology, vascular, trauma, cardiothoracic, and pediatric) during Shackford's time. Additional rotations in critical care, emergency medicine, endoscopy, and other sub-specialties were instituted as staffing permitted. R.W.P. Mellish's former secretary, Louise Hamel, provided resident support as Program Coordinator. Judy McGivney succeeded her, and was followed by Diantha Langmaid. The trio's efforts were much appreciated by the housestaff.

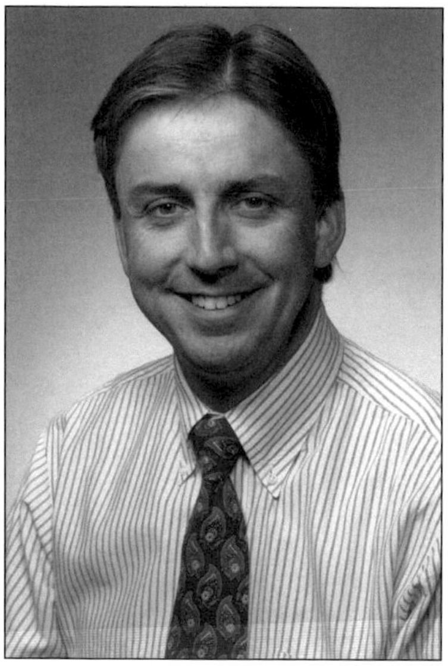

Deciding how to reward professors (and later, depart-

FIGURE 11-4. James Hebert replaced Gamelli as Residency Program Director. He was intimately involved with UVM's curriculum reform.

Chapter Eleven: Tragedy and Transition: Rebirth of the Department ments) for teaching students and conducting research had been an ongoing problem. The College of Medicine, under Dean John Frymoyer, instituted the "Faculty Teaching and Rewards System" during the mid-1990s. The program quantified teaching hours and then adjusted each Department's share of the general funds accordingly. Frymoyer's successor revised the plan once the VIC was implemented.[26]

Shackford took a different approach. Patient care, teaching, research, and service were the foundations of his surgical philosophy. Thus, he established annual departmental awards in these fields to galvanize faculty awareness and to recognize excellence. The honors were named after prior faculty members who had made their mark in each respective area: the Albert G. Mackay Surgical Clinician Award (later renamed for H. Gordon Page), the Jerome S. Abrams Teaching Award, the James E. DeMeules Surgical Research Award, and the John H. Davis Service Award.

Surgical Outcomes and Complications

Saturday mornings started with an eight o'clock Morbidity and Mortality (M&M) conference during the Mackay years. Attending and resident participation was virtually one hundred percent. Residents presented all of the preceding week's complications, which were then adjudicated by the group. The attendings of record preferentially remained mute during the initial reviews, but were permitted to defend their actions at the end of the discussions. Unfortunately, the residents' memories and perceptions often differed from those of the attendings. Spending time watching the attendings correct the residents was hardly beneficial for the rest of us.

The Vermont presentations, at least, always had a certain honesty and integrity to them. Koplewitz, in his brief practice venture in New York, was struck by the lack of scruples at a local hospital. He remembers discussing a patient with colon cancer who had died after undergoing a colectomy. The staff doctors wrote it off as a death due to cancer before proceeding to the next case. When Koplewitz asked, "But why did he die?" he was met by a wall of silence.[27]

Davis' M&M conferences were preceded by a more formal grand rounds presentation. The meetings were moved to Thursday mornings shortly after his arrival in order to reduce the weekend workload. Curtailing the Department's available operating room time ensured full attendance. The residents briefly recounted the week's complications, and then focused their attention on a single case. The conferences were an educational highlight for the attendings and residents alike, largely due to the charismatic yet respectful manner in which Davis conducted the proceedings.

Shackford continued the Thursday morning sessions, book-ending them with basic science lectures and formal attending floor rounds. These two additions led to a completely "academic" morning. Distressed by the lack of sub-specialty surgeon attendance at M&M conferences, Shackford posted announcements throughout the hospitals and clinics. He also reviewed every case with the presenting resident ahead of time. This kept the discussions focused on the pertinent issues resulting in better overall organization. Long-term participation swelled, thanks to the presentations' educational value and Shackford's constant tutelage.

The chief resident of each division presented on a rotating basis. The format eventually consisted of: 1) A list of the division's complications since the previous conference, 2) A radiographic "puzzler" directed to a junior house officer, 3) A detailed case presentation (which usually involved a death) interspersed with relevant teaching points, 4) A brief review of the underlying disease process and/or therapeutic problem, and 5) An accounting of case-specific complications with opportunities for improvement.

A high level of preparation and presentation was expected and achieved. As a result, the M&M conference was a model of excellence. Shackford set a great example for the housestaff and the students with his insight and conscientiousness. He urged the audience to listen to the "little man" sitting on their shoulder. As gender neutrality became an issue, he changed the metaphor to "little person" whenever he remembered.

Shackford's appreciation for the value of outcomes accuracy was contagious. Channeling the spirit of surgical "end results" advocate Ernest Codman, he enthusiastically developed a reporting system that identified, categorized, and quantified untoward events.[28] The data collection forms (dubbed "Shack Sheets" by the residents) listed and defined general and specialty-specific complications. These, in turn, were classified as technical, judgmental, or diagnostic errors, failures in equipment or policy, or patient disease. Complications were then determined to be either avoidable or unavoidable. The "Surgical Activity Tracking System" was widely embraced for its ability to objectively identify problems and assess the impact of corrective measures.[29, 30]

Non-Clinical Innovations

Shackford, to his credit, also worked to create a collegial atmosphere. His rigorous military-based leadership style became more conciliatory and cooperative with time, although he maintained a certain degree of toughness. He applied the same principles to patient care. New interns sat through a mandatory screening of the movie "The Doctor", starring William Hurt, every year to gain awareness of patient sensitivities.

Several new team-building traditions were started. Noteworthy among these were the yearly football/volleyball game and chili cook-off. Fierce competitions arose between the attendings and the housestaff as the games unfolded in Shackford's back yard. Athletes and neophytes joined forces, ringers were inserted, and outcomes were disputed. A scrape on the nose was a badge of honor, and lame surgeons were the rule the following day.

The chili submissions were judged in the kitchen. Samples from each entry were placed in Styrofoam cups that had been secretly numbered by Shackford's daughters. Shackford's wife Ellen, my (DBP) wife Suzanne, an experienced dairy foods evaluator formerly affiliated with the UVM dairy science department, and ENT resident Debbie Gonzalez served as judges. Plastic surgeon David Leitner won the inaugural event with an outstanding venison-based recipe. When I asked Suzanne why I didn't even place, she simply replied "tough beans." The next year, I soaked my beans for two days. On the morning of the contest, I found that I still had tough beans. I picked each one out of the chili, added two cans of store-bought pre-cooked beans, and took the top prize.

Shackford also instituted an annual winter conference at a Stowe mountain resort entitled "Current Concepts and Controversies in Surgery." UVM surgeons and families, community

FIGURE 11-5. Vane (left) and Shackford officiating at the Stowe winter surgery retreat.

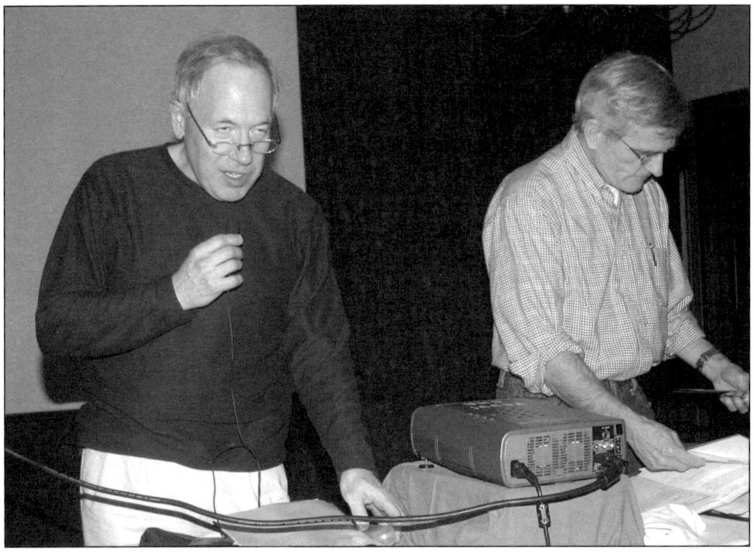

FIGURE 11-6. Steven Shackford, Mrs. Fred (Mimi) Rogers, and Ellen Shackford enjoying clam chowder during the winter retreat.

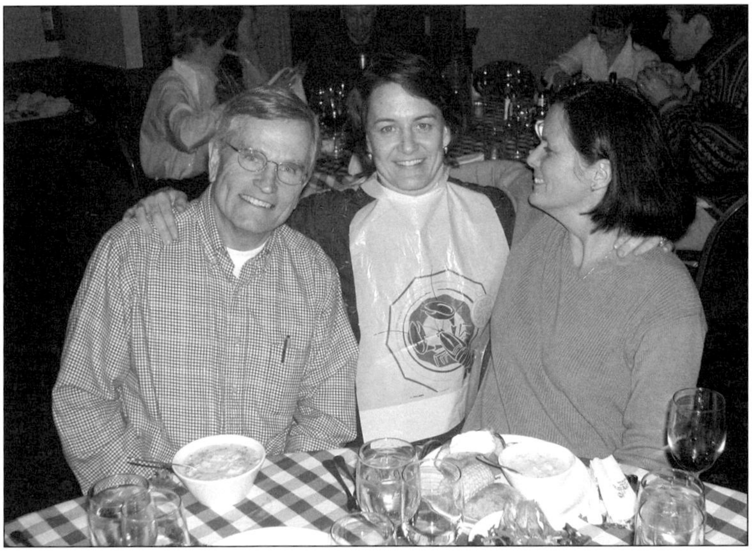

FIGURE 11-7. Leavitt and Shackford finally came up with a trophy for the winter retreat's annual ski race.

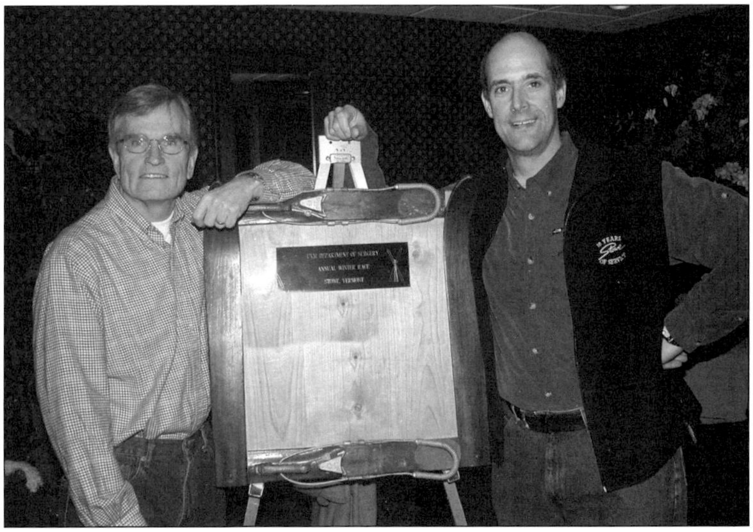

180 CATAMOUNT SURGEONS

surgeons, visiting professors, available housestaff, and medical students on the service attended the two-and-a-half day seminar. Scientific sessions were held from 8-10 am and 4-6 pm with an intervening "break". The event's final day featured a faculty and resident ski race. Stowe Ski Patrol member and medical advisor Bruce Leavitt was appointed race manager. Former collegiate champs Seth Harlow and Philip Camp usually clocked the fastest times, while Neil Hyman, in a position befitting a colorectal surgeon, usually brought up the rear. The race was preceded by divisional meetings and followed by a faculty and family lobster dinner.

The affair was reminiscent of earlier gatherings conducted by the Western Trauma Association (WTA) — an organization to which Shackford not only belonged, but also eventually presided over. Although the WTA met in the Rockies, a skiing rivalry emerged between the Universities of Colorado and Vermont. Prior UVM resident Eugene Moore led the contingent from Denver General Hospital alongside his brothers Fred and John, while Bishop McGill and his son John represented Vermont. Shackford maintained the good-natured but spirited competition upon his move to UVM.

Shackford initiated an academic liaison with the Maine Medical Center (MMC) that was organized by Leavitt, a native of Maine and a former MMC general surgery resident. MMC's Chairman, Carl Bredenberg, embraced and fostered the relationship. Our faculty lectured and administered oral exams to UVM students rotating through Portland, while Maine's attendings were given UVM appointments. At the program's height, our staff practically begged Leavitt for the opportunity to enjoy Maine's hospitality, which usually included great lobsters. Sadly, leadership changes at MMC led to the cessation of this dynamic interaction after several years.

Another innovation was the inception of the "UVM Surgery" newsletter in July of 1990. The idea was to inform alumni and friends of the Department of Surgery about the activities of its members. Shackford told readers that, "I asked Doug McSweeney to edit our inaugural issue. Doug as many of you know, has a long Burlington history and, as such, he knows many of you personally. In addition, he has a real penchant and talent for writing."[31]

McSweeney's stories were interesting, as were his occasionally irreverent and candid editorials. Shackford caught wind of one particular diatribe directed against the Department of Medicine after the newsletter had already been mailed. Secretaries scurried to retrieve the controversial issue, which was subsequently rewritten and redistributed (although a few uncensored contraband copies still exist). Other UVM departments eventually followed surgery's lead by establishing their own newsletters.

McSweeney, sadly, had to retire in 1992 after suffering a massive heart attack, although he lived for another decade. Frank Ittleman, who had nurtured McSweeney through emergency cardiac surgery, assumed the newsletter's editorship with a new, but equally entertaining style.

The department's surgeons had volunteered their services at home and abroad for years. Nights off were spent in local clinics, and vacations were used for sojourns to underserved areas such as Haiti, Peru, and Nepal. These endeavors were recognized with a "Giving Back" program in 2002 that provided each willing surgeon with three weeks of leave per year for charitable work that was not charged as vacation. Trip expenses were still left up to the individual, and yearly salary and budget projections were not modified accordingly. Nevertheless, the model reflected another novel UVM approach to outreach care.

THE LAST WORD

This issue is a report card on the performance of the Department under the stewardship of its new chairman. It is long and detailed but we feel we owe our readers a documentary, replete with statistics: a recapitulation of our academic output. Literature citations are given so that readers may directly and personally assess the quality of the research published. With this information in hand, our efforts can be gauged and judgement rendered on the work.

Surgeons are a strange breed. The College (ACS) and our specialty societies have not risen up in revolt as the RBRVS and HCFA fee schedules are imposed. An excellent study in a recent JAMA (Vol 226, No. 24, pp 3453-58) by Maloney shows that the perception that surgeons are reimbursed at a higher rate than cognitive practitioners is in error; surgeons simply put in an average of 17.2 more hours of work in a week. Surgeons shift charges for cognitive work hours to the 18 percent of their time spent in the operating room. The RBRVS provides equal pay for unequal work. There is no recognition of the hours of professional effort, post graduate specialty training or differences in the nature of the physician's work.

I mention this because you could fire an artillery piece down any of the halls of the Medical Center at 3 a.m. (or for that matter, after 4:30 p.m.) on any given day; I guarantee the cannon ball will not dismember an ▆▆▆▆. There will be many dead procedurists: surgeons, orthopods, obstetricians, angiographers, endoscopists, and anaesthesiologists, but no ▆▆▆▆.

Beyond the academic accolades is the clinical work of the Department in the mileau of a tertiary care comprehensive treatment center. If the average surgeon works 87.8 hours per week, imagine the effort and hours put out by our surgical house staff. Their hours are in the 100's and the cannon ball referred to above will count as its victims mostly residents and the odd attending. The leaking aneurysm, the dead leg, the perforated viscus, the

(continues on page 11)

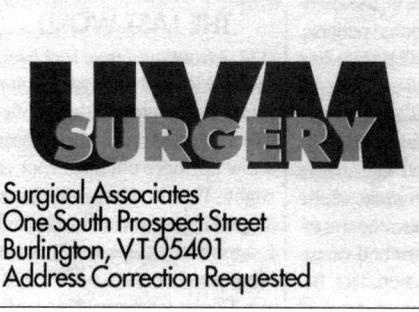

From your editor...

Dr. Doug McSweeney

UVM SURGERY
Surgical Associates
One South Prospect Street
Burlington, VT 05401
Address Correction Requested

BULK RATE
U.S. POSTAGE
PAID
BURLINGTON, VT
PERMIT NO. 200

FIGURE 11-8.
A contraband copy of the "UVM Surgery Newsletter" that contained McSweeney's inflammatory editorial. The offending column was hurriedly rewritten before re-mailing.

All of these activities built an esprit de corps unique among academic surgery departments. This was further enhanced by the development of a departmental "coat of arms" in 1997. This emblem currently adorns paper products, PowerPoint presentations, and patches attached to the breast pockets of surgeons' white coats.

The Great Ice Storm of 1998

On the evening of January 7, 1998, a massive ice storm blanketed upstate New York and northern Vermont. By the time it was over, the entire region had been coated with at least three inches of ice and a state of emergency had been proclaimed. Power was out across much of Chittenden County, and rural parts of the state were without service for more than a week. Luckily, the warm weather that had caused the storm persisted for several days.

Anticipating a disruption in service, the following day's elective surgery schedule had been cancelled. The hospital's emergency electrical system was excellent, but it had never faced such a severe test. Power fluctuations were seamlessly handled as generators kicked in. Emergent operations were delayed only if personnel were unable to reach the hospital. Shackford was never late, even under the most trying of circumstances. He managed to perform a femoral-femoral arterial bypass while others were still struggling to leave their driveways.

My (DBP) scheduled carotid endarterectomy patient showed up at 7:15 am. This took me by surprise, as he hailed from Potsdam, New York — a town more than one hundred miles away. He too had anticipated the storm, and had come to Burlington the preceding day. The O.R. staff had dutifully tried to call him at home the night before about the change in plans. He, of course, was not at home, but nicely tucked-in at the local Sheraton.

I lived on a dirt road, two miles from the closest highway. The road itself was totally blocked by a series of fallen trees. Plastic surgeon Phil Trabulsy lived on the same road and faced a similar predicament. After four hours of spirited chain saw cutting, we managed to

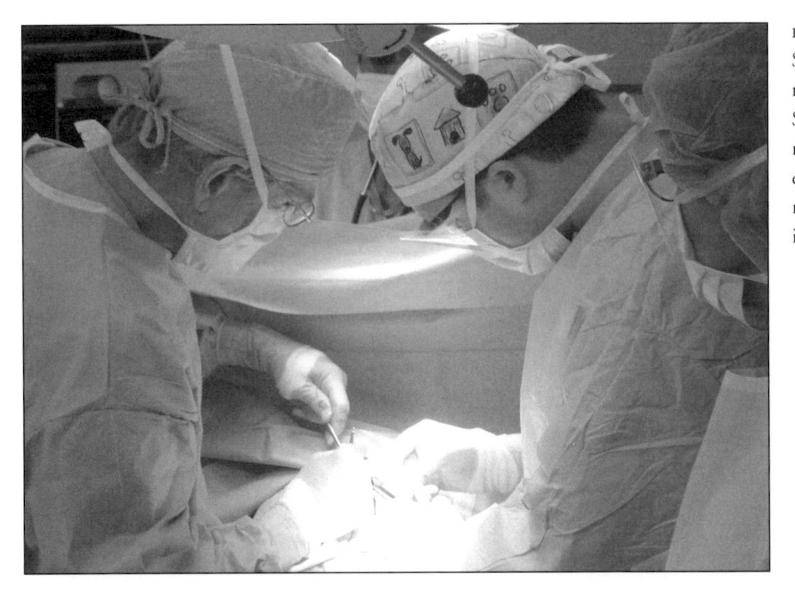

FIGURE 11-9. Shackford (L), and resident John Schneider, and nurse Betty Gilbert excise recurrent thyroid tumor in Haiti in 2008.

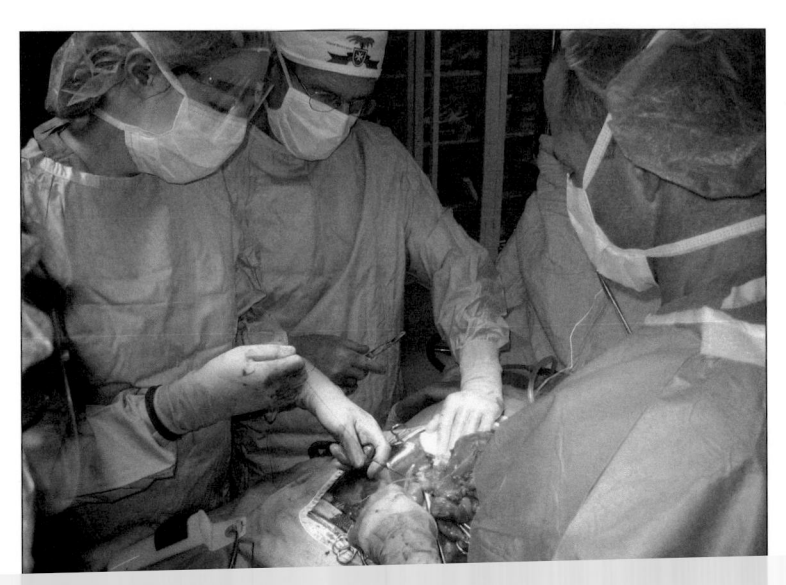

FIGURE 11-10. Surgery resident Alicia Privette, Shackford, and Cataldo performing a colectomy in 2006 as part of the Department's Port-au-Prince, Haiti outreach program.

hack our way out. Upon reaching the hospital, I found my resourceful patient calmly awaiting his operation. I brushed off as much sawdust as possible, changed to sterile scrubs, and proceeded with the otherwise uneventful case.

Fletcher Allen Health Care

The same economic pressures that had forced the Mary Fletcher/DeGoesbriand Memorial merger came to the fore again with the advent of managed care. As a result, the leaders of the Medical Center Hospital of Vermont, the University Health Center, and the Fanny Allen Hospital agreed to combine forces in January of 1995. Following a popular trend of the day, the newly integrated entity was named "Fletcher Allen Health Care" (FAHC). MCHV and UHC maintained the status quo, but the Catholic run Fanny Allen hospital was relieved of its acute care responsibilities. Although the FAH operating rooms remained open, their services were limited to a purely outpatient population. After 100 years, the Fanny Allen ceased to exist as a Catholic Hospital.

In the meantime, the DeGoesbriand Memorial Unit had begun to show its age. Its mechanical systems were outdated, its handicapped access violated building codes, and its parking remained abysmal. A major investment was unavoidable. Instead of sinking money into the DMU, however, the decision was made to start afresh. FAHC unveiled plans for its $356 million "Renaissance Project" in 1999. At its heart was an Ambulatory Care Center (ACC) that encompassed much-needed clinical, educational, and surgical space.[32]

Expansion took its toll, however. Before the project, a resident parking lot had been carved from an unpaved patch of land between the old Burgess Nurses' Residence and the staff

FIGURE 11-11.
The light and spacious lobby of the new Ambulatory Care Center contains a gift shop, seating areas, and most important, an elevator that goes to the underground garage.

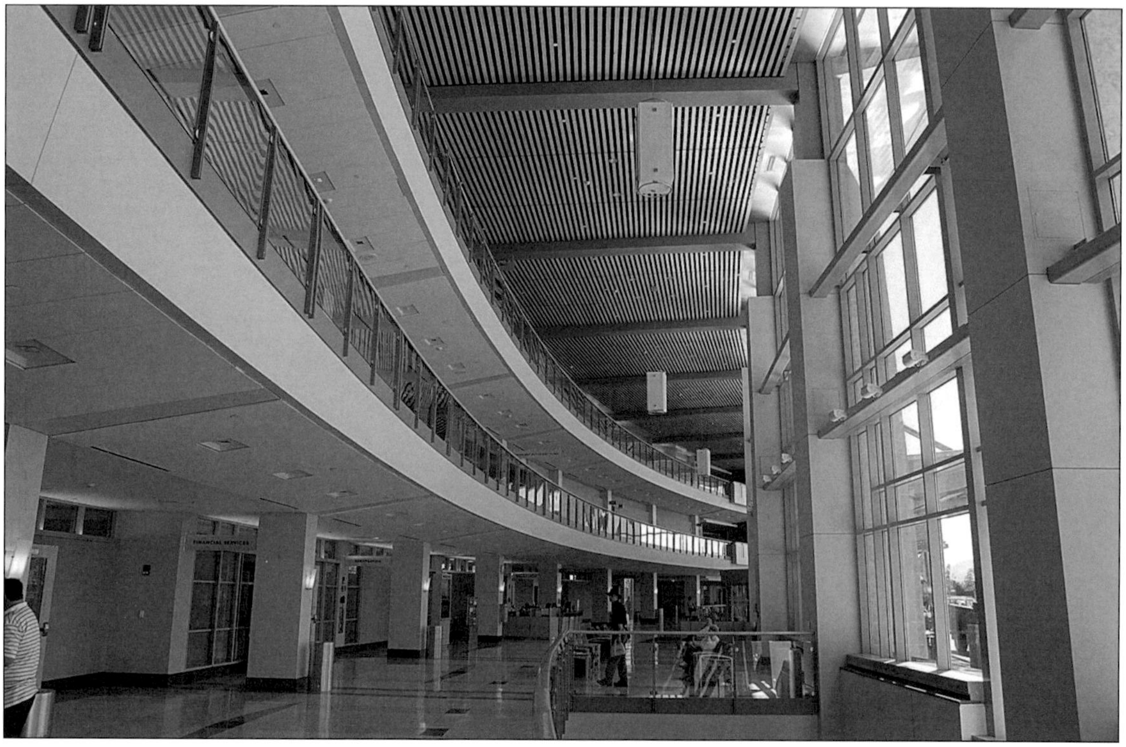

physician lot. Spots were taken on a first-come, first-served basis. Surgical residents usually secured the best positions, thereby ensuring themselves a short walk to the Adams House entrance. Later-rising residents were consigned to the far reaches of the employee lot. Then the "Renaissance Project" began. The Burgess and Adams buildings were demolished to make way for a five-story underground parking garage. Residents were banished to the medical student lot on the far side of the Given Building. The students — ranking even lower in status — were assigned parking at the Gutterson Field House lot and then were bused back to the hospital. The inconvenience was forgotten once the garage was completed and indoor parking became a reality. Medical student parking improved, but is still not within the garage.

Despite alleged scandals surrounding the Renaissance Project's rumored lack of disclosure of its financing and irregularities of its permitting, (which led to resignations and criminal charges filed within the administration) the end result was a success. Adjacent to both the hospital and the College of Medicine, the ACC is home to the Department's clinical offices as well as eight outpatient operative suites. The days of waiting for the DMU shuttle bus or driving to the Timber Lane annex are just a memory.

The World of the 80-Hour Work Week

In the wake of the Libby Zion-resident fatigue case, the Accreditation Council for Graduate Medical Education (ACGME) capped resident workloads at 80 hours per week effective July 1, 2003.[33] Shackford introduced the restrictions in the spring of 2003 so that the changes were in place before the summer's new residents arrived. The attendings worried about sign-outs between covering teams, and the residents fretted over the future of their surgical experience. Improving patient handoffs and obtaining operative simulators allayed most of those fears, although some attendings ended up first-assisting each other. An informal UVM survey showed that, three years after the fact, both parties felt that the number of patient errors were either the same or greater.[34]

The use of physician and surgical assistants expanded from cardiothoracic surgery and orthopaedics into the divisions of plastic, vascular, minimally invasive, and general surgery. Residents were required to focus their efforts on the core disciplines of gastrointestinal, laparoscopic, endocrine, surgical oncology, thoracic, vascular, trauma, and critical care surgery. Emphasis on cardiac, pediatric, and transplant surgery was significantly reduced.[35] Fortunately, UVM's long-standing lack of fellows resulted in a largely adequate in-house resident hands-on experience.

Given the level of Shackford's integrity, there was no question that the rules would be followed. The work ethic that had been instilled in the residents, however, came to the fore. When surveyed by the ACGME, over half of the residents thought that their time in the hospital had remained the same in spite of the new regulations.[36] "The ACGME mistakenly perceived that our program was not in compliance with the new rules. An inadequate number of certain index cases didn't help matters. The ACGME placed the UVM surgical program on probation in 2004. The work hour issue was not felt to be valid by our residency directors. The lack of index cases, regrettably, was. In fact, the problem had been pointed out during previous inspections."[37]

dedicated head and neck specialist, and the ENT surgeons (who had their own case number problems) were reluctant to share. An inadequate volume of penetrating trauma and hepatic surgery was also a problem. Blunt trauma prevailed in UVM's rural setting, which inherently lacked the so-called "knife and gun club" of the inner cities. And of course, today's standard of care for blunt hepatic trauma is non-operative management! Nevertheless, efforts were under way to rectify these deficiencies.[38]

Shackford Steps Down at His Peak

FIGURE 11-12. Shackford relinquished the Chair to his running partner Frank Ittleman on an interim basis, as the Search Committee continued its deliberations.

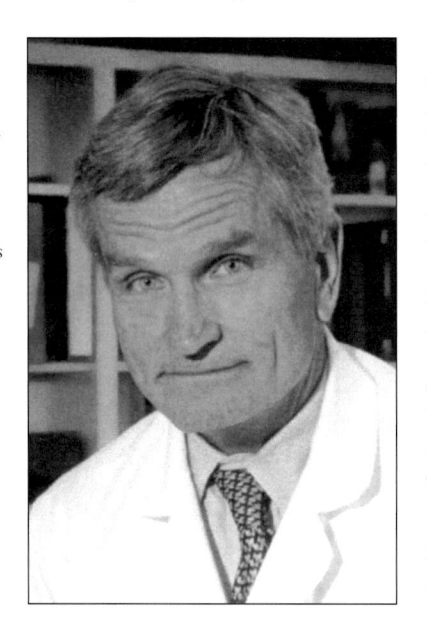

Shackford was asked to oversee FAHC's Institute for Quality and Operational Effectiveness in the fall of 2004.[39] He accepted the position of Chief Quality Officer (CQO) with some reluctance, but ended up becoming so immersed in the role that he considered taking a sabbatical. Unfortunately, the hospital, strapped for cash following the financial difficulties of the Renaissance Project, was unable to provide the support needed to accomplish its own goals. A year after the appointment, Shackford announced that he would step down as CQO, and — in a move worthy of John Pomeroy circa 1822 — as Chair one year hence.[40]

In one of his last acts as Chairman, Shackford issued the following call to arms during his 2005 Presidential Address to the AAST:

"... real innovative change is needed, requiring both a personal and an organizational commitment. The changing demographics of the medical workforce, a loss of altruism, the continuing finite specialization of surgery, increasing public awareness and expectations about the quality of care, resident work hour limitations, an aging and more fragile patient population, and more societal intrusion into the explicit practice of medicine have catalyzed a process of dramatic change that has presented us with a tremendous opportunity. Unless we proactively respond, our social contract with patients is threatened, and the art that is surgery will be transformed to the job that is surgery."[41]

The College of Medicine found itself in need of a new Dean and a new Chief of Medicine and a new Chief of Surgery at the same time. The search committee's energies were devoted to filling the departmental spots first, so that the new chairpersons could help select the new dean. When the search extended beyond Shackford's one-year mark, Frank Ittleman was appointed interim Chair of Surgery. Ittleman kept the members of the department happy, making few, if any, major changes.

In the final analysis, Shackford had essentially done everything that had been asked of him. The department had grown from 32 surgeons to more than 75, and annual gross billings had risen nearly tenfold to more than $120 million.[42] Davis' teaching and research standards had been maintained, and quality care assurance had taken a quantum leap. The Department continued on an even keel under Ittleman's guidance, awaiting its next Chief.

CHAPTER 12

The Future Will Be History

A new chief, David McFadden, arrived as the Stanley S. Fieber Professor and Chair of Surgery in January 2007. McFadden, a Virginia native who performed his surgical training at Johns Hopkins, had previously served as Chief of General Surgery at the University of California at Los Angeles and Chair at West Virginia University. His clinical and research interests are in gastrointestinal disease and oncology.

McFadden joined a strong department that anticipated, yet was anxious, about change. His vision includes the development of subspecialty residencies in Urology, Ophthalmology, and Emergency Medicine, surgical service outreach into Vermont's community hospitals, and the development of multidisciplinary cancer clinics to streamline patient care and increase the College of Medicine's profile as a regional tertiary center for cancer care.

The residency deficiencies addressed by Shackford, Ittleman and McFadden were rectified and UVM's probationary status was lifted following the 2008 site visit.

The need for leadership, research, and junior faculty recruitment, functioning under the existent and looming local and global financial circumstances, the maintenance of excellence in the surgical residencies in the presence of work hour restrictions and a changing work force are all imminent challenges. As with all challenges, opportunities exist. Only time will tell, but we hope that the successes of the past are mirrored by the triumphs of the future.

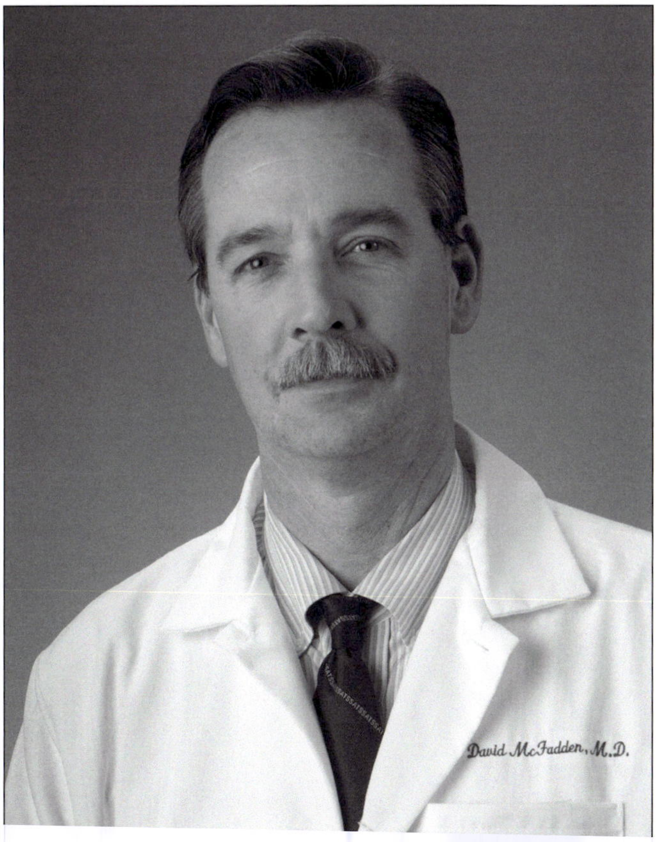

FIGURE 12-1. David McFadden has led UVM's Department of Surgery since January, 2007.

Mario Trabulsy examines trauma victim in the Emergency Department. (UVM med photo).

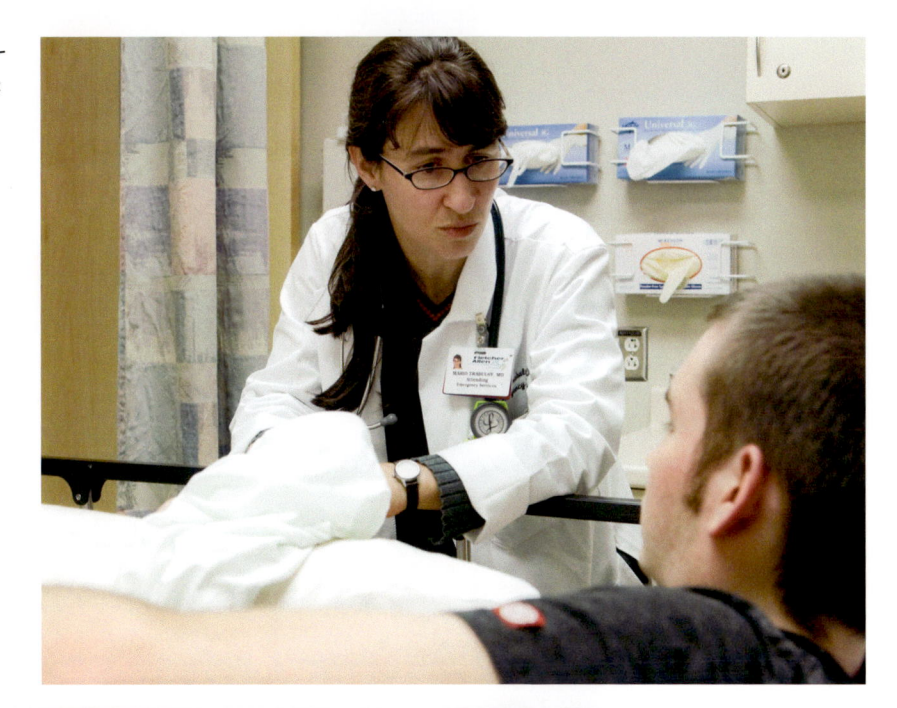

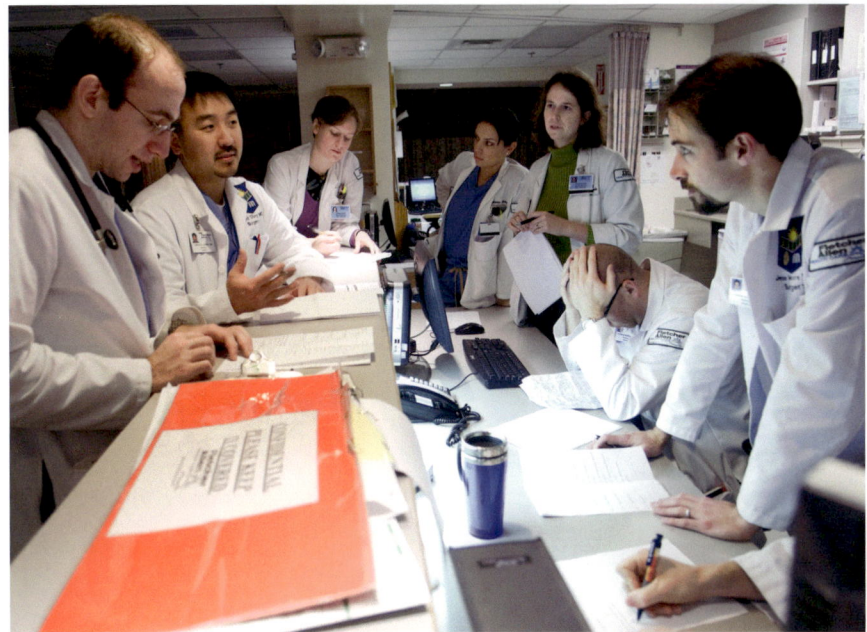

Chief resident Arnold Chung (2nd from L) conducts patient rounds with l to r: Daniel Greenlane, anesthesia resident, medical students, and surgical residents Patrick Mannal (2nd from R), and Jesse Moore (far R). (UVM Med Photo).

The author (DBP) stands with his sons at his 2003 retirement party. L to R: Christopher Pilcher, MD, Infectious diseases UCSF, DBP, Warren Wulff, MD, Orthopaedist, Syracuse, NY, and Jonathan Pilcher, MD, Emergency medicine,

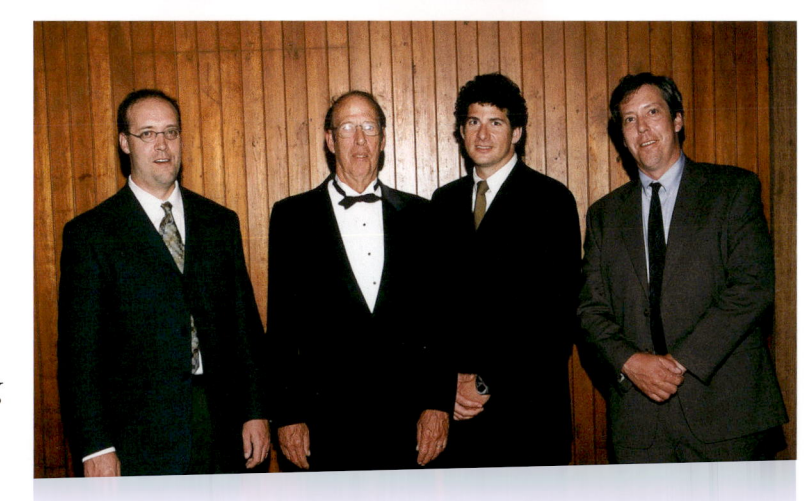

Philip Trabulsy's original tree house (non handicapped accessible) is the precursor of the many handicapped accessible tree houses to come. (DBP photo).

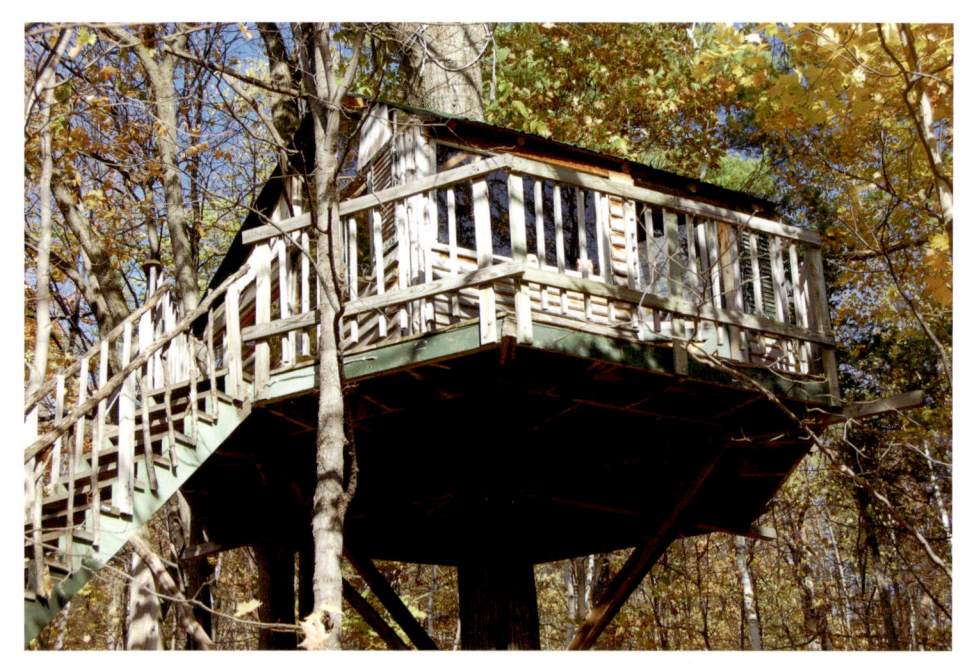

The patient with the salvaged BK amputation discussed in Chapter 25, here demonstrates her mobility in tree climbing. (Courtesy of Linda Horn).

The dedication of the John Davis textbook at the 1979 AAST meeting was absent its primary author as he was still adapting to life as a paraplegic. L to r: William Drucker, Roger Foster, George Sheldon, Richard Gamelli, Basil Pruitt, and Donald Gann. (Courtesy of Roger Foster).

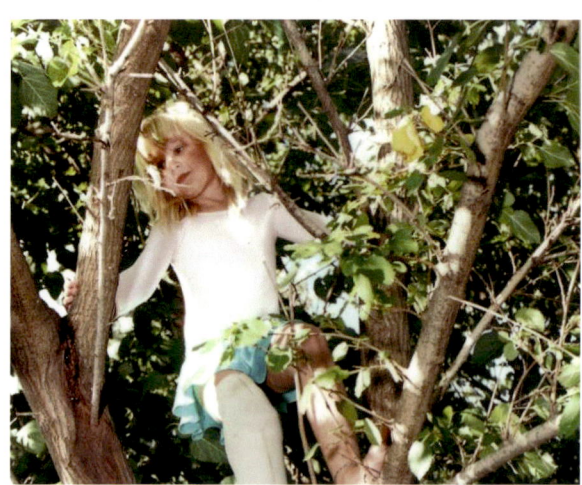

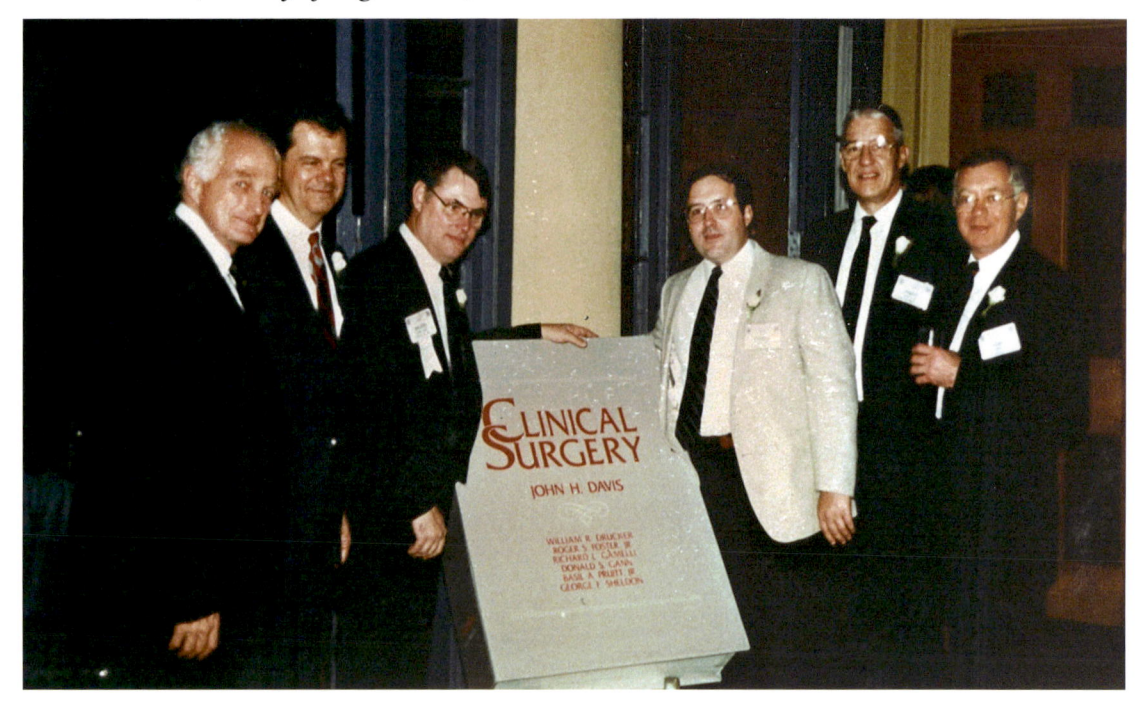

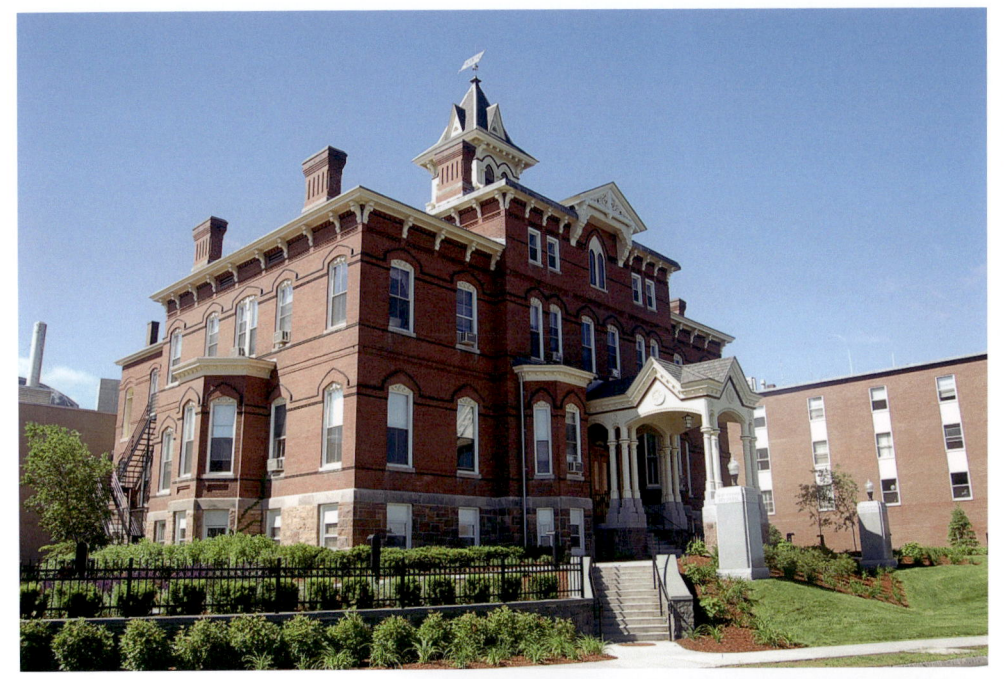

The restored Fletcher House in 2008 retains its original features. (DBP photo).

The newly opened Ambulatory Care Center, here pictured in 2008, features an underground parking garage beneath the green lawn foreground. (DBP photo).

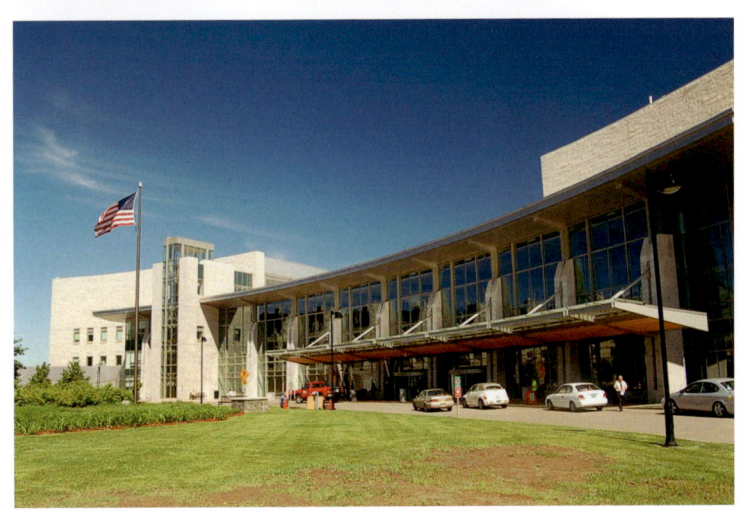

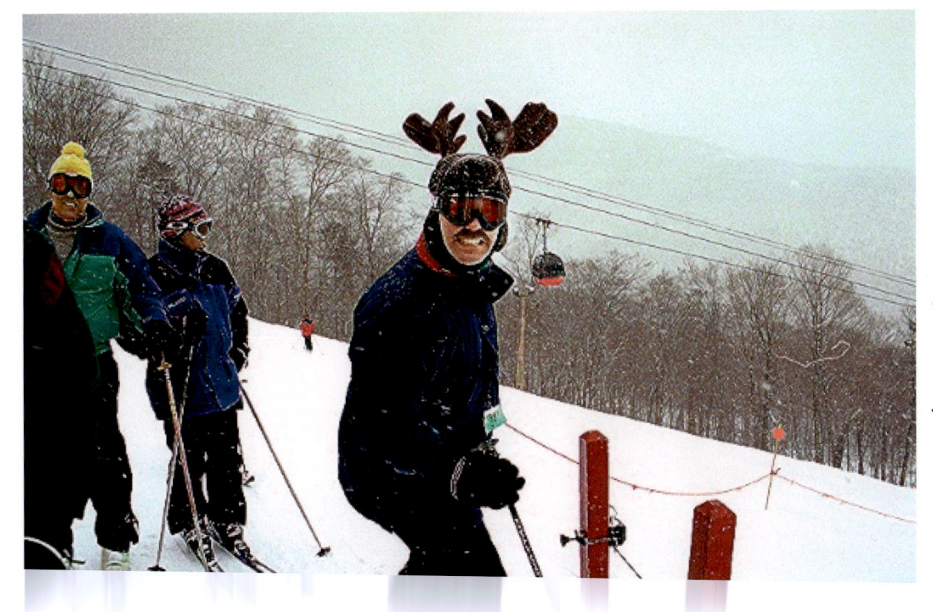

Neil Hyman (R) here entering the race course at Stowe provides comic relief at the Annual surgery ski races. The author DBP is at left with yellow cap. In 1997 the helmet revolution had not yet reached surgery. (Courtesy of

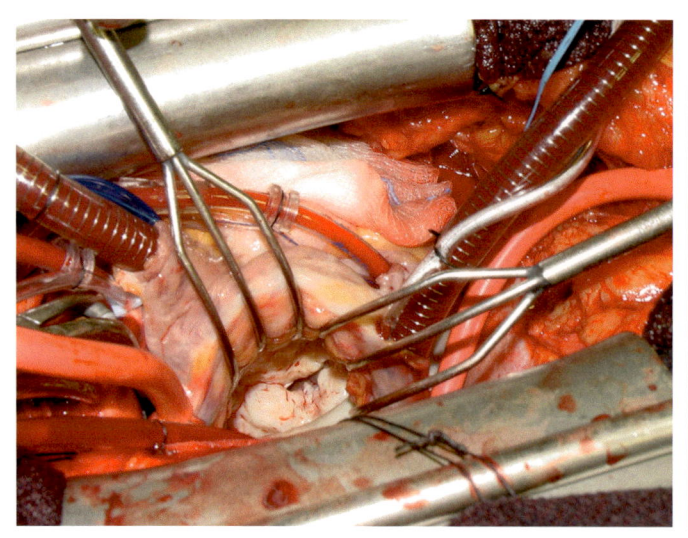

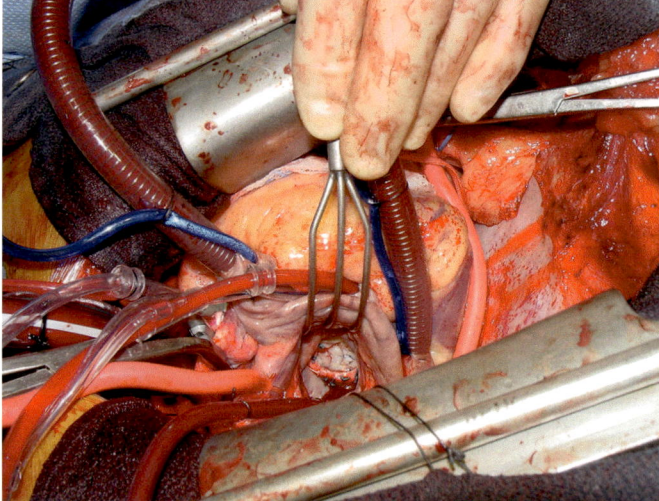

Mitral valve before (a) and after (b) repair by Bruce Leavitt using the French Correction. (Courtesy Bruce Leavitt).

Geoff Tabin on "Top of the World" 1988 (Photo Dawa Tsering Sherpa. Courtesy of Geoff Tabin).

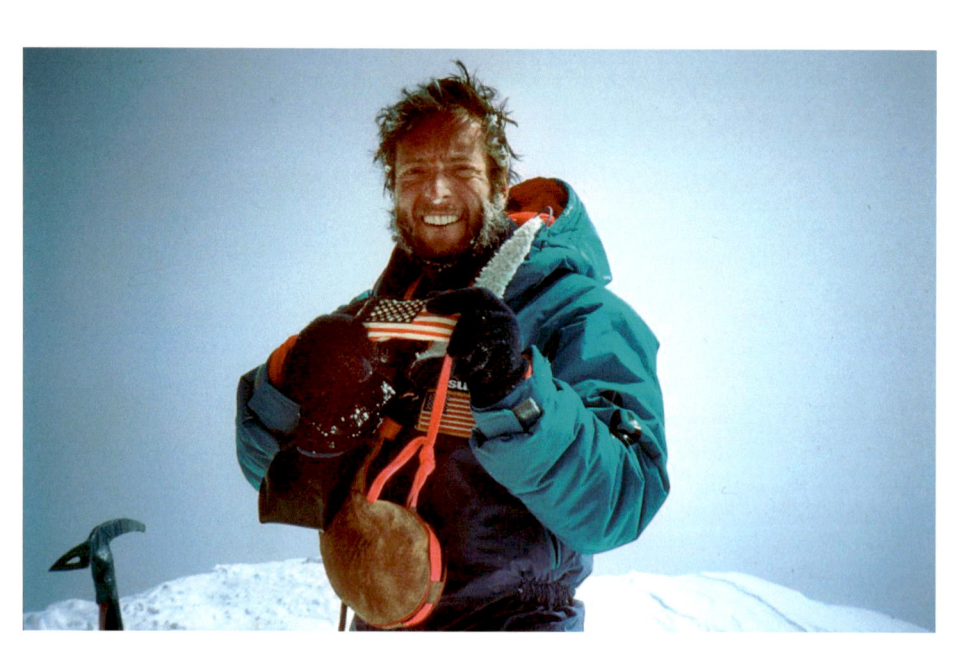

Geoff Tabin happily greets his postoperative cataract patients at a Nepalese Cataract Camp. (Courtesy Geoff Tabin).

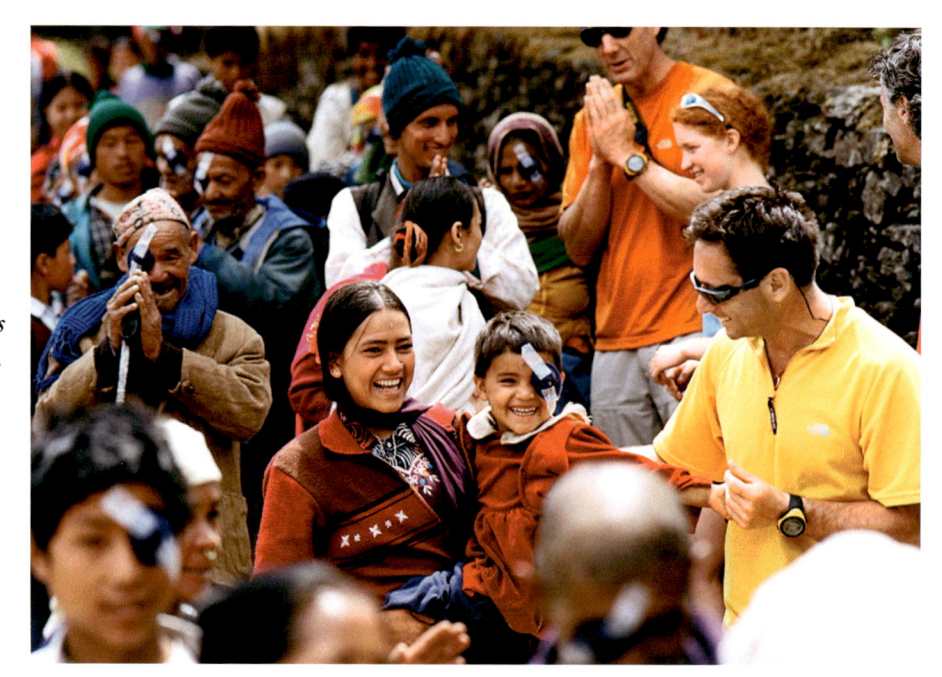

Stephen Leffler reviews Emergency Department x-rays with medical student (UVM med photo).

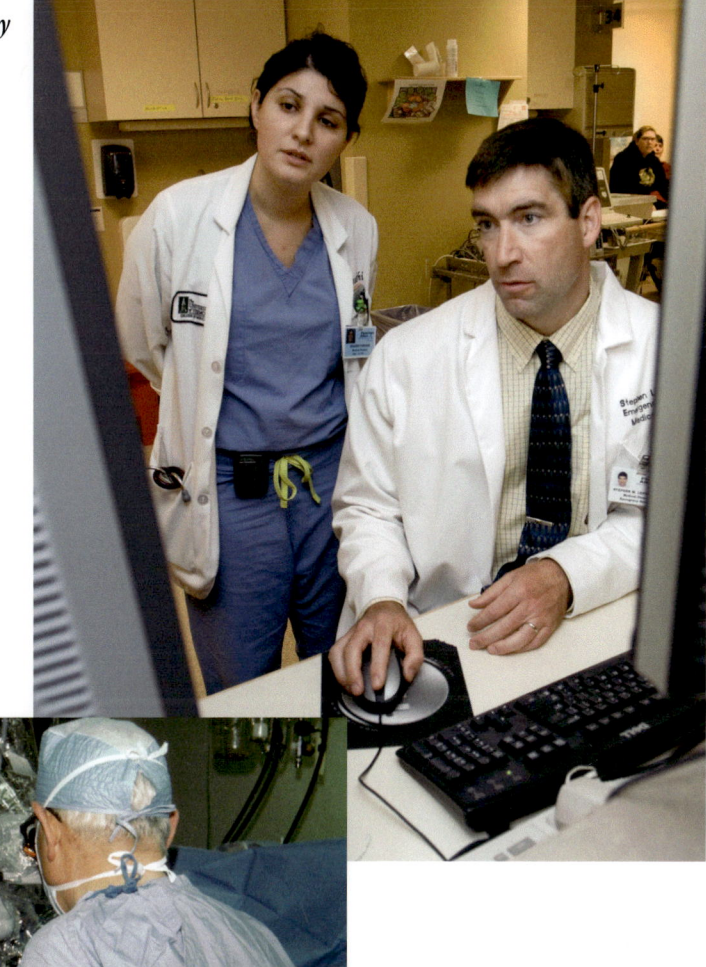

Alan Irwin operates with his father Edwin Irwin this one final time. (Courtesy of Alan Irwin).

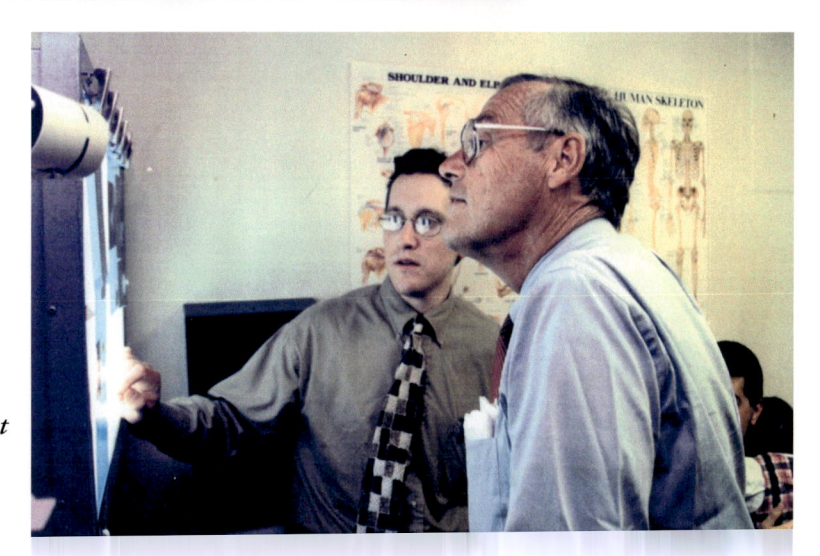

Patrick Devanney orthopaedic resident reviews a case with John Frymoyer in 2001. (UVM Med

Christopher Abajian wearing his Huggable Scrubs, soothes his patient with music. (Christopher Abajian photo).

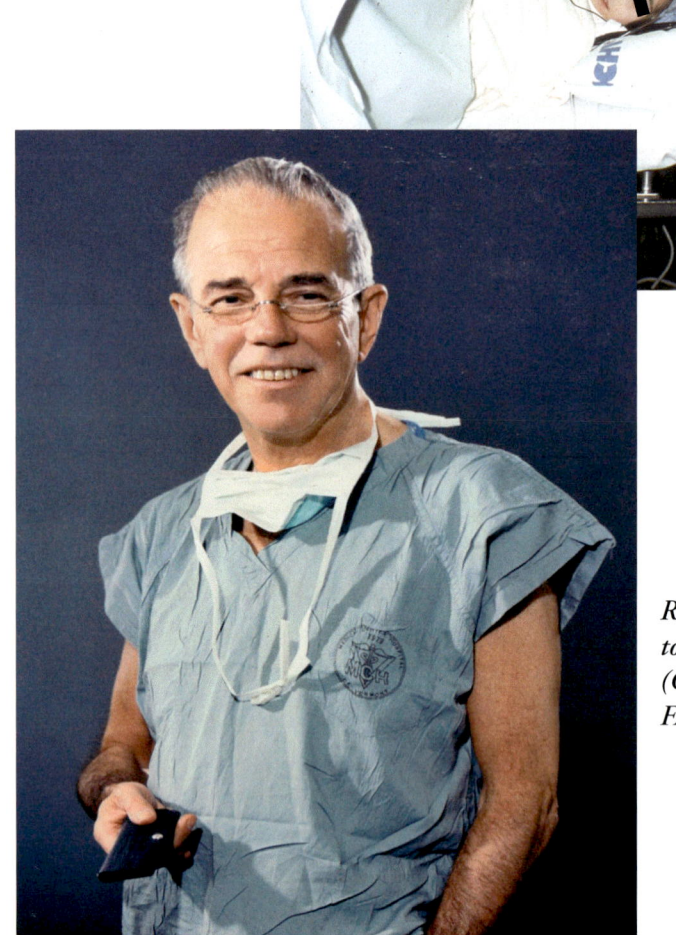

R.M.P. Donaghy in his research laboratory scrub shirt, always had a smile. (Courtesy of Neurosurgery archives, FAHC and UVM).

Vascular teaching rounds always had excellent attendance. Here L to R. DBP, resident Brad Jimmo, resident Dino Visioni, Steven Shackford, Andrew Stanley, Wallace Tarry, and Michael Ricci convene. (UVM Med photo).

The Department of Surgery Coat of Arms

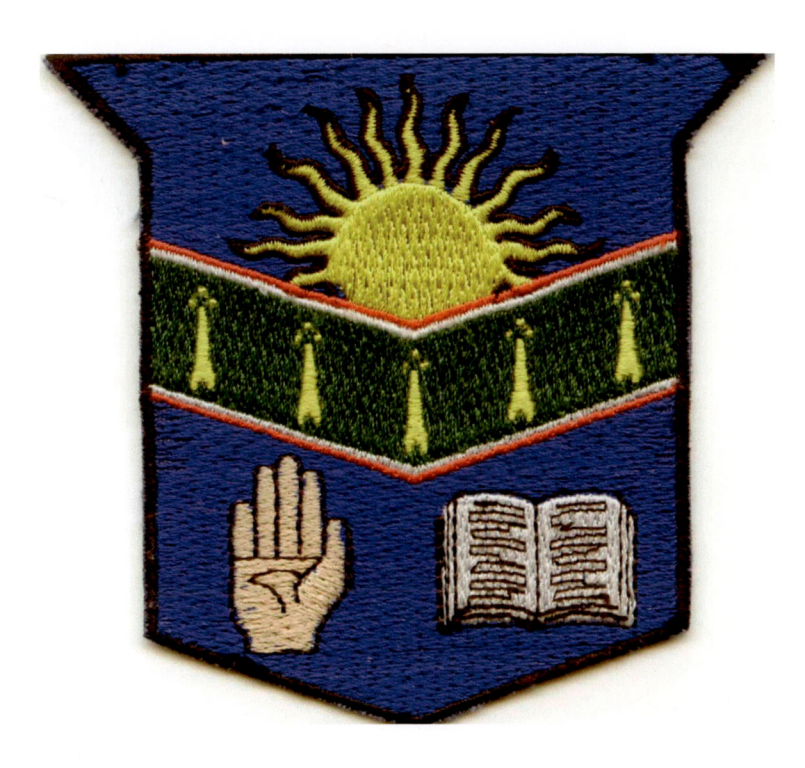

The Department adopted its unique crest in 1996. Designed by Philip Camp under Steven Shackford's direction, it embodies the core attributes of a successful surgeon.

The sun signifies wisdom, strength of character, and personal warmth.
The reverse chevron implies that rank (hierarchy) is integral to the profession.
The upward ermine arrows within the chevron indicate that the art of surgery is noble.
The hand reflects the dexterity and technical skill required of surgeons.
The open book symbolizes the knowledge that is available to all.
Blue exemplifies renown and beauty.
Green is the traditional color of both medicine and Vermont.
Gold represents the four virtues of nobleness, goodwill, vigor and magnanimity.
Silver stands for the five virtues of humility, beauty, clarity, purity and innocence.[1]

The author (left) performing splenectomy in a tent with temperature 105°F, in Duc Pho, Vietnam, with the 101st Airborne Division in 1967. Gary Roman, UVM trained anesthesiologist is in the center. (DBP photo)

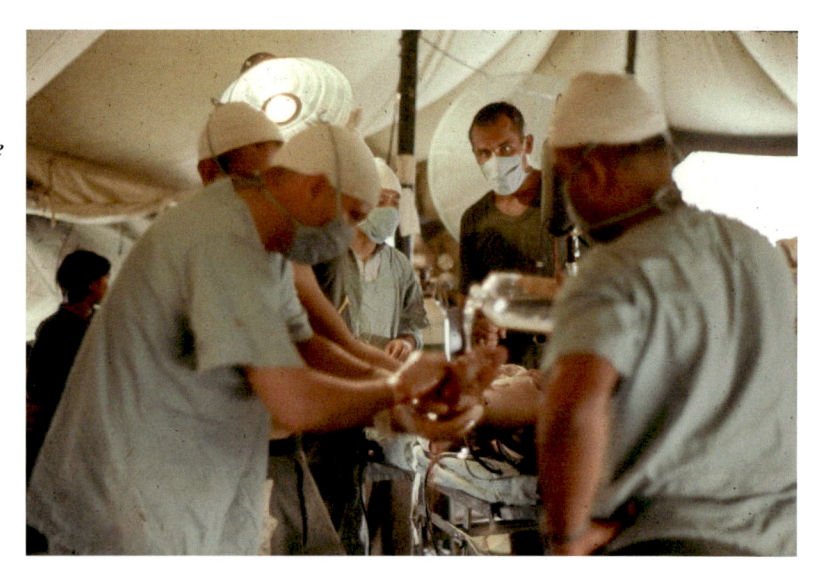

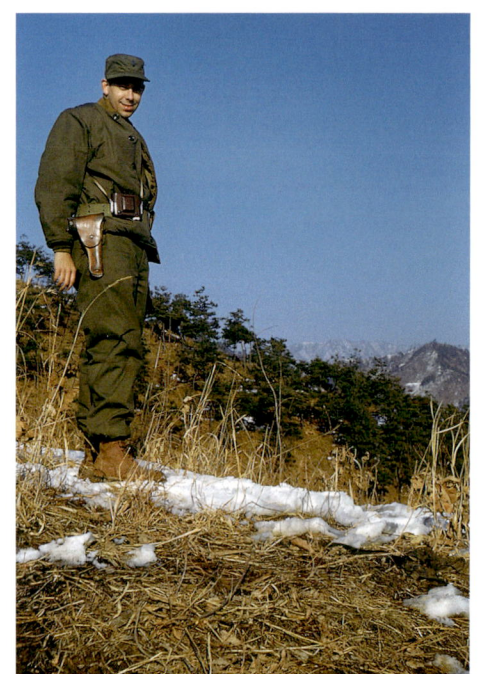

John Davis in Korea modeling for Hawkeye? (courtesy of John Davis).

A simulated accident victim is splinted by C. Earl Gettinger Jr (orange coat), Emergency Medical Services Coordinator of the State of Vermont. David Modica, head of the ambulance service of the Burlington Fire Department, (far L) guards the airway in this scene from the 1973 movie "Emergency Care". (DBP photo).

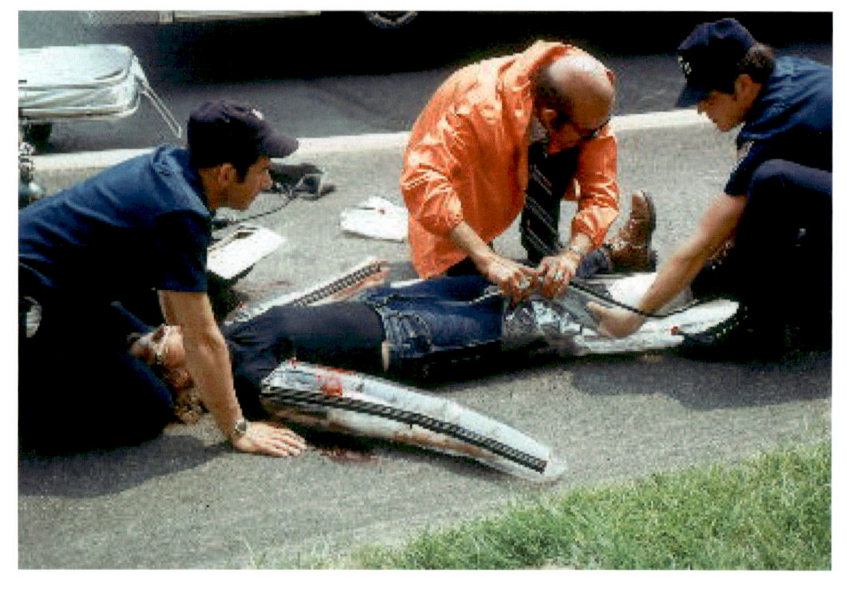

As sub-specialist groups split off from general surgery to become divisions or departments of their own, general surgery continued to grow. Graduates of our programs who migrated to rural areas were required to do many procedures themselves, especially in emergencies. Caesarean sections, repair of blood vessels, and care of fractures that otherwise would be handled by specialists in a major center, needed to be performed by general surgeons in many outlying areas.

At UVM, all subspecialties save Anesthesia and Orthopaedics continue to be part of the Department of Surgery. The lack of fellowships or residencies in many specialties leads to broader general surgery training at Vermont than in many other academic centers.

The timelines overlap, and events and personalities are at times featured in several parts.

PART VII

THE DIVISIONS OF THE DEPARTMENT OF SURGERY

CHAPTER 13

Anesthesia

UVM's John Abajian revolutionized military anesthesia during World War II by using regional techniques, saving thousands of lives in the process. Anesthesiologists at UVM pioneered similar methods for adults and infants.

The perfection of precision vaporization, and the publication of UVM's favorable experience with more than 5000 patients led to the widespread use of halothane in the United States.

Groundbreaking work on respirators and arterial pressure monitors belied the group's status as a Division of Surgery, an oversight that was finally addressed with an elevation to independent Department standing in 1991.

Anesthetics Arise During the 19th Century

The "discoveries" of nitrous oxide, ether, and chloroform revolutionized surgery overnight (see Chapter 4). The task of administering these new agents was assigned to fellow surgeons, dentists, or nurses. Interns poured ether for tonsillectomies and simple laparotomies. If an operation was performed in a patient's home, then a medical student or an interested bystander was sometimes recruited.

It was an age of experimentation. Former Professor of Surgery John Brooks Wheeler described an 1886 case in which he used local regional anesthesia (an eventual UVM forté) for the first time:

> "A seventeen-year old girl came to me with an osteo-myelitis of the cuboid bone of her left foot, the result of an injury. I thought it was a good case for cocain and the patient was glad of a chance to avoid taking ether, so cocain was used. I injected down to the bone ten drops of a four percent solution of cocain in each of three places around the place where I proposed to cut. Ten minutes after making the injection I sat down opposite her, took her foot on my knee, and made a two-inch cut down to the bone. The patient watched the proceedings with great interest and said she felt no pain at all."[1]

The specialty of Anesthesiology arose as manual open drop administration gave way to machines capable of mixing anesthetic agents and oxygen, and as the role of regional techniques expanded.

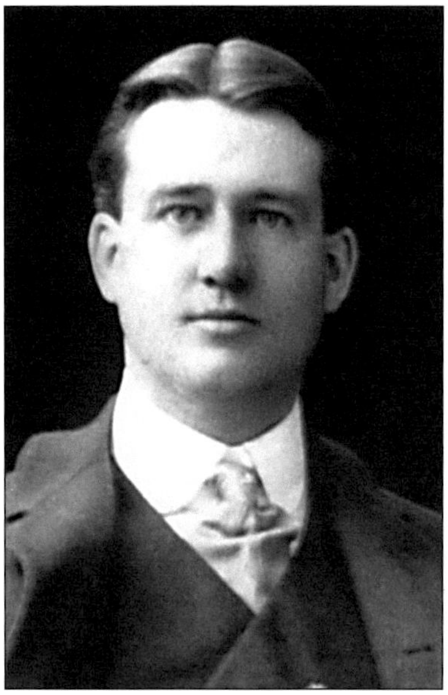

FIGURE 13-1.
John Dodds was UVM's first "Instructor in Anesthetization".

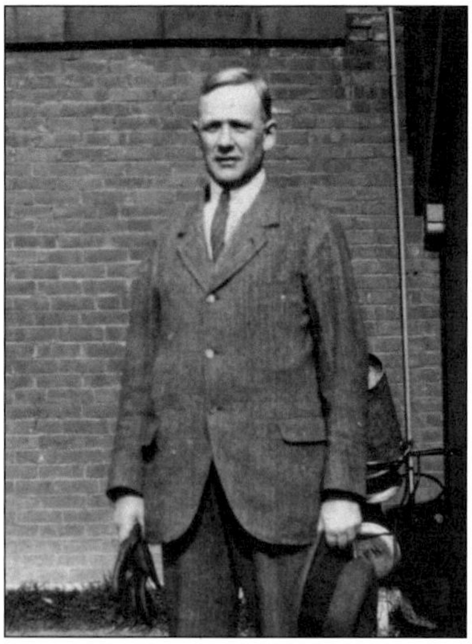

FIGURE 13-2.
George Sabin introduced spinal anesthesia to UVM.

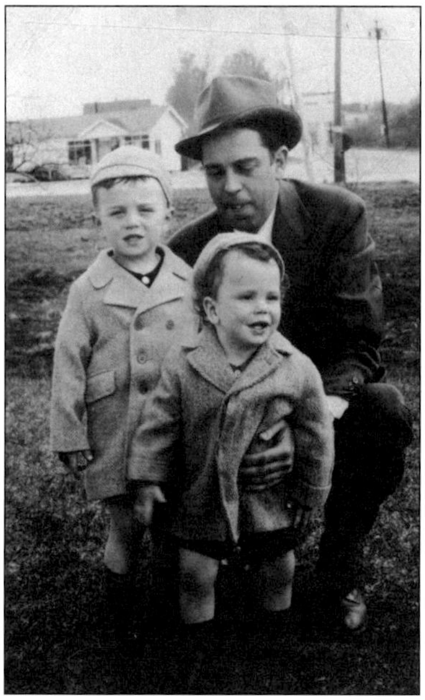

FIGURE 13-3.
Christopher Terrien, Sr. gave anesthesia at all three Burlington hospitals during the War. Here he poses with sons (and future UVM doctors) Timothy and Christopher Jr. in 1944 at the Terrien home and office on the corner of Patchen and Williston Roads. (the later site of Gracey's Store)

UVM's Original Anesthetists

John Hazen Dodds (1873-1964) was UVM's first (and only) "Instructor in Anaesthetization" from 1906 until 1933. The 1898 College of Medicine graduate and general practitioner obtained his training through New York City courses and working with Burlington dentists.[2] The "Dodds Routine" was described by E.L. Amidon, quoted by Betty Wells as follows:

"No pre-op medication for the child, [who] usually crying was placed on the O.R. table. As a deep breath was taken in preparation for another yell, the intern would place the gauze cone soaked with ether over the child's face so he would get the full benefit. Not too many breaths were required before sleep mercifully took over. The trauma to both patient and 'anesthetizer' probably lasted a lifetime."[3]

George M. Sabin popularized the use of spinal anesthesia at UVM during the 1920s. Surgeons usually administered the spinals themselves and then scrubbed while nurses monitored the patients. Former General Surgery Chairman A.G. Mackay noted that Sabin "was quite criticized if any of the spinals got too high and the paralysis was uncontrollable, although it may have saved a lot of lives which would have been lost otherwise from an inhalation anesthetic."[4]

Edward John Ford of Philadelphia was UVM's "Instructor in Anesthesia" from 1937 to 1939. Ford advocated cyclopropane over ether. The use of this highly explosive agent obviously led to a great deal of apprehension.

At the same time, the Fanny Allen's legendary Christopher M. Terrien, Sr. (1910-1994) was looking for a way to augment his income. "I took a postgraduate course in anesthesia in New York." Upon completion, "I did anesthesia from 1939 until after World War II." Terrien also taught anesthetic technique and procured equipment. "One of the first gas machines that Fanny Allen ever had was a Foregger, which I went down and bought from Dr. Foregger in New York City early in 1940s."[5]

Terrien recalled being an anesthesiologist at all three Burlington hospitals during the War. "I would start out early in the morning at the FAH, where we had nurse anesthetists, go to the MFH, where we had nurse anesthetists, go to the DeGoesbriand Hospital, where I worked mostly as an anesthetist, and I would end up working with about 20 anesthetists in the morning." Terrien stopped administering anesthesia in 1947 after becoming a board-certified internist with a specialty in cardiology.[6]

John Abajian Recruited as Chief of Anesthesia

Today's Department really got its start under John Abajian, Jr. (1912-1996). Abajian had entered college in Rhode Island, but was whisked off to New York City by an appalled visiting grandfather who found him "gambling" instead of studying. After completing his studies at Long Island University, Abajian attended New York College of Medicine. He then finished a one-year "preceptorship-type" anesthesia residency at New York's Gotham and Lennox Hill Hospital.

Abajian's preceptor mentioned that UVM's College of Medicine was going to establish an anesthesia division. The intelligent, energetic, and ambitious Abajian looked into the situation and took the job. Years later, he had this to say about his 1939 arrival:

"I remember arriving in Burlington on the old Colonial Airlines one cold December, and having left New York with the lights and seeing the bleak snow, I felt that I had been banished to Siberia ... but perhaps that was the greatest day of my life."

Abajian asked the taxi driver to immediately take him to the nearest pub. It was there that Mackay found him. As Abajian put it:

"The medical school had been advised following the Flexner report to bring in some outside blood and the first person in was two-gun Hardy Kemp as Dean of the medical school, from Texas. Dr. Kemp [who literally kept two pistols on his desk] brought up two other foreigners — Wilhelm Raab with his Viennese accent, and the other, myself with a New York accent."[7]

Abajian was given permission to hire a nurse that he could train as an anesthetist. His selection, Betty Wells, recounted the process:

"I had been asked by [MFH] superintendent Brown if I would like to be an anesthetist. I said I didn't know anything about anesthesia and didn't care much for the operating room. Brown said Dr. Abajian preferred a nurse who didn't know anything; so I felt that I qualified."[8]

Abajian quickly "earned the respect of UVM surgeons for his use of innovative regional techniques, especially peridural anesthesia, a skill he learned from New Orleans surgeon, Charles Odom."[9] Respect was the major thing that Abajian actually earned, however:

"In 1940 there was no charge for anesthesia. It was given to the person as part of the operating room charge, and I

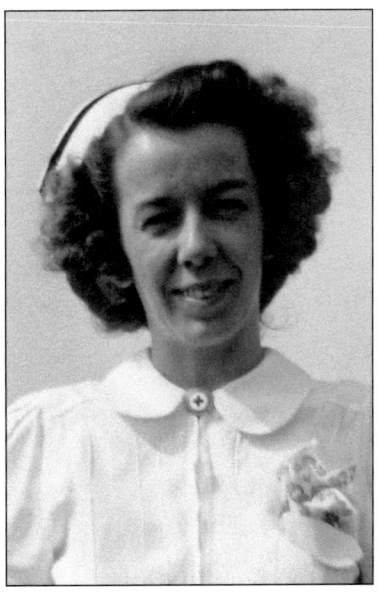

FIGURE 13-4. Nurse anesthetist Betty Wells started her long UVM career before WWII.

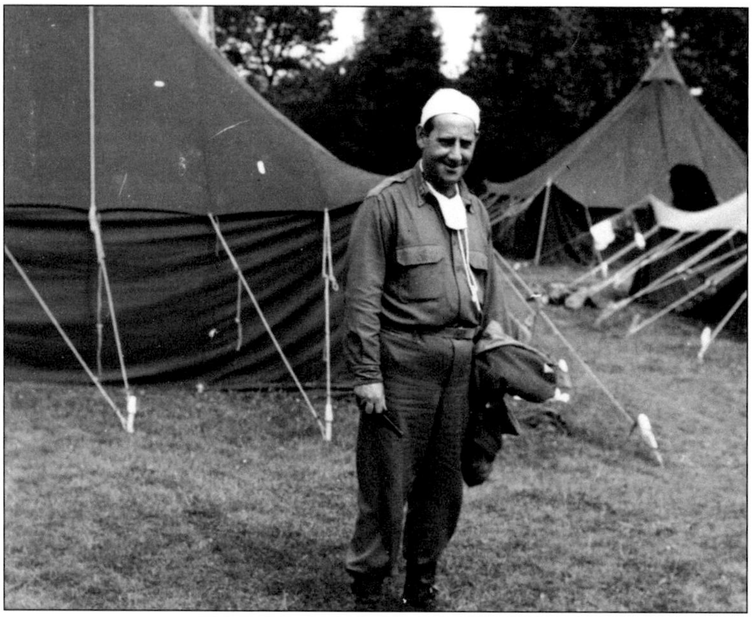

FIGURE 13-5.
John Abajian, pipe in hand, bivouacked with Patton's Third Army.

was employed as an employee of the hospital for $3,000 a year. At the end of one year I was promoted for satisfactory performance to $3,600 a year." [10]

Abajian Goes to War With Patton

Odom, as George Patton's surgery consultant, called on Abajian a few years later:

"As 1942 approached and people were going into the service, Dr. Wally Rees was the first to volunteer to go. I was rather young but felt that I too should volunteer, although we were all exempt because of our medical school connection. I found myself, at the age of 31, as the consultant anesthesiologist for Patton's Third Army. My job was to break the bottleneck in getting soldiers anesthetized fast enough to keep the surgical evacuation chain moving. The usual table of organization of each evacuation hospital was one anesthesiologist and two nurses for each shift. With three anesthesiologists trying to handle twelve tables it became rather hairy, and the solution ... was teaching corpsmen to inject Pentothal.

The natural consequence of this was a rather high mortality rate. I immediately began to take steps in local regional anesthesia, in which I was somewhat adept thanks to the help I received from Keith Truax and other people in Vermont prior to going into the service. There were real anatomists in those days in the medical school, and anatomy is all you need to know to teach local regional anesthesia. It wasn't long before we had the anesthesia picture for the Third Army changed from 85% Pentothal to 85% local regional." [11]

Abajian was recommended for the Legion of Merit for his endeavors. He also engaged in a few extra-curricular activities during this time:

"We traveled over the European theater of operations with a six-by-six [truck] confiscating German material (radios, cigars) which we disseminated to everybody. During one of those episodes I was in a warehouse which was guarded by some Polish soldiers, and on the

way out in my command car I jokingly stood up and gave the Hitler salute (just in case we lost), and these people took me seriously and began shooting at me. I had the scare of my life! I remember getting down in the bottom of my command car and scooting out of there in a hurry."[12]

Abajian's departure had left UVM shorthanded at the worst possible time — the beginning of the new intern year. Luckily, the first intern on the anesthesia service was Ernest L. Mills, who had been a senior medical student under Abajian's charge. Mills was proficient in general anesthesia, as well as epidural, spinal and other blocks.

Mills shared his knowledge with the interns that followed him on the service. This supplemented the nurse anesthetists that Terrien had trained to give spinal anesthetics. Mills was called into the Army in 1943 and sent to the Mayo Clinic for a six-month surgery and anesthesia course courtesy of Uncle Sam. Payback came in the form of a South Pacific deployment.

Anesthesia After the War

Despite his military accomplishments, Abajian was not exactly welcomed back to UVM with open arms. The reason was obvious even to Abajian. "Like a safety valve, I blow off steam easily. Maybe some of the patient souls around me get singed now and then, but it sure prevents ulcers!"[13] Mackay relates that others were less kind:

"Two men came to me from the medical faculty, to say that John Abajian was such a loud-mouthed bombastic individual, and so disruptive of faculty affairs, that he must not be allowed to return to Burlington to work. My answer to them was the fact that every veteran who had served his country, of course, would be accepted back at his old desk to work as he was before the War, but that if these gentlemen would return to me with their complaints after Dr. Abajian had been back on duty for a minimum of six to nine months we would then have a hearing and decide whether or not their wishes could be carried out"[14]

Needless to say, such a hearing never occurred. Abajian worked hard in the laboratory publishing studies on curare, hypothermia, and blood volume. He organized the Vermont-New Hampshire blood bank, which was the second of its kind in America. He even started his own cable TV company. Somewhere along the way, he also found time to establish UVM's anesthesiology residency program.

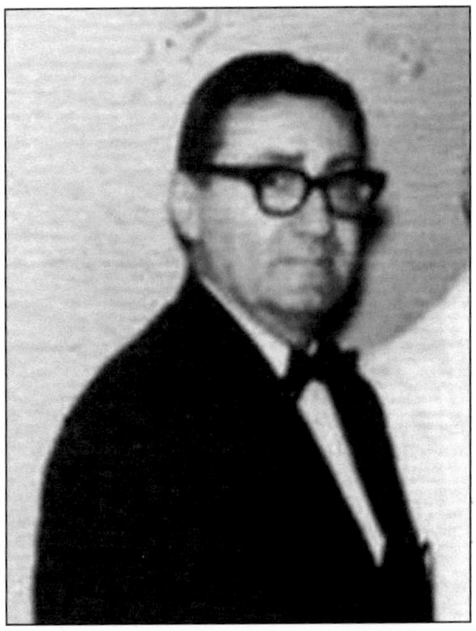

One of Abajian's first residents was Gino Dente. The Barre native graduated from the College of Medicine in 1941 as a civilian, but finished his Brooklyn internship nine months later as an "administrative lieutenant" in the Army. The rank came with a big paycheck, a snazzy uniform, and a looming military assignment. Sent to the Pacific as an infantry company medical officer, Dente eventually assumed the role of anesthesiologist. He usually ad-

FIGURE 13-6. John Abajian recruited Gino Dente from the White River Junction VAH after WWII.

ministered open drop ether. Regional anesthetics (spinals) were rarely used in the Pacific Theater.

Dente returned to Vermont after the war and went to work at the White River Junction VA Hospital as an anesthesiologist. Abajian approached him during a visit and said, "Why don't you come to Burlington and be a resident with me? You don't want to stay in the VA."[15] Dente agreed. He later recalled his first day at the DeGoesbriand:

> *"I found Abajian conducting a dental case under endotracheal cyclopropane anesthesia. He welcomed me and said he had to go to the Fletcher to do another case, and I should stay with this case until it was completed. I had never seen a case under endotracheal anesthesia and when the procedure was completed I did not know what to do. Helen Finnegan was the operating room nurse in charge and she told me: 'take the damn tube out!' All went well."*[16]

Dente stayed on after completing his UVM residency in 1949, joining Abajian and Mills. The trio covered anesthesia at the Mary Fletcher and DeGoesbriand on a regular basis, and the Fanny Allen when needed. Nurse anesthetists and general practitioners filled the gaps, especially at the FAH.

The Shift to Regional Anesthesia

Abajian was convinced that regional anesthesia was safe and reliable based on his military experience. UVM soon became one of the foremost proponents of this technique. It was an unusual approach, since most hospitals relied solely on general anesthesia.

For example, there were 497 inhalation and 593 spinal and block anesthetics administered at the MFH in 1948. Open drop ether or cyclopropane was used for adult "above the waist" surgery, while ether was the sole choice for pediatric cases. Intercostal nerve blocks were used in combination with general anesthesia for poor risk patients. Spinals were preferred over general for lower abdominal or lower extremity surgery. Upper extremities were covered with brachial or other types of blocks.

Rectally administered Pentothal® or Avertin® were used for pre- and intra-op sedation. Although other hospitals were using intravenous Pentothal, Abajian steered clear of this method, as it had been associated with high mortality rates during his Army days. Similarly, chloroform, which was also used elsewhere, was banned by Abajian: "Anyone giving chloroform was guilty of malpractice ... with ether there's plenty of warning but with chloroform there isn't even time to say goodbye."[17]

Dente described a typical O.R. day during this period thusly:

> *"Because of the dangers of explosions with cyclopropane, our mornings started with the whirling of the hygrometer to check the relative humidity in the operating rooms. If it was low, we would open the doors of the steam sterilizers ... until the humidity was acceptably high. The breathing bag and tubing were rinsed with water ... and the Horton inter-coupler was attached. A non-explosive mixture was promoted in the mid '40s, with a cyclopropane-nitrous oxide-oxygen mixture. Abajian was fond of lighting a match at the pop-off valve to*

prove nothing would happen. Others in the room weren't particularly enthused or amused by this demonstration — even though everyone knew he was right![18]

The trend toward regional anesthesia continued. In 1950 there were 2,299 operations at the MFH with 923 inhalation anesthetics and 1,031 spinal blocks. The agents used for inhalation were: ether 512, cyclopropane 120, nitrous 104, cyclo-nitrous 187, and endotracheal 87.[19]

UVM Leads the Nation in Halothane Administration

Dente learned of a new agent called halothane (AKA Fluothane®) from a visiting English medical student. Intrigued, he wrote investigator James Raventos in November of 1956 and asked for more details. Raventos obliged by sending Dente two bottles from England. Dente and Mills found that the liquid allowed higher oxygen concentrations, was non-flammable, and was free of the post-op emergence problems and nausea associated with ether. Dente noted: "I had forgotten to ask Dr. Raventos for the instructions. Initially we tried to give it open drop, like ether, and that was a mistake."[20]

It was a mistake because halothane was very potent and thus very difficult to precisely control. Abajian thought that a semi-closed circuit with the existing copper kettle liquid vaporizer might work, but did not know how temperature fluctuations would affect output. This seemed like an ideal problem for Edward Brazell, the new director of anesthesia research. Brazell had done some engineering work for Abajian, and then entered the College of Medicine at his mentor's urging. Abajian immediately hired Brazell in 1956 upon the completion of his protégé's anesthesiology residency.

FIGURE 13-7.
Abajian working on his "Abajian Scales."

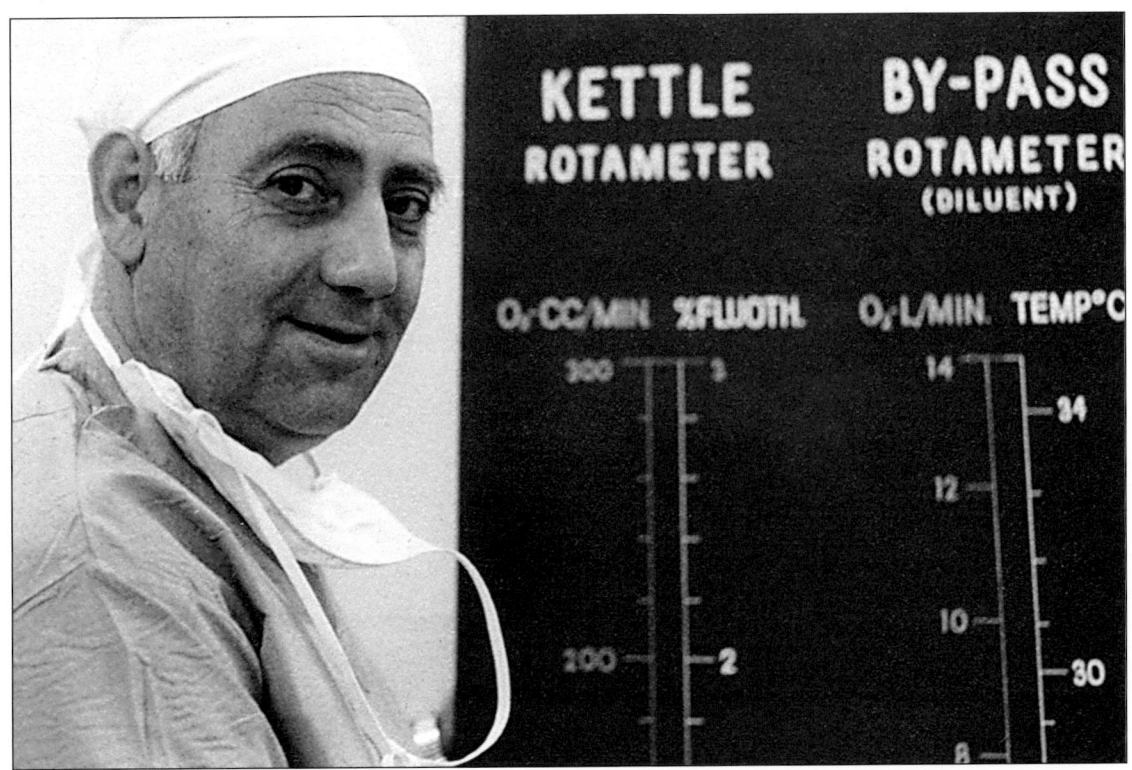

Brazell set to work. He calculated exact halothane concentrations at various kettle flow rates, and then created a set of temperature-corrected flow meter markings. The resulting "Abajian Scales" allowed even the most inexperienced anesthesiologist to accurately control flow based on desired concentration and ambient temperature.

Halothane became UVM's preferred agent for general anesthesia long before it gained popularity in the rest of United States. Within a year, nearly every inhaled anesthetic given in Burlington utilized a pure halothane-oxygen technique. Abajian presented supporting evidence that halothane approached the ideal anesthetic in 1958, followed by the results of more than 5000 cases in 1959.[21, 22] UVM was at the leading edge of halothane administration, an edge that cut badly when the first reports of "halothane hepatitis" arose. The claims were eventually disproved, but not before halothane had fallen out of favor.[23] It nevertheless remains the first choice of inhaled anesthetic in the third-world due to its safety and simplicity of use.

John Mazuzan, the Division's "De Facto Chief"

John E. Mazuzan, Jr. wanted to be a newspaperman until a 1944 case of rheumatic fever and bacterial endocarditis derailed his plans. Mazuzan's Northfield, Vermont family physician secured a two-week supply of the new (but wartime restricted) drug penicillin. The fourteen year-old recovered, became interested in medicine, and started reading borrowed medical books. His efforts were later rewarded with a College of Medicine diploma.[24]

Mazuzan was one of 12 general or "rotating" Mary Fletcher interns in 1954-55. Anesthesia was one of the rotations. The 36 hour on, 12 hour off schedule resulted in coverage by six interns per night. Mazuzan joined the Air Force in 1955 and was sent to Georgia where he served as a general medical officer and obstetrician for the next two years. When the surgeons complained to the Army brass about the poor quality of their nurse anesthetist, she was transferred and not replaced. Mazuzan, who had the most anesthesia experience (one month), became the anesthesiologist by default.

FIGURE 13-8. John Mazuzan, a native of Northfield, Vermont, was recruited to UVM by Abajian in 1959.

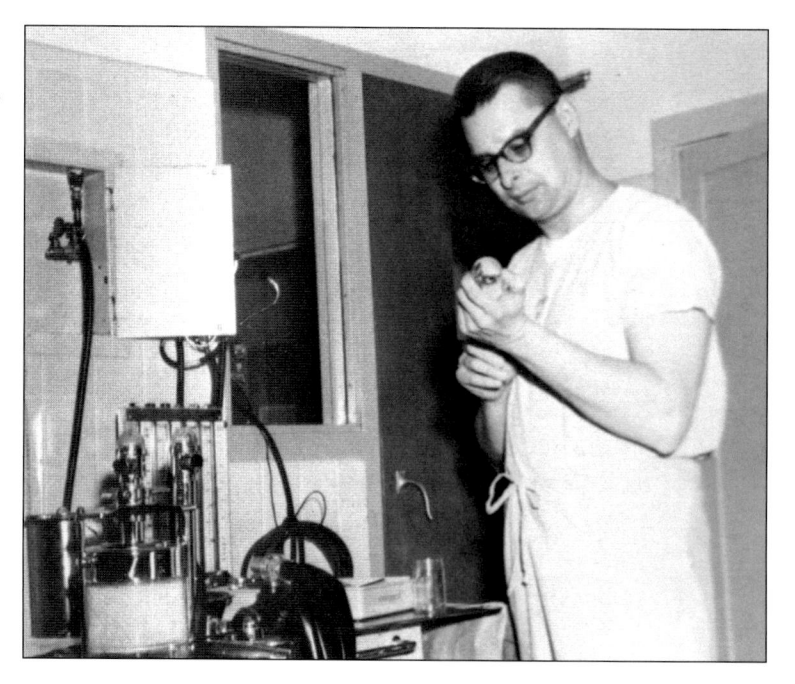

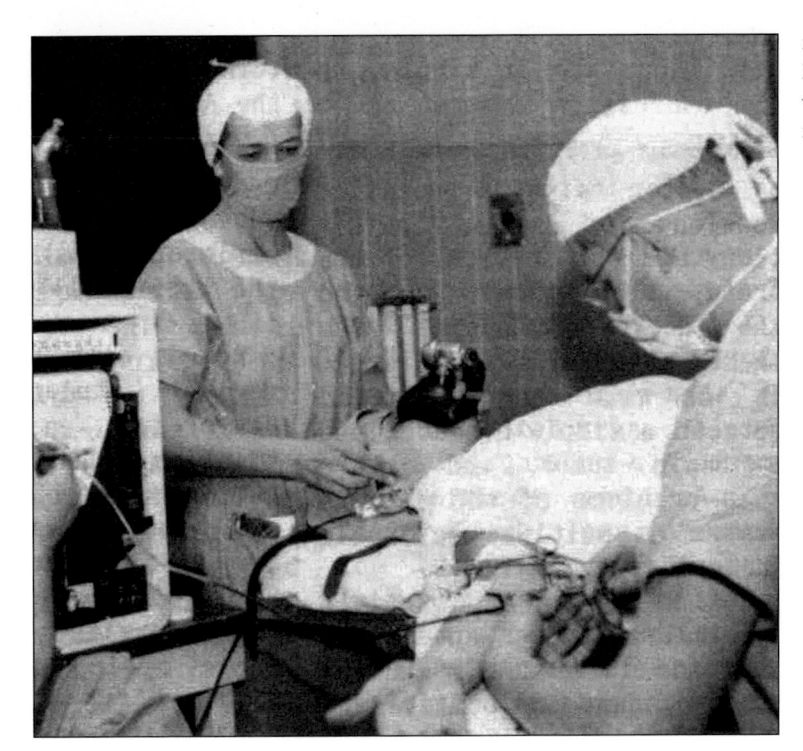

FIGURE 13-9.
Mazuzan working with Betty Wells in 1961.

He almost stayed in the Air Force, but left in 1957 to start an anesthesiology residency at the Massachusetts General Hospital (MGH). The MGH sent its anesthesia residents to either the Boston Lying-In Hospital or Yale for obstetrics, as it did not have its own obstetric service. Mazuzan reasoned that he could complete an "obstetrics rotation" at UVM and simultaneously learn about the new agent halothane, which was not being used at the MGH. He relocated his wife and children to the old Northfield family home, thereby taking a bit of a vacation in the process. He took anesthesia call every weeknight so that he could spend weekends in Northfield with his family.

Mazuzan returned to the MGH after finishing his UVM-based rotation. He was sitting in the O.R. during his chief year, administering anesthesia when Abajian called with the following news: "Dr. Brazell is moving to California, and we have an opening for you." Mazuzan's 1959 arrival heralded the Division's expansion and the publication of many scientific papers.[25]

Research Remains a Part of Abajian's Division

The 1955 polio epidemic had aroused Abajian's fertile imagination. At the time, patients with paralyzed diaphragms were supported either temporarily or permanently with negative pressure ventilators. Such an individual was placed within a sealed metal cylinder that left their head exposed to room pressure. A pump increased and decreased the pressure around the chest cavity, which moved air in and out of the lungs through the patient's mouth and nose. While effective, these "Iron Lungs" or "Drinker Respirators" (after their inventor) were cumbersome and confining.

The Mary Fletcher kept its original "Iron Lung" near the Operating Room. The machine served as a reminder of the WW II anesthesiologist shortage, when more than a few patients received inadvertent "high" spinals at the hands of inexperienced interns who injected the

FIGURE 13-10.
Abajian and his ever present pipe with Tom Shinozaki in 1966.

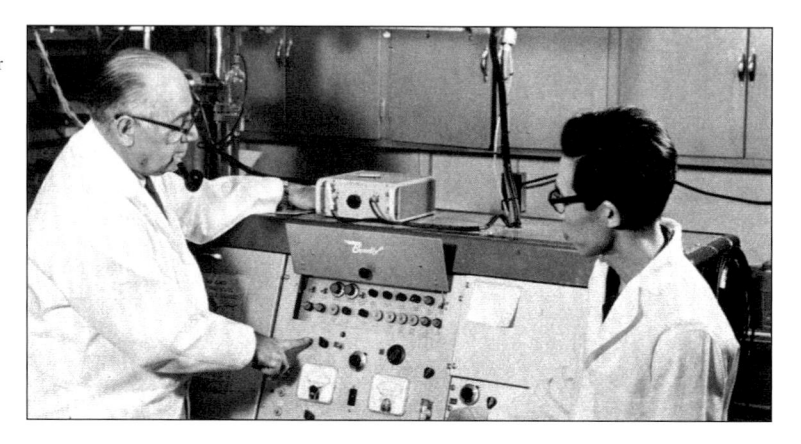

larger doses intended for epidural injection inadvertently into the spinal canal. Epidurals were essentially banned after the War in the interests of safety and peace of mind.[26]

Abajian knew that positive pressure ventilators, which blew air into patients' lungs via intubation or long-term tracheostomy, had been successfully deployed during a European polio outbreak a few years earlier. The concept was directly applicable to the O.R. as a potential replacement for the old open drop technique. Abajian sent Mills to Rhode Island to learn more about advanced ventilatory support.

Abajian and his team started to modify respirators to suit the demands of the O.R. This led to a collaborative design project with Forrest Bird, the originator of the "Bird Respirator", after Abajian befriended the inventor. Burlington's two main hospitals eventually shared ten of the useful little green boxes, one or two of which remained in service well into the 1990s.

Abajian recruited Tamotsu (Tom) Shinozaki, a doctor with an engineering background and inventive mind, to help with his research endeavors. UVM, already flush with anesthesiologists such as Michael Burfoot, Roy Bell, and Harold Jacobs, had to prove that Shinozaki's presence was essential in order to satisfy immigration policies. Abajian got around the issue by supposedly convincing Louis Thabault, the Fanny Allen's Chief of Surgery, to attest that the new hire was desperately needed at the FAH. Thabault thereafter received enhanced anesthesia help at the Fanny Allen!

Abajian and Shinozaki invented a machine that measured pulmonary nitrogen washout with the aid of a desktop computer. The device was manufactured by the pair's "Vertek Company®", which was acquired by Hewlett Packard in 1972. They then developed the "JATS" (John Abajian Tom Shinozaki) arterial pressure monitor. Shinozaki remained at the vanguard of computer implementation throughout his career, especially with respect to his work in the cardiac room and ICU.

UVM Finally Gets an ICU and a Recovery Room

Abajian thought that a post-op Recovery Room was an excuse for poor anesthesia administration and poor nursing care. He had, after all, been awakening patients in the O.R. since his Army days. But some individuals were kept in the O.R. longer than necessary when they did not rapidly emerge from anesthesia. At other times, patients were returned to the wards prematurely in order to keep the schedule moving. It was not a huge problem, since UVM used more regional blocks and halothane than elsewhere. And it did give the floor nurses experience with awakening/recovering surgical patients.

Other large academic medical centers, however, were not as "enlightened" as UVM. So when inspectors from the Joint Commission on Accreditation of Hospitals (JCAH) came to the MFH and DeGoesbriand, they always asked to see the Recovery Room — only to get a long explanation as to why neither hospital had a Recovery Room.

The hospitals were also without Intensive Care Units as well. This changed in 1961 when a UVM Trustee (who was also a prominent member of the community) came into the MFH with status asthmaticus and died. The surviving Trustees decided that UVM should immediately implement a respiratory support team. Pulmonary Medicine was approached, but declined since "they had no manpower to start such a service." When Anesthesia was asked, Abajian replied "Mills can do it part-time." Mazuzan put his foot in his mouth by saying: "It won't work part-time, we've got to do it right ... let him develop a proper service."[27]

Mills had been running anesthesia at the DeGoesbriand, so Abajian replaced him with Dente (who stayed there until retiring in 1987). The job of managing the MFH O.R. was then assigned to Mazuzan, leaving Mills free to organize and run the new Intensive Care Unit. It was an eleven-bed affair located in previous pharmacy space between Smith 2's Operating Suites and Patrick 2's patient wards. Medical and surgical patients were cared for in the unit, with an emphasis on respiratory problems. An office between the ICU and the O.R. just large enough for two beds became the first Recovery Room.

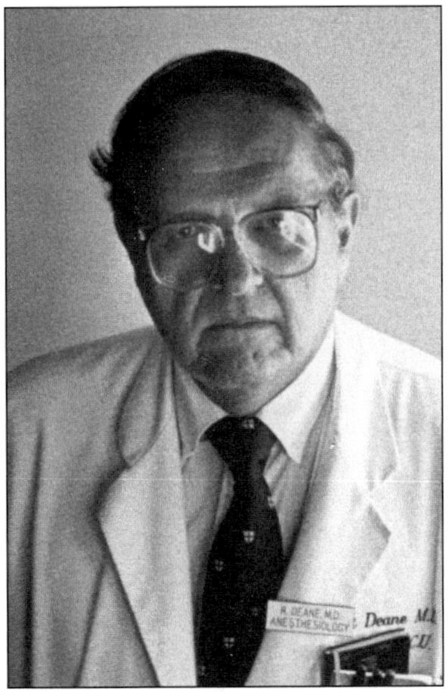

Robert S. Deane stepped in to fill the post when Mills retired in 1965. The always affable South African directed the Surgical ICU alongside the reserved Shinozaki for the next 30 years. The pair oversaw the unit's expansion and eventual relocation into the McClure building. SICU leadership was transferred from Anesthesia to Surgery at the time of Shackford's arrival, which made sense in light of his background in trauma and critical care management. Deane and Shinozaki adapted, serving until their mid-1990 retirements. Anesthesia continues to maintain a strong and collegial role in the SICU. This relationship remains one of the strengths of the UVM anesthesia residency.

FIGURE 13-11. Robert Deane (pictured here in 1988) had a long tenure in the ICU after his arrival from South Africa.

A New Chief and Department in Name Only

Abajian spent increasingly more time in the research laboratory developing his inventions, delegating his clinical and administrative responsibilities to others. Much of that work fell to Mazuzan, who considered himself the "de facto chief" of the Division — even though he didn't have such a title. When Abajian finally retired in 1977, Dean William Lughinbuhl sent a letter to Mazuzan naming him "Interim Chief." Mazuzan angrily refused the appointment, replying that he considered it a demotion from the "de facto" position he had held for years.

Lughinbuhl got the message, and appointed Mazuzan permanent Chief one month later without further discussion.[28]

Mazuzan carried on many of Abajian's policies. He had no reason to challenge the status quo, since he and John Davis had such a cooperative arrangement. Davis let the anesthesiologists maintain their business and financial management, while still giving them the authority to run the O.R. as they saw fit. Davis' successor Shackford thought otherwise, so the Division of Anesthesiology became the Department of Anesthesiology in 1991 with little fanfare.

UVM Leads the Nation in Pediatric Spinal Anesthesia

Abajian's son John Christian followed in his father's prominent footsteps. After graduating from the College of Medicine, "Chris" completed an internship in Montreal, an anesthesiology residency in London, and a fellowship at Toronto's Hospital for Sick Children. He subsequently returned to UVM in 1974 as its first formally trained pediatric anesthesiologist.

A few years later, pediatric surgeon Paul Mellish asked the younger Abajian to evaluate a premature infant with a huge inguinal hernia. Mellish had already determined that the defect was too large to repair under local. Chris felt that the baby was too sick for a general, so Mellish floated the idea of using a spinal. After conferring with Dente, a dosage of 1 mg of tetracaine per year of patient age was selected. Chris then successfully administered the spinal as a NICU nurse talked him through the procedure. He became enamored with the technique and went on to publish 1,500 cases during the 1980s. UVM has since continued as a world leader in pediatric regional anesthesia.[29, 30, 31]

Chris Abajian, unlike John Dodds, was keenly aware of the need to provide a calming environment in which to sedate his pediatric patients. He started by designing a line of O.R. scrub clothing that featured kid-friendly designs and characters. These Huggable Scrubs® are

FIGURE 13-12. Chris Abajian specialized in pediatric anesthesia, and adapted spinal anesthetic techniques for use in pediatric cases.

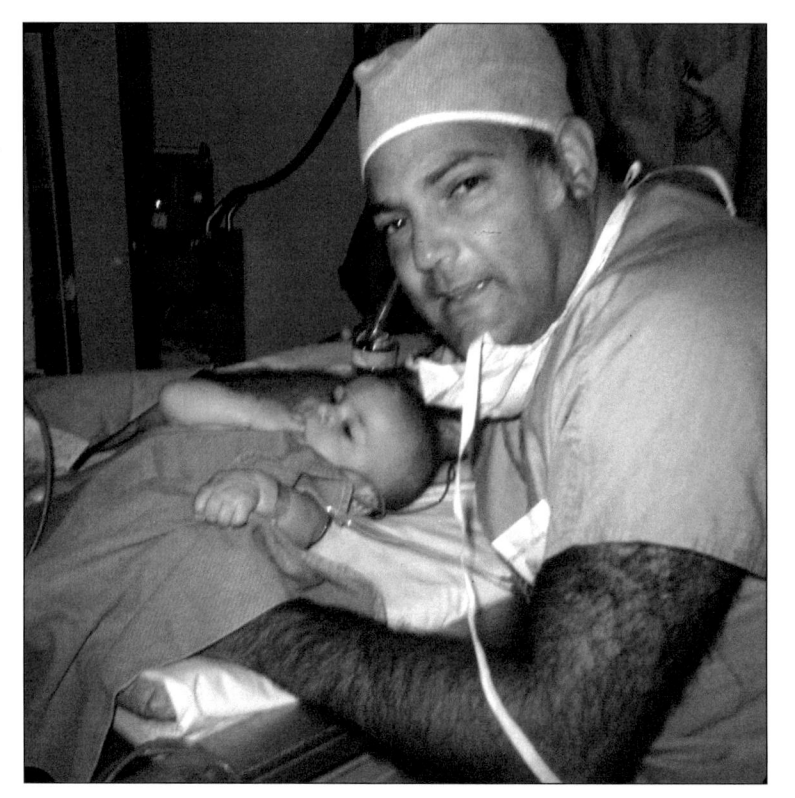

still manufactured and distributed through a company managed by Abajian and his wife. Abajian has also developed toys that deliver inhaled induction anesthetics as a means to pacify otherwise excitable children.

Abajian's partner, Rob Williams, runs an innovative outreach program called "PHAT" (Protect your Head at All Times) that promotes helmet use among young skiers and snowboarders. The Critical Care specialist started the venture after surviving a major bicycling accident thanks to his helmet. Progress has been made as more than 80% of Vermont's children now wear head protection, up from a previous level of 50%. Even seasoned skiers proudly sport the helmets that they once shunned. Williams spreads his message firsthand every winter as medical advisor to the Smuggler's Notch Ski Patrol.

Music in the Operating Room

Operating Rooms are filled with all kinds of strange noises, many of which are misunderstood by anxious patients. Fragments of a conversation may be mistakenly interpreted as an impending disaster or a malignant diagnosis when neither exists. With this in mind, Chris Abajian started a system in which comforting music was played via headphones during the induction of anesthesia or the duration of a regional block.

Of course once such a system was in place, the O.R. teams wanted to listen to music themselves. This created certain challenges, as former UVM surgeon Julius H. Jacobson noted:

> "Introducing music into the operating room seemed logical for the calming influence it would bring into an otherwise stressful environment. This was soon abandoned [at New York's Mt. Sinai Hospital]. We discovered that the music often took over without our conscious realization. For example, one day the rhythm of a polka was discovered to be dictating the speed of the operation. On another occasion, the lilt of a waltz was completely inappropriate to stanching the flow of a major hemorrhage."[32]

Several of UVM's surgeons felt the same way; namely that they performed better with minimal distraction. Frank Ittleman has never allowed music in his cardiac room (although he does direct some lively conversations). Former orthopaedic surgeon Charles Rust banned talking altogether, claiming it prevented spreading germs through the mask!

Nonetheless, the tunes originally chosen to soothe patients' nerves were supplanted by each attending's individual preferences. Courteous surgeons asked their nurses and patients for suggestions, while others imposed their own questionable tastes on all. One surgeon even answered the question, "What do you do when the patient doesn't like your choice of music?" by humorously (I hope) responding, "Sedate him."

Music was initially piped into the rooms through the overhead speakers. Bulky yet versatile portable tape decks soon arrived on the scene. Up to three different such "boom boxes" could travel through one room during the course of a day. The CD player that had been "donated" to the cardiac group by a corporate supplier, on the other hand, moved from room-to-room during the night shift. CDs have since given way to the 21st century's iPods®, which play through synchronized docking stations.

I (DBP) usually played Mozart during carotid endarterectomies. Less stressful procedures called for selections from Jimmy Buffett, the Phantom of the Opera, or Allison Krauss. Other surgeons played hard rock, show tunes, and even recordings of whales singing. The scene from the movie "The Doctor", however, in which the O.R. team gleefully dances to surgeon William Hurt's "closing music" (a particularly raunchy Jimmy Buffett number) has never been re-enacted at UVM.

No matter how long or difficult the case, I always felt better after remembering that home and a loving family were awaiting my return. Despite long hours of separation, a wife's unconditional love is inspirational. To this end, I frequently selected Bette Midler's "Let the world stop turning. Let the sun stop burning ... the only dream that mattered had come true: In this life, I was loved by you."

The Department Nearly Falls Apart

Unfortunately, no amount of music could compensate for the turmoil that followed Mazuzan's 1995 retirement. The specialty was already in an uproar nationwide. Health care reformers maintained that there were too many doctors, and that there were specifically too many anesthesiologists. Residency applications plummeted on fears that nurse anesthetists were going to replace physicians. Skyrocketing malpractice coverage and declining reimbursement added more fuel to the fire.

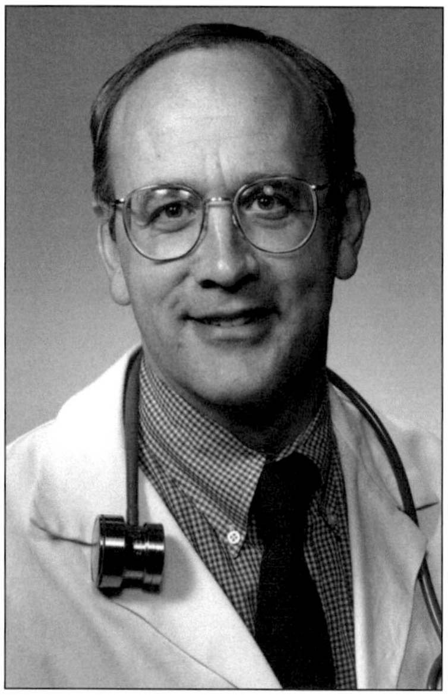

FIGURE 13-13. Thomas Poulton became Chief of Anesthesia in 1995.

UVM conducted a nationwide hunt for Mazuzan's replacement after a suitable internal candidate failed to materialize. The Search Committee selected Thomas J. Poulton, an excellent anesthesiologist with a strong background in both Critical and Palliative Care. His prior affiliation was with a large community hospital in Topeka, Kansas.

The anesthesiologists at UVM had continued to function as a stand-alone entity despite their elevation from divisional to departmental standing. They maintained their own practice structure and billing format. And while they did pay the Dean's tax and part of their residency program expenses, the arrangements were no different than when they were part-time faculty. Thus, one of Poulton's main assignments was to integrate the Department with the College of Medicine.

Conflicts arose which can perhaps partially be understood by the following quote from the 1999 American Society of Anesthesiologists Newsletter:

"In September, Anesthesia Associates of Burlington (AAB), Vermont, and Fletcher Allen Health Care (FAHC) agreed to pay $3.2 million to settle the U.S. government's claims of improper billing. ... As the U.S. attorney noted, both the anesthesiologists and the health system denied any liability under the False Claims Act, but they agreed to resolve the matter at this stage in order to avoid the costs of litigation.

According to the U.S. Attorney's press release, at issue were several allegedly incorrect billing practices.

The lawsuit originated as a qui tam, or "whistle blower" action. The former president of the practice group, who was also the health care physician services leader, and the chair of the department of anesthesiology for the University of Vermont College of Medicine, filed the suit under seal in 1997. Under the false claims act if the government decides to intervene in a qui tam action, the whistle blower may be entitled to up to 35% of the United States' recovery. In its press release announcing the settlement, AAB indicated that its erstwhile president "had lost his officer's position because the members of AAB were not satisfied with his leadership." A separate claim alleging illegal retaliation for filing the False Claims action is still pending; so are claims against the independent billing service used by AAB."[33]

Anesthesia briefly reverted to divisional status during the battle. Staff members were discouraged, and several actually quit. It was left to those who stayed behind to resurrect the program.

Howard Schapiro Rebuilds the Department

Howard Schapiro had followed his 1980 College of Medicine graduation with three years of UVM surgical residency. After shifting to anesthesiology, he broadened his background

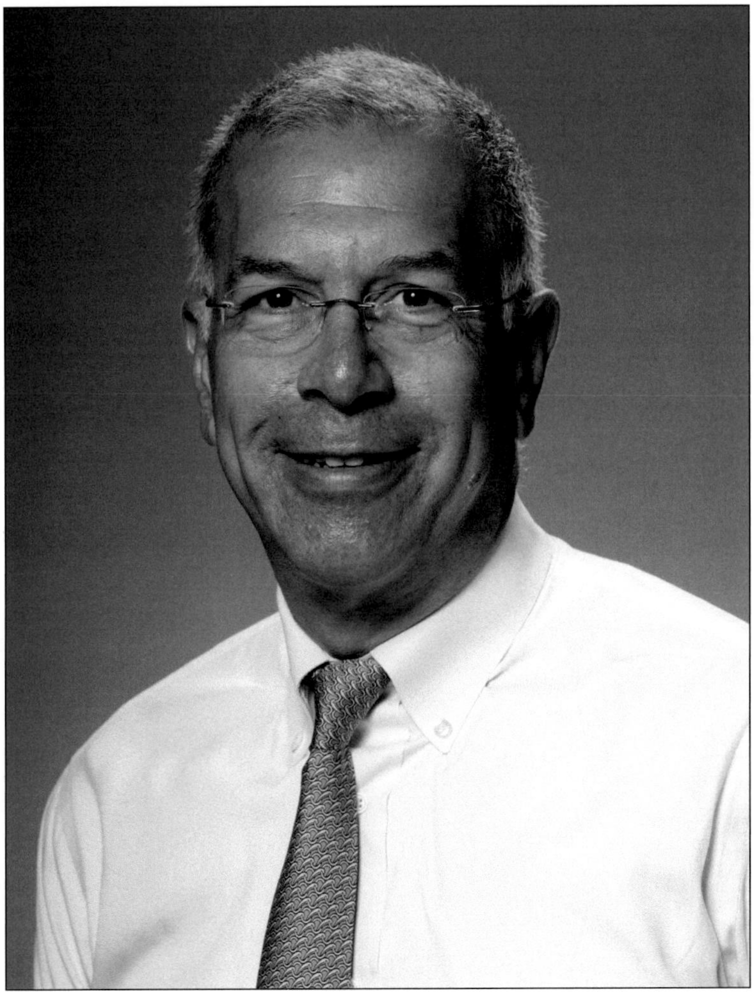

FIGURE 13-14. Howard Schapiro rebuilt the Department upon succeeding Poulton in 1996.

through an Ob/Gyn fellowship at New York's Columbia-Presbyterian Hospital. Mazuzan recruited Schapiro to fill the position that Heidi Kristensen was vacating, but had to reconsider when Kristensen decided to stay. Luckily, a spot was found so that Schapiro could be brought back for good.

Schapiro became the acting clinical chair of the reconstituted Department of Anesthesia in 1996, and was appointed permanent chair shortly thereafter. The problem then became one of stabilizing and re-staffing a department in disarray. Schapiro responded by reassuring the faculty that had remained, and rehiring the best of those that had abandoned the sinking ship. The residency program was totally revamped with an eye toward recruiting and teaching excellence.

Sub-specialization and shared responsibility have been integral parts of Schapiro's leadership. The team of Bruce Vianni and Jim Rathmell have built a model outpatient pain clinic. Rathmell has also led a strong clinical research effort, one that has been taken up by the residents as well.

The Department of Anesthesia has separated from the Department of Surgery in name, but is joined at the hip, and remains a prime example of close teamwork.

CHAPTER 14

Orthopaedic Division / Department

Chapter written jointly with John W. Frymoyer, MD

When Orthopaedics split from Surgery at UVM, the new department took great pride in their independence, and believed that being in charge of their own destiny would surely help them succeed and achieve national recognition.

Starting early in the 20th century, UVM was known for expertise in spinal disease. Later, three editions of "The Adult Spine"[1] were originated and edited in Vermont, adding to the group's prestige. Sports medicine also caused UVM to be internationally known, particularly for innovative research in the epidemiology of ski injuries, the prevention of binding related ski accidents, and biomechanics of the knee. In these areas, UVM clearly succeeded in its aspirations.

Less well known is the fact that microsurgical hand surgery had its roots in Vermont. Other sub-specialties developed, and had their own successes, some durable and others transient. There have been notable achievements in foot and ankle surgery, contemporary management of skeletal trauma, and the biomechanical attributes of scoliosis.

A pioneering foray in 1960 into knee arthroscopy fell off the road, following veto by departmental leaders, and came to a halt, despite its innovation.

Orthopaedists Are Found in Vermont in the 19th Century

The Civil War Casebook of Henry Janes devotes major attention to fractures and extremity injuries. Because plaster of Paris casts were yet to be invented, wooden splints were used for fracture immobilization. Of special interest in Vermont is the splint used by Henry Janes in the civil war era, which resides in his museum in Waterbury, Vermont. During the civil war, yellow pine from the South was no longer available for splints. The only supply in the

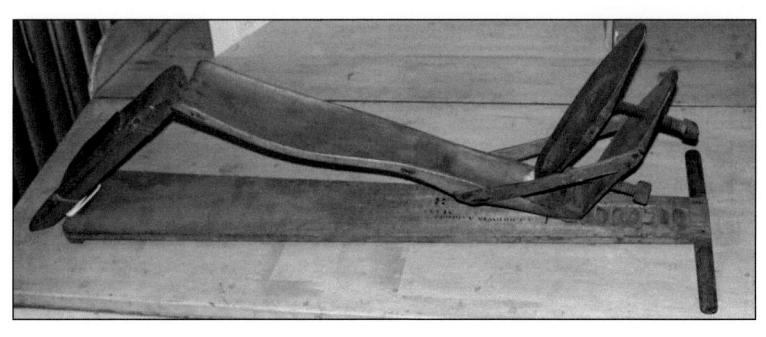

FIGURE 14-1. Civil war splint in the Janes Museum in Waterbury, VT was built from yellow pine supplied by the Estey Organ Co.

North was the Estey Organ Company of Brattleboro who converted pipe organ wood to splints for the war effort![2]

The first recorded orthopaedist at UVM was Milton J. Roberts of New York, listed as a Special Professor of Orthopaedics at UVM in 1884. He is best remembered as describing an electro-osteotome.[3]

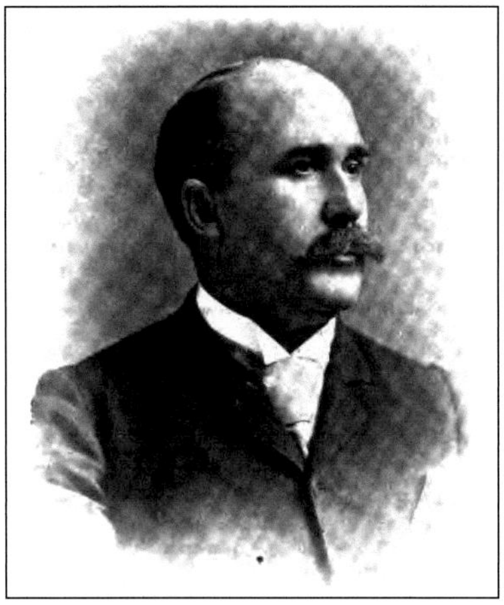

FIGURE 14-2. Abel Phelps served as UVM's Special Professor of Orthopaedics and then as Professor of Surgery.

In 1886 Abel M. Phelps who had been born in 1851 in Alburg, VT, was appointed Special Professor of Orthopaedic Surgery. He had just returned from Germany, where he was reputed to have organized the Orthopaedic Department at Allegemeines Krankenhaus. In 1889 he was advanced to Professor of Surgery (and Chief of Surgery) at UVM while he simultaneously held an appointment with the New York Post Graduate Medical School. Among his publications was the description of the "Phelps" operation for treatment of clubfoot.[4]

Phelps was a bold and rapid operator who always seemed in a hurry. For example several times he excised a knee joint in 10 minutes. Few arteries were tied, instead relying on pressure for hemostasis. One Saturday morning he did one of his knee joint excisions for tuberculosis, telling the class that he would show them how rapidly and easily the operation could be done. He had a train to catch to return to NYC. Later that day a nurse found the patient with a blood soaked cast. Dr. Bingham who was the surgeon on duty at the time, reoperated and controlled the bleeding. The patient made a good recovery, but Phelps thereafter took a little more time with his knee-joint excisions.[5]

By 1899, the faculty in Vermont opined he should resign because the focus of his interest was in New York, and not Vermont. In 1900 Phelps took their advice.

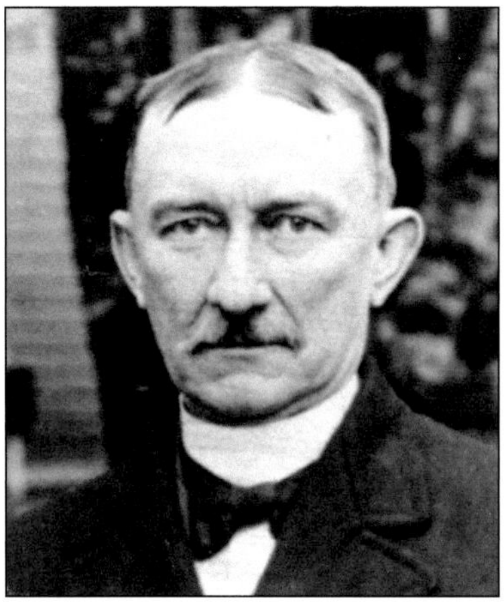

FIGURE 14-3. Aurelius Shands of Philadelphia succeeded Phelps as Professor of Orthopaedics.

His successor, Aurelius Shands in 1901 continued the tradition of people coming up from the city (Philadelphia in his case) to teach and operate as visiting professors at Vermont for two week sessions. He was an expert on childhood musculoskeletal diseases. His work was recognized when the Dupont Family established the Shands Institute in Delaware as one of the premier pediatric orthopaedic centers in the world.

UVM's relationship with New York was reestablished when one of the foremost orthopaedists of the world at that time, Fred Albee, Chief of Orthopaedics at the New York Post-Graduate Medical School, was appointed Special Professor of Orthopaedics at UVM in 1911. He held this position until 1925.

The First Spine Fusion by a Vermont Orthopaedist?

The first major surgical breakthrough in treatment of spinal diseases occurred in 1911 when another New York surgeon, Russell Hibbs, and Albee separately described successful lumbar spinal fusions. Albee and Hibbs were rivals. Hotly contested was the question: Who was first to make the discovery? Both articles were published in the same year, Albee's in the JAMA[6], and Hibbs' in the New York Medical Journal.[7] Hibbs' article came out first, but Albee thought he trumped Hibbs when he noted his article was published previously in the Journal of the Vermont State Medical Society. Hibbs countered with: "Nobody has ever heard of that journal." The Hibbs and Albee techniques for lumbar fusion were quite different. Hibbs feathered the lamina, a technique still used, but did not employ additional bone grafts. Albee split the spinous processes, and in his later cases inserted an autogenous tibial bone graft. Perhaps the bone graft techniques were adapted from Albee's childhood grafting in the apple orchards of his home farm in Maine.

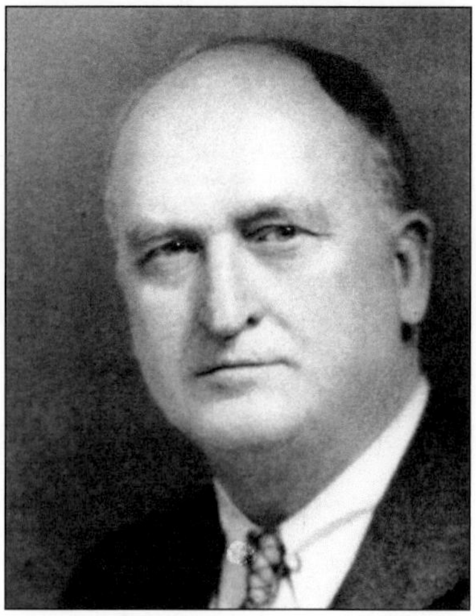

FIGURE 14-4. UVM's Special Professor of Orthopaedics Fred Albee was the first to describe successful lumbar spine fusion. The article appeared in the Journal of the Vermont State Medical Society in 1910.

For a patient with spinal tuberculosis, and other serious spinal conditions, spinal fusion for the first time offered hope their disease could be ameliorated, controlled and function restored.

Albee was both an inventive and colorful surgeon. He developed a special oscillating saw to obtain tibial bone graft which had many of the characteristics of modern cast saws.[8] He also pioneered a table for performing hip surgery, and insisted the Mary Fletcher Hospital buy one for $1,000, a major investment for that era. His stock-in-trade opening remark in the operating room was: "Bring out the Albee table."[9] Like many surgeons faced with suboptimal anesthesia, he was fast, often cutting from skin to bone in a single swipe of the scalpel. In February 1916 Albee gave a postgraduate course in Orthopaedics in Vermont ... the first postgraduate course of which we have a record.

David Bosworth Starts a 47 Year Career as a Teacher at UVM College of Medicine

As Albee continued his work at UVM, another future star in spine surgery was starting his training. David Bosworth was a native Vermonter, son of a Baptist minister in Bristol, Vermont, and graduate of the UVM Medical School Class of 1921. He then became an Instructor in anatomy at UVM. In 1926 Bosworth took his orthopaedic training under Hibbs at New York Orthopaedic Hospital where he then started his practice. It was inevitable that two enormous egos would come into conflict. Because his income was so meager, Bosworth played the flute professionally when not working at the hospital. Hibbs berated him for such non-professional behavior, and soon thereafter Bosworth left to become an attending surgeon at Saint Luke's Hospital in New York, and later chair of its Department of Orthopaedics. Bosworth was a surgeon, who, like Albee, was particularly interested in spinal fusions. He and his associate, Mather Cleveland, developed a technique called the "H-graft" which compressed an iliac bone graft between the adjacent spinous processes. He also invented the circumferential spinal fusion which allowed surgery to be performed successfully for the first time on tuberculous patients with actively draining sinuses.

FIGURE 14-5. David Bosworth with his tractor and boat on Gardner Island, VT.

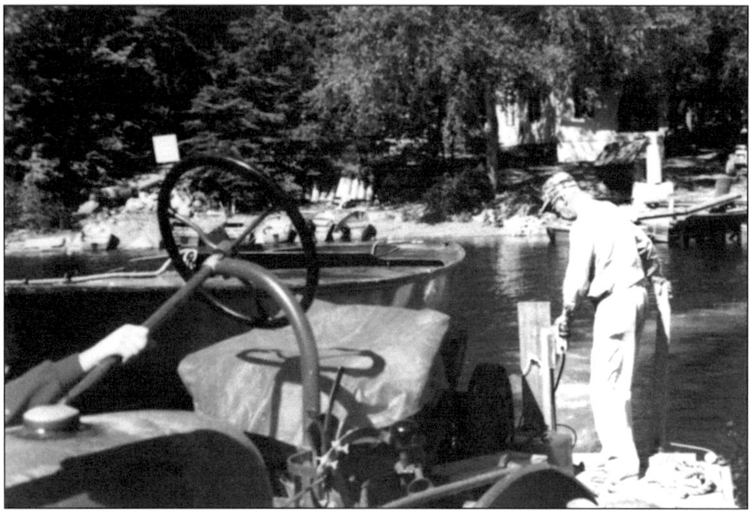

Like Albee, Bosworth served as Visiting Professor at the University of Vermont. Every Friday, accompanied by his secretary, he took the train from New York or flew from Teterborough Airport in New Jersey to Vermont, where he had a home on Gardner Island in Lake Champlain. Saturday morning he would see 60 patients in the Durfee clinic. His only tool was a pair of sharply pointed scissors which he used both to test sensation, and as a reflex hammer. In the afternoon, he would perform five or six major operations, and then take the operating team to Burlington for dinner at Marietta's. He would retire to Gardner Island, and return to NYC on Sunday. Bosworth was a facile, fast, totally self-confident, cigar-chomping surgeon, and something of a local character.

On one occasion he was performing a lumbar osteotomy on a "lady of the night" whose spine spontaneously had become fused from ankylosing spondylitis, such that she was totally bent forward and could only walk with the aid of prism glasses. Within an hour Bosworth had performed an osteotomy and put her into a two legged spica cast which went from her chest to both her knees. Then he took her neck and twisted it rather violently. This was accompanied by a loud "craaaack." He quickly checked her ankle reflexes, and Babinski sign, which if positive would have signified damage to her spinal cord, and was gratified the sign was negative. When asked "What if the Babinski had been positive? he was reported to have said jokingly: "Twisted her neck harder."[10]

Bosworth's New York Office was on Park Avenue, identifiable by gold plated doors. His waiting room was set up with bridge tables and cards so that society patients waiting to see him (often for hours on end) had a diversion.

Bosworth was reputed to have told the story of an orthopaedist of that era who treated the daughter of a very wealthy industrialist for a congenital hip dislocation. A shelf arthroplasty was performed — but as the doctor inspected the surgery it became apparent he had operated on the wrong side. What to do? He proceeded to operate on the affected side. Then, he reported to the parents "Good news, not only did we fix the bad hip but that surgery went so well, I decided to do the other hip to prevent future problems." Talk about, chutzpah![11]

Bosworth had a notable career and achieved considerable acclaim for his spine surgery techniques. He was particularly popular in Japan, and trained many Japanese orthopaedists in his residency program at St. Lukes in NYC. He also organized the first meeting between

Japanese and American orthopaedists following WW II. These efforts were recognized by the Japanese government by the "Order of the White Elephant." On his retirement in 1968 he moved to Vermont, but on the basis of his age was denied surgical privileges at the DeGoesbriand and Mary Fletcher Hospitals. He was granted privileges at the Fanny Allen Hospital, even though he was past 75 years old. Later one of his adoring Japanese acolytes wrote a biography of Bosworth entitled "Dr. Japan." In that biography the author berated the Vermont orthopaedists and the Hospitals of Vermont for denying the great man privileges.[12]

With Bradley Soule (chair of radiology) he spent hours cataloguing radiographs of interesting orthopaedic cases. He also continued to perform surgery, often as an assistant to one of his former residents, Richard Nesti. Often frustrated by his role as assistant, he was known to grab the scalpel from Nesti, and without a trace of his usual tremor, complete the surgery.

In 1969 he performed his last operation (assisted by Frymoyer): the removal of calcium from the rotator cuff of his secretary. The operation took exactly 5 minutes.[13]

Orthopaedic Handicapped Children's Clinics

While visiting professors were an important part of UVM's development in orthopaedics, a separate group of visiting orthopaedists from Boston were critical to the care of children in Vermont. Before World War I, Robert Lovett of Boston had visited Vermont and studied the

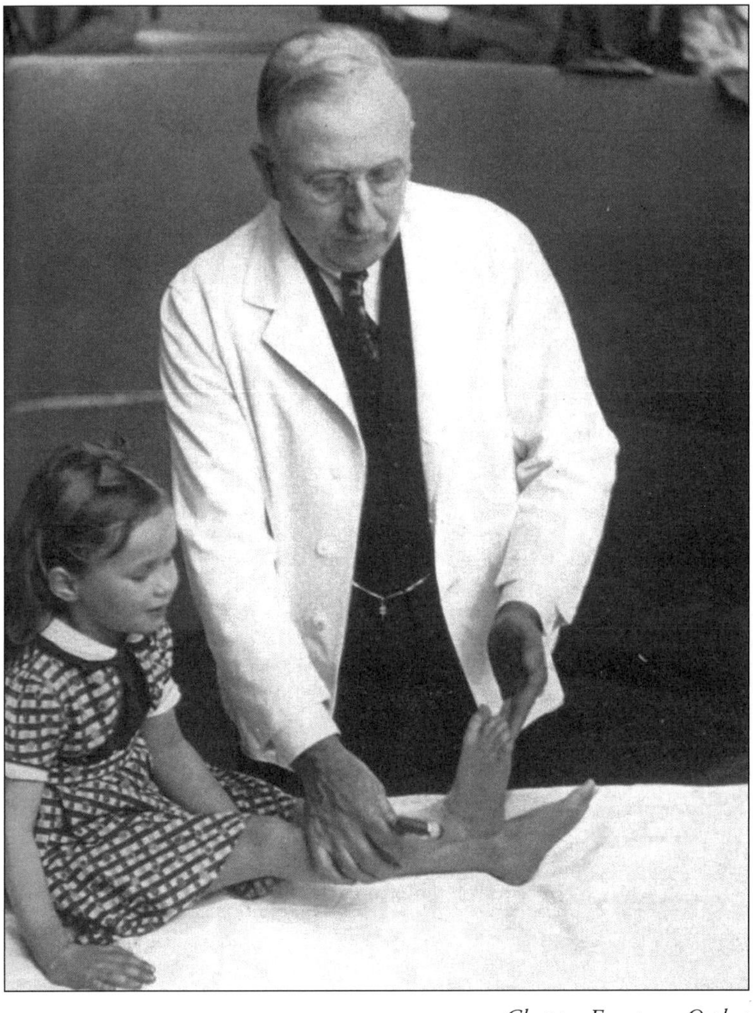

FIGURE 14-6. Frank Ober conducting one of his UVM Children's Clinics.

epidemiology of poliomyelitis. Published as a book in 1916,[14] this is still considered a classic example for modern epidemiological studies. It is not surprising that soon after the end of the war, another Boston orthopaedist, Frank Ober, started coming to Vermont to conduct children's clinics throughout the state. Once the two weeks of clinics were complete, a special train would go from town to town picking up the children, who were then taken to Boston Children's Hospital. When all of the surgeries had been completed, all the children were brought back by train to Vermont. They were then cared for by specially trained nurse/physical therapists, or in a hospital called the Caverly Preventorium near Proctor, Vermont. At one time that institution had over 200 children in residence, the majority for orthopaedic conditions.

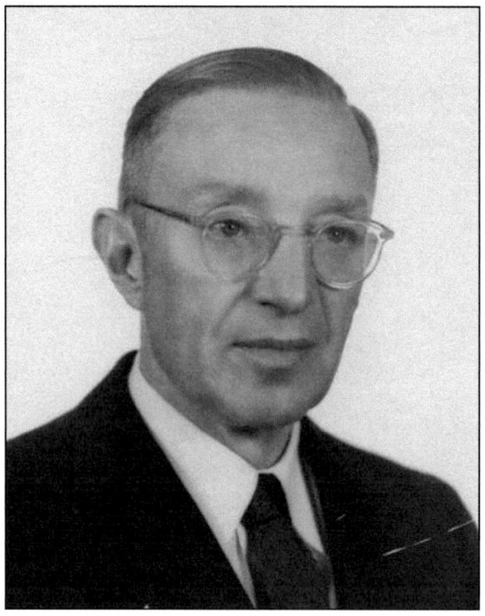

FIGURE 14-7. Joseph Barr (pictured) and William Mixter described lumbar disc herniation in a Vermont skier.

One of the young residents who accompanied Ober was Joseph Barr, later to become famous for his discovery of the syndrome of lumbar disc herniation. When Ober retired, Barr continued the tradition of the clinics well into the 1950s. That longstanding involvement also led to the recruitment of John F. Bell, a Harvard trained orthopaedist to head the Vermont Orthopaedic Handicapped Children's program. This later was a factor in Raymond Kuhlman's choice of Burlington as a place to establish his practice.

The First Recognized Ruptured Disc Removal

While Albee and later Bosworth were developing new insights about spinal fusion, another seminal event in the understanding of spinal disorders was taking root in Vermont. One of the diagnostic enigmas at that time was the cause of sciatica in some patients with low back pain. The discovery of the cause started in Vermont.

In 1928 a young Vermonter by the name of Newton went skiing, twisted his back and experienced severe pain. With bed rest his symptoms improved, but a year later he again twisted his back, followed by excruciating left leg pain. He was admitted to the Mary Fletcher Hospital under the care of "Moose" Maynard who treated him as was the practice of that era with one month of bed rest in the hospital. His symptoms were unimproved and he was transferred to Joseph Barr, a young Boston orthopaedist at the Faulkner Hospital. Numerous consultations were obtained, and finally, it was concluded the most likely diagnosis was a spinal tumor. Jason Mixter, a prominent neurosurgeon at the Massachusetts General Hospital was consulted, and he determined to explore the lumbar spine with the presumptive diagnosis of neural tumor. At L5-S1 he discovered a mass under the nerve root which had the typical appearance of a "Chordoma." A chordoma was then thought to be a fairly rare, benign tumor. This was removed. During the operation a number of transfusions were required, and blood was obtained from orthopaedic residents — a test of their real commitment to the indications for an operation!

Newton was relieved of his leg pain, and had an uneventful recovery. The pathologists dutifully reported "Chordoma." Like so many great discoveries in medicine, serendipity intervened. Barr was studying a collection of lumbar disc specimens amassed by Schmorl and Junghans in Germany. He also was looking at specimens obtained from spinal operations. In a moment of insight, he identified the similarity between the "chordoma" removed from Mr. Newton and lumbar disc specimens and concluded the lesion was not a tumor but a herniation of lumbar disc material. This finding stimulated Mixter and Barr to review all of the specimens of chordoma removed surgically at the Massachusetts General Hospital. The result of their inquiry was the publication in the New England Journal of Medicine of lumbar intervertebral disc herniation wherein they described the clinical history, physical findings, operative findings, and pathology of what they observed.[15] Although others had described disc herniations, none had recognized the entire clinical syndrome and its importance. This was indeed a profound discovery which fundamentally altered the treatment of back disorders.

That Newton was the first case in the United States seems indisputable. In 1946 he had a recurrent episode of back and leg pain, and was seen by the then new chief of neurosurgery at UVM, Donaghy, who wrote to Mixter giving him follow-up. Mixter's reply includes this memorable quote: "There is no doubt Newton is the first patient where we recognized a lumbar disc herniation as such, and thus he is the man who started all the damn trouble!"[16]

Vermont Gets Orthopaedists After WW II

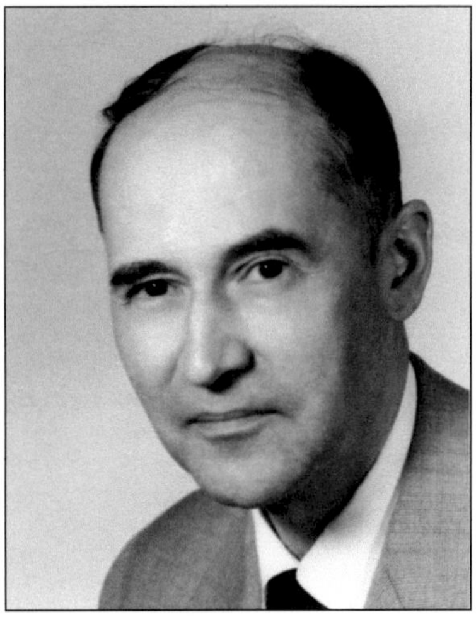

Following World War II, the Department began to grow with orthopaedists who set up their practices in Burlington. Each new faculty member had a linkage to one of the earlier Vermont leaders. The first was John Bell who was trained in Boston by Barr. Bell was appointed as associate professor of orthopaedics in 1947, and was first described as Chair of the Division of Orthopaedics in 1954.[17] Charles Rust, a 1939 graduate of UVM Medical School, had done his Othopaedic training at St. Lukes in New York with Bosworth, and for his entire practice career fused all patients with lumbar disc herniations using the H-graft. Initially Bell and Rust practiced together, but their styles were antithetical. Rust like his mentor, Bosworth, could pin a hip in 15 minutes, while Bell took much longer. Rust saw 60 patients a day, whereas Bell would spend an hour with a child with flat feet.[18]

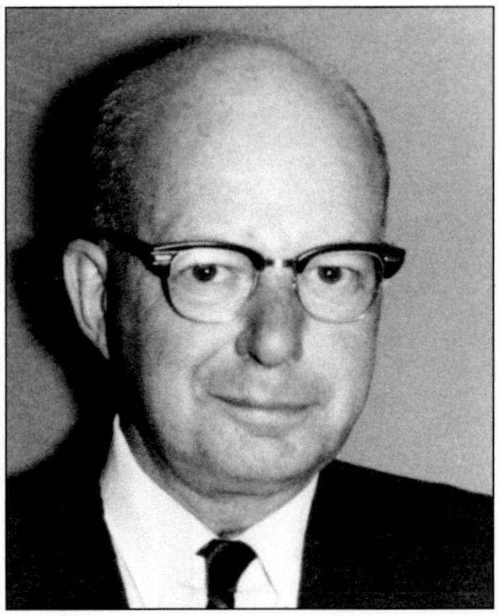

Bell became a legendary figure around Vermont. He traveled wearing a railroad engineer's hat, drove 40 miles an hour, and stopped at every diner along his route. Inevitably he was known by someone in the diner whom he had cared for. It was not unusual for a trip from Burlington to Rutland to take four hours. Bell eventually went to work as a consultant for the Handicapped Children's Services of the State of Vermont, and gave up private practice.[19]

FIGURE 14-8. John Bell became UVM's first Chair of Orthopaedics in 1954.

FIGURE 14-9. Charles Rust returned to UVM as Bosworth's protégé.

FIGURE 14-10.
Raymond Kuhlman became Co-Chair of Orthopaedics with Rust in 1960.

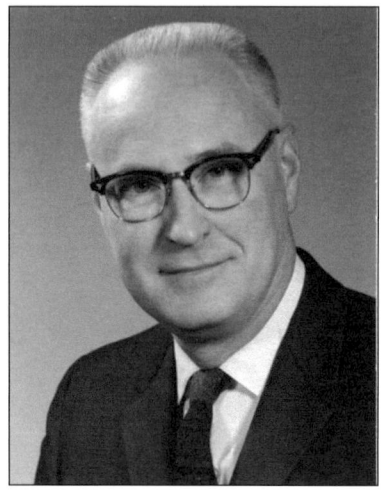

FIGURE 14-11.
Ed Simpson introduced the intertransverse process fusion to UVM.

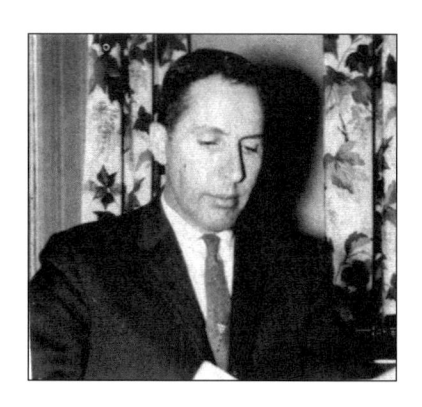

FIGURE 14-12.
Phil Davis specialized in hand surgery, becoming an expert in microvascular and microfascicular nerve grafting techniques.

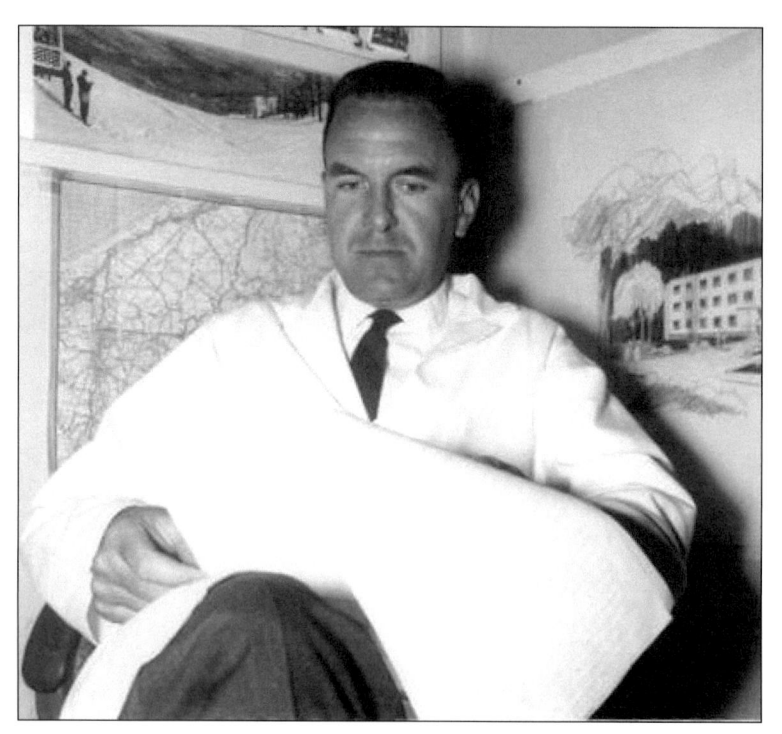

Soon thereafter, Raymond Kuhlman who had trained with Barr in Boston, came to Burlington. He had entered the Army after internship at the University of Minnesota, and was assigned the hardship post of Aruba for the duration of World War II. This Army experience was followed by an orthopaedic residency at the Massachusetts General Hospital in Boston. In Boston he worked with Barr and Ober at the MGH.

As was the practice in Boston, the discs were removed by the neurosurgeon, and the fusion performed by the orthopaedist. James E. Simpson, following completion of an orthopaedic residency in Memphis, TN, had spent a fellowship year, under the aegis of Nachlas and Barr, doing the first long term analysis of the results of disc excision alone, compared to excision with lumbar fusion. Simpson was a talented surgeon who liked to try new procedures. In 1967 he introduced the intertranverse process fusion to Vermont, and that technique has remained the mainstay of lumbar fusion.

In 1958, Philip Davis, who had gone to UVM Medical School, and then served in the Navy as a medical corpsman, trained at Northwestern University with specialty training in hand surgery. He returned to Burlington as the first orthopaedist interested in research. Stimulated by Jacobson's pioneering work at UVM, Davis quickly applied microsurgical techniques to hand surgery. He had also developed a collaborative research project with his neurosurgical colleague, Donaghy, to perfect microfascicular repair of peripheral nerves. In 1965 he was asked to put on a course at the AAOS meetings and he for many years trained hand surgeons who adopted the technique. Vermont, with little heavy industry, had few traumatic amputations suitable for replantation. As a result, those he trained got more acclaim than Davis for his innovation.

Davis also worked on a new hip nailing technique in the laboratory, and studied biomechanics of the hip. He worked one day a week in research, and pushed the idea of an orthopedic residency.

By 1960, Kuhlman and Rust were co-chairs of the division. At that time unassigned orthopedic cases (fractures and trauma mostly) were divided equally between general surgery and the division of orthopaedics.

Orthopaedics Seeks Departmental Status

Mackay reminisced: "Orthopedic surgery has wanted to be a separate department, and this move is largely on a political basis. The American Board of Orthopaedic Surgery has felt that to gain stature they would do better if they were represented on a full departmental basis when they send academic men into a new faculty. This may be true. On the other hand, it fragments surgery in such a way that we no longer have them in our counsels of general surgeon makeup, and I think it detrimental both to the development and interchange of the orthopedic surgeons themselves as well as the overall picture of surgery."[20] One can hear reverberations of this argument throughout subspecialization arguments in surgical specialties throughout the ensuing years.

Initially the "negotiations" were conducted by Mackay, Rust and Kuhlman. Rust, a well known poker player, and believer in Cal Coolidge's axiom: "Silence is golden," would sit for minutes refusing to respond to Mackay. Eventually the debate reached the dean, George Wolf, who acceded to departmental status, and a residency program. A search was initiated for a new chief. The orthopaedic residency was started with two residents, John Frymoyer and Fred Lippert.

The New Chief of Orthopaedics Starts Out by Taking a Sabbatical Year

The search for a chairman was completed in 1965 and Frank Hoaglund from Johns Hopkins medical school and the University of Rochester orthopedic residency was selected, but accepted contingent to going on a year sabbatical prior to assuming the job. This sabbatical was in Hong Kong studying tuberculous spines. This left Kuhlman and Rust as co-acting chairs, with Frymoyer a second year resident and Lippert a first year resident.

Officially at this time the Division of Orthopaedics of the Department of Surgery, now became the Department of Orthopaedics and later Department of Orthopaedics and Rehabilitation.

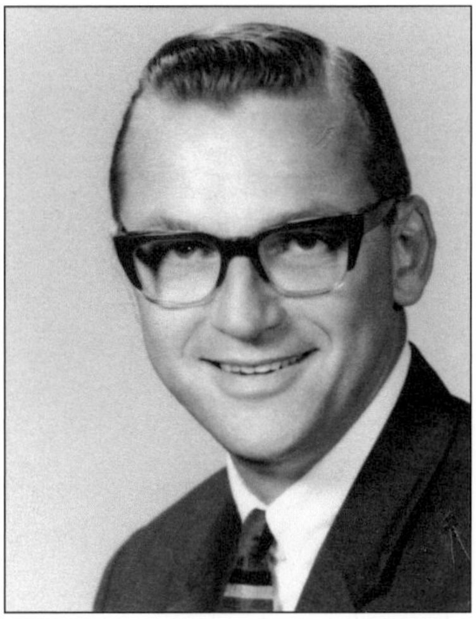

FIGURE 14-13. Frank Hoaglund became the first Chief of the Department of Orthopaedics in 1965 with a ticket to Hong Kong already in hand.

Hoaglund was in Hong Kong, never having served in Vermont. There were some funds accumulating available for outside rotations and research startup from clinic patient fees. The resident was in charge of the clinic patients. There were not enough clinic patients for a residency program, so private patients comprised a significant part of the residents' patient care and operative work experience.

Once in Vermont, Hoaglund began a concerted effort to build an academic orthopaedic department. He almost immediately began to revamp the rounds, insisted the residents be given time weekly for basic sciences, and personally conducted walking rounds which were a model for clinical teaching. He also encouraged research activities, and started his own projects, including work on the epidemiology of osteoarthritis.

As a result of these efforts, the residency program began to attract a larger pool of applicants. Space was made available for research activities in the Medical Alumni Building. Space for seeing patients was a different problem. Eventually Hoaglund wrangled virtually subterranean space in the basement rooms of Fletcher House. To say the space was barely adequate was no exaggeration. The patient waiting room sloped to a drain in the center of the floor, a design originally used for hosing down psychiatric patients who were violent. There was no x-ray, and patients had to be wheeled down a narrow basement corridor, past the machine shop, to radiology and back.

Clinically, Hoaglund was interested in the emerging field of total hip replacement which had been spearheaded by John Charnley at Oxford, England. Soon after his arrival he received a phase III FDA approval to use methylmethacrylate as the "grout" to hold the prosthetic components. Harlan Amstuz, a well known Hospital for Special Surgery orthopaedist, came to Vermont in 1969 and taught Hoaglund and the chief residents the new techniques.

The great fear with total hip replacement, was infection. Charnley had developed a vertical laminar air flow system and demonstrated that using it reduced infections. The magnitude of this reduction was hotly debated. John Davis as Chief of Surgery was of the opinion that most infections came from within the patient by hematogenous spread, and that airborne infections were secondary, if of any importance at all. Initially he would not approve the laminar air flow device for UVM's operating rooms. A grateful patient of Hoaglund donated some of the funds, and a laminar flow system was purchased.

John W. Frymoyer, First Orthopaedic Resident at UVM

Under Hoaglund's leadership, the residency training program gained in academic excellence. The first, John Frymoyer, had gone to the University of Rochester Medical School from Amherst College where he took a year "out" in the research lab of Ralph Jacox (a rheumatologist) who was developing an animal model, and studying the metabolism of steroids and Isoniazid®. He attended rheumatology clinics with the orthopaedists, but thought he might go into medicine or even obstetrics and gynecology. The medical department at Rochester had a career mapped out for Frymoyer which consisted of going to the NIH, then to Johns Hopkins, and returning as an attending at Rochester. When he decided to take a rotating internship at UVM, they told him he was doomed to obscurity.

Frymoyer became the first orthopaedic resident who, as a 2nd year resident, got credit for a year spent in medicine residency! Fred Lippert started at the same time having graduated from Annapolis prior to UVM medical school. He, however, started as a G2 and finished a year later than Frymoyer.

The first three residents, Frymoyer, Lippert and Edgar Holmes, were responsible for covering all attendings in the operating rooms, as well as operating the clinics. They managed in-patient services at the Mary Fletcher and DeGoesbriand Hospitals as well as covering both emergency rooms. At that time each inpatient unit had as many as 50 patients. Patients with spine fusions routinely were kept in hospital on bed rest for three weeks. Patients with meniscectomies rarely went home before a week, and it was not unusual for a hip fracture patient to stay six weeks. A fractured femur in traction might well be in hospital for three months. Lippert rode a bicycle between the two hospitals regardless of weather conditions. He estimated he might have biked more than 4000 miles during his residency!

By 1969 the Department was thriving under Hoaglund's leadership and the possibility of growth was entertained. Hoaglund recruited Frymoyer at an initial salary of $14,800/year as

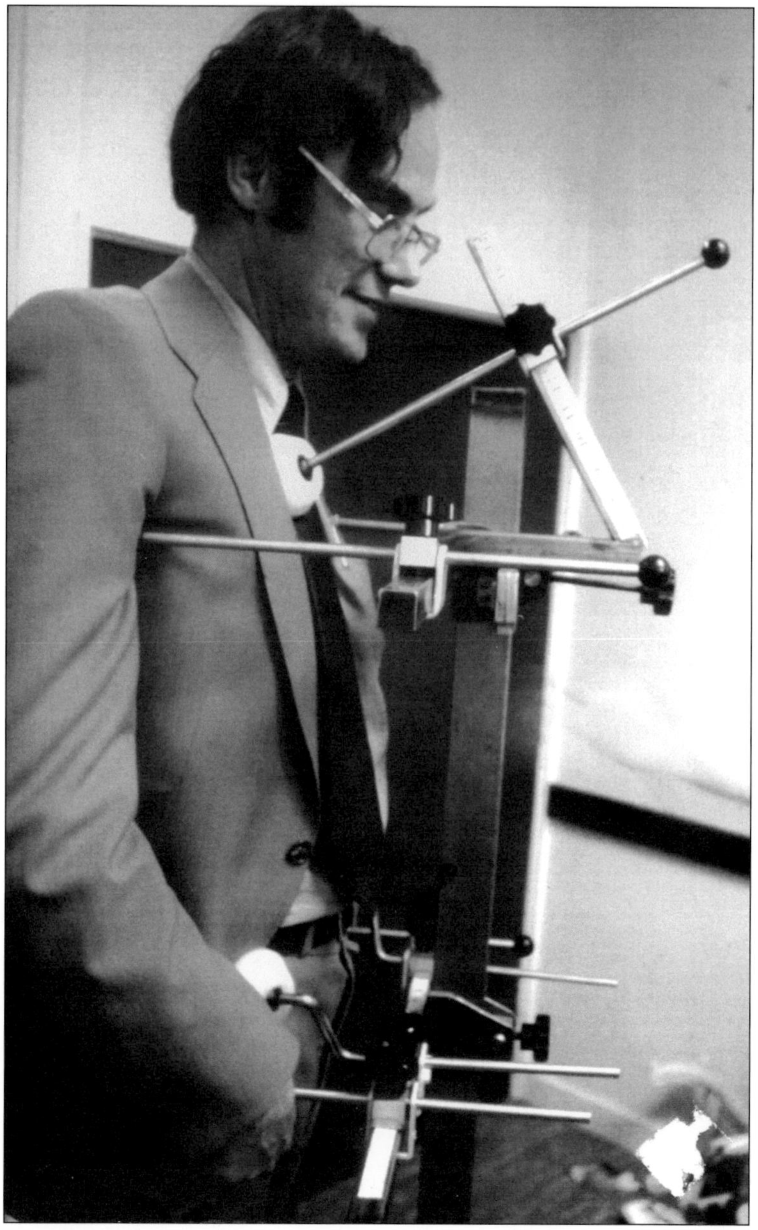

FIGURE 14-14. John Frymoyer, UVM's first orthopaedic residency graduate, researched spine vibrations here and in Sweden.

Chapter Fourteen: Orthopaedic Division/Department

Assistant Professor. His responsibilities included setting up an outpatient office, teaching residents, and gradually building a surgical practice. However, the message was clear: "Do not step on the toes of the men in private practice."

Soon after Hoaglund's arrival, Maureen Molloy came to Vermont to head the Orthopaedic Division of the Vermont Handicapped Children's service. She had trained in Boston with Barr, and as part of her Masters thesis had done a major follow-up evaluation of his patients in an attempt to answer the question: "Is disc excision with accompanying spinal fusion more successful than disc excision alone?"

Given the history of Vermont, the above debate, and interests of the attending staff, it is not surprising that a number of students and residents became interested in lumbar spine disease. In 1972, as a young attending, Frymoyer started a minimum 10 year follow-up study of patients who had undergone disc excision with or without fusion. A resident, Richard Matteri, and two medical students, Ed Hanley and Jim Howe, became interested in the project. One of the unusual aspects of this study was a plan to obtain planar spinal radiographs, as well as flexion-extension radiographs to evaluate the long term effects of spinal surgery on spinal degeneration. This required developing new techniques which would be reproducible. Encouraged by Hoaglund, a recently minted PhD in Bioengineering, Malcolm Pope, was looking to create linkages to Orthopaedics, and this led to his initial involvement with the Department. With Pope's help the new techniques were developed and the study was completed in 1976. It remains to this day the longest follow-up study of lumbar spine fusion. It suggested there was no or minimal clinical benefit to fusion in patients with lumbar disc herniations. Although fusion may increase adjacent level degeneration, that radiographic finding was rarely associated with pain.[21, 22]

It is interesting that three of the giants in the history of spinal disorders (Barr, Albee and Bosworth) had Vermont connections; and that the three largest studies of spine fusion in the treatment of lumbar disease were conducted by Vermont orthopaedists (Simpson, Molloy, and Frymoyer.)

Sports Medicine Assumes Priority and Prominence at UVM

Another major initiative at Vermont was the development of research in skiing injuries. When Hoagland came to Vermont he correctly assumed one fruitful area for research would be skiing injuries, an area of interest as he had published a paper on tibial fractures. Since ankle and tibial fractures were the most common skiing injury in the days of low boots, this seemed a natural starting place. The plan was to set up a clinic in Stowe. Two surgeons at the Copley Hospital in Morrisville objected to the "competition" of a clinic at Stowe, and Hoaglund was forced to look elsewhere, in the process learning about the politics of rural Vermont. He noted there was no one in the Valley (Mad River/Sugarbush/Glen Ellen) area. The Waitsfield general practitioner, Shep Quimby, had a good working relationship with UVM's Philip Davis, who often covered weekends to take care of injured skiers from Mad River. Hoaglund now felt ready to hire someone interested in sports medicine and in 1971 successfully recruited Robert Johnson from the University of Iowa with an interest in sports medicine and the knee.[23]

Johnson's father and uncle were doctors in Iowa, and he always knew he would be a doctor. He was scrubbing in surgery at age 14! He finished his orthopaedic training at Iowa and entered the air force with the Berry Plan, planning to return to Iowa as a sports medicine orthopaedist. Iowa in the interim lost its funding for that position and he was recruited by Vermont in 1971. The newly arrived Johnson, not yet an expert skier, started up a clinic at Glen Ellen in Dec 1971 and later at adjacent Sugarbush. Later, Cleveland Clinic orthopaedic residents did a rotation and came to help staff the clinic. UVM residents weren't ever excited about staffing the ski clinic.[24]

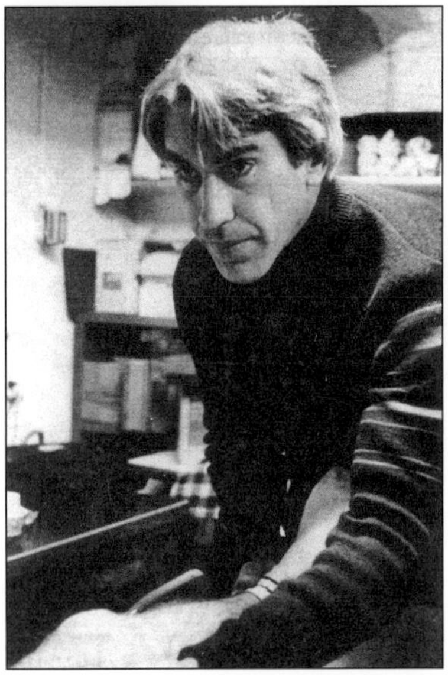

FIGURE 14-15. Robert Johnson revolutionized skiing safety by promoting binding innovations and later focusing on knee injury prevention during skiing.

In 1973, Johnson started working with Carl Ettlinger a researcher and epidemiologist. They began an epidemiologic study of ski injuries with an equipment and accident registry which has continued for over thirty years. Decreases in ankle injuries starting in the 60's were related to changes in ski boot height and rigidity. The remarkably low rates of tibia fractures by 1980 were due in large part to ski binding improvements. This was scientifically proven by the studies of Johnson and Ettlinger. The 1974 seminal article by Johnson, Pope and Ettlinger showed that more expensive bindings and better binding maintenance was associated with fewer equipment related injuries, as were sole friction pads.[25] The twenty year results of these equipment-related studies were published in 1998 with adult tibial fractures decreasing 89% and overall rates of injury decreasing 43%. The distressing finding was an increase of 280% in anterior cruciate injuries, with that becoming the commonest skiing injury for adults.[26]

Johnson and Ettlinger devoted their attention to the knee injuries, studying the mechanism with videotapes of cruciate injuries actually occurring. They termed the mechanism of injury as "the phantom foot ACL injury" and defined the skier as being "off balance to the rear, with all of his or her weight on the inside edge of the tail of the downhill ski ... the injury is sustained in each case by the downhill leg."[27] Using a training program viewing the tapes, now educated ski patrollers had a decline of knee cruciate injuries of 62%.

Scoliosis Becomes a Vermont Focus

The next addition to the staff was Morey Moreland, a graduate of the University of Rochester School of Medicine and Dentistry. On completion of his residency at UVM, he spent a year at the Nuffield Orthopaedic Center in Oxford, England. During that time he studied the effects of twisting (torsion) on animal growth plates. This was one of the first demonstrations that long bone growth can be modified in torsion. On his return to UVM, he joined the faculty to assume the care of a large volume of the orthopaedic problems in children.

Moreland's focus became scoliosis, including the new screening techniques called Moire Fringe Topography. Ian Stokes, an engineer from Oxford, collaborated. Together, they later developed a number of animal models and mathematical modeling techniques for scoliosis which attracted national attention. His successor, David Aronsson picked up the collaboration with Stokes, and that work continues to this day.

Aronsson had trained in San Diego, France and Germany and had been in practice in Michigan. He was attracted to UVM by the presence of Stokes in the research lab and the internationally recognized faculty at UVM including Frymoyer, Per Renstrom from Sweden, and Leon Grobler from South Africa. The work on minimally invasive and non operative treatment of scoliosis has been internationally recognized[28], and was the recipient of numerous awards, including the American Academy's highest research prize, The Kappa Delta Award. This was the fourth time the Department received this award. Others include Pope and Wilder for research in the effects of vibration on the spine and Johnson and Beynnon for their work on knee ligaments. Stokes and Aronsson have been funded with NIH RO-1 grants since 2000.

Physicians' Assistants Start at UVM in Orthopaedics

The rapid growth in the clinical practice during the 1970s put significant strains on the Department, particularly in making time available for faculty members to carry out research. For that era, a radical plan was developed. One of the operating room nurses, Robert Lavalette, had been a medic in Vietnam, where he had responsibility for many aspects of patient care. He was anxious to develop his skills further, but to do so would require further formal education as a Nurse Practitioner. Given his prior experiences this seemed like a poor use of his time. As an alternative, he was brought into the orthopaedic offices where the attending surgeons taught him diagnostic techniques, particularly in fractures and sports medicine, as well as skills in cast application. This "hands on" experience was amplified by attending all of the training sessions for residents, as well as nationally at the American Academy of Orthopaedic Surgeons. Over time he became sufficiently well known in the community that primary care physicians were comfortable referring patients directly to him.

A number of years later Carol Blatspieler, a radiology technician, elected to go to nurse practitioner school with sponsorship of the Orthopaedic Department. On her return she became yet another physician extender. Both she and Lavalette were charter members of the American Academy of Orthopaedic Surgeons Nurse Practitioner programs. Both left the Department in 1996, and eventually went to work for private practice orthopaedists in the community. At the time the program was started it was indeed radical to entrust care of a patient to anybody other than a medical doctor.

Hoaglund Takes a Second Sabbatical

By 1975, the Department had many of the attributes of larger orthopaedic programs, particularly with the emphasis on research. Hoaglund had been in Vermont for almost six years and was determined to take another sabbatical to Hong Kong. This left an administration void, which Frymoyer attempted to fill. He took steps to improve the business operations of the practice, became involved with a newly emerging university practice group (UHC), and worked on improving department communications.

With Hoaglund's approval, Frymoyer hired David Seligson who had trained at the Massachusetts General Hospital to fill the gap in trauma. There were plenty of orthopaedists

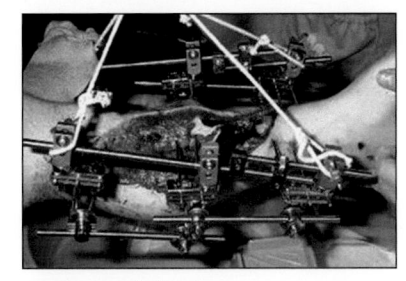

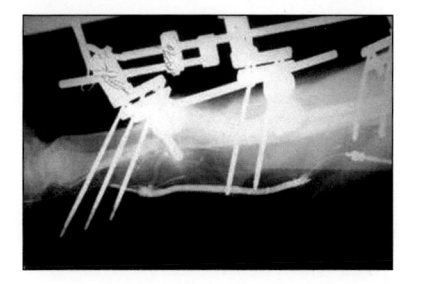

FIGURE 14-16 A&B.
David Seligson used fixateurs at UVM for the first time to treat injuries such as this associated with vascular injury. This limb was salvaged after many surgeries.

doing trauma cases, but they were reluctant to move forward with newer techniques of fracture treatment, which involved plating and screwing and applying fixateurs. These new approaches were revolutionizing trauma fracture care, and were now possible because of improved asepsis, antibiotics, and metallurgy. UVM was being left behind. Seligson turned out to be the proper catalyst and rapidly launched UVM into the forefront of innovative trauma care. He prevailed over the old guard partially by bringing a parade of international trauma experts to Vermont. Naturally the establishment didn't give up easily, and Seligson certainly was a controversial and dynamic figure.

Seligson also launched a significant research program to evaluate surgical implants. Although the residents moaned and groaned about his demands and high standards, he inspired a number of them to launch trauma careers. Tom DeCoster became head of trauma at New Mexico. Ray White became head at Maine and Gary Jones at Concord, NH. Seligson moved on to Louisville KY as Chair of Orthopaedics and Chief of the Fracture Service, where he continued to pursue further innovation in trauma.

UVM Forays Into Foot and Ankle Surgery

In 1977, Hoaglund hired Nathaniel Gould as foot and ankle specialist. A native of St. Johnsbury, VT, and a UVM graduate, he brought a large referral base with him to UVM from his practice in Brockton, MA. Brockton was known as the "Shoe Capitol of the World." He had been sought by many of the companies to help them develop more comfortable shoes, marketed with the reminder: "These shoes were designed in collaboration with an orthopaedist." This further developed his interest in foot surgery, and by the time he came to Vermont, he was well recognized as a leader in foot and ankle surgery and a founder and early president of the "Foot and Ankle Society." Gould announced he was coming to Burlington within or out of the full time group. Hoaglund grudgingly accepted him into the full time group, and foot and ankle surgery quickly became one of the busiest and well known programs in the department. Gould was famous for complex procedures performed on patients with rheumatoid arthritis. This often involved artificial joints, tendon transfers and fusions ... and were referred to by the residents as "blue plate specials." Two young surgeons, Saul Trevino and Richard Alvarez, were attracted to Vermont as fellows and stayed on in the group for a number of years. Alvarez left in 1987 and Trevino in 1993. Gould also attracted an array of national and international visitors who came to learn his techniques for treating complex foot and ankle problems.

Frymoyer Takes a Sabbatical to Begin Spine Research

Frymoyer took a sabbatical at the Neufeld Orthopaedic Center in Oxford England in 1977. During that year a grandiose plan took shape. During the sabbatical year, Frymoyer and Pope developed a large epidemiologic study, which if funded, would become the first such study in the United States and launch the department as a major spine research center. As part of that planning both Frymoyer and Pope spent time in Gothenburg, Sweden, widely acknowledged as the world's center for spine research. The head of that program, Alf Nachemson, had become famous for his work in measuring pressure within discs, and (with Volvo) designing for the first time, seats engineered to reduce back stresses.

Frymoyer Returns From Sabbatical With UVM in Crisis

While Frymoyer was in England, a battle between Orthopaedics and the Dean's Office emerged. Like many medical schools, UVM was facing a critical strategic moment. Should it grow a larger full time faculty, and thereby become more competitive with those in private practice? Under John Davis' leadership, the Department of Surgery already had moved aggressively in that direction. The decision involving all Chairs was to build a clinical practice facility. As part of that decision, the central leadership of UHC would take over many of the financial management and billing functions heretofore performed by the individual specialty practice groups. Rallying around the banner of "Quality Care," a new facility would also feature a single integrated medical record system. At that juncture, a critical event occurred. The Catholic Diocese of Burlington led by Bishop James Joyce agreed to sell the DeGoesbriand Hospital (DMU) to the University. In turn the University would arrange a long term lease with the newly formed University Health Center (UHC) and its confederate practice groups. Over time it was contemplated that the hospital functions of the DMU would be integrated into the Medical Center Hospital. Spurred by a large grant from the Given Foundation, this complex agreement was successfully negotiated. Its success, and to a real degree the future of the medical school, depended on the involvement of all the practice groups, particularly the surgeons who had the largest financial operations.

What exactly happened during those months is uncertain, but it is certain Orthopaedics had entered into negotiations with the owners of the Red Cross building. An architect was employed and plans drawn up for a free standing orthopaedic building which would include its own radiology services. UHC amalgamating all the full time doctors had decided to use the DeGoesbriand Hospital buildings for its clinical offices. Orthopaedics going off on its own obviously didn't fit the plan. Davis was dispatched to have a big brother discussion with Hoaglund in the latter's office. Exactly what was said has never been revealed, except that during the conversation, Davis leaned back in a UVM chair, which broke. The meeting was ended!

When Frymoyer returned from his sabbatical, he rather summarily was given a copy of the architect's drawings, and it was intimated it would be necessary for him to put up money if he wanted to be a part of the new building. Soon thereafter the Medical College of South Carolina approached him to be Chair of Orthopaedics. A number of UVM orthopaedic faculty indicated their interest in making that move with him. Dean Luginbuhl now had an

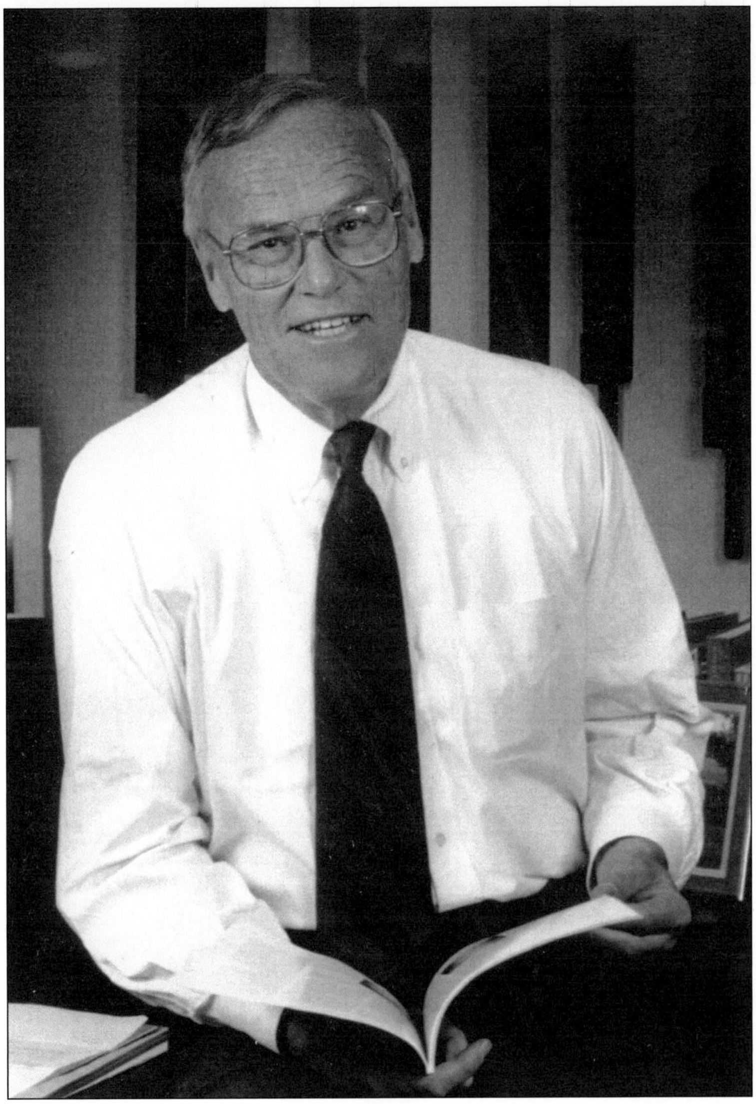

FIGURE 14-17. John Frymoyer assumed the Chair of Orthopaedics from 1978 to 1988, resigning to become Dean of the College of Medicine.

opening. He pronounced the move would "gut" the department clinically, and be detrimental to its research programs. As such he would have no recourse but to return the Department to Divisional status. The result was the Department voted to request Hoaglund's resignation, which shortly followed. He had successfully transformed the department from a small division to a nationally recognized orthopaedic department.

Frymoyer became acting chair, and after a national search two years later, Chair of the Department of Orthopaedics. Hoaglund left to become professor in residence at U.C. San Francisco, and head of the VA Program there.

In the chaotic aftermath of these events, the Dean agreed in a complex move to give Orthopaedics a significant amount of space for its research and teaching programs. This became a time of opportunity. The faculty, and residents rallied around the department. The major research programs started to grow rapidly.

Research Grows at UVM

By 1978, the Department of Orthopaedics was well positioned to become a major force in bio-engineering. Malcolm Pope PhD had completed his doctoral work under an engineer,

Dr. John Atwater, well known for his work on fracture biomechanics. Although he had been hired as a junior faculty member in Engineering, Pope was already heavily involved in the spine and knee ligament research programs of the Department of Orthopaedics. Hoaglund had promoted this relationship by giving him a joint appointment in Orthopaedics, where increasingly Pope was spending more time.

As part of his appointment as acting chair, Frymoyer had successfully negotiated for Pope to become tenured in the Department of Orthopaedics. Again this was considered a radical departure by most universities. After consultation with Vermont, the University of Iowa later tenured engineers in that department, and a national trend was started. Pope was instrumental in the growth and development of the Department into a national force in bio-engineering. Eventually the importance of this program was recognized by endowment of a chair and the creation of a musculoskeletal research center by Warren and Lois McClure.

The McClures were well known Burlington philanthropists. In the mid 1980's "Mac" was seen by Frymoyer with persisting complaints of back pain which despite seeing many doctors in Florida had gone undiagnosed. He was convinced it must be cancer. That diagnosis was not supported by the history. Examination revealed an area of point tenderness at a muscle insertion, and Novocaine® and a steroid were administered with immediate relief of the chronic pain. As he left McClure said, "Thanks a million." Over the next months he and Lois became intrigued by the work of the Department in bio-medical research, and eventually they endowed the Chair as well as the naming of new research space as "The McClure Musculoskeletal Research Center" with a two million dollar gift. Much later they donated an additional one million dollars to the College of Medicine for the "Frymoyer Scholars."

FIGURE 14-18. Warren and Lois McClure endowed the McClure Musculoskeletal Research Center and an orthopaedic chair that supported the Department's rapidly growing research.

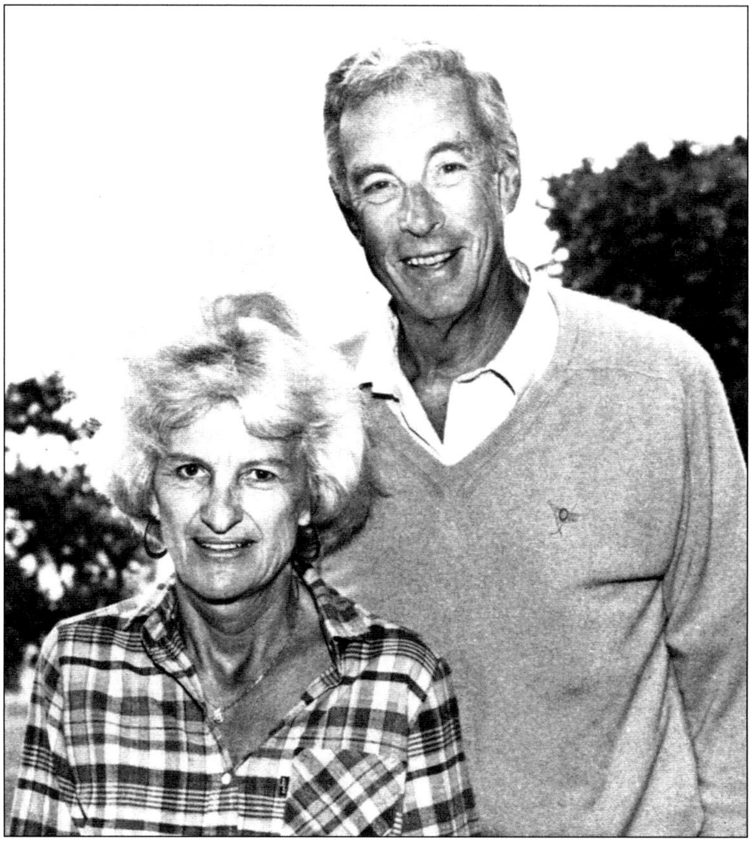

This overall growth of bio-engineering was promoted in 1978 when the Department of Orthopaedics received a large grant from the Government, and undertook an epidemiologic study involving more than 3000 individuals. A team was assembled now including two additional bio-engineers, David Wilder, and Ian Stokes recruited from Oxford; a psychologist, James Rosen, statisticians, and graduate students. One of the major findings of this study was that smoking and driving vehicles were significant risk factors for low back pain and sciatica. Both of these research findings were pursued, this included building a large vehicle simulator which allowed measurements of spinal stresses under a variety of vibrational inputs. A striking finding was that automobile seats, under conditions simulating road time, caused the spine to resonate (the phenomenon of a soprano breaking a glass.) This work clearly was of interest to the automobile industry, and was a natural place now to collaborate with the team in Gothenburg and Volvo. Pope took his sabbatical in Sweden, and with their team developed yet another machine for vibration simulation, which was then used to optimize car seat designs. In the tractor trailer the entire cab is dampened, while in the bus, the drivers seat is dampened. The effect is the same, to convert vibration from the roadway so that resonant frequencies are eliminated.

At the same time this work was occurring a number of other major developments involved other members of the orthopaedic faculty.

Martin Krag had trained at Yale and was intrigued by the work being done in Vermont by Frymoyer and Pope. The job opening in Vermont centered around the development of a rehabilitation center headed by Raymond Milhous which would be a division of orthopaedics. Krag went to Rancho Las Amigos Hospital Rehabilitation Center for 9 months, with his fellow's salary supplemented by UVM orthopaedics. He then came on the UVM faculty in 1981 initially to help the new division of rehabilitation medicine, but his heart was really in research and spine surgery.

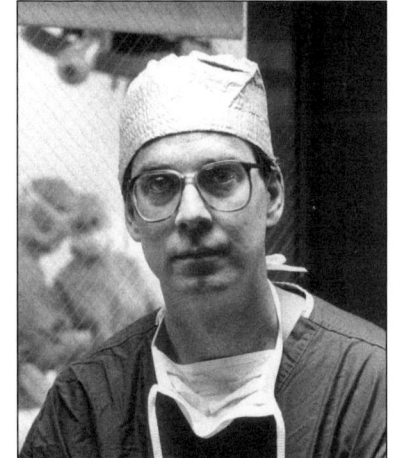

FIGURE 14-19. Martin Krag developed the Vermont Spinal Fixateur at UVM.

In the winter of 1985, a skier severely injured his back (L-5 to S-1) when he hit a tree. The existing hardware (Harrington Rods) was totally inadequate for fracture reduction and repair, and Krag remembers being extremely frustrated. External fixateurs for extremity fractures were becoming widely used, and Krag decided there was a need for an external fixateur type of device for spine fractures, which could then be somehow internalized. Krag's review showed there was work in Switzerland and France with spinal external fixateurs, and he visited both countries but failed to find already developed techniques for the problem. Laboratory work initially focused on the stress and design of screws and plates, leading to a design with only 3 moving parts. The tools were complicated, but the device he developed was versatile and effective. Pope, and a graduate student, Bruce Beynnon, collaborated. Later, Beynnon became director of research at UVM Orthopaedics. The Vermont Spinal Fixateur worked well and its principles led to future evolutionary developments in spinal fixation.[29] This research into the relevant anatomy of the spine, and methods and pitfalls in screw placement, remain the standard today.

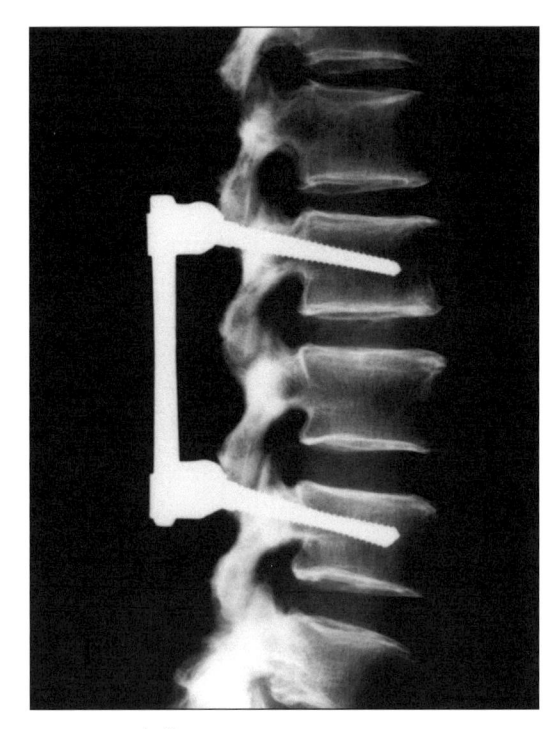

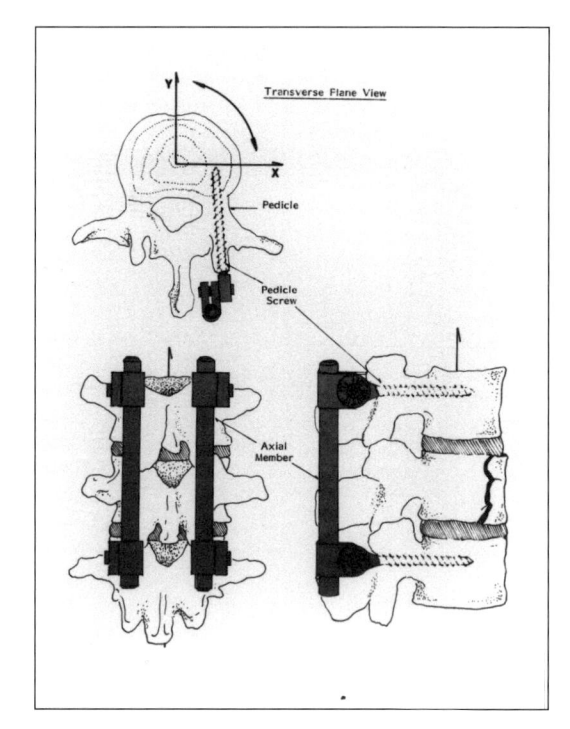

FIGURE 14-20 A&B.
X-ray and diagram showing application of a Vermont Spinal Fixateur, the principles of which have endured to this day.

Rowland Hazard was recruited to start a spine rehabilitation program, the second of its type in the United States. Using new techniques, the rate of successful rehabilitation was increased from 20% to 70% as measured by the ability of the patients to return to work.

As a result of all of these developments, by the mid-1980s, the department was recognized as one of the two leading centers for spine research in the world. In 1988 the American Academy of Orthopaedic Surgeons and the National Institutes of Health co-sponsored a symposium on "New Perspectives in Low Back Pain" which resulted in a publication by that name in 1989. In that year, Lippincott-Raven Publishers approached Frymoyer to determine if he would be interested in editing the first major academic text related to spinal disorders. He assembled a team of Associate Editors and over 100 authors which resulted in the two volume text "The Adult Spine", now in its third Edition.[30] It is of interest that when the International Society for Study of the Lumbar Spine started its "Career Achievement Award" the first four recipients were Nachemson, Frymoyer, Anderson (Nachemson's co-investigator) and Pope.

Leon Grobler was brought in from South Africa as a spine surgeon, and UVM then had its first spine fellow (Kevin Gill.) The spine fellowship was abandoned after several years because it was thought having fellows detracted from the resident clinical experience.

During the Frymoyer years, the residency program expanded to the current level of three residents per year. The department became more engaged with student teaching and coincidentally merged with the Department of Rehabilitation Medicine. Pope and Frymoyer published a text on occupational low back pain.[31] Clinically, the full-time people ruled the orthopaedic world in Burlington. Their billings grew from about $450,000 in 1978 to 12 million 8 years later.

Trauma Finds a New Leader in Thomas Kristiansen

Thomas K. Kristiansen, originally from Potsdam, NY, had completed medical school at Syracuse, and was in a residency at West Virginia, where the orthopaedic department was undergoing a change in leadership. Kristiansen had taken an acting internship at UVM, and when openings developed he jumped at the chance to come to Vermont for orthopaedic residency. The residency included a four month away rotation, and Kristiansen was sent to Berne, Switzerland for 2 months and Paris, Brussels, and Vienna for another two months.

He was planning on opening a private practice of orthopaedics, but was asked by Frymoyer if he would join the group as a trauma surgeon as Seligson was leaving in 1983. Kristiansen said he would do it for two years, but is still at it in 2008, 25 years later.

He became director of the orthopaedic trauma service (and its only physician) until Craig Bartlett joined the group in 1996. Bartlett brought new horizons to UVM as an innovative trauma surgeon who was a wizard at dealing with pelvic fractures. Kristiansen was active in research[32, 33] until Fletcher Allen's emphasis on billing goals in 1993 made clinical practice a priority. Joseph Abate also joined the group. It seemed there was limitless orthopaedic trauma.

Sports Medicine Continues to Grow at UVM

A 6 1/2 month sabbatical in Sweden by Johnson followed the precedent set by Hoaglund and Frymoyer. Per Renstrom from Gothenburg, Sweden, who was a prominent authority in sports medicine, got to know Johnson. In 1983, Renstrom took a sabbatical and chose to come to Vermont. Johnson's Swedish connection was instrumental in getting Renstrom to Vermont. Renstrom returned to Sweden for two years, but then came back to Vermont as a full time faculty member in 1989. He returned to Sweden in 1996 to become chair of the Sports Program at the Karolinska Institute in Stockholm, where he continues to be one of the internationally prominent experts in that field. He left his mark on UVM as a center of excellence for sports medicine.

In the mid 1990s, Frymoyer became the founding editor of the "Journal of the Academy of Orthopedic Surgeons."

Frymoyer Moves Up to Be CEO of UHC

John Davis, chair of surgery and CEO of the University Health Center (UHC — the full-time practice group for all of UVM) became ill and Frymoyer was tapped to become the head of UHC. He stepped down from the chair of Orthopedics. Jim Howe became the acting Chair, and then Chair.

Howe was going to be a vascular surgeon "because his mother said so." During medical school at UVM, he worked with Frymoyer on spine research. He then went to the Medical College of Virginia to do a surgical residency with David Hume. Hume ran a dynamic one man department, until he died in a plane crash. Meanwhile, Howe had seen the light and was looking for an orthopedic residency. He was talking with Hoaglund who had just had a G-2 resident drafted for the Vietnam conflict in 1975. He came back to Vermont and finished the residency in 1978. Luckily the Vietnam conflict was ending or he would himself have

FIGURE 14-21. Dean Frymoyer continued to practice non-operative orthopaedics in order to remain clinically active.

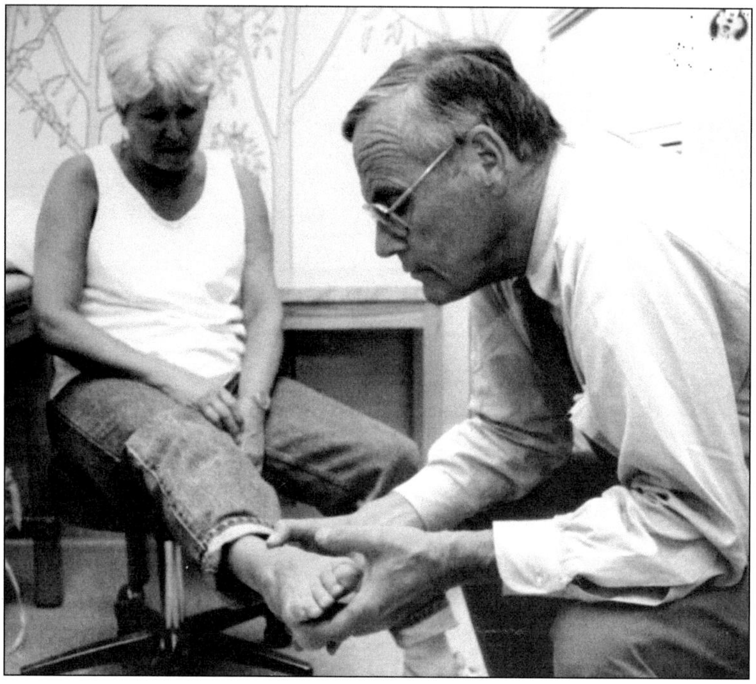

faced military duty. The department sent Howe to the Mayo clinic for a fellowship in total joint replacement, and he came back to fill that need at UVM.

Howe joined enthusiastically with the orthopaedic staff. This was a time when reimbursements had dropped. Orthopaedics ran an open book system with all members seeing billings and compensation for all department members. At this time there was a huge problem with lack of space for patient office visits. UHC was talking of building an Ambulatory Care Center (ACC), but if orthopaedics saw patients there, there wouldn't be space for the rest of the UHC doctors. The offer was tendered to have orthopaedics see patients at the soon-to-be renovated Medical Office Building at the Fanny Allen. Finances were a problem and this was solved by Orthopaedics buying the ground floor (where their offices were to be.) They were assured this was on the fast track, but Orthopaedics was afraid the ACC would never get built.

Steven Incavo had started training at Syracuse in Orthopaedics, and was brought to UVM for a "fellowship" with Howe and Frymoyer in total joint replacements and stayed on as an attending. Incavo worked in the operating room and in the laboratory and shouldered much of the total-joint load. He left in 2007 for Texas.

Howe Steps Down as Chair of Orthopaedics and Nichols Takes Over

The ten years that Howe had planned on being chair were over, and he wanted to step down. Fletcher Allen was at a critical juncture in its formation, and Frymoyer as dean, asked him to stay for an additional two years to give stability to the transition. Claude Nichols was appointed interim Chair. Two years later, a national chair search was conducted, and Nichols was appointed Chair in 2001.

Nichols was brought up in Harrisburg, PA on the second floor above his physician father's office. He thought, however, he wanted to be a chemist while at Brown. He saw the light and

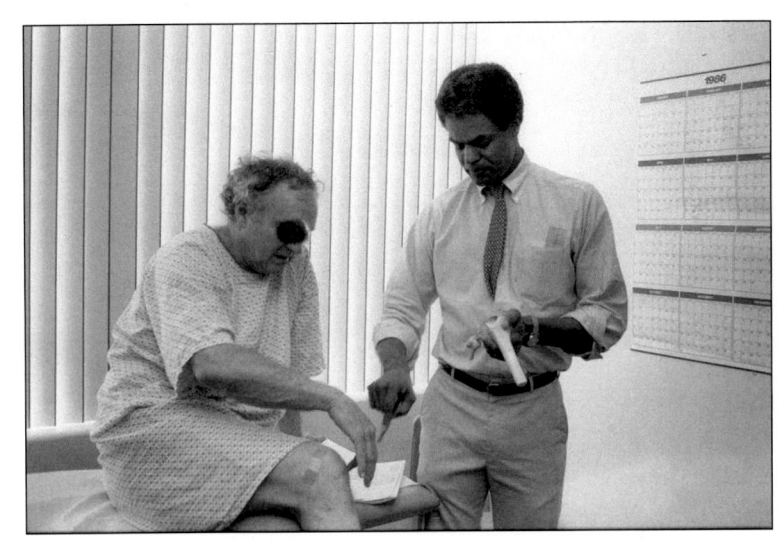

FIGURE 14-22. Claude Nichols assumed the Chair of Orthopaedics in 2001, and has continued to foster UVM's expertise in sports medicine and research.

attended Temple Medical School. While a first year medical student he tore his ACL and went through multiple procedures but not ACL repair. This led to a shift from running to bicycling, and perhaps was the start of his interest in orthopaedics and sports medicine. Orthopaedic residency at the University of Pennsylvania was followed by a sports medicine fellowship. A friend told him UVM was looking for a sports medicine specialist and he joined the UVM staff in 1985.

Nichols started doing ACL studies in the lab with Pope. Bruce Beynnon came as a graduate student and stayed on, and Renstrom returned. The sports medicine group became a powerful force in UVM orthopedics. Two surgeons (Nichols and James Mogan) were sharing the shoulder surgery, but Mogan left to enter private practice in Burlington. His practice focus shifted to hand more than shoulder.

Under Nichols' regime, the decision was made to accept space for surgery and offices at the Fanny Allen, rather than move to the new ambulatory care facility. But there wasn't sufficient room for the whole full time staff. So orthopaedics remained situated in divided sites.

Knee Arthroscopy Comes to Vermont

Knee surgery at UVM and elsewhere has changed dramatically since Bob Johnson's own open repair in 1982. This entailed excruciating pain and swelling during recovery, and being in a cast for seven weeks after the repair. Vermont was on the cusp of pioneering this change to endoscopic surgery years before the revolution took orthopaedics by storm.

In 1962, fifteen years before orthopaedists became interested, a rheumatologist, Richard Lipson had read of Watanabe's device in Japan, and worked with Carl Zeiss Inc. to develop the optics. He needed someone with a surgical interest to work out the operative techniques. Frymoyer and Lipson developed a technique for insertion of a scope into the knee joint, and for biopsy through the instrument orifice. In 1966, this work was published in an obscure journal under the title: "A telescope for the knee." This was the first paper on the topic in the United States. Rust, who was co-chair of the Division, thought the technique risked infection. What could have been a blaze of glory was cut short according to Frymoyer. Lipson continued to do diagnostic arthroscopies for many years but never again published.

Later Johnson became the area knee specialist, and went to Boston to observe knee arthroscopic procedures. He had a visiting expert come and assist him in his first cases here. In those days (1987) this was all that was required to start new procedures.

Rebirth of an Orthopaedic Hand Section

Brian Adams was recruited as a hand surgeon as Mogan left for private practice. He was to stay only two and a half years and make great progress in developing a total prosthetic wrist, among other things, when he was at his new home in Iowa.

Meanwhile, Michel Benoit was about to join the UVM team. At age seven, in 1967, Benoit attended a movie "Man and His Health" at the expo in Montreal. The movie was about heart surgery, and inspired Benoit to go into medicine and surgery. In medical school, still in his native Montreal, the orthopaedic residents were inspirational in their mastery of anatomy, and Benoit made his career decision. He trained in Ottawa and Syracuse, and was ready to return to Montreal. The Canadian government underwent budget cuts, eliminating the job promised to Benoit. He cast his net looking for a hand surgery job, and UVM called him and requested an interview the day before his phone was to be disconnected. When he came in September 1992 to join Adams, he found Adams had accepted a job in Iowa, leaving Benoit alone in the hand surgery division! Howe (as chair) wanted an additional hand surgeon, but the decision was made to hire a double hitter, Philip Trabulsy, to help plastic surgery and orthopaedic hand surgery under a dual appointment.

When Trabulsy became ill and unable to operate, Donald Laub was hired to fill the dual appointment. Finally … Shafritz was hired as a hand surgeon with shoulder training to bolster the orthopaedic hand service.

The hand service offers a full complement of services with six certified hand therapists in the office. Replantations are done by hand surgeons as well as by some of the plastic surgeons.

Struggles to Restart Foot and Ankle Surgery

When Trevino left in 1993, Kristiansen took on the additional load of foot and ankle surgeon for the orthopaedic group. Relief was a long time coming. In 1999 James Michelson came to give the Nathaniel Gould Lecture at UVM on an invitation from Nichols (with whom he had been a resident at the University of Pennsylvania.) Michelson had been raised in Baltimore in the shadow of his father, a thoracic surgeon who was rarely at home. He originally thought he would be an engineer, but ended up in orthopaedics on the staff at Johns Hopkins in 1988. Because of a need for foot and ankle specialty work at Hopkins, he took a fellowship in that specialty in New York (Hospital for Joint Disease-Orthopaedic.) Nichols finally convinced Michelson to move to Vermont in 2000, but his family couldn't be transplanted and he returned with them to the Baltimore area. He came to Burlington to teach everything the residents needed to know about foot and ankle orthopaedics in one week each June. Finally in 2007, Michelson assumed a four day work week (Monday though Thursday) in Vermont doing foot and ankle orthopaedics. He also worked on developing an electronic medical record system for UVM. He spent Fridays at his Baltimore area home doing research.

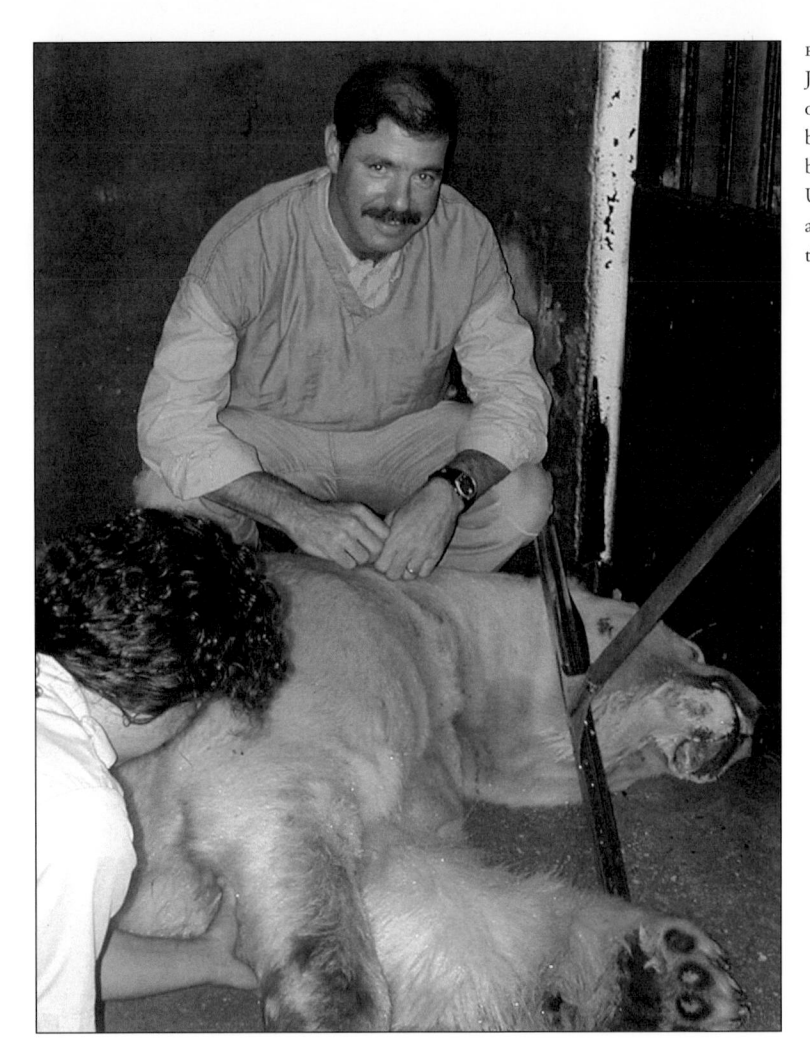

FIGURE 14-23. James Michelson operates on a polar bear (Magnet) before rejuvenating UVM's foot and ankle service here in the North Country.

Help finally appeared on the horizon with the arrival of a new foot and ankle surgeon Mark Chadson, whose arrival coincides with the writing of this book.

Orthopaedic Research Continues

Research continues with Bruce Beynnon Ph.D. as director of research. He won national research awards in 2005 for anterior cruciate knee ligament and ankle ligament injury research. He has become deputy director of the Journal of Orthopaedic Research.

Krag continues his focus on research with development of the basic science relative to halo vest fixation for cervical spine problems.[34] Krag is currently the national P.I. for a multicenter randomized study of a new technique for lumbar spinal fusions, using a synthetic bag containing bone graft pieces inserted into the disc space through a small incision. (Optimesh®)

CHAPTER 15

Cardiothoracic Surgery Division

Cardiac surgery started early at UVM, but was halted after results were suboptimal. Attempts to restart the program failed when research credentials didn't translate into clinical expertise.

Laurence Coffin, a physician who switched from marine architecture to medicine, rescued the program. His tireless work in the research laboratory and clinical arena was carried on by a series of surgeons with Vermont connections.

The Division currently participates in an innovative, groundbreaking, outcomes improvement group and conducts state of the art research. Its success is also reflected by the large percentage of surgical graduates that have pursued cardiothoracic fellowships.

Thoracic Injuries Were Treated By Surgeons for Years

UVM's surgeons had treated traumatic thoracic injuries for decades, usually with varying degrees of success. Former Chairman Benjamin Howard had published a detailed approach to penetrating chest wounds as early as 1863 (see Chapter 4). Of course, he got the physiology completely wrong, recommending the snug closure of entry sites and the application of airtight dressings. As a result, "infection was common, and a high case fatality rate was inevitably associated with this type of treatment."[1]

The discipline eventually came into its own in 1943 with the arrival of Richard Overholt (1901-1990) as part time "Consultant in Thoracic Surgery."[2] Overholt's work at the Lahey Clinic and his own Boston-based thoracic center was impressive; he had pioneered tubercular surgical therapies, had developed segmental lung resection techniques, and in 1933, had conducted the world's first successful right-sided pneumonectomy for cancer.[2] Vermont's physicians were soon performing many of his pulmonary procedures, but heart surgery was a decade away.

Overholt, however, always felt that his biggest contribution to medicine was his anti-smoking campaign. He launched the crusade after observing that the lungs of non-smokers healed faster than those of smokers. A society, though, in which cigarettes were fashionable and tobacco consumption was on the rise, did not want to hear about smoking cessation. Overholt was actually laughed off the stage when he presented his initial anti-tobacco work in 1934.[4] His impact at the Mary Fletcher Hospital (where the patient lounges usually choked visitors with smoke) was also limited. In fact, post-cardiac surgery patients in Vermont could still smoke in their rooms well into the 1970s!

Cardiac Surgery Begins at UVM in the 1950s

Overholt, busy with his clinic and his academic responsibilities at the Lahey Clinic, stopped visiting UVM in 1947.[5] The School's first dedicated thoracic surgeon, Donald Miller (1916-1995), took his place in 1951. Miller — a graduate of Johns Hopkins and a flight surgeon during World War II — had completed additional specialty training at the Bronx Veterans Administration Hospital. Miller did both thoracic and "closed" cardiac surgery in Burlington. He accomplished the latter by incising the left atrium, placing a finger or knife into the beating heart, and then dividing the stenosed mitral valve leaflets. He also initiated a diagnostic cardiopulmonary laboratory that performed cardiac catheterizations.[6]

FIGURE 15-1. Henry Minot, a student of Walton Lillihei, helped Miller with the first open heart case.

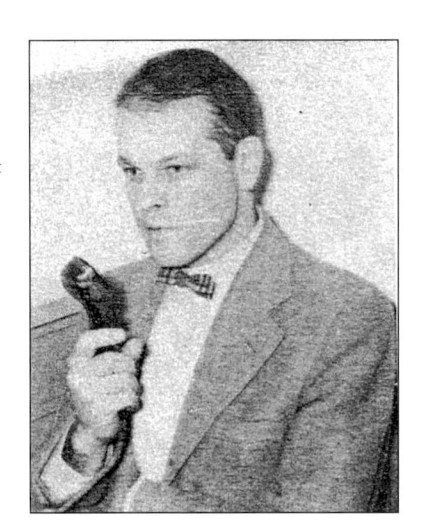

The University of Minnesota's F. John Lewis and C. Walton Lillehei carried out the first "open" cardiac operation in September of 1952, slowing the heart and giving cerebral protection with whole body hypothermia. This method, however, was limited to cases of less than ten minutes duration. In March of 1955, the Mayo Clinic's John W. Kirklin used a modified version of John Gibbon's pump oxygenator to repair a ventricular septal defect. Lillehei followed suit shortly thereafter with a slightly different setup.[7] Miller took an immediate interest in cardiopulmonary bypass after reading their landmark reports. He hired one of Lillehei's pupils, Henry D. Minot, Jr., in 1956 and started studying open-heart procedures.[8]

Miller recruited Clement Comeau (1927-2004) to run the bypass machine the same year. Comeau, a former DeGoesbriand Memorial Hospital operating technician, was "part mechanic and part medical technologist." He learned the pump's intricacies in the cardiac

FIGURE 15-2. Clem Comeau checks the heart lung equipment in 1959.

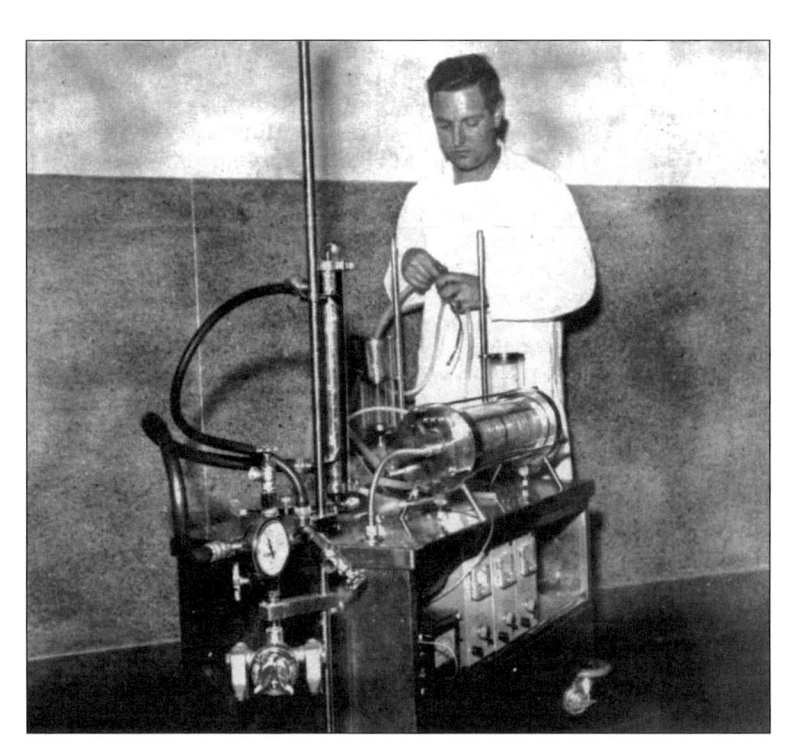

236 CATAMOUNT SURGEONS

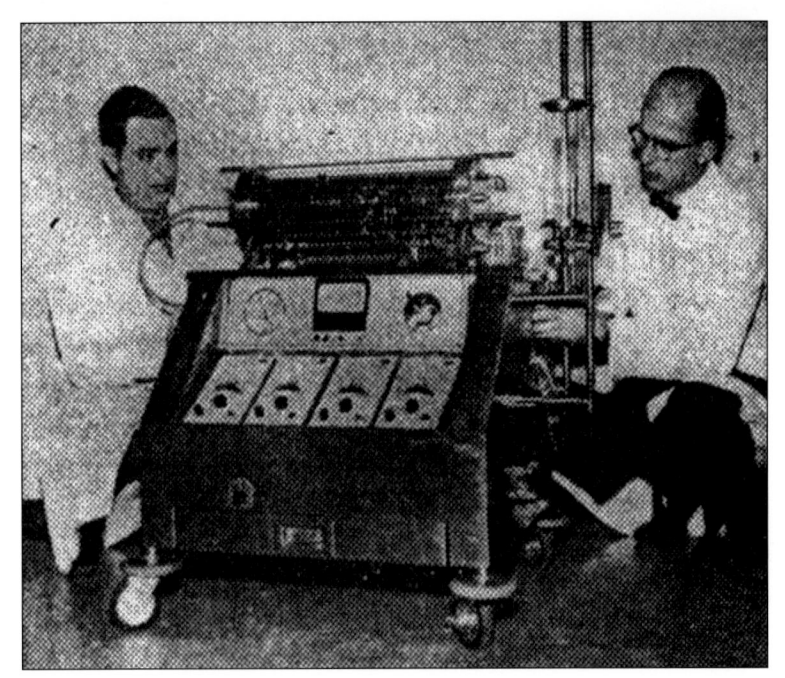

FIGURE 15-3. Miller and Comeau improved their cardiac bypass equipment in the lab and in the operating room.

research lab, becoming highly competent through his work with large animals during Julius Jacobson's tenure. Comeau remained Chief Research Technician and Clinical Perfusionist until his retirement in 1990.[9]

UVM's first open-heart operation was performed by Miller in 1959 on B.W., a patient with a complex 3 cm atrial septal defect. The six-hour long surgery went according to plan, and the patient did well (the O.R. nurses having been flown to Boston for training in surgical technique and post-operative care beforehand). His discharge "less than a month later" was hailed as a remarkable event by the local newspaper, which also praised the hospital's progress.[10] B.W., still thriving 36 years later, spoke in gratitude at Miller's 1995 memorial service.

In spite of its rural setting, UVM ran a cutting edge cardiac surgery program with a first-rate team. Miriam "Parky" Parkinson devoted herself to cardiothoracic surgical nursing.

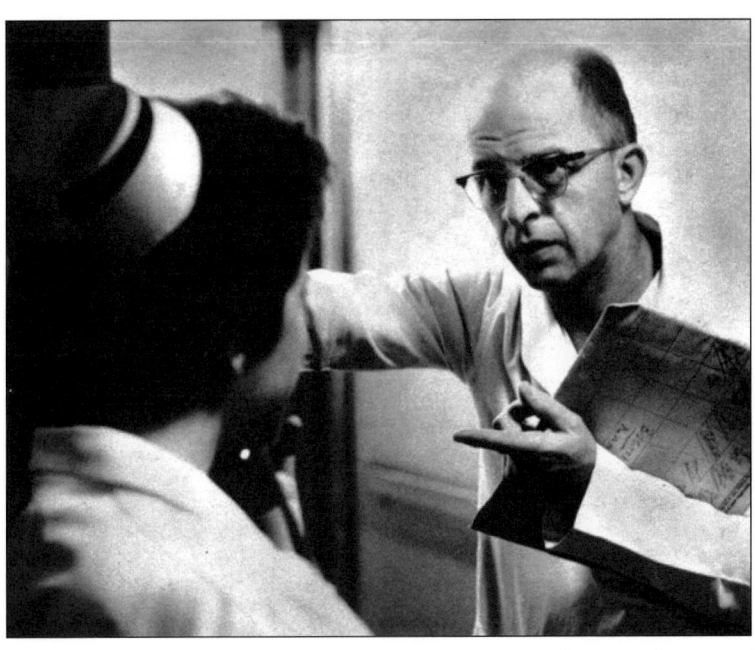

FIGURE 15-4. Miriam (Parky) Parkinson specialized as a cardiothoracic surgical nurse and assistant.

Chapter Fifteen: Cardiothoracic Surgery Division

FIGURE 15-5. Parkinson later ran the cardiac bypass machine, alternating with Comeau for many years. (1983 photo)

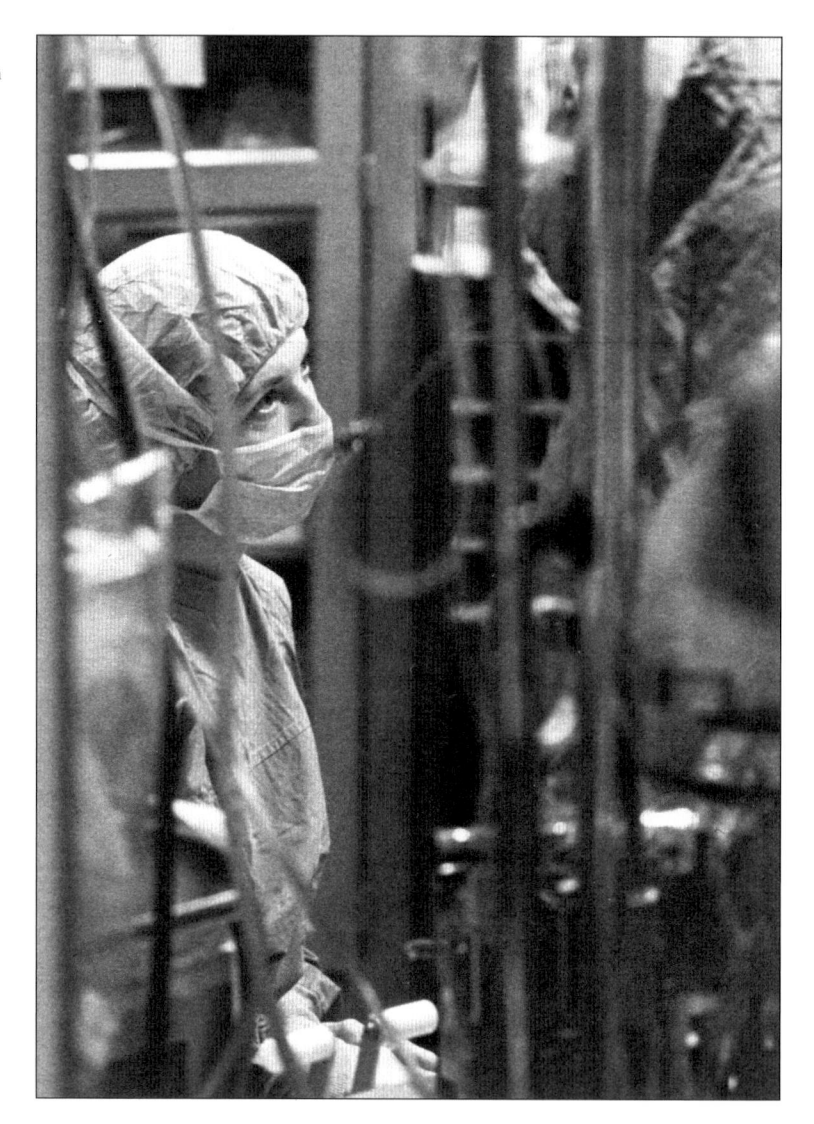

Tamatsu "Tom" Shinozaki provided the anesthesia for the early cases. Jacobson essentially took over for Minot (who had moved to Connecticut and gone into private practice right after the first pump procedure) in 1960. Jacobson assisted Miller on occasion, and even performed a few cases himself.

Sixteen septal defect and aortic valvuloplasty cases were carried out with good (but not spectacular) results over the next four years. This was despite a head injury Miller suffered flying himself to a medical meeting. A mitral valve replacement was succesfully completed in 1961, although it did require nine units of blood! Stanley Christie (1928-1994) arrived in 1963, following Jacobson's departure. He had been a resident at New York's Bellevue Hospital under Jacobson's successor, William M. Stahl, and had completed a cardiothoracic fellowship with Denton Cooley in Houston, Texas.[11]

Several aortic valves were replaced in 1964. In 1965, a combined aortic and mitral valve replacement was successfully performed. Christie, as the junior partner, felt constrained by Miller and — his friendship with Stahl notwithstanding — left Vermont for independent practice.[12] Miller's next assistant, Alexander Geha, was hired in 1967. Geha, fresh from an extended fellowship at the Mayo Clinic, brought additional expertise from the land of Kirklin and company.

Cardiac Surgery is Halted Twice at UVM

Unfortunately, the heart-lung bypass equipment wasn't fully developed yet, and overall valve surgery statistics were not satisfactory. Miller, Mackay, and the Chief of Anesthesiology, John Abajian, subsequently called for a moratorium on open-heart procedures. Geha left in 1969 for a distinguished career, eventually serving as the Chairman of Cardiothoracic programs at Yale, Case Western, and the University of Illinois at Chicago.[13] Miller, undaunted, continued performing thoracic cases.

With the open-heart program at a standstill and research director Stahl on his way back to New York, Mackay decided to address two problems by making one appointment. His attention turned to the University of Maryland's Emil Blair (1922-1998), an established researcher and thoracic surgeon. Blair, a native of Satu Mare, Romania, came with an impressive resume and a high profile.[14] Unfortunately, his clinical skills at UVM were not as evident. Blair's blunt thoracic trauma experiments were not fruitful. In addition, clinical mortality was high following the few open-heart cases that he did attempt. As a result, the program was suspended yet again. Research expertise without sufficient clinical experience was not the solution.

UVM Gets a New Cardiac Leader and Transiently a Thoracic Surgery Residency

Miller was still doing thoracic cases when John Davis became chairman, but cardiac surgery was at a standstill. Davis brought one of his Cleveland acquaintances, Laurence Haines Coffin Jr., onboard to revive Vermont's program. Coffin successfully righted the Division and put it back on a stable course.

Coffin had dreamed of being a naval architect, but left the Massachusetts Institute of Technology with a degree in bio-chemical engineering instead. He developed an interest in medicine as an undergraduate, and frequently sneaked into the nearby Massachusetts General Hospital's (MGH) observation dome to watch surgery. Coffin enrolled at Cleveland's Western Reserve Medical School in 1955. He capitalized on his engineering background as a first-year student, securing a role in the design and construction of the school's original heart-lung machine under the direction of his mentor, Jay Ankeney.[15]

Three years later, Coffin ran the pump oxygenator during Western Reserve's first open-heart operation. At the end of the procedure, he pushed the bulky device through the tunnel back to the animal laboratory for the following day's research. The trek was then reversed 24 hours later for the second hospital pump case. Since intensive care units were not fully developed at Western Reserve, Coffin and his fellow medical students spent their nights in the recovery room monitoring the post-operative cardiac patients.

After taking a clerkship at the MGH, Coffin was pressured to return to Boston for his internship. Interns, though, did not receive a salary from MGH — just room, board, and laundry service. Moreover, interns could only bring their families to dinner on Sundays. Coffin had been married for a year at that stage and thought that he should at least earn something for his efforts. He therefore wisely chose to stay in Cleveland for both internship and residency. During this interval, Coffin joined the Navy and spent two years at Camp Lejeune, North Carolina. While there, he worked in the research lab studying the effects of burn shock on canine cardiovascular systems.[16]

FIGURE 15-6. Laurence Coffin rejuvenated the open-heart program upon his arrival from Cleveland, and did UVM's first CABG in 1971.

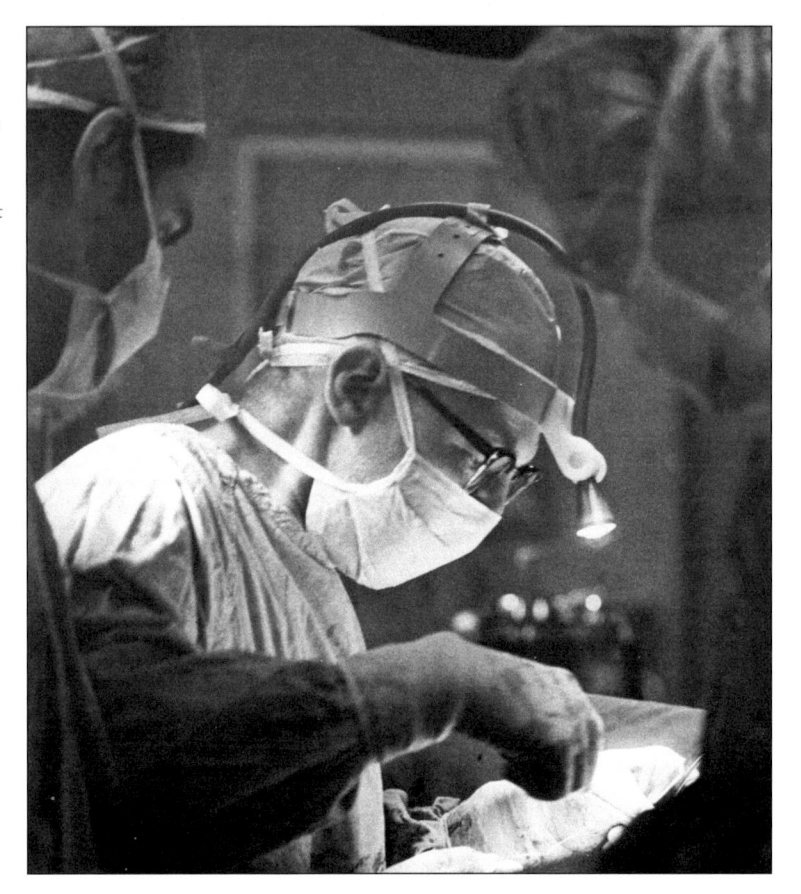

Coffin remained in Cleveland at the completion of his residency, becoming a junior partner at Western Reserve. In 1967 he was assigned to the Veteran's Hospital. Across town at the Cleveland Clinic, Renè Favaloro had just done the first coronary artery bypass graft (CABG) in the United States. Coffin, ever the innovator, went and watched Favaloro reroute blood around coronary lesions with segments of saphenous veins. He then teamed with Ankeney to conduct the same procedure at the VA; a remarkable accomplishment considering that the operation was done without the aid of the pump. Coffin also learned how to use the left internal mammary artery as a conduit for left anterior descending (LAD) and right coronary artery bypasses.

Coffin was vacationing in Maine when Davis called with an invitation to visit Vermont. Coffin had never applied for a job before and hadn't even considered leaving Cleveland, but he was intrigued by his former chairman's offer.

Coffin wrapped up his obligations in Cleveland, and prepared to come to Vermont. Burlington, in the meantime, had received its largest snowfall ever from a single storm — 29.8 inches from December 25th to 28th, 1969. Coffin recalled arriving on January 1, 1970 in the midst of another raging storm. Snow was four feet deep in places and oxygen tanks were being delivered to the hospital on military halftracks. He thought that was normal for Burlington!

Coffin accepted Davis' challenge to restart the UVM cardiac surgery program. He assiduously worked with the equipment in the dog lab, making use of the improvements in angiography along the way. He repaired an atrial septal defect on-pump in March of 1970. This was

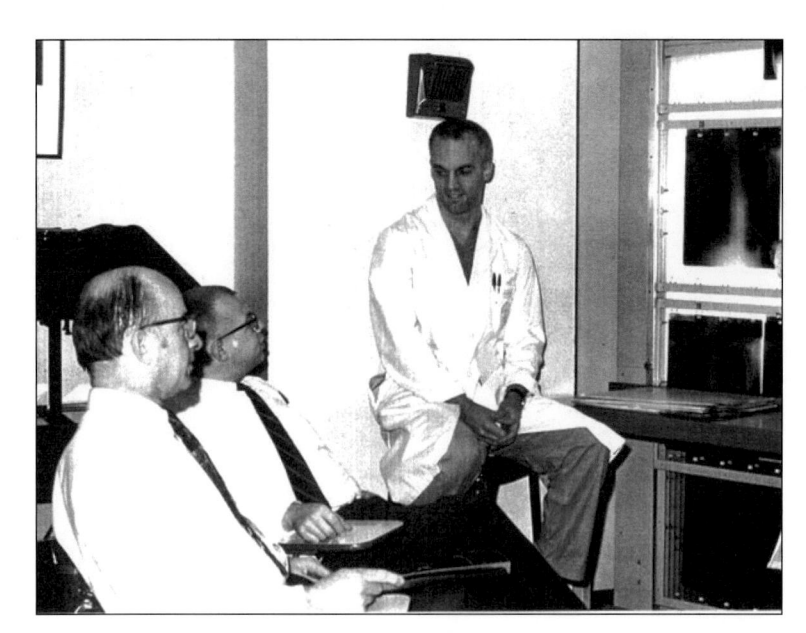

FIGURE 15-7. John Soeter (R), UVM's first thoracic surgery resident, discussing cases with Miller (foreground) and Coffin in 1971.

followed by Vermont's first coronary bypass operation that summer — a successful LAD graft on a patient who subsequently lived without angina for many years.

The American Board of Thoracic Surgery had approved Emil Blair's request for a sub-specialty residency in 1969 on a provisional basis, but Blair was unable to start a program. Coffin took advantage of the situation, and appointed graduating MCHV surgical resident John Soeter to fill the first slot. Soeter performed thoracic cases with Miller and assisted Coffin with cardiac cases. Fellow MCHV resident David Brodie followed Soeter. Brodie supplemented his thoracic residency with additional training in pediatric cardiac surgery. It became apparent though that there were not enough cases for a residency — especially if the Division was to continue providing adequate experience for general surgery residents — and the idea was abandoned in 1973.

Double-Teaming Cardiac Surgery

James Eugene DeMeules (1938-1988), another Western Reserve alumnus, joined Coffin in 1972. DeMeules was dedicated to his patients. His successor, Frank Ittleman, said of him:

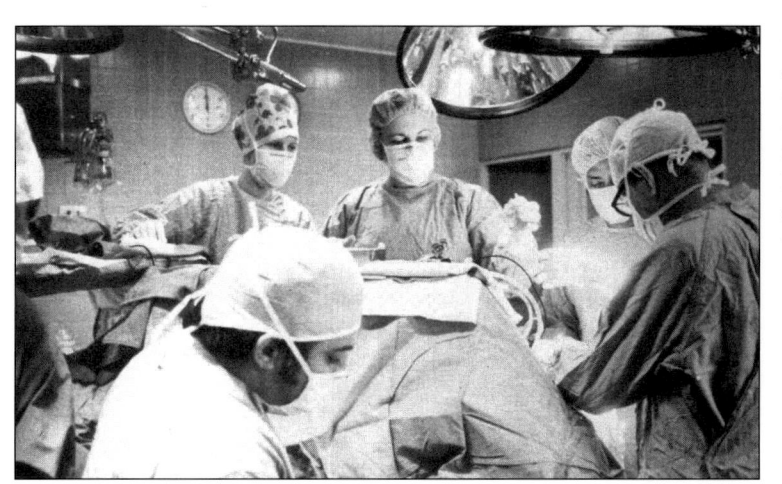

FIGURE 15-8. Jim DeMeules (R) operates at the Mary Fletcher in 1980 while John Hartford (foreground) gives anesthesia.

"Jim radiated an energy when he was working that drew you to him. It was a force, a unique quality that few people possess. When asked some years ago what surgeon you would like to have with you if you were on the end of a limb, the residents uniformly said Jim DeMeules ... he would never leave you there alone. He was the same way with his patients. I never saw a man will a patient to live the way Jim did. With skill and care, and yes sweat, he did beautiful work." [17]

DeMeules was devastated when a patient (who was also an MCHV nurse) couldn't get off the respirator. No one knew what was destroying the nurse's ability to breathe. DeMueles, in desperation, performed an open lung biopsy in the ICU. The specimen revealed the presence of *Legionella pneumophila*, the bacterium responsible for Legionnaires' disease. His team tried everything, including extracorporeal membrane oxygenation (ECMO), an experimental lung bypass machine that essentially oxygenated the patient's blood.[18] DeMueles didn't save her life, but he did go the extra mile trying.

The 1977 MCHV outbreak occurred within months of the July 1976 outbreak in Philadelphia among attendees at a convention of the American Legion. The source of the still mysterious disease at UVM was eventually traced to the cooling towers atop the Given Medical Building. Airborne bacteria gained entrance to the Fletcher Unit's Operating Room air intakes, infecting several workers and patients in the process. Immunosuppressed individuals were hit especially hard.[19]

Coffin and DeMeules assisted each other with open cardiac cases whenever possible. The absence of good help was problematic though, especially when on-call residents were occupied elsewhere. DeMeules was summoned on one such evening to a crashing post-op patient's bedside. True to form, he dropped everything and raced to the ICU. It was thus that a soaking-wet, half-naked DeMeules appeared on the scene, fresh from his shower. Suds flew everywhere as the patient was resuscitated. DeMeules' towel, thankfully, stayed in place for the duration of the event.

Richard Overholt's anti-tobacco warnings, unfortunately, were lost on the heavy smoking DeMeules. He sustained a massive heart attack at the age of 42 that left him a cardiac cripple unable to operate. DeMeules' biggest regret, naturally, was that his condition couldn't be improved through cardiac surgery! DeMeules struggled with his transition, but swallowed his disappointment and diligently plunged into research. Disaster struck again a few years later, however, when he was diagnosed with lymphoma.

Coffin had successfully resuscitated UVM's cardiac surgical program with the help of DeMeules, to become a first rate program which would continue to the present. A remarkable achievement.

UVM's Future Cardiac Surgery Leader Emerges

Frank Ittleman was a UVM resident during the Coffin and DeMeules years. He was on-call every night as a pediatric surgery intern and his car was unreliable. His solution was to sleep in the Adams House. The young bachelor found it so convenient that he never left; he basically lived there his entire residency. Free time was spent suturing vascular grafts to one another and to the bedspread. An occasional basketball game was augmented with a long run

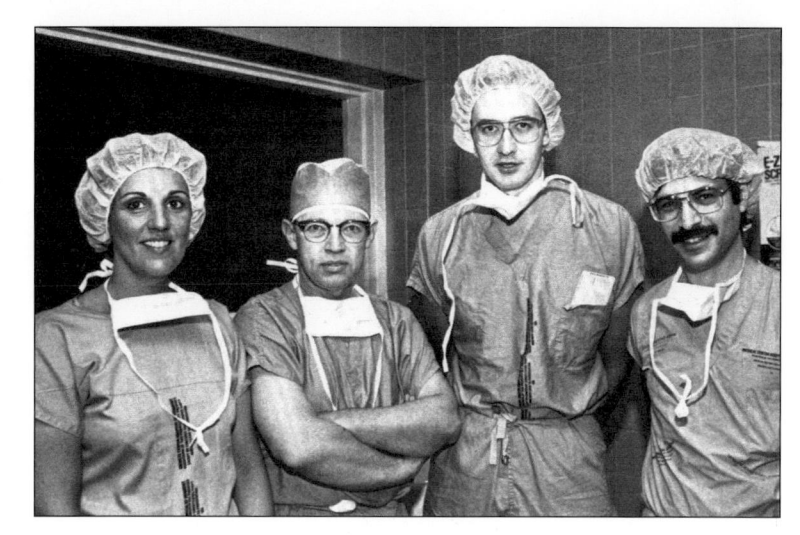

FIGURE 15-9. The team after a 1984 CABG (left to right): cardiac nurse Jan Atkins, Coffin, G-2 resident Paul Kispert, and G-4 resident David Zeiler.

— enough training to complete the Boston Marathon in a very respectable 2 hours and 47 minutes.

Even though the Adams House did not have a kitchen, Ittleman managed to creatively acquire meals after hours. He kept track of the late afternoon discharges since patients often left before eating supper. And he was always present when a tray "mistakenly" arrived for a comatose ICU patient. It seemed a shame, after all, to waste good food. Ward refrigerators were another source of nourishment; at least until the Baird 3 nurses set a trap with cat food sandwiches.

Ittleman, like Coffin and DeMeules before him, went to Western Reserve for his cardiothoracic fellowship. He joined the staff at Cleveland, but yearned to return to New England. Coffin called following DeMeules' 1980 heart attack and offered him a position. Ittleman opted for Vermont without hesitation and left Ohio the next day. Ittleman insisted on surgical independence. Gone were the days of attendings assisting each other. Ittleman's surgical productivity seemed to have no limits. As a result, the fourth-year residents gained terrific exposure and responsibility.

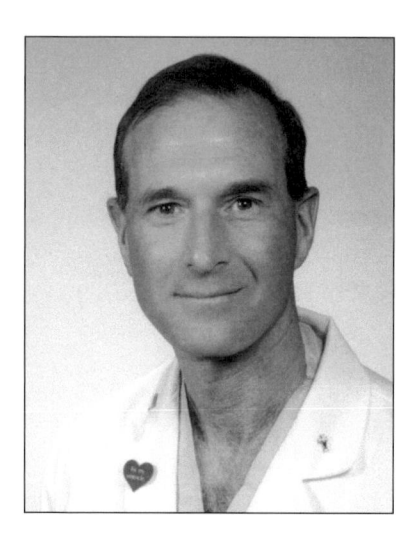

FIGURE 15-10. Frank Ittleman came back from Cleveland in 1980.

UVM Requires a Couple of Transfusions

Advances in anesthesiology, perfusion, and critical care led to ever-increasing numbers of cardiac cases. By the early '80s, the volume finally exceeded Coffin and Ittleman's ability to keep up, especially with DeMeules out of the picture. This was compounded by diminished thoracic coverage following Miller's 1981 retirement. It was clear that the Division needed a third full-time clinician; the problem was that the sub-specialty was in demand throughout the country. Fortunately, a newly trained surgeon with Vermont ties was readily available.

Recent MCHV surgical graduate Richard Jackson had just completed his cardiothoracic training at Tufts' New England Medical Center. He left Boston and returned to practice with Coffin and Ittleman in 1982. Jackson's attention to detail in the operating room was enhanced

FIGURE 15-11. Two rooms large enough to accommodate the extra equipment needed for cardiac surgery were produced after an early 1970s operating room renovation. Here we are looking from room 8 (used for complicated non-cardiac cases) through the equipment storage area into room 7 (used mainly for cardiac cases).

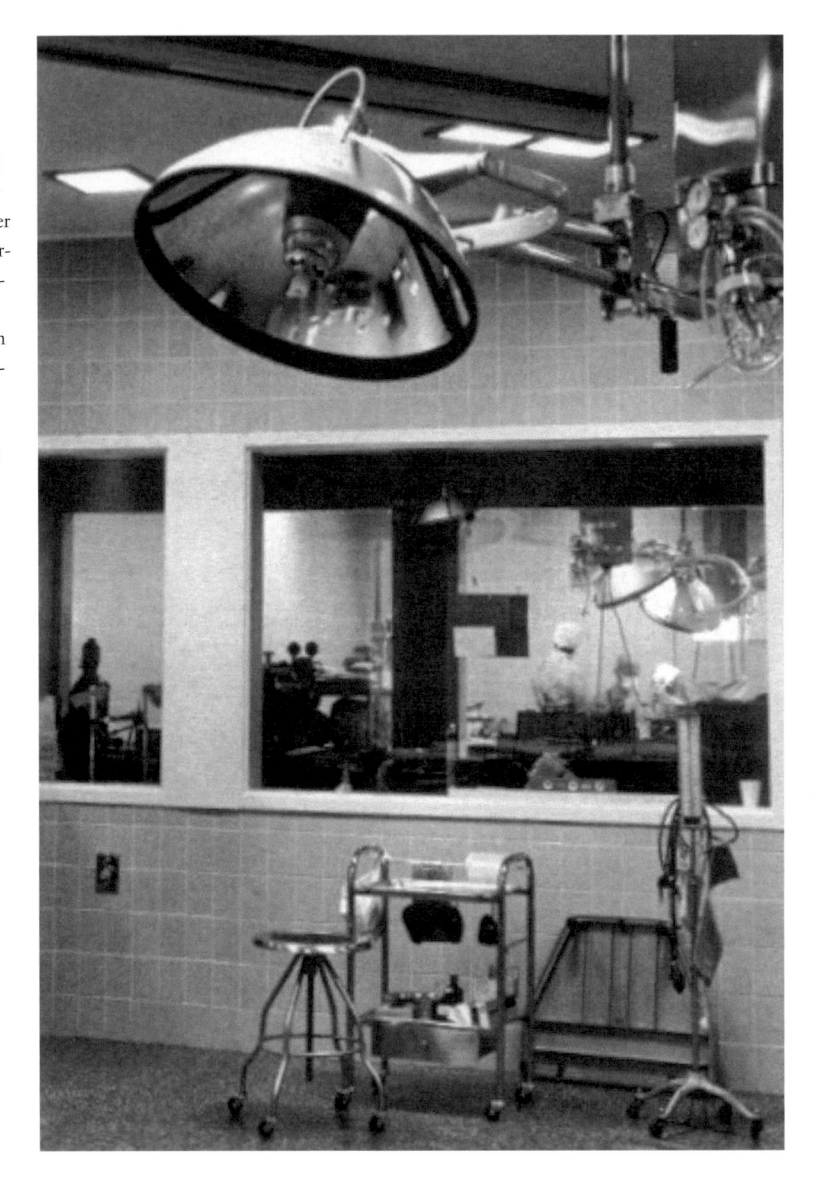

by his compulsive post-operative care. He was almost always on hand whenever one of his patients took a turn for the worse. His vigilance paid off though; Jackson's aortic dissection patients enjoyed a considerably above-average survival rate of 85%.

In addition to his cardiac surgery responsibilities, Jackson shouldered a major part of the thoracic and critical care teaching load. He dutifully took on the additional role of Surgical Core Course Director, shepherding the third-year medical students as they rotated through the surgical services. He single-handedly upgraded the clerkship, mentored the students, and initiated the clinical preceptor program.

Changes at the end of the decade opened the door for yet another surgeon. Coffin decided to stop doing cardiac surgery and focus on thoracic procedures and pacemakers. DeMeules, in the meantime, was losing his battle with lymphoma. UVM's subsequent hire, Bruce Leavitt, was thus expected to perform pump cases and find time to conduct research. DeMeules agreed to provide laboratory mentorship, but died within two months of Leavitt's arrival in June of 1988.

Leavitt, the grandson of Lithuanian immigrants, had been raised in Waterville, Maine. His father wanted him to go into dentistry, but Leavitt saw the light as he performed adrenalec-

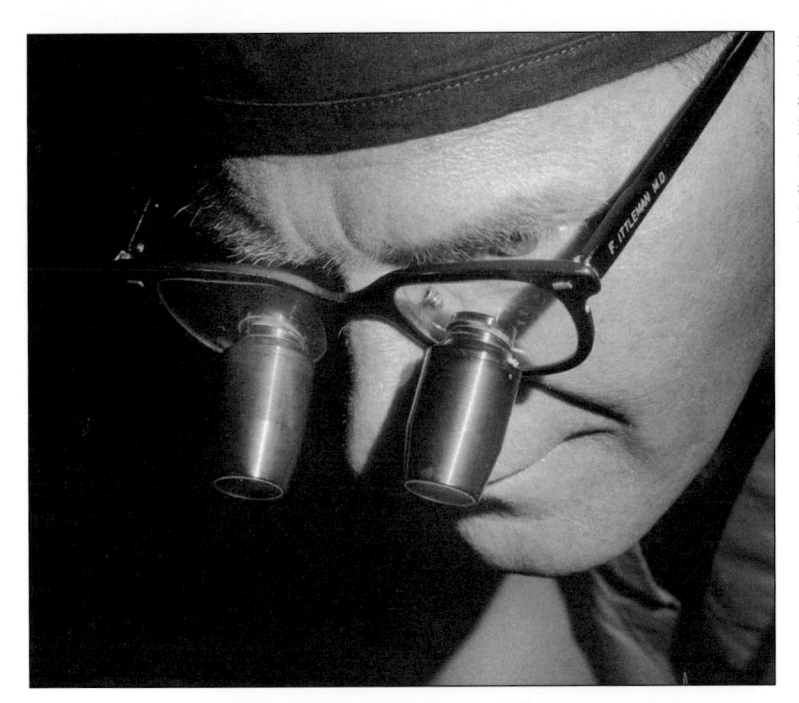

FIGURE 15-12. Ittleman, with his steady head and hands, is a study in total concentration as he looks through his loupes.

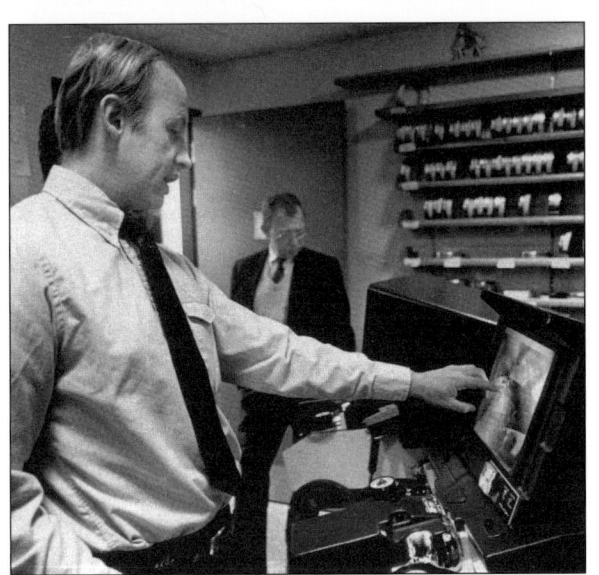

FIGURE 15-13. Jackson and Coffin review a coronary angiogram in the cardiac catheterization laboratory during 1988.

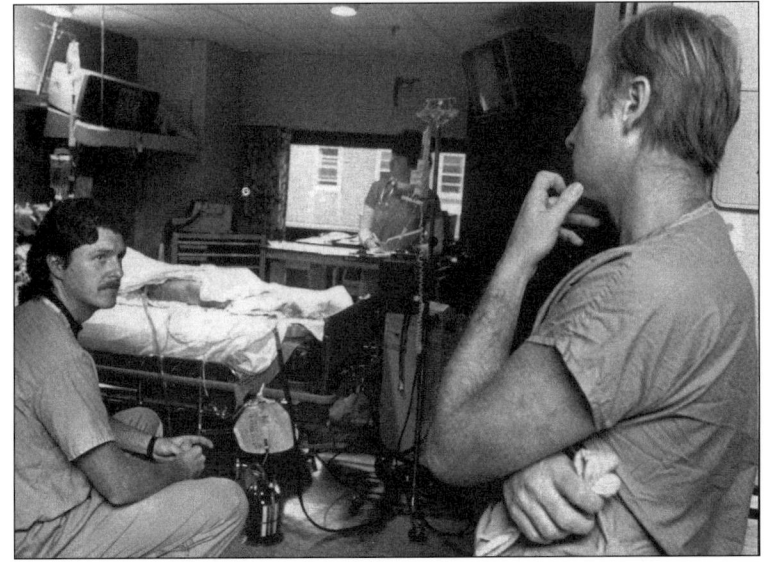

FIGURE 15-14. Richard Jackson supervising post-op care with G-2 resident Greg Dostal in 1988.

Chapter Fifteen: Cardiothoracic Surgery Division   245

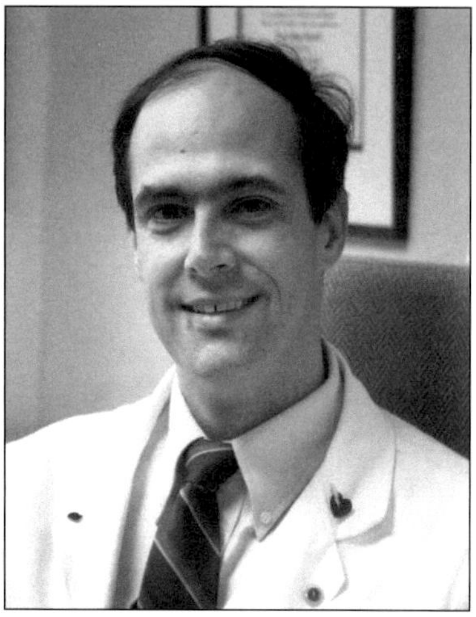

FIGURE 15-15.
Bruce Leavitt arrived in 1988 to help with the expanding caseload and to initiate bench top research.

tomies on mice during a University of Maine research project. He set his sights on medical school, coming to UVM as a "contract" student. The State of Maine paid Vermont $6,000 a year with the expectation that Leavitt would return to Maine and enter general practice.[20] A good deal, but not good enough to abandon a surgical career.

Leavitt finished his residency at the Maine Medical Center (MMC), and then traveled to Syracuse for his cardiothoracic fellowship. He had planned to work with MMC surgeons Clem Hiebert and Jeremy Morton upon graduating, but the Maine faculty had just voted to limit the number of new practitioners in various fields, thus eliminating his potential job. Although these practice restrictions were later deemed illegal, Leavitt was left hanging. Around the same time, one of his wife's friends was getting married in Burlington. Luckily, Frank Ittleman was also at the wedding. The two got to talking, and before long, the UVM group had its newest recruit.

Leavitt was expected to be productive in the research lab, but was not given much support. Left to his own devices, he did some work on an isolated rat heart preparation with resident help. This was difficult, as he was frequently called away from the lab. Leavitt later worked with cardiologist Martin LeWinter and his lab technicians studying the mechanics of heart failure.[21] Despite these efforts, Leavitt's bench-top cardiac surgery research initially struggled at UVM.

Leavitt Leads a New England Registry and Learns a French Valve Repair

The cardiac surgery programs of Vermont, New Hampshire, and Maine entered into a voluntary data-collecting consortium in 1987. The resulting Northern New England Cardiovascular Disease Study Group evaluated the quality, safety, effectiveness, and cost of medical intervention among patients undergoing CABG, valve replacement, and angioplasty. Coffin participated from the outset, with Leavitt soon taking the lead. Leavitt spearheaded studies examining the use of internal mammary arteries and the influence of diabetes and

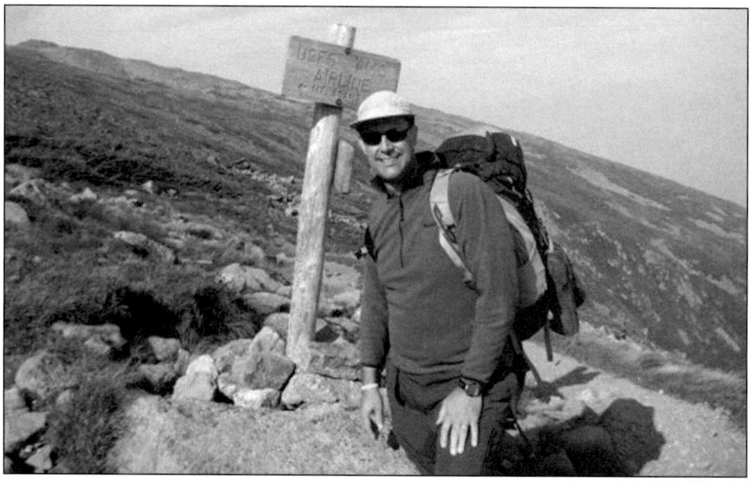

FIGURE 15-16.
Leavitt enjoys climbing, although not as high as Ophthalmology's Geoff Tabin.

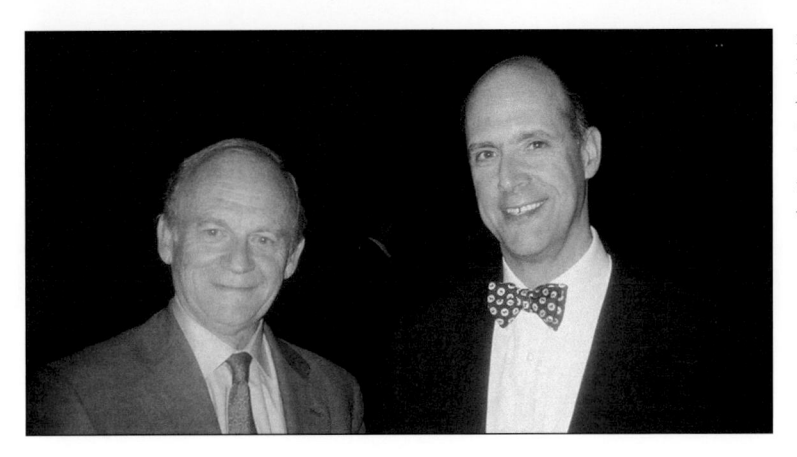

FIGURE 15-17. Leavitt visited with Alain Carpentier (left) to learn the "French Correction" technique of mitral valve repair.

COPD on long-term survival after CABG.[22, 23, 24] The group has used such data to steadily improve cardiac surgery outcomes throughout New England. The carefully studied prospective registry has become a model for the rest of the country.

Leavitt also improved patient care through a novel technique in which leaking but otherwise healthy mitral valves were repaired with prosthetic rings, rather than replaced with mechanical devices. Such repaired valves functioned better and did not require the lifelong anticoagulation associated with clot-prone mechanical valves. He spent a week in Paris during 1990 learning "The French Correction" from its inventor, Alain Carpentier. Leavitt has done over 200 repairs at UVM since then. A 15-year follow up revealed that 87% of these valves were still functioning.

Physicians' Assistants

The Division had grown into a large, busy service by 1990. Although most major cardiac cases called for an assistant, the old model of one surgeon helping another surgeon was not cost effective. The absence of a fellowship-training program gave the service's three rotating residents plenty of operative experience, but those opportunities came at the expense of perioperative patient care. Even worse, the procedures usually didn't count toward graduation requirements.

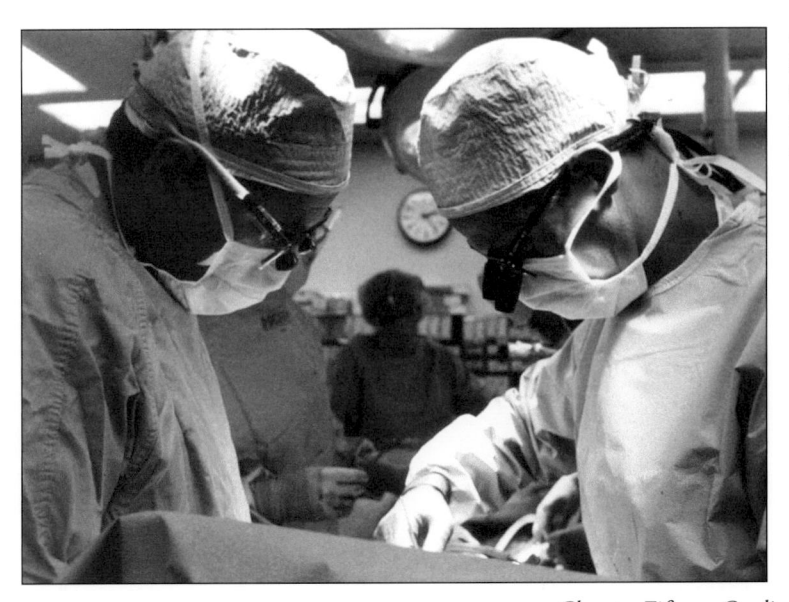

FIGURE 15-18. Steve Colmenero first-assisting Leavitt with a CABG.

Chapter Fifteen: Cardiothoracic Surgery Division

The hiring of a Physician Assistant (PA) solved the staffing shortfall. Steve Colmenero had held a similar position at New York's Montefiore Medical Center for years. He came to Vermont in 1990 for an improved lifestyle, one without night or weekend call. It was also a lifestyle that came with a 40% pay cut. Colmenero assisted in the Operating Room, helped the residents with rounds, did patient workups, and placed chest tubes.

Dale Bundy and Kevin Casey joined the group as Nurse Clinicians. The Division sent Casey to PA school with the expectation of a reciprocal payback. Bundy and Casey eventually moved on and Steve Marcus, a colleague of Colmenero's at Montefiore, took their place. He helped bring endoscopic saphenous vein harvest to town after attending an industry-sponsored training. The technique has since become the surgical gold standard, and is unique in that it is one of the few procedures at UVM done solely by a PA.

1997 Brings a New Face to Cardiac Surgery

The open-heart program was doing about 800 cases a year at the time of Coffin's June 1993 retirement. Ittleman, Jackson, and Leavitt carried on shorthanded for the next several years. The transition between MCHV and FAHC was underway, and the hospital's advisory group had issued a hiring freeze. It was more than a hiring problem, though. The financial difficulties were perceived to be so bad that the administration pinched pennies by squeezing vendors for surgical supply discounts and controlling the size of cafeteria sandwiches. It didn't change the fact that a fourth cardiac surgeon was needed.

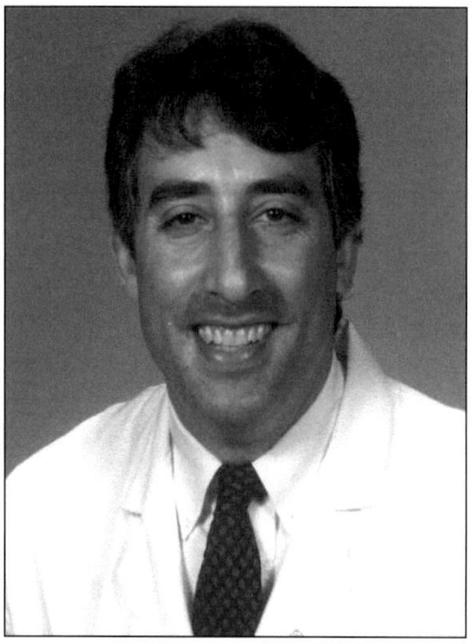

FIGURE 15-19. Mitch Norotsky had to wait for a hiring freeze to end before returning in 1997.

Mitchell Norotsky couldn't wait to get out of Boston after graduating from Harvard. Although initially wait-listed at UVM's College of Medicine, he was accepted at the last minute. Massachusetts (like Maine) still contracted with UVM for medical education, which enabled Norotsky, to pay a more favorable in-state tuition. During both medical school and his ensuing MCHV residency, he was torn between careers in either vascular or cardiothoracic surgery. UVM's professors felt that the prospects for vascular innovation were limited at that time, according to Norotsky, so he pursued a cardiothoracic fellowship at Yale. He was anxious to return to Vermont at the end of his training, but Ittleman suggested that he get a temporary job elsewhere since the hiring freeze was still on. Norotsky worked for a year on Staten Island before finally returning in 1997. The fact that he had been the star on Ittleman's basketball team was an added bonus to the UVM team.

Jackson left for other opportunities within months of Norotsky's arrival. The resulting vacuum once again spotlighted the need for a fourth surgeon. Fortunately, another former MCHV resident was ready to step in.

Schmoker Adds Research and New Talents to the Cardiac Program

Joseph Schmoker had grown up on a large rural Iowa farm. He made the transition to university life at Iowa's Central College without difficulty, but the inner city environment of St. Louis University's medical school came as a bit of a culture shock. Another shock was in store when Shackford replaced Davis during the middle of Schmoker's residency at UVM. A mandatory research year was announced, which was to be filled by one of the current residents. Schmoker volunteered and ended up working with Shackford on secondary brain injury for the next three years.[25]

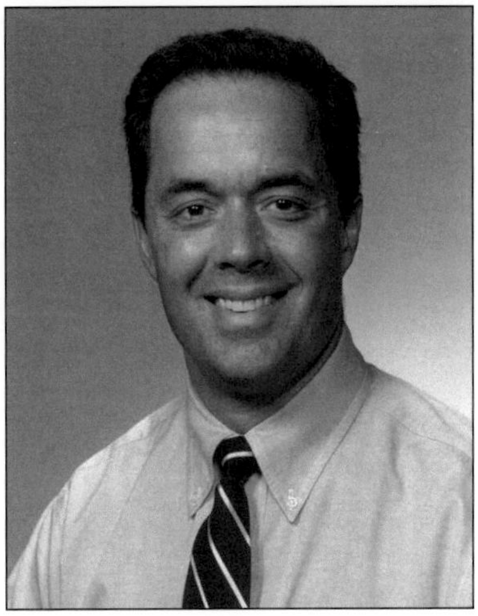

FIGURE 15-20. Joseph Schmoker spent three years in the lab during his UVM surgical residency; he returned from Stanford with new techniques and research ideas.

Schmoker chose to do his cardiothoracic fellowship at Stanford, spending an extra year learning thoracic aortic and cardiac transplant surgery. He came back to Vermont in 1998 with the aim of conducting his own bench-top research. It was a challenging time to proceed with such an agenda, especially since Fletcher Allen funding was still a problem. As a result, money to cover the $300,000 startup cost was postponed for nearly two years. In addition, the Given Building was short on lab space, so Schmoker was relegated to a cramped, remote facility in Colchester. His persistence has since paid off, and he is now able to spend one day a week studying thoracic aortic injuries.[26]

Thoracoabdominal aortic aneurysm surgery had been suspended at UVM prior to Schmoker's return due to suboptimal results. Schmoker made use of his extensive experience in this area and, in conjunction with vascular surgeon Andrew Stanley, resumed the procedure. The pair's superb teamwork has rejuvenated the program and led to superior repair results. Questions regarding transplantation and ventricular assist devices have also been largely channeled to Schmoker because of his background.

New Frontiers

UVM has kept up with latest advances in cardiac surgery. Today's bypass pump oxygenators are a world apart from those of 1959. Pumps that had been primed with six units of blood are now primed with Ringer's Lactate alone. The majority of FAHC's cardiac patients do not receive a perioperative blood transfusion, as it has been demonstrated that such an intervention is associated with more complications.

Saphenous veins were customarily harvested through lengthy vertical leg incisions. Since patients undergoing coronary bypass surgery often had some degree of lower extremity arteriosclerosis, their leg wounds at times healed poorly. It was always depressing to see these wounds lingering long after the heart had been repaired. Most veins are now retrieved with an endoscope through a series of much smaller incisions. This approach has decreased leg wound complications by 75%.

Minimally invasive techniques have been applied elsewhere. Open chest surgery incisions between the ribs are notably painful. Video-assisted thoracic surgery (VATS) is an exciting new field in which operations are done through half-inch ports with the aid of a thoracoscope. Both Leavitt and Norotsky have performed VATS lung biopsies and resections. The discomfort of a traditional thoracotomy has also been alleviated through the delivery of local anesthesia through epidural catheters.

FIGURE 15-21. This successful open-heart valve replacement patient received 13 units of blood intra-op in 1961.

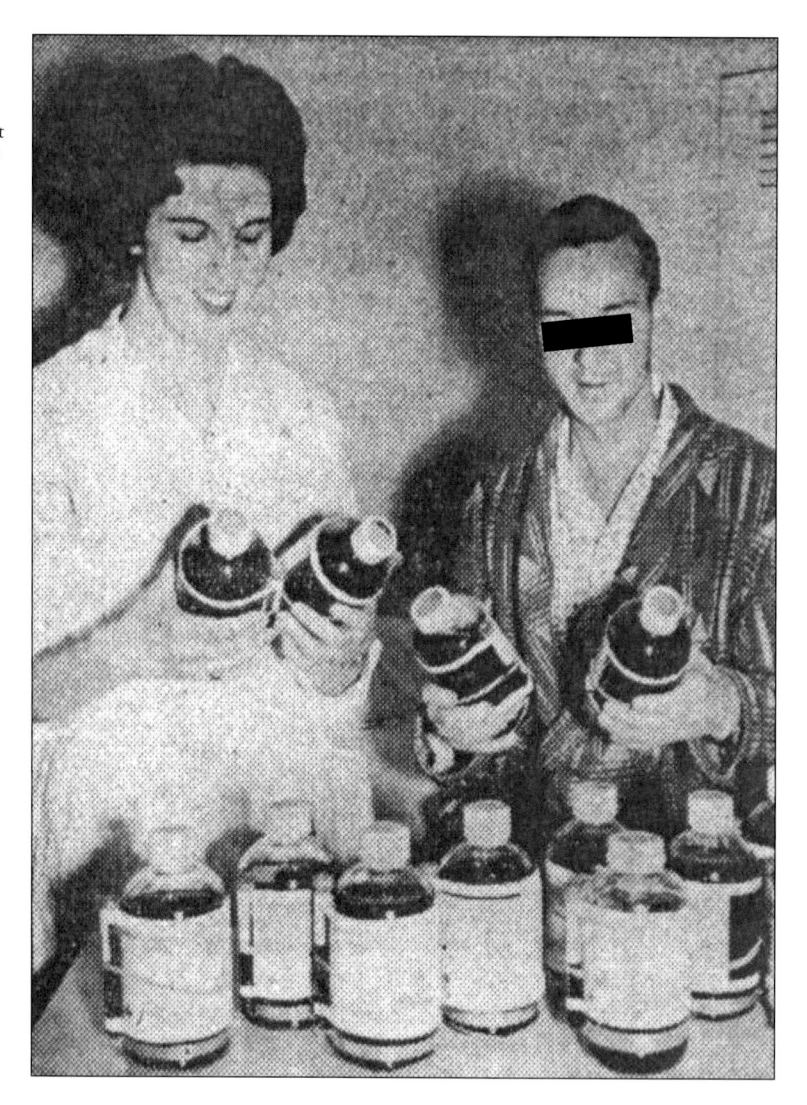

In addition, selected patients suffering from atrial fibrillation can now be treated surgically. The "maze" procedure uses a cryoprobe to obliterate the heart's errant conduction pathways, thereby restoring normal sinus rhythm. This allows the heart to pump more effectively, reduces the need for anti-arrhythmic medications, and eliminates the possibility of embolus formation. Chronic anticoagulation is avoided in the process, along with its inherent risk of hemorrhage.

One of Miller's former patients was a firsthand witness to this transformation. F.L. had undergone an atrial septal defect repair on cardiopulmonary bypass in 1961. The procedure required thirteen units of blood, all of which had been drawn from donors the day before and cross-matched with the patient. He was on a ventilator overnight, stayed in the ICU four days, and remained hospitalized for two weeks. Norotsky performed a significantly more complicated mitral valve replacement on F.L. in 2005. The Carpentier-Edwards valve consisted of bovine pericardium leaflets suspended on Titanium struts — a truly futuristic device by 1961 standards. There were no blood transfusions. The patient was extubated on the evening of surgery, went to the ward the next morning, and left the hospital in four days. As F. L. later remarked, things sure had changed.

CHAPTER 16

Dentistry, Oral and Maxillofacial Surgery Division

UVM's oral and maxillofacial surgeons have run a General Dentistry program for more than 40 years. Collaboration with the Department of Surgery has led to state-of-the-art treatment for facial fractures, temporomandibular joint disorders, and other craniofacial abnormalities such as cleft lips and palates.

Dentists Are Supplanted by Oral and Maxillofacial Surgeons

Unlike other New England academic medical centers, UVM did not have its own dental college. It did, however, have an undergraduate School of Dental Hygiene. Established in 1949, it was directed for decades by Wadi I. Sawabini. The dentist of Lebanese origin oversaw the care of indigent patients at the School's Dental Clinic, which eventually moved to the DeGoesbriand Hospital. The Clinic provided students with a steady stream of grateful patients, most of whom were otherwise unable to obtain such excellent care.

Oral and maxillofacial surgery was regularly performed at all three Burlington hospitals during this time. Sawabini was the nominal chief at the DeGoesbriand, while Harvard-trained N. Noel Cenci held a similar position at the Mary Fletcher. Alexander Lavalle supervised affairs at the Fanny Allen.

Major change came with the arrival of John E. (Jack) Farnham in 1962. Farnham had been born at the DeGoesbriand, and had done his undergraduate work at Vermont's Norwich University. He served in Korea after dental school, and then worked for two years as a dentist before completing additional studies in oral surgery at Tufts and Boston City Hospital. Farnham thus held the distinction of being Vermont's first board-certified oral and maxillofacial surgeon at the time of his return to Burlington.

UVM's General Dental Residency

Farnham's sub-specialty was still relatively new, as the American Board of Oral and Maxillofacial Surgery had only been formed in 1946. Certification required a dental degree plus four-to-six years of additional specialized instruction. Many board diplomates also had MD degrees, although this was not a requirement.

FIGURE 16-1. Jack Farnham brought UVM oral surgery to new levels, which have been maintained by his successors.

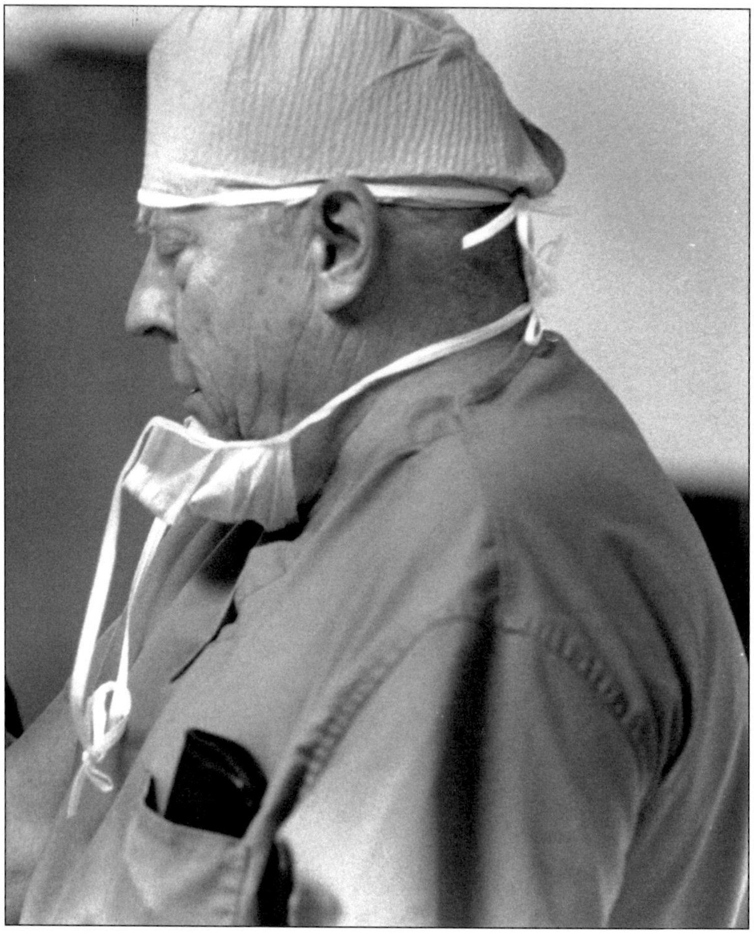

UVM had started its own American Dental Association-approved General Dental residency around the time of Farnham's certification. There have been three to seven dental residents every year since then. The one-year program teaches its graduates about comprehensive case management and routine dental emergencies. It has grown over the years to include hospital-based exposure to oral surgery, maxillofacial trauma, and anesthesia.

Farnham became chief at all three UVM hospitals in 1964. He quickly instituted a number of steps to improve the residency program. Farnham also performed most of the facial trauma surgeries in league with plastic surgeon Bernard Barney. This case sharing was more a division of responsibility than a collaborative adventure. Oral surgery received unassigned Emergency Room patients and consults every third day. Plastics and ENT covered the other two days, respectively.

This system continues, though maxillofacial surgeons now care for all mandibular fractures. External fixation was the treatment of choice for these fractures in the 1960s. The next decade introduced internal fixation with transosseous wires. Plates and screws replaced wires as of the early '80s. These have since evolved into more technologically advanced micro-plates.

Farnham was eventually elected Medical Center Hospital of Vermont Medical Staff president, the first non-MD to hold the position. His invitations to Father Paul St. James-sponsored Caribbean cruises joined by faculty members such as cardiothoracic surgeon Laurence Coffin, anesthesiologist Bob Deane, and cardiologist Chris Terrien, Jr. were additional evidence of his acceptance by the staff.

The Faculty Grows During the 1970s

More change came about in 1971 with the additions of oral surgeon Charles R. Bowen and orthodontist Richard R. Reed. The pair brought orthognatic surgery to UVM for the first time. This technique, in which bones are cut, realigned, and then held in place with either screws or plates, was used to correct a variety of conditions. Among these were mid-face skeletal deformities, temporomandibular joint (TMJ) disorders, cleft palates, and severe orthodontic problems not amenable to braces.

Paul A. Danielson joined the group in 1978 after studying at Tufts, UVM, and Connecticut's Hartford Hospital. He implemented leading-edge TMJ treatments, such as total joint replacement. This procedure uses CT-guided acrylic skull modeling and sophisticated computer-assisted design to create perfect titanium and polyethylene prosthetic implants. Danielson also pioneered the performance of office-based orthognatics under general anesthesia, being only the second oral surgeon in the country to achieve such certification.

Thomas W. Connolly came on board in 1981 following his training at the Massachusetts General Hospital. He brought expertise in distraction osteogenesis, the process through which bones are lengthened by means of controlled, intentional fractures. UVM became the

FIGURE 16-2.
A perfect bite has been highly sought after throughout the ages, as this Mayan sculpture demonstrates.

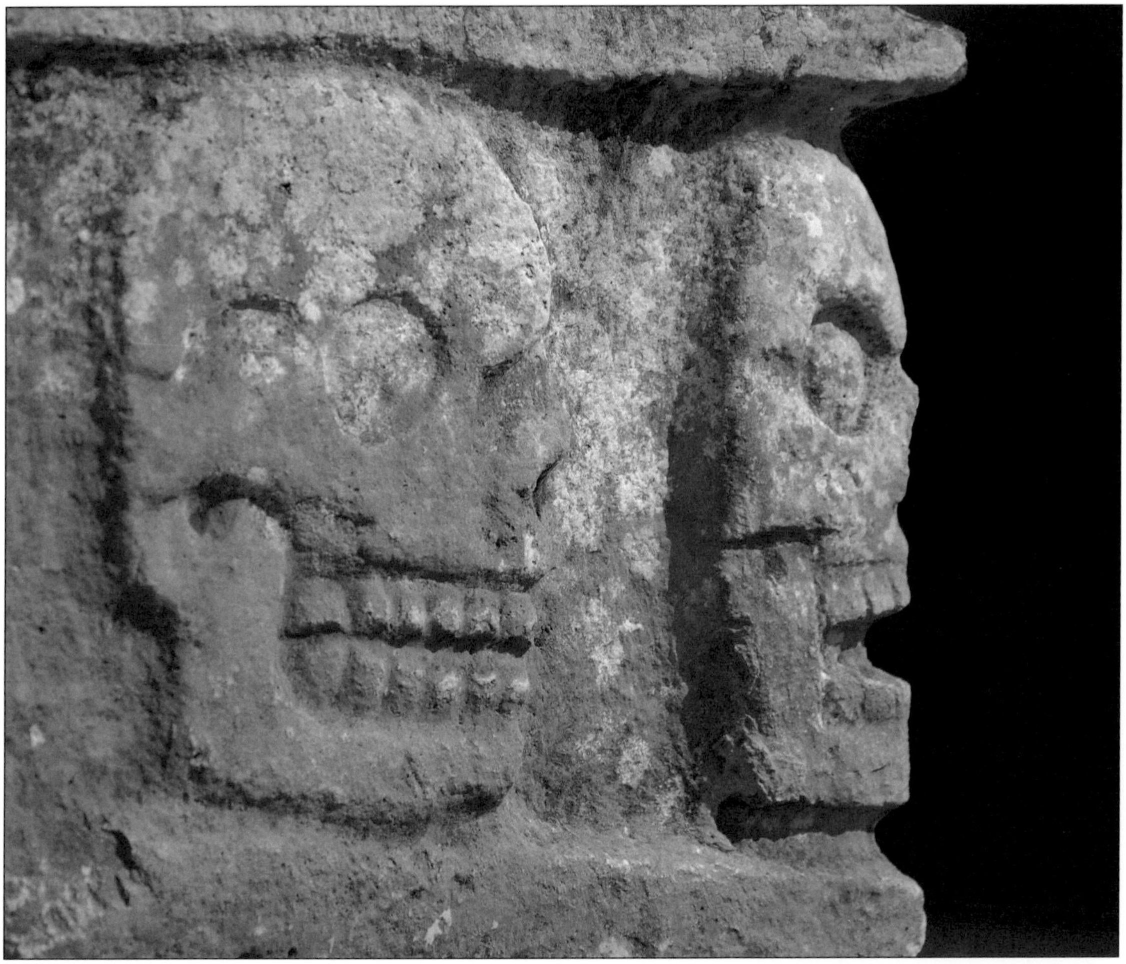

only rural New England medical center to offer this technique. Connolly has since specialized in craniofacial abnormalities, and has helped plastic surgeon Donald Laub repair dozens of complicated cleft lip and palate defects.

Relocation and Adaptation

The Methadone Clinic and other drug dependency programs displaced the oral surgeons from their long-standing DeGoesbriand space in the late 1990s. Bowen, Danielson, and Connolly relocated to South Burlington, where they established Champlain Valley Oral and Maxillofacial Surgery, PC. The Dental Clinic, still managed by Farnham, relocated to Burlington's Community Health Center. The UVM undergraduate school of Dental Hygiene was discontinued in 2002, although similar training continues under the auspices of nearby Vermont Technical College.

The current residency program continues under Danielson's able leadership. He is an advocate for program and procedure certification, and is the past president of the American Board of Maxillofacial Surgery (1999-2000). He has also followed in Farnham's footsteps as the 2008 president of the Fletcher Allen Health Care Medical Staff.

FIGURE 16-3. Paul Danielson leads the Division of Oral & Maxillofacial Surgery and has been president of the Medical Staff.

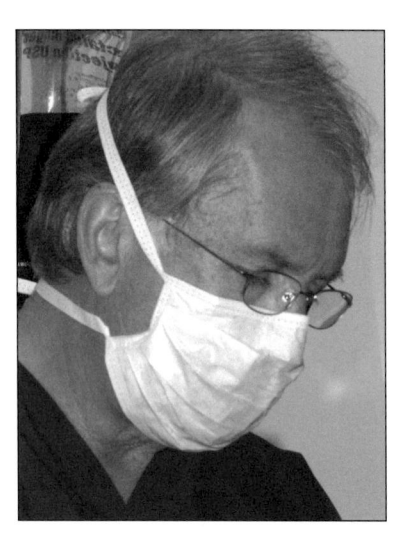

Paul A. Danielson validated UVM's philosophy of training dentists in additional surgery and anesthesia by the following personal experience in 1980. He was filling his tank, minding his own business, when a car crashed in front of the Taft's Corners gas station. The unrestrained driver suffered severe facial fractures and was unable to breathe. Danielson grabbed the razor used to scrape inspection stickers from windshields, ran to the scene, and successfully performed an emergency cricothyroidotomy.

UVM's oral and maxillofacial surgeons carry out complicated procedures on a regular basis. The cooperative effort among UVM's maxillofacial, plastics, ENT, and trauma teams is a unique success.[1]

CHAPTER 17

Emergency Medicine Division

UVM's emergency room capabilities slowly evolved over fifty years. Commitment to emergency care training, however, was present almost from the start.

Ambulance reform, EMT training courses, and drunk driving prevention programs were championed throughout the 1970s. UVM's ambulance review conferences were a national model for quality assurance.

The Division of Emergency Services is currently a leader in the use of focused abdominal sonogram for trauma assessment. It is also on the cutting edge of electronic record keeping and digital radiographic imaging.

Early Emergency Room Care

Prior to World War II, emergencies were treated in patients' homes, at the scenes of accidents, or in doctors' offices. Cases that reached the hospital were directly admitted with or without a side-trip to the Operating Room. While the Mary Fletcher Hospital did maintain specific "emergency" rooms in the old Surgical Wing and original Women's Pavilion (today's Shepardson South), they were primarily devoted to "accident work" and "minor surgery."[1]

Formal Emergency Rooms were created at both the Mary Fletcher and Bishop DeGoesbriand Hospitals during the expansions of the early 1950s. The MFH complex was on the first floor of the Smith building, one flight down from the operating suites, whereas

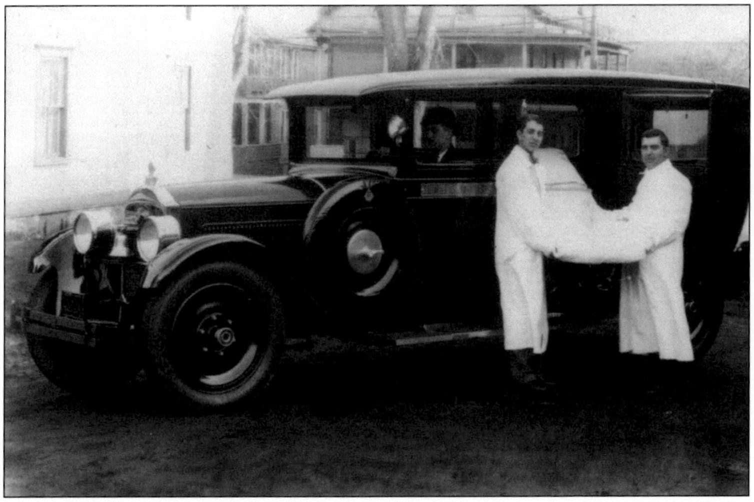

FIGURE 17-1.
A 1927 Winooski, VT based Packard ambulance/hearse.

the DeGoesbriand's equally competitive unit was in the St. Joseph's Pavilion. Patients were still on their own with respect to transportation.

Once a patient had arrived at one of these emergency rooms, a nurse quickly assessed the severity of their injury. They then called the intern on duty, based on what they deemed appropriate for the situation. The attending on call from the corresponding specialty was sometimes called directly. Surgeons and specialists were summoned for even the most minor complaints. Patients without insurance usually received their primary care at the hands of an intern. The Fanny Allen Hospital had no interns, so nurses (and sometimes even medical students) provided initial triage and care.

Full-service emergency departments were in place at the MFH and DeGoesbriand by the 1960s. Two attending surgeons were assigned to each hospital, usually for a week at a time. The "senior" surgeon chose the hours or days for which he was responsible, along with the hours or days that his "junior" associate was on duty. For example, the senior attending might see non-trauma emergencies, such as acute cholecystitis (an admission that almost surely resulted in a later well compensated abdominal surgery). The junior attending was then left on call every day and night for trauma!

Resident coverage was light, with a senior resident at the Mary Fletcher and an intern at the DeGoesbriand. An intern assigned to the emergency room was physically present for 24 hours, then off for 24 hours. The chief resident covered both hospitals from home, independently picking and choosing cases of interest.

The Medical Society's Bright Idea

As E.R. volume increased, emergency-related house calls declined. The Chittenden County Medical Society responded to public complaints with a 1963 policy under which ALL members were to provide house call services. The Society had 150 members, so it was expected that each physician would take two or three days of call a year. But the policy encompassed pathologists, psychiatrists, and other physicians that had not treated medical problems for years. And although everyone had voted for the proposal, many didn't relish the idea of dealing with these types of emergencies.

The solution was to "hire" other doctors to take their places. Pretty soon, residents were taking emergency house calls for Society members. Surgical residents, in particular, seized upon the opportunity to make the going rate of $10 a day. And the money didn't stop there, since residents were also allowed to bill patients directly for the visits. Residents took emergency house call on their regular call days, obtaining temporary coverage from their colleagues whenever they had to leave the hospital.

Eventually, more than 50% of the emergency house call days were farmed out to surgical residents. Some of these calls were dispatched from the Burlington jail, as Sheriff McLaughlin found it easier to have a physician come to the jail than to transport a guarded, handcuffed prisoner to the emergency room. Such abuses, along with overall Society apathy, led to the discontinuation of the service.

Multiple Emergency Rooms Eventually Merge

A total of 15,736 cases were serviced at the MFH and the DeGoesbriand in the year leading up to their 1967 merger. Surgical residents covered both hospitals, though the medical resident staffing was entirely separate as a result of UVM politics. John Davis consolidated the emergency rooms when he took over the Department of Surgery in 1969, closing the DeGoesbriand and unifying the resident services in the process.[2] The Fanny Allen E.R. responded by increasing its staffing. It stayed open until 1981, at which point it became a walk-in care center.

The "new" MCHV Emergency Room of 1969 remained in its old Smith 1 location. It featured an enclosed ambulance bay and an x-ray machine. The former was a tremendous advantage during the winter, while the latter was useless for anything more than the simplest of films. More complicated studies always had to be sent to the X-Ray Department, one floor above. The E.R. also contained the ambulance radio control system. This was staffed in conjunction with the Poison Control Center and the Health Care Information Center. The combination, I always thought, was put in place to justify the expense of the ambulance radio system to the hospital's administrators. Joseph Mailloux, a dedicated and committed manager, oversaw the area.

Davis told me at the time: "Since you have been in Vietnam, Dave, you can do vascular surgery as you requested, but you will also be the director of the Trauma Service and the surgical side of the emergency room." Richard Ryder was the medical co-director for a couple of years, but surgery took over when he left. I reviewed cases, set policies, organized teaching conferences, and coordinated the call schedule.

Beside the Lake in the Winter of 1970

Patients usually came to the Emergency Room under their own power, or with the help of family and friends. Townspeople who absolutely needed an ambulance called the Burlington Fire Department. Local undertakers, whose hearses doubled as ambulances, provided transportation from beyond the city's limits. One such establishment was run out of the back room of a Winooski hardware store!

I still remember the black Cadillac hearse as it backed into the MFH ambulance bay. It was my first year as an attending surgeon at UVM, and I was on call for trauma. The "ambulance" held a hysterical young mother whose car had hit an icy corner, slid off the road, and come to a rest near the frozen surface of Lake Champlain. The two attendants got out of the front seats, walked around the hearse, and opened its rear door. Nurses in starched white uniforms wheeled the injured patient, strapped to the stretcher with a single lap belt, into the emergency room.

A trauma victim does not come with a label, and when first encountered may be in any condition from uninjured to critical. The patient's airway and breathing need to be rapidly assessed, since inadequate respiration can quickly lead to death. Checking the circulation for signs of shock comes next followed by a neurological assessment. This was where our patient failed, having no sensation or motor control below her waist. It was indicative of a spinal cord injury that had caused permanent paralysis.

FIGURE 17-2.
A 1969 Cadillac ambulance in the Mary Fletcher's enclosed E.R. bay. Head nurse Jay Jones and surgical resident Ed Hixson are receiving the patient.

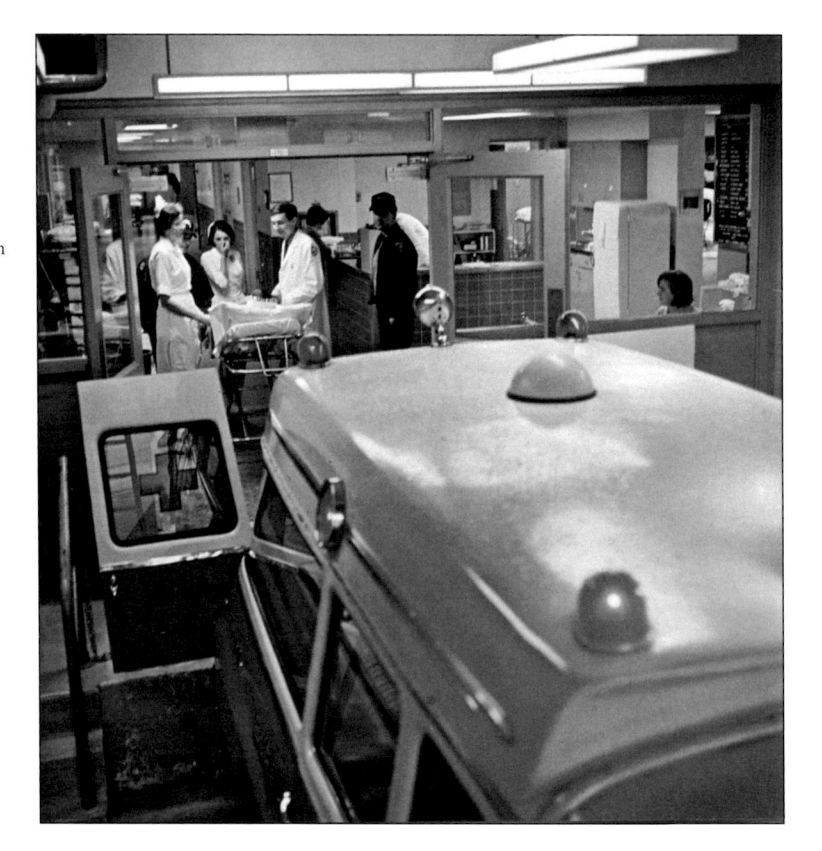

The police, however, reported that the patient was definitely moving her legs when they arrived on the scene. The patient also confirmed that she was able to move her legs when she was put feet-first into the ambulance. She said that the vehicle, with its lights flashing and siren blaring, had come to an abrupt halt at an intersection. This had caused her to jerk forward into a sitting position, doubled-up over the stretcher's lap belt. After she flopped back onto the board, she could no longer feel or move her legs.

I was appalled — and angry. This woman had not been experiencing any airway or breathing difficulty and was not in shock, so there was no need for the attendant to have driven so recklessly. The patient should have been anchored to a backboard with multiple straps, and she should have been placed head-forward. And the other attendant should have been at the patient's side, not seated up front while she was left alone in back!

In fairness, the attendants had not been trained beyond the level of standard Red Cross first aid. The two held this position because they ran a morgue, and thus had a vehicle that could hold a stretcher and serve as an ambulance. Unfortunately for our patient, the revolution in ambulance standards and training sweeping the nation at the time had not yet reached the Green Mountain state.

Davis, with his connections to the American Association for the Surgery of Trauma (AAST) and the American College of Surgeons (ACS) Committee on Trauma, pushed for improved emergency care in Vermont, largely assigning the project to me later that same year.

Surgery Teams with Epidemiologist Julian Waller

Horrified by a similar incident involving one of his family members, orthopedic surgeon Joseph D. "Deke" Farrington applied medical lessons learned in World War II and Korea to civilian practice. Working with the Chicago Fire Department, he taught the country's first pre-hospital care program in 1957. He continued to promote the use of controlled extrication and spine boards after retiring to rural Wisconsin. His landmark 1967 paper "Death in a Ditch" led to the nationwide push for better emergency services.[3] Farrington then helped the ACS Committee on Trauma and the American Academy of Orthopedic Surgeons develop the original Ambulance Care and Emergency Medical Technicians (EMTs) training course.

UVM had its own emergency care pioneer in the person of Julian A. Waller. One of the epidemiologist's more alarming findings was that funeral homes had provided 72% of Vermont's ambulance services in 1967, a number that had only dropped to 45% by 1970.[4] The study dramatically pointed out the need for proper ambulance training and certification. Waller also studied preventable deaths, helped revolutionize highway design, and defined and waged war against drunk driving.[5]

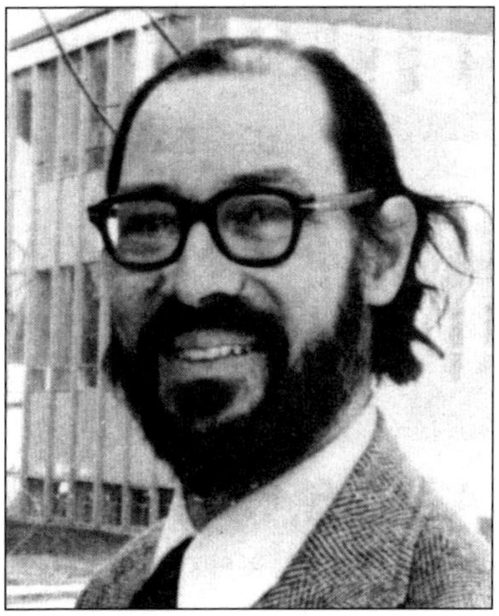

Vermont launched the "Project CRASH" deterrence program in 1970 with Waller's assistance. The outreach was desperately needed, as proven by an encounter that I had one night in the DeGoesbriand E.R. A patient had caught my eye as I was treating the victims of an automobile accident. He was so drunk that he could barely stagger from wall to wall. The police turned the other way as he stumbled towards his car. When I complained that they shouldn't let him drive in that condition, they replied that they weren't going to stop him because he hadn't committed a crime!

FIGURE 17-3. The Department of Epidemiology's Julian Waller worked closely with Surgery. He was ahead of his time when it came to addressing accident prevention, alcohol abuse measures, and pre- and post-hospital emergency care.

Waller and I taught UVM's first EMT course in 1972 to more than 155 students. He gave one of the lectures, while I conducted the rest with the help of the orthopaedic and neurosurgery faculty. We taught from the ACS text during the evenings, staying one chapter ahead of the students in our own learning. Extrication experts from Connecticut showed us how to dismantle an automobile. UVM even agreed to give credit to undergraduate students who took the course, a policy that continues to this day.

As time evolved, the ambulance personnel became proficient enough to teach the classes themselves with minimal physician supervision. In time, I attempted to integrate a similar course into the first year medical students' curriculum, but was shot down by the Dean's office. It was a shame, since College of Medicine graduates were otherwise not taught appropriate pre-hospital emergency care.

Ambulance Movies and M&Ms

The State of Vermont, using 50% matching funds from the U.S. Department of Transportation, hired C. Earl Gettinger, Jr. as Emergency Medical Services Coordinator in 1970. Gettinger helped support and direct the revolution in ambulance care throughout the state and at UVM.[6]

One of the projects on which he and I worked together was an educational film for the ACS. The Davis and Geck® surgical supply company had sponsored the production of similar movies throughout the '60s and '70s. The finished products were available to surgeons free of charge through the ACS film library. We started by filming some actual ambulance scenes. A film crew was then assigned and dispatched to Burlington to shoot some simulated scenarios.

The best of these took place in an Essex Junction field. One vignette demonstrated a long board extrication set against the backdrop of Davis' top-down convertible. We strategically placed broken glass near the car, and created a realistically bloody face for the actor. In another scene, the Essex Fire Department foamed an abandoned wreck under the hood to simulate fire containment techniques. We also demonstrated short-to-long board extrication, with simultaneous two-way radio communication between Essex Rescue, EMTs, and the hospital. Participation by some Vermont State Police officers added a bit of realism.

Our real-life ambulance shots were interspersed with the simulated scenes during the final cut. I edited the whole thing at Davis and Geck's impressive Danbury, Connecticut movie studio. The 16 mm film was screened during the 1973 ACS annual meeting, and then distributed through the ACS film library for many years thereafter. The library, unfortunately, no longer exists.

The film itself, however, survives. It becomes obvious on repeat viewing that precautions against infected fluids were never considered and that an inordinate amount of time was spent on spine immobilization. But the movie's main points: airway management, bleeding control, backboard immobilization, and rapid transport have become key goals in the EMT treatment of severe trauma.

Gettinger also helped me conduct a weekly "Ambulance Critique Review." Physicians and emergency coordinators gathered interesting cases from ambulance report forms and then reviewed them in detail. Outstanding examples of care were highlighted and opportunities for improvement were discussed. This variation of a surgical Morbidity and Mortality (M&M) conference became a national model.[7] We settled on an early morning meeting time, since it gave volunteer EMTs an opportunity to attend before going to their day jobs. Unfortunately, ambulance M&M lost its impetus and effectiveness after I stepped down as Emergency Room Director in 1981.

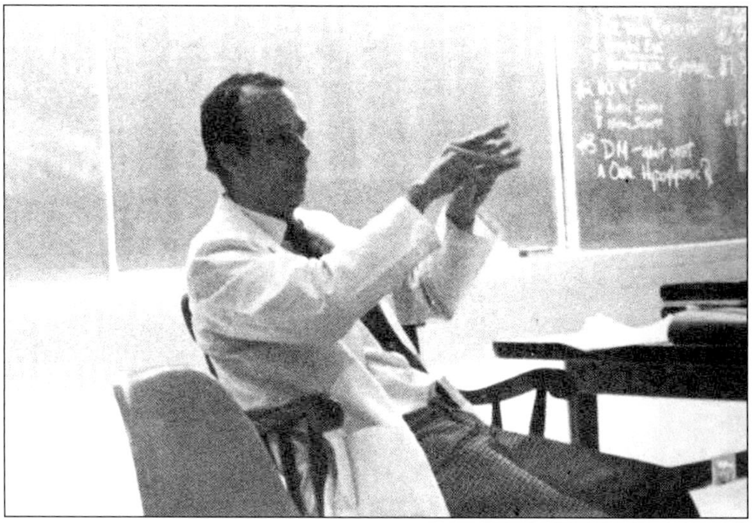

FIGURE 17-4. Ambulance critique sessions were very popular. They were held in the early morning to accommodate volunteer squads. Here I (DBP) am talking with my hands as usual.

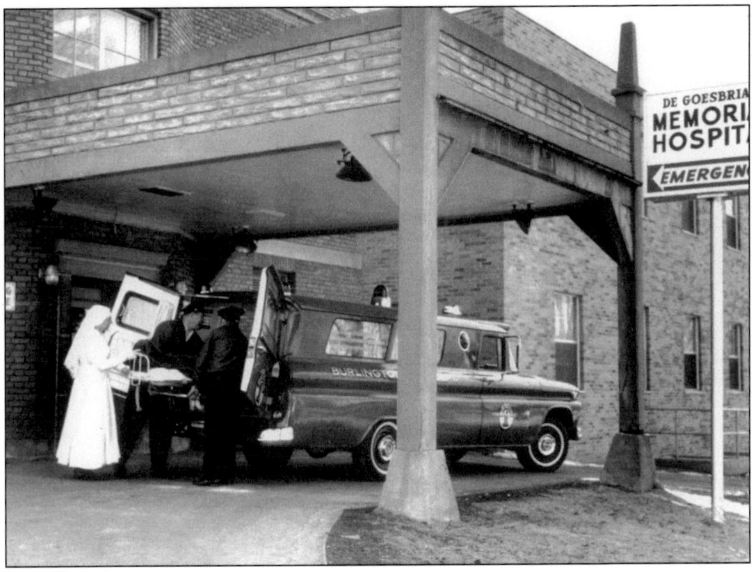

FIGURE 17-5. A portico sheltered the DeGoesbriand's Pearl Street ambulance entrance. Burlington Fire Department Rescue 1 had not yet evolved into its larger, boxier 1970s incarnation.

Burlington Fire Department Ambulance and College Student Ambulance Services

Although the Burlington Fire Department (BFD) ran the city's ambulance service, it regarded its attendants as second-class citizens. New recruits were assigned to the crew almost as an initiation, becoming firefighters only after gaining seniority and experience. They reverted to their ambulance roots during active fires by caring for victims and injured comrades. The BFD ambulance attendants are highly respected today, even though the same is not necessarily true in other urban fire departments.

BFD ambulance chief David Modica and I were sent to Lansing, Michigan in the early '70s as part of an effort to upgrade the ambulance service. Lansing was home to John Wiegenstein, a community-based physician who essentially invented the specialty of Emergency Medicine. With his encouragement, the Lansing Fire Department had embraced Deke Farrington's teachings. Observing their methods in action proved to be of inestimable value to both the BFD and me.

However, when I suggested that MCHV ought to manage the ambulance service, I was met with coolness by the hospital and ice-coldness by the Fire Department. The two institutions were apparently very comfortable with the status quo. It seemed obvious to me that if the hospital ran the ambulance, attendants could obtain ongoing emergency care training whenever they weren't on calls. The idea is revived on a regular basis, only to be squelched time and again by politics and financial considerations.

Administrators at St. Michael's College felt differently, as evidenced by the 1972 establishment of an undergraduate-staffed volunteer ambulance service. UVM followed suit several years later. The region's rescue services, in turn, were markedly improved as EMT-trained college graduates relocated to the surrounding countryside. Vermont's volunteer system and the college programs that supported it were models for their time.

The State was eventually divided into ambulance districts, each with a defined primary catchment area. Local unaffiliated units sprung up in Shelburne, Richmond, Essex Junction,

FIGURE 17-6.
The Mary Fletcher Emergency room was tucked behind Smith 1 in 1966. The operating room was one floor up.

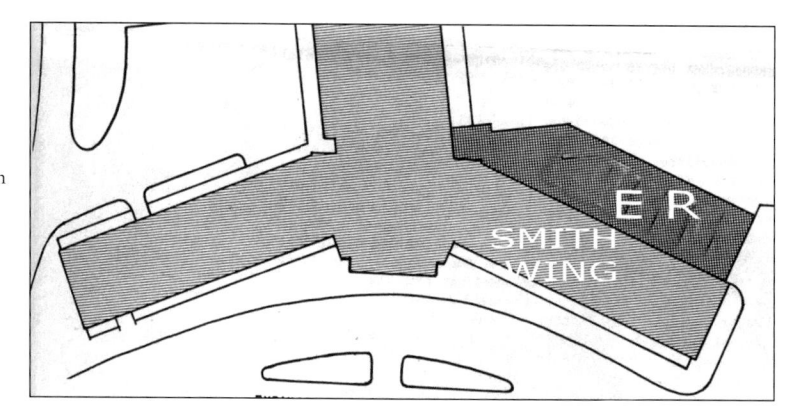

Colchester, and South Hero/Grand Isle. Each outfit was staffed by volunteers, and supported through donations or insurance billings whenever applicable.

Advanced EMT Training at UVM

In the winter of 1974, a Mad River Glen skier ruptured his liver after hitting a lift tower. Although the responding ambulance carried Ringer's lactate and intravenous (IV) tubing, the EMTs were neither trained nor authorized to give IV fluids. They stopped at a physician's office, but the doctor refused to start an IV. He instead urged rapid transport to MCHV. As the ambulance negotiated the Burlington exit ramp, the young skier went into cardiac arrest. When he finally arrived, he could not be resuscitated.

FIGURE 17-7.
Head nurse Jay Jones, the one constant on the ever-changing E.R. personnel scene.

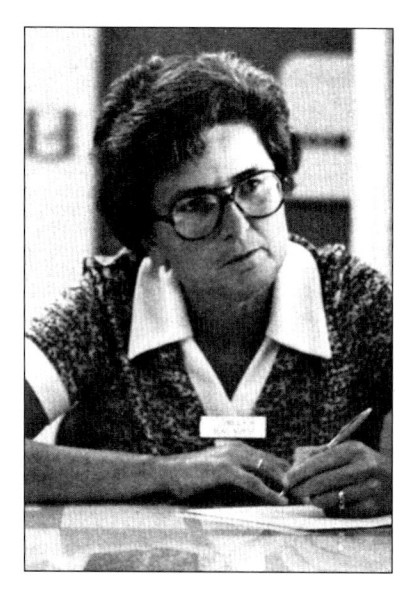

I was outraged once again, and immediately made plans for an EMT-level IV training module. At the conclusion of the first course, I personally watched every student start an IV on either a classmate or me! Twelve EMTs were certified IV capable in June of 1974. My colleagues warned that I was setting myself up for a lawsuit, but their fears were unfounded. There has only been one complaint in 30 years, and that was from an IV nurse who thought that her injured son didn't need an IV!

Vermont EMT Course Has an Animal Cardiac Model

UVM's EMT training was unique in that it included an animal laboratory. I thought that the students should have a clear idea of what ventricular fibrillation was and how cardiac massage worked, since EMTs administered CPR to cardiac arrest patients on a regular basis. We anesthetized a dog, connected it to a blood pressure strain gauge, opened its chest, and chemically stopped its heart. As the students squeezed away, we showed that cardiac massage created adequate blood pressure. The dog's heart was then defibrillated, its chest was closed and it was allowed to recuperate.

The students saw the dog alive and without deficits at the following week's class. We felt that the example gave them an appreciation for the efficacy of cardiac massage during cardiac arrest. Someone, however, complained that this "cruel animal surgery" was totally unnecessary. The Dean of the medical school challenged us to "document that this surgical experiment is beneficial or else stop doing it." He claimed that we were putting the research efforts of the entire University in jeopardy, so we deleted the animal lab from the course.

During the early 1980s, we started to train the next level of EMTs (EMT-I, intermediates) in advanced assessment, IV administration, and esophageal airway procedures. The latter were substitutes for the endotracheal intubation skills that were really needed, but not taught secondary to physician reluctance. UVM was ahead, but only just ahead, of the rest of the country in these initiatives.

Defibrillation, Combitube® airway management, and Narcan™ administration have since been added to the EMTs' treatment repertoire. The Fletcher Allen Coordinated Transport (FACT) teams at UVM and in upstate New York continue to provide state-of-the-art EMT instruction.

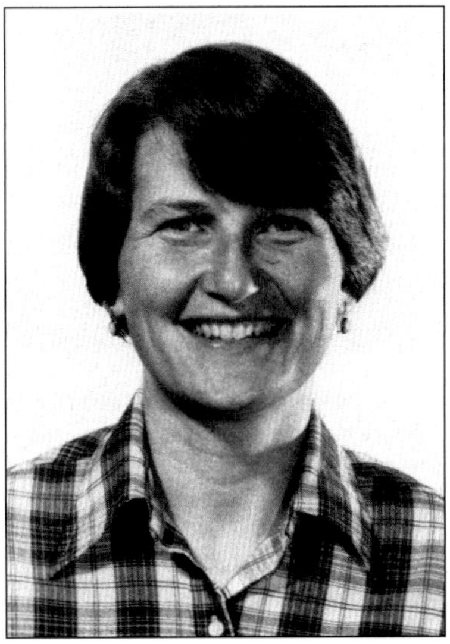

Emergency Room Physicians Arrive at UVM

UVM conducted a search for a new Director after I relinquished my E.R. duties in 1981. Emergency Medicine had just attained national board status, thanks in no small part to Lansing's Wiegenstein. Ruth E. Uphold, a young graduate of the newly organized UCSF Fresno Emergency Medicine Residency, was invited for consideration.

Uphold asked orthopaedic surgeon David Seligson to douse his cigar during her interview in his 8x8 foot office. Upset by the request, he retaliated by announcing that he had to do an emergency case in the operating room. Seligson dragged Uphold along, and had her change into scrubs. When she came into the O.R., she found him removing a Steinmann pin — a three-minute procedure that could have been done in an exam room. Uphold held her own with the rest of UVM's surgery staff, and was hired.

FIGURE 17-8. Ruth Uphold, UVM's first residency trained emergency physician, arrived in 1981.

Uphold was "surprised" to see how the E.R. functioned at the time of her arrival:

> "The two interns would be actively seeing patients on the floor and the upper level residents would be downstairs in the lounge waiting to be consulted on difficult cases. It was not uncommon for patients to wait four or five hours to be seen. The first thing that I instituted was that all the residents, regardless of level, would be actively seeing patients to improve patient flow. The transition occurred rapidly, although there was initial disgruntlement on the part of the G-2s who felt that they had paid their dues as G-1s."[8]

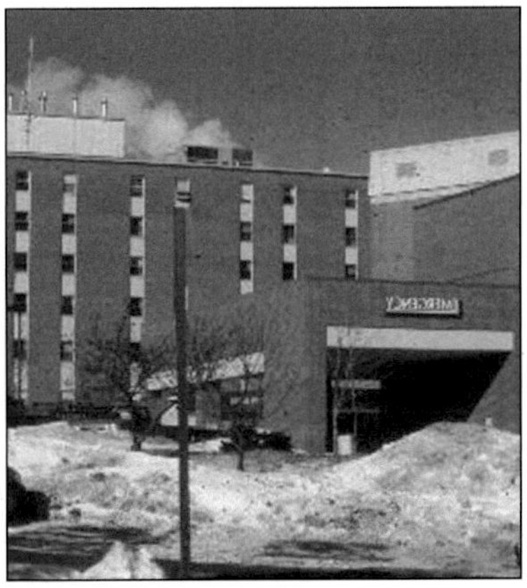

Uphold had come expecting to recruit a full staff of similarly trained E.R. doctors. A few months later, she pro-

FIGURE 17-9. The E.R. with single enclosed ambulance bay and two stretcher sized trauma rooms served from 1966 thru 1985.

FIGURE 17-10. Amazingly, there were only five fatalities following the 1984 Amtrak derailment.

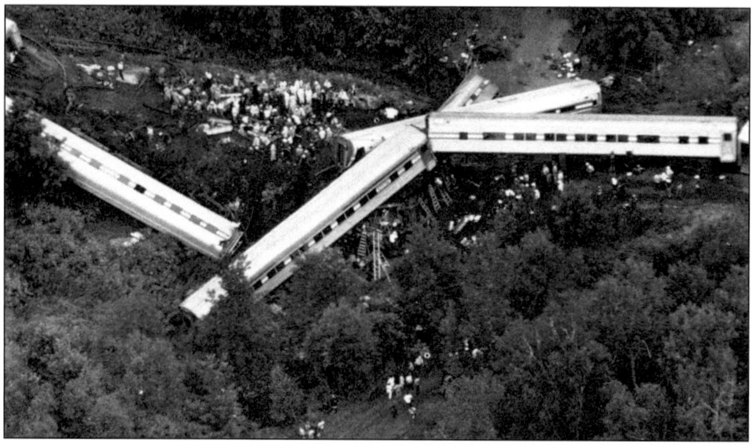

posed that the hospital employ another physician for the 8 A.M. to midnight shift. Seven long years later, she was given permission to hire Wayne J.A. Misselbeck, an Emergency Medicine trainee out of Akron, Ohio. At that point, the entire staff consisted of two E.R. attendings, four interns, and four residents. The evenly divided surgical and medical housestaff took shifts of 24 hours on and 24 hours off.

The emergency physicians were initially paid by the hospital, even though they were part of the Department of Surgery. Emergency room staff didn't even bill patients directly for their services until 1990. The Emergency Division has remained under Surgery's control, as UVM doesn't want too many diverse departments in its organizational structure.

The Vermont Amtrak Disaster: Spring 1984

All hospitals conduct disaster drills. We had done a few at MCHV, although probably not enough. Part of our drill dictated that a team of experienced physicians went to the disaster scene. Upon arrival, they were to perform triage and render lifesaving care including using IV solutions and intubation equipment. These provisions were apparently forgotten when a real-life call came on Saturday July 7, 1984.

Amtrak's "Montrealer" had derailed after hitting a section of washed-out track near Essex Junction. The accident either destroyed or heavily damaged two locomotives and the seven forward-most cars. For whatever reason, two G-2 residents coming off a 24-hour E.R. stint

FIGURE 17-11. This crushed, upside down railcar produced some challenging extrications and tested MCHV's disaster plan.

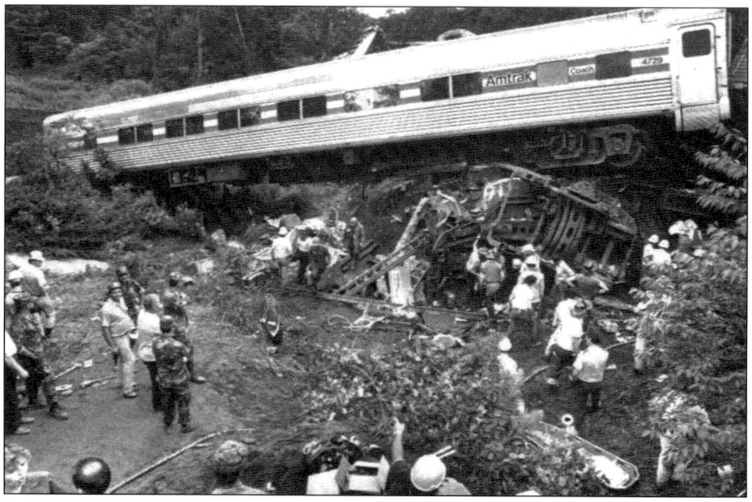

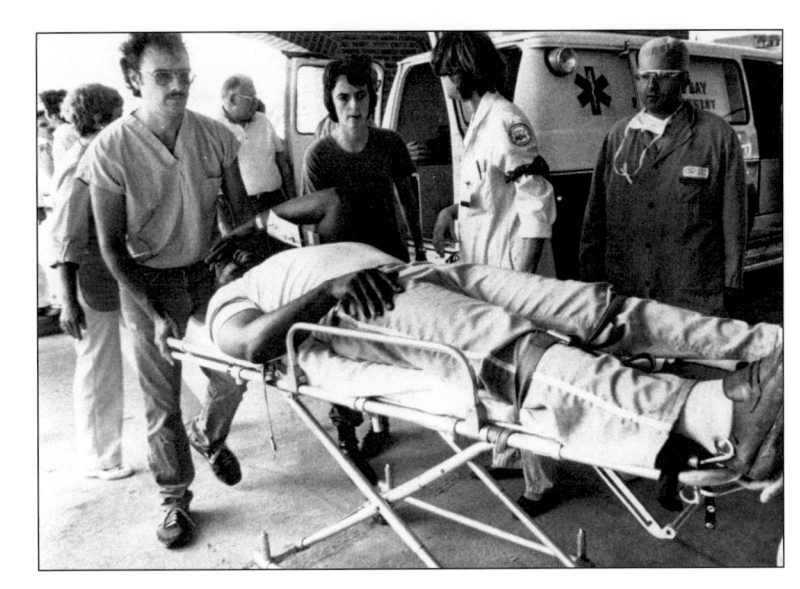

FIGURE 17-12. Chief surgery resident Tom Schwartz helps unload an ambulance on the day of the Amtrak derailment, while McSweeney (white shirt in background) assists and Gamelli (next to ambulance) supervises triage.

were dispatched to the scene. Surgery's Steve Payne and medicine's Bill Kalwait thus found themselves carrying the "trauma trunk" towards the wreckage that soggy morning. As Payne recalled:

> "MCHV security rushed us to the scene and it was about the eeriest thing I had ever seen. We traipsed through the wet woods into a clearing where the wash out occurred. There were literally dozens of stunned people milling around in the mud and the grass in front of the crumpled train cars. Bill and I thought we were going to an in-the-field drill, but knew it was the real thing when we got there. Bill turns to me after looking at an overturned smoking train car and says to me: 'Boy Steve, they went all out for this drill!' Bill and I worked like Trojans freeing people from particularly the dining car where they were jammed into one end like a plug of humans covered with scrambled eggs, coffee, and bacon. What an experience. We were damn glad when about a hundred rescue and National Guard personnel showed up!"[9]

Meanwhile, the entire staff had been mobilized back at the hospital. Residents and attendings took turns unloading ambulances and triaging patients. The orthopaedists set up a portable fluoroscope in a conference room to screen for fractures. The radiologists were highly critical of this efficient system, since it lacked hard copy documentation. The grumbling died down when they discovered that the chief of orthopaedics was one of the major participants.

In the end, 118 of the 275 people onboard were hurt (29 seriously) in the worst train accident in Vermont history. Four people were killed instantly and one died within three hours of the crash.[10] Everyone who made it to the hospital survived. Thankfully, UVM's revised and strengthened disaster plan has yet to be implemented again.

1985 Emergency Room Remodeling

A new emergency room was to be constructed as part of the 1985 MCHV remodeling and expansion. The E.R. had been treating around 25,000 patients a year at that time. Uphold,

FIGURE 17-13. The front of Smith 1 contained offices, clinical laboratory space, and the Dental Clinic. The Emergency Department section had three connecting trauma bays that held two stretchers apiece. An x-ray room was immediately adjacent. There were five other exam rooms and a cast room. One of the exam rooms was used for sigmoidoscopies.

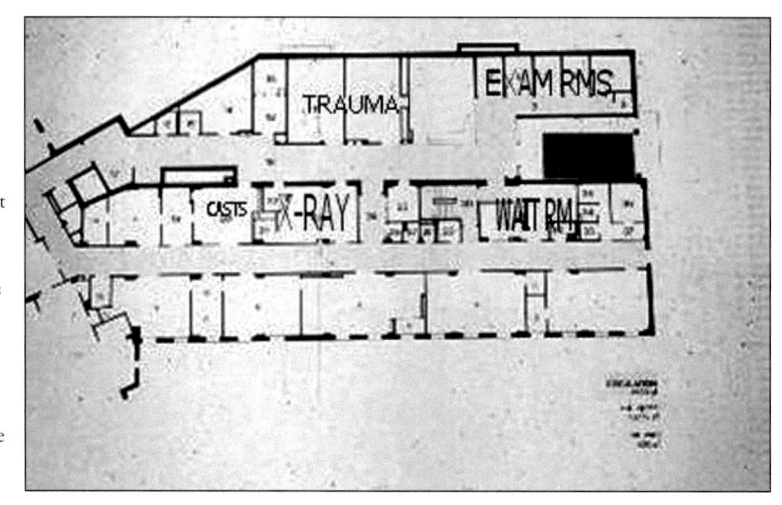

head nurse Patricia Rock, and I worked on the initial stages of planning. Our goals were an enclosed two-vehicle ambulance bay, separate acute and ambulatory patient care areas, and a nearby X-ray Department, preferably on the same floor. We hoped that these reasonable requests could be met.

The hospital planners, in what seemed like an arbitrary decision, decreased the size of our space by 50% (other departments suffered similar fates). A dedicated elevator to the operating room, a helipad, and adequate room for growth were axed. The new McClure Wing's two enclosed ambulance bays, trauma resuscitation rooms, and patient flow patterns were vast improvements over Smith 1, but the space itself remained far too small. The E.R. was overcrowded almost from the day it opened, and was unable to cope with the ever-increasing number of annual visits.

Nine additional emergency room physicians had come on board by 1991. Included among the new hires were David Claus, Maj Eisinger, and Ray Keller. The around-the-clock coverage provided by the eleven attendings led to more consistent levels of patient care. Resident shifts were reduced from 24 to 12 hours and staggered across morning, evening, and overnight blocks. Aside from the addition of a few interns, overall housestaff coverage remained the same.[11]

Clinicians Perform Trauma Ultrasounds

Steven Shackford, Davis' successor as chairman, brought additional changes. Recognizing the usefulness of the focused abdominal sonogram for trauma (FAST), he asked Radiology to train UVM's surgeons and emergency physicians in the technique. When that failed, he went to Germany to learn FAST exams from clinicians. Shackford also studied at an Atlanta "knife and gun club" emergency room. He then taught the method to the rest of the Department of Surgery's staff himself.

It became a family affair when the hospital wouldn't pay for a dedicated emergency room ultrasound machine. The women's auxiliary, under president Ellen Shackford's leadership, generously donated a device to the emergency department. The Emergency Division subsequently replaced this early '90s unit with a more advanced model using its own funds.

Shackford also led the nationwide ACS-sponsored movement to teach and credential sur-

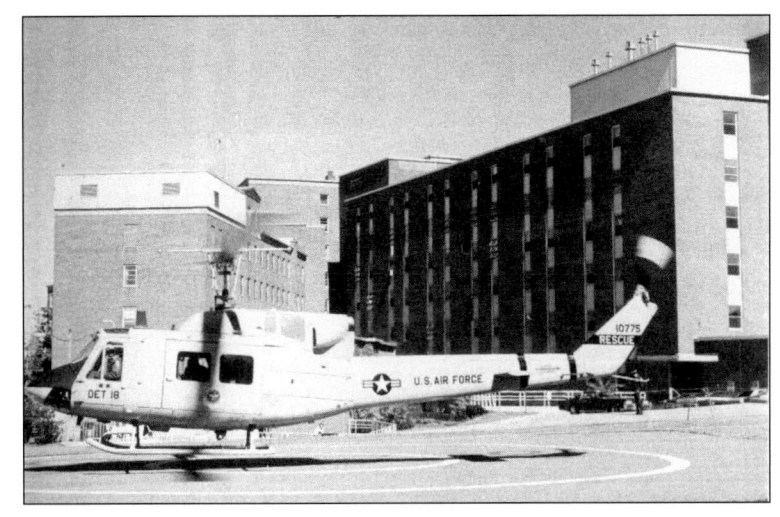

FIGURE 17-14. The MAST helicopter landed on a temporarily blocked road across from the emergency room. This left a short stretcher ride to the emergency entrance.

geons in the use of ultrasound. This work was done in collaboration with trauma surgeon Grace Rozycki and breast surgeon Edgar Staren.[12] Shackford's efforts led to the creation of the ACS's "Ultrasound for Surgeons" course, which is currently offered on DVD. Shackford even appears as one of the disc's presenters.

Helicopter Ambulances in Vermont

Congress had authorized the use of military helicopter rescue units for civilian missions in 1970. The resulting program was called Military Assistance to Safety and Traffic (MAST). UVM had a most successful MAST helicopter service in cooperation with Plattsburgh AFB's 380th Bombardment Wing from 1973 until the air rescue unit's departure during the 1980s. A helicopter ambulance service was then coordinated through the Vermont Air National Guard for a while.

One would think that Vermont was ideally suited for helicopter transport, given the presence of the Green Mountains to the east and Lake Champlain to the west. Weather constraints and cost considerations, however, suggested otherwise. That didn't stop our surgeons with past military helicopter evacuation experience from advocating for a lost cause. UVM ultimately did not start its own hospital-based helicopter transport service.

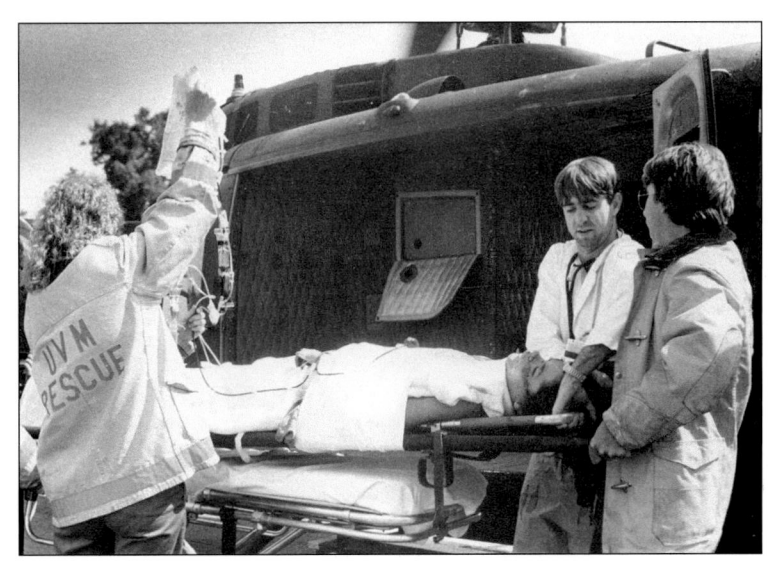

FIGURE 17-15. Surgery resident Bill Wilson and UVM rescue personnel unload an immobilized patient from the helicopter.

Chapter Seventeen: Emergency Medicine Division

Dartmouth, perhaps because of its deeper pockets, went ahead and developed such a system. Today, patients are brought to UVM in helicopters run by the Dartmouth-Hitchcock Advanced Response Team (DHART) and the New York State Police Helicopter/Aviation Unit. The efficiency of these helicopters is somewhat reduced by the remote location of UVM's East Avenue helipad, which necessitates an additional land ambulance trip before a patient can reach the emergency department.

A New Emergency Room and a Changing of the Guard

The Emergency Department went completely electronic in December of 2003 thanks to a gift from an anonymous donor. The change is almost unfathomable to those of us accustomed to paper charts. Digitized X-Rays are presented through state-of-the-art electronic technology and can be compared to old traditional films at the click of a button. This places UVM at the leading edge of emergency care in this country.

By 2005, the Division of Emergency Services was bursting at the seams. Its 17 emergency doctors and ten physician assistants were seeing 50,000 patients a year in a facility designed for half that many. The Division finally obtained the space that it needed and deserved as part of the "Renaissance Project," the massive remodeling of the entire medical complex. The emergency rooms still aren't on the same floor as the operating suites, but at least there is a private elevator between the two. The new emergency room is, however, adjacent to a cutting-edge 64-slice CT scanner.

The College of Medicine has also finally seen the light, inserting a mandatory one-month emergency medicine rotation into its latest curriculum. An average of 15 UVM graduates a year currently seek careers in emergency medicine, although the University still lacks its own residency program.

Uphold continued as chief of the Division until 2006, when she passed the reins to Stephen Leffler. The Vermont native whose father had run a general store in Brandon, had graduated from the College of Medicine. He returned to UVM for good in 1993 after completing an emergency medicine fellowship in New Mexico. Leffler has been an enthusiastic teacher and promoter of the electronic medical record system.

The Emergency Department continues as an administrative division within the Department of Surgery, but clinically functions as a separate Fletcher Allen Health Care unit. This is somewhat unique, as virtually every other large teaching hospital has an independent Emergency Department. Nevertheless, the combination works well at UVM.

CHAPTER 18

Colorectal/Bariatric/Minimally Invasive Surgery Division

Colorectal surgeons were among the Department's first sub-specialists. The discipline, however, remained under the control of the general surgeons until Neil Hyman and Peter Cataldo brought it into prominence.

Bariatric surgery, while a still relatively new field, has been performed in one form or another at UVM for decades. Today's program is nationally recognized for its surgical excellence.

Advanced minimally invasive surgery, on the other hand, has only recently come to the Green Mountain state. Nevertheless, UVM is now on the front lines of the latest technology and procedures.

UVM's First Colorectal Surgeons

Joel Williston Wright, UVM's chief of surgery from 1885 to 1889, wrote one of the first specialized anorectal disease textbooks in 1884. Among the popular treatise's topics were fistula in ano, hemorrhoids, pruritus ani, anal fissure, anal stricture, and rectal prolapse. The work advocated "extirpation of the rectum" (proctectomy) for the cure of rectal cancer and "colotomy" (colostomy) for its palliation.[1]

Interest in colorectal matters waned after Wright's premature retirement, but was revived twenty years later by Benjamin D. Adams. The College of Medicine graduate and self-taught proctologist was a decent surgeon, but a "lousy instructor" (according to Gladstone).[2] Fortunately, this didn't dissuade student Arthur Gladstone from pursuing the subject.

Gladstone built on his experience with Adams to become UVM's first trained colorectal specialist. He did this by completing a general surgery residency at Mt. Sinai Hospital in 1939. While there, he studied with gastroenterologist Burrill B. Crohn, and the three surgeons who pioneered the operative treatment of Crohn's Disease, John H. Garlock, Leon Ginzberg, and Gordon D. Oppenheimer.[3]

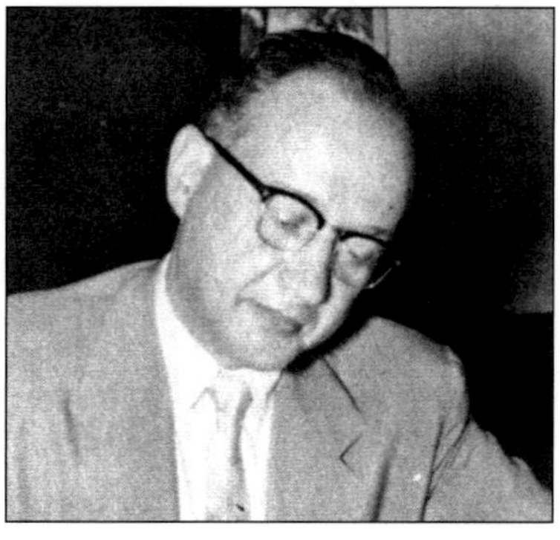

Gladstone recognized the importance of post-op patient

FIGURE 18-1. Arthur Gladstone was THE colorectal surgeon until Abrams arrrived.

FIGURE 18-2. Gladstone's 1979 autobiography, "Beyond the Scalpel".

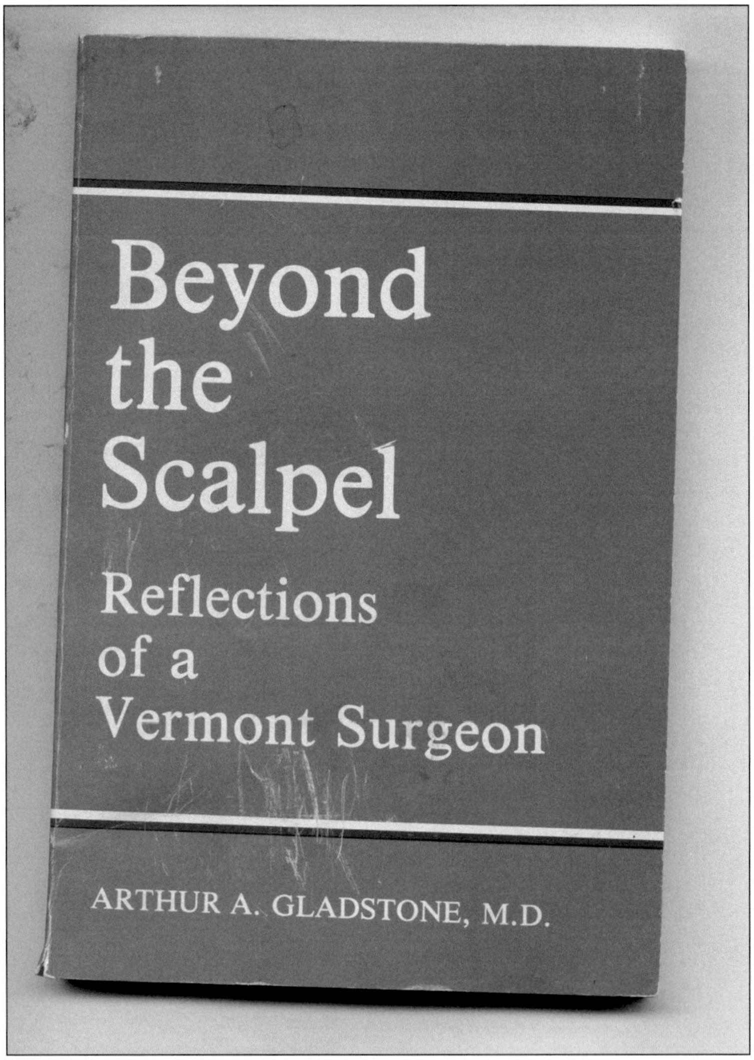

education and follow-up care. He was inspired to form the "Vermont Ostomy Club" after an encounter with a patient who had undergone a Hartmann's procedure for a low rectal cancer:

"We found Frank at his Winooski home, withdrawn into his bedroom with the shades down, apparently feeling himself an outcast. A strong fecal odor pervaded the room. Feeling himself to be offensive, he refused to join his devoted family for meals. With no medical support or instruction, Frank was at a very low ebb, regarding his life as futile. When we visited him, he was told for the first time that his external apparatus should be a water- and airtight protection against leakage and odors. At our request, his personal physician arranged for a Visiting Nurse to instruct him in colostomy care and the details of hygiene. A week later he greeted us at the door cheerfully, declaring himself ready to resume employment."[4]

Gladstone became Chief of Surgery at the DeGoesbriand shortly after his return to Vermont. He had held the position for nearly thirty years at the time of the 1967 merger with the Mary Fletcher. Gladstone's title disappeared overnight, however, when A.G. Mackay was appointed Chief of Surgery of the resulting Medical Center Hospital of Vermont.

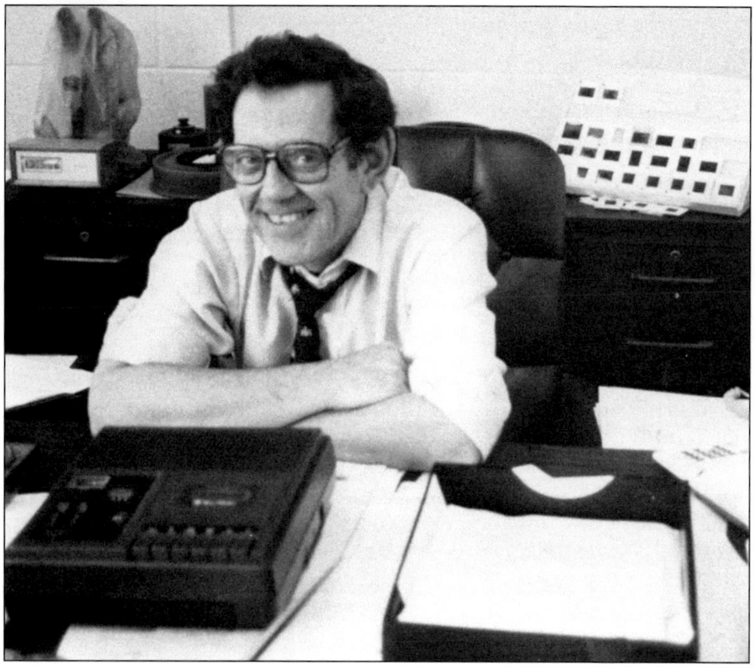

FIGURE 18-3. Jerry Abrams, John Davis' right-hand man, developed and managed the colorectal group.

Gladstone and Koplewitz Join Forces

Although colorectal surgery was a distinct sub-specialty, many general surgeons still treated colorectal problems. Such was the case when John Davis succeeded Mackay in 1969, bringing Jerome Abrams along with him from Cleveland in the process. Abrams was a general surgeon without formal colorectal training, but saw the need for further development of colorectal surgery and endoscopy at UVM.

Martin Koplewitz had returned to Burlington around the same time that Davis and Abrams had arrived. Koplewitz, another College of Medicine graduate and former UVM surgery resident, had left his private practice in St. Albans to become Gladstone's partner. Koplewitz grew interested in colonoscopy after reading the original articles on its use. After convincing Gladstone of the procedure's potential, Koplewitz went to Mt. Sinai for a week where he learned the new technique from pioneering colonoscopist Hiromi Shinya.[5] Gladstone, in the meantime, raised funds for the purchase of a colonoscope specifically anticipating Koplewitz's future use.

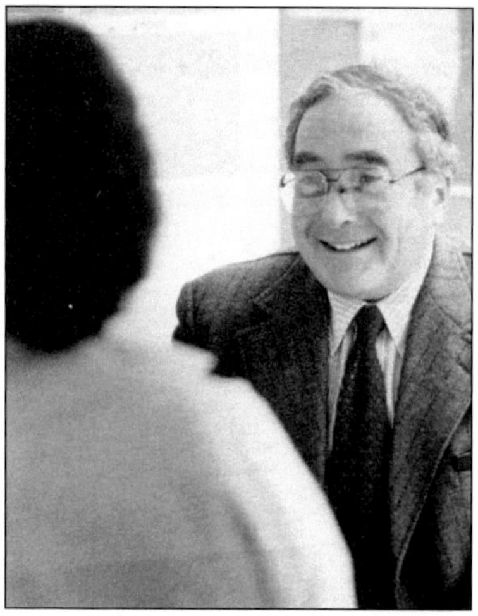

FIGURE 18-4. Martin Koplewitz left St. Albans in the 1960s to join Gladstone.

The colonoscope, according to Koplewitz was acquired through MCHV in 1971. He said "this proved to be an error on Gladstone's part, as Abrams immediately restricted its use to full-time faculty." Koplewitz and Gladstone had not yet joined the Surgical Associates' fold, and were thus considered part-time staff despite their UVM teaching appointments. "Koplewitz had to wait ten more years before the Department let him perform a colonoscopy!"[6]

Another of Abrams' colonoscopy rules involved billing. He decreed that the charge for colonoscopic polyp removal should be the same as that for traditional open abdominal polypectomy. Abrams thought that this would prevent surgeons from performing the more invasive operation unnecessarily. His decision seemed to ignore the fact that colonoscopy was a 30-minute outpatient procedure, whereas open polypectomy required a spinal or general anesthetic as well as pre- and post-op care. The precedent, once established, remained in place for many years.

Hyman and Cataldo Usher in a New Era

Davis, pre-occupied with his own health issues, did not hire another colorectal specialist after Abrams' untimely 1985 death. It was thus left to Davis' replacement, Steven Shackford, to fill the staffing void in 1990. Shackford's choice was Neil H. Hyman, a former UVM medical student who had subsequently completed a residency at Mt. Sinai, and a colon and rectal fellowship at the Cleveland Clinic. Hyman brought such procedures as low anterior resections and pull-through ileo-anal anastomoses to UVM as an alternative to abdomino-perineal resections with their resultant permanent colostomies.

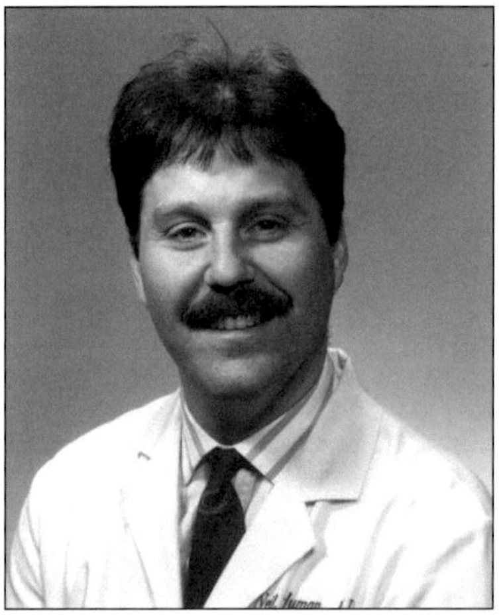

FIGURE 18-5. Neil Hyman was recruited from the Cleveland Clinic to lead the colorectal section.

Hyman has since looked at the quality of life among inflammatory bowel disease patients and helped establish practice parameters through the American Society of Colorectal Surgeons. He has also worked with surgeons across the state in an attempt to improve colon cancer treatment.[7] Under Hyman's leadership, numerous UVM residents have pursued colorectal fellowships. Many of them have gone on to academic careers.

Peter A. Cataldo joined Hyman in the section of colorectal surgery in 1995. Cataldo had been an undergraduate at UVM, and had roomed with Seth Harlow (who went on to join UVM's staff as a surgical oncologist). Cataldo ended up in the Air Force, teaching at Wright State University, after a Tufts medical school education, a Baystate residency, and a colorectal fellowship at Michigan's Ferguson Hospital. Hyman recruited Cataldo right out of the military after meeting him at a colorectal gathering on Nantucket Island.

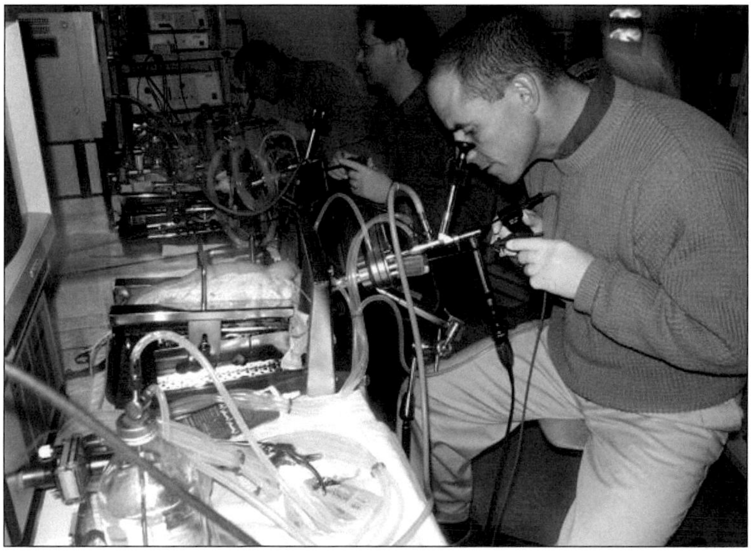

FIGURE 18-6. Peter Cataldo learning trans-anal endoscopic microsurgery in Germany.

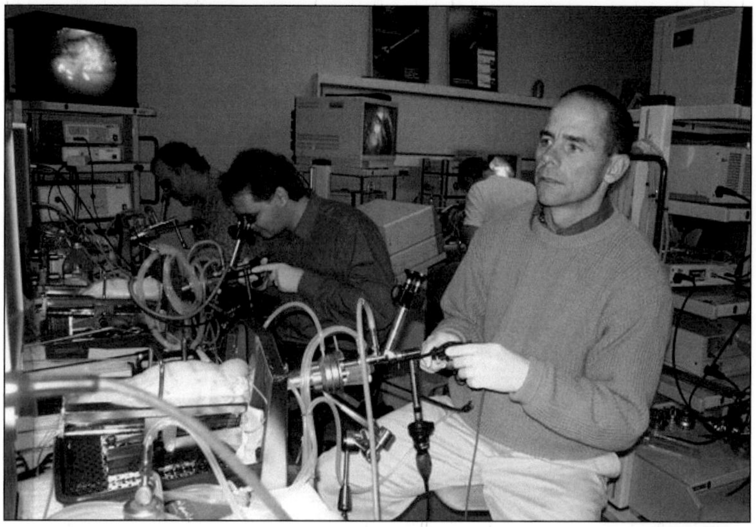

FIGURE 18-7. Cataldo at the phantom, training for robotic endoscopic surgery.

Cataldo brought needed laparoscopic skills to UVM, doing Vermont's first laparoscopic Nissen fundoplasty in 1995. He went on to perform the State's first stapled hemorrhoidopexy in 2001 after learning the technique in Europe. He has since enrolled the largest number of patients in this procedure's national trial. Cataldo has also popularized the use of transanal ultrasound at UVM and co-authored one of the definitive volumes on stomas.[8]

Another of Cataldo's trips took him to Germany, where he learned how to perform transanal endoscopic microsurgery. The technically demanding procedure is dependent on access and visualization. Instruments are parallel to each other, as opposed to laparoscopy, where the instruments are at different angles. The equipment is expensive as well. Nonetheless, UVM has now done more cases than any other center in the country.[9] Cataldo teaches the technique in multiple venues here and abroad. He expects to publish the world's first textbook on microscopic transanal surgery soon.

The Community Surgeon Connection

Cataldo's arrival coincided with that of another colorectal surgeon, although the latter was here to retire, not start a career. Samuel B. Labow had graduated from McGill, been a resident at Beth Israel and Bellevue, and then finished a colon and rectal fellowship in Muhlenberg, New Jersey. He settled at Long Island's North Shore University Hospital, worked hard, and before long established a very successful practice. During this time, Labow served as the president of the American Society of Colon and Rectal Surgeons and on the Board of Governors for the ACS.

Labow had always loved to ski. Six years into practice, he bought a vacation home in Stowe. Labow had also planned from the start to retire before age 60. At age 58, he promptly moved to Stowe for good. Hyman met Labow at his front door in 1996 as he was unpacking and invited him to help teach at UVM. Shackford offered Labow a clinical appointment and a weekly teaching session with the students.

Martin H. Wennar, who had practiced in St. Albans and had also served on the ACS' Board of Governors, joined Labow within a year. Wennar was a familiar face, as he had been attending UVM's surgery conferences for more than twenty years. Their instruction has

FIGURE 18-8. Samuel Labow voluntarily taught at UVM after retiring from his large Long Island practice. He and his wife Michelle have generously funded a surgery chair and a lectureship.

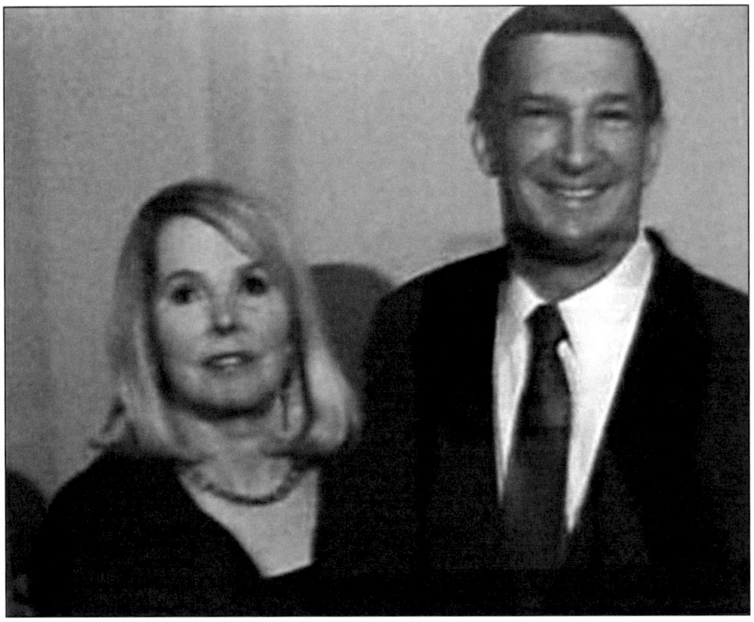

proven to be a bonus for the surgery rotation's medical students. The pair's one and a half hour sessions continue the UVM tradition of post-retirement service previously established by Davis.

Labow and Wennar have also contributed to the Department in another, more substantial way. Labow and his wife have endowed the "Samuel B. and Michelle D. Labow Green & Gold Professorship in Colon & Rectal Surgery" (which is currently occupied by Hyman), along with the "Samuel B. and Michelle D. Labow Lectureship in Colon & Rectal Surgery," and the "Labow-Shackford Lectureship in Quality." Wennar, meanwhile, has endowed the "Martin H. Wennar Lectureship in Professionalism."

Bariatric Surgery Section Slowly Grows

Morbid obesity unresponsive to diet has been treated with surgery for years. The operation of choice during the '70s was the jejuno-ileal bypass. This procedure produced weight loss through malabsorption. Diarrhea was a frequent side effect, liver dysfunction was a life-threatening complication, and long-term weight loss was an elusive goal. Nolan Cain did a handful of these bypasses in Burlington. Vascular surgeon Rodger Weissman performed such cases at Dartmouth in conjunction with arterial bypasses in order to control hyperlipidemia. Richard Hornberger, better known to all as the author of "MASH", also did many of these surgeries at his rural Maine hospital.

Richard Gamelli did a few intestinal bypasses in the 1980s. He also reversed a fair number due to liver problems. Gamelli then embraced the next trend, vertical banded gastroplasty (VBG). This operation created a restrictive stomach pouch using a plastic band and staples. Complications were mainly restricted to reflux, obstruction, and pouch expansion. Long-term weight loss, however, was successful for compliant patients. Bariatric surgery volume increased substantially, at least until Gamelli's 1991 departure.

One of Gamelli's residents during this period was Laurie Spaulding. She had been a UVM medical student and an MCHV intern before spending two years in Alaska with the Public

Health Service. While there, she performed more surgical cases than she had even seen in Vermont. Having left Vermont considering a career in ENT, she returned as a dedicated general surgeon. She finished her residency in 1991, just as many of the old guard were moving on or retiring. Shackford hired Spaulding at Koplewitz' behest, and gave her office space at Timberlane alongside Gladstone's former partner.

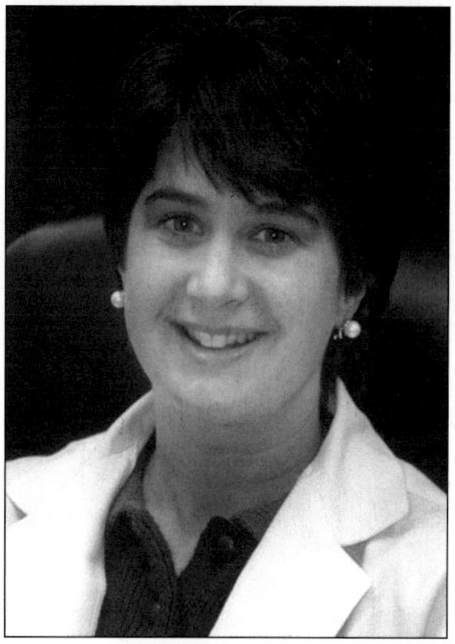

FIGURE 18-9. Laurie Spaulding almost settled in Alaska, but returned to her native Vermont to expand and revolutionize bariatric surgery at UVM.

The demand for bariatric surgery continued, so Spaulding took on the challenge. She was somewhat unfamiliar with the operative details of VBG, but had seen many of the reflux complications. Spaulding reviewed the literature and decided that roux-en-y gastric bypass was a better option. This procedure also created a small stomach pouch, but then connected it to a distal portion of small intestine. It was thus restrictive and malabsorptive, but without the dangerous electrolyte imbalances or reflux of the other two operations.

Spaulding did weeklong "mini-fellowships" with Harvey J. Sugerman of the Medical College of Virginia and Walter J. Pories of East Carolina University. Sugerman had written one of the classic papers on roux-en-y bypasses, while Pories was not only an expert in the procedure, but also the father of one of Spaulding's senior UVM residents, Susan Pories.[10] Spaulding subsequently started the UVM program in 1992.

Under Gamelli, the medical service had screened patients pre-op and assumed their care post-op. Spaulding found that this medical "program" was nonfunctional, so she created her own program within surgery. Psychologists, dieticians, and nurses were recruited to evaluate, educate, and encourage patients throughout the medically and emotionally fraught process. The combination of an effective procedure and intense patient support led to improved results and a dramatic increase in bariatric surgeries.

Aware of this, the American College of Surgeons now designates bariatric surgery centers of excellence. UVM, based on its large volumes and favorable outcomes, became a Level I Bariatric Surgery Center (the ACS' highest rating) in 2006. It is the only such center in Northern New England.[11]

Bariatric surgery was originally done only for those with life-threatening obesity-related medical conditions. Today, thanks to reductions in surgical risk and long-term complications, it is performed on patients who may not have qualified for such procedures under older guidelines. Having observed friends and faculty members undergo these procedures, I can attest that this surgery opens up a new life for these individuals.

Minimally Invasive Surgery Comes to UVM

Laparoscopic and minimally invasive surgeries have taken center stage during the past twenty years. Urologists, however, have been resecting bladder and prostate tumors through small tubes under direct cystoscopic visualization since 1900. Gynecologists have been performing simple laparoscopic procedures for nearly as long. Others have advocated diagnostic "celioscopy," "organoscopy," "peritoneoscopy," or "pelviscopy" for decades. Crude instruments that were often improvised from devices designed for other purposes limited acceptance. Visualization was barely adequate, at best.

The introduction of fiber optics and solid-state video cameras unleashed the late '80s revolution. Improved clip appliers, staplers, and insufflation equipment followed. General surgeons saw that large abdominal wounds could be avoided through the use of laparoscopy's smaller incisions. UVM's established surgeons learned their laparoscopic skills through industry-sponsored seminars, animal lab work, and direct observation. Cataldo's training had come in the Air Force. The staff's repertoire was mainly limited to cholecystectomies, but Cataldo and Hebert also performed Nissen fundoplications.

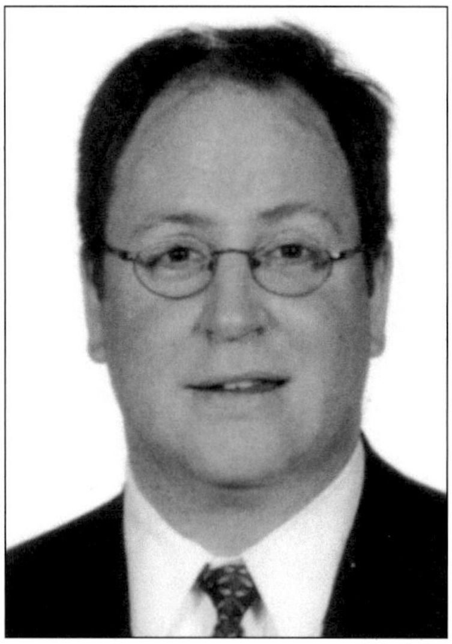

FIGURE 18-10. Edward Borazzo brought new minimally invasive laparoscopic surgery techniques to UVM at the time of his 2001 arrival.

Edward C. Borrazzo, meanwhile, was still deciding on which career to pursue. He had earned a Masters in mechanical engineering at Cornell, but medicine seemed more intriguing. After graduating from SUNY Stonybrook, he wrestled with general versus orthopaedic surgery. Residency at Jefferson in Philadelphia was followed by yet another choice. He thought that he might stay at Jefferson for a bariatric surgery fellowship, but the discipline was "on the outs there," so he returned to his Cornell roots to learn advanced laparoscopic techniques at New York Presbyterian Hospital.

Borrazzo answered UVM's advertisement for a "laparoscopist" and was hired in 2001. His arrival, like Hyman's, infused the Department with a wide array of new procedures. Among these were laparoscopic appendectomies, splenectomies, incisional and paraesohpageal hernia repairs, and adrenalectomies. Borrazzo has worked to improve endoscopic training for the residents in both the minimally invasive lab and a practice course. He also looks forward to using natural orifice transluminal endoscopic surgery (NOTES) and robotics at UVM.

The Next Generation

Additional staffing needs across all three sections have been met by a couple of recent UVM alumni, Gino T. Trevisani and Patrick M. Forgione. Trevisani supplanted his residency, like Hyman, with a Cleveland Clinic colon and rectal fellowship. He came back to UVM in 2002 with a few years of private practice under his belt. Trevisani introduced laparoscopic colectomies and leading-edge treatments for anal incontinence upon his return. He also found a niche alongside Spaulding caring for the super-obese. Trevisani has managed to do all of this while serving several tours of duty in Afghanistan and Iraq (see Chapter 29).

Forgione, on the other hand, followed a little more closely in Borrazzo's footsteps by taking a laparoscopic fellowship at Labow's old haunt, North Shore University Hospital. Forgione returned in 2005, and introduced laparoscopic roux-en-y gastric bypass, as well as the latest treatment for those with less severe obesity, gastric banding surgery. The Lap-Band® is a restrictive device that is wrapped around the top of the stomach and then adjusted through a small port under the skin. Unlike other weight-loss procedures, it does not alter normal anatomy, and can be removed without significant difficulty.

Forgione taught Spaulding and Trevisani the new techniques. Within a few years, however, Spaulding decided to return to her general surgery frontier roots. She resigned as a full-time faculty member in 2008 in order to engage in locum tenens and medical mission work. Trevisani and Forgione carry on the bariatric program in her absence. The two also remain true to their fellowship training, participating in colorectal and minimally invasive research respectively. This is but one of many examples of the continuing collaboration between the Department of Surgery's sections.

CHAPTER 19

Oncology Surgery Division

UVM's early surgical oncologists participated in a number of groundbreaking breast cancer trials. Real innovation, however, came with the appointment of David Krag.

Krag revolutionized breast cancer surgery with his development of sentinel lymph node biopsy. He and Seth Harlow restored UVM's national prominence with their validation studies.

The division remains out front with intra-operative ultrasound localization of non-palpable breast masses, complex liver resections, and total laparoscopic esophagectomies. Breast cancer research continues at micro-metastatic and microbiologic levels.

UVM's Early Breast Cancer Research

Cancer has been one of the surgeon's greatest challenges from the beginning. John Pomeroy wondered, "whether cancers differed from other complaints" as early as 1793.[1] Nathan Smith went further, telling his medical students:

> *"It is difficult to define cancer. There is considerable variety in its appearance. There are but few parts of the body [that are not] subject to it. It occurs in skin, bone, glands, cellular substance, and in many of the viscera ... It takes place in the rectum, urinary bladder, prostate gland, lips, glans penis, etc. which parts are particularly liable to it. Sometimes cancers almost immediately ulcerate, a scab at first appears and then when this is rubbed off an ulcer forms and spreads rapidly and extensively."*[2]

By the first half of the 20th century, surgeons attacked cancer by widely excising the primary site en bloc along with the corresponding region of lymphatic drainage. The Halsted radical mastectomy, with its removal of the overlying skin, pectoral muscles, and deep axillary nodes, was an example of just such a philosophy. Cleveland's George Crile questioned the necessity of radical excision without exception. He felt that cancer was a systemic process and suggested that patient immunity might play a major role.

Early surgical resident Carleton Haines was UVM's first formally trained surgical oncologist. He directed Vermont's Division of Cancer Control and UVM's tumor clinics and registry from the early 1950s to the early 1970s. Haines also participated in a number of National Cancer Institute (NCI) cooperative cancer study groups. Most focused on the role of androgens in the treatment of metastatic breast cancer.[3]

FIGURE 19-1. Roger Foster, director of the Vermont Regional Cancer Center, enters his office. Foster brought research and a scientific approach to UVM as an NASBP member.

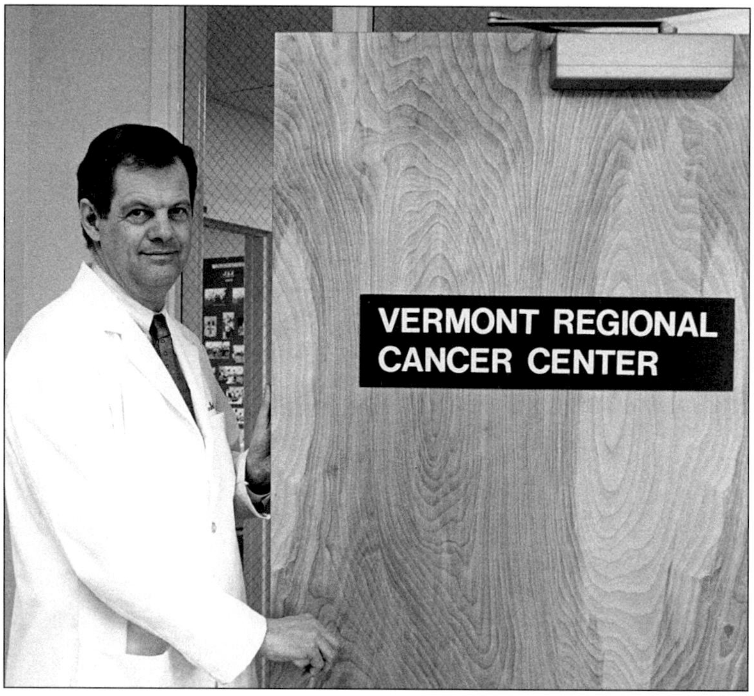

Roger Foster was brought to UVM by John Davis. He was named the Vermont Cancer Center's (VCC) director in 1974. The collaborative research, treatment, and education venture became very successful under his leadership. Foster (who had married George Crile's daughter) continued Crile's pioneering ideology at UVM. Perhaps it was no coincidence that fellow oncologic surgeon Caldwell Esselstyn, the husband of Crile's other daughter, promoted similar beliefs at the Cleveland Clinic.

Foster's research centered on breast cancer and, not surprisingly, immunology. His work on breast self examination was widely noted and respected. He had entered into the study thinking that breast self examination was not advantageous, but ended up proving the opposite to be true.[4]

Foster also kept UVM relevant by participating in the National Surgical Adjuvant Breast and Bowel Project (NSABP) B-06 study of 1976-84. The trial compared modified radical mastectomy and axillary dissection to lumpectomy and axillary dissection with or without radiation. Of note, 90% of Foster's patients elected to join the NSABP project, while only 10% of the other UVM surgeons' patients participated. Obviously, a certain amount of bias was communicated during the study's explanation!

The efficacy of self-breast exam and breast-conserving surgery became central tenets in the treatment of breast cancer among oncologists. The question of whether extensive lymph node dissection was of benefit, however, remained.

The Sentinel Node Ignites UVM

Oklahoman David N. Krag had learned about UVM from his orthopaedic surgeon brother Martin. Foster, eager to hire another surgical oncologist after Haines' 1989 retirement, recruited the younger Krag at the time of Martin's wedding. Krag came in 1991, under the impression that he would be working alongside Foster. The need for clarification was reasonable, as Foster had been a candidate to succeed John Davis as chairman. As it turned out, ultimately Foster decided to pursue a chairmanship elsewhere.

Shackford, meanwhile, designated "oncology surgery" as a division. Krag, as the only physician, became its chief by default. Krag found himself with a clinical practice that was larger than he wanted from the start. He also felt he was overburdened with follow-up patients from previous NSABP studies. In addition, the new Breast Care Center was now part of another NSABP preventive trial that had been launched under Foster's watch.

Basic research had always been Krag's major interest. He had pursued a number of studies during his medical school days at Loyola, his residency at the University of California at Davis, and his John Wayne Cancer Institute (JWCI) fellowship. One such project had been to inject patients with radioactive tumor antibodies and then use a gamma probe to locate the tumor intra-operatively.

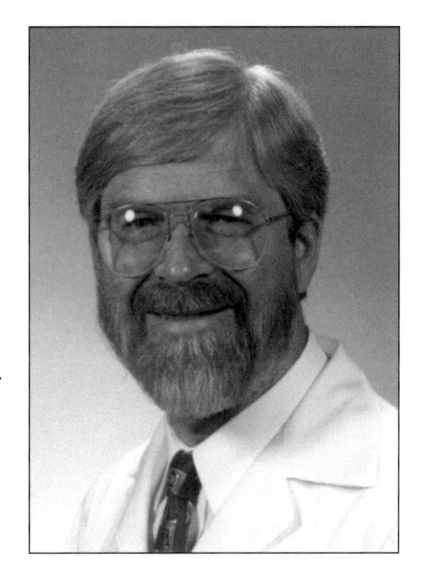

FIGURE 19-2. David Krag was walking to the Operating Room when a "light came on" and he came up with the idea for sentinel lymph node biopsy.

Krag was on his way to the operating room one spring day in 1992, when he happened to read an abstract from the Archives of Surgery. Written by Donald Morton, one of the JWCI's founders, the seminal article outlined a technique to map lymph node drainage using blue dye.[5] In Krag's words "a light came on." The implication was that if the first node in a drainage bed could be identified and shown to be cancer-free, then it would be unnecessary to remove the rest of the nodes. The blue dye's drawback was that the lymph channels had to be dissected, visualized, and then followed in order to find the node.

Krag immediately realized that a radioactive tracer could be substituted for the blue dye. Nodes could then be identified directly through the skin, obviating the need for a lengthy dissection. ENT resident James Alex, in the meantime, had been making preparations for his research year in Krag's lab. Alex and Krag came up with new plans at once. "Bingo!" — The radioactive tracer worked better than expected in a cat model, so the research moved directly to humans.[6]

Krag's initial work (like Morton's) focused on melanoma. Pretty soon, though, it shifted to breast cancer. Momentum grew with a generous start-up grant from William and Carol

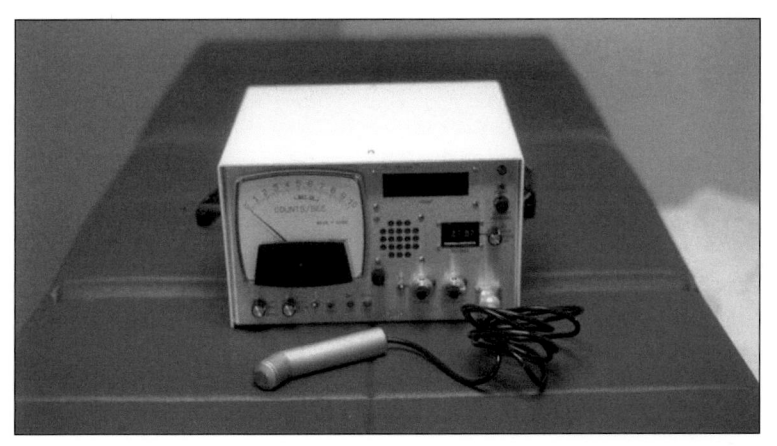

FIGURE 19-3. The gamma probe that Krag used during UVM's initial sentinel node biopsy experiments.

Hauke of Burlington. Krag, knowing that the NCI was sponsoring laparoscopic research, pitched the sentinel node project as a minimally invasive procedure. The NCI swung, and the sentinel node venture has been funded ever since. Emphasis then turned to confirmation and quality control. Krag personally trained fourteen surgeons in the technique for the 1998 multi-center validation study.[7] The success brought Krag and UVM into national prominence.

Help Arrives Just in Time

Krag continued to essentially carry the load of two clinicians during this time. Fortunately, another surgeon with a Vermont connection came to the rescue. Seth P. Harlow had been colorectal surgeon Peter Cataldo's college roommate at UVM. The magna cum laude graduate went on to the University of Massachusetts for medical school, then Northwestern University for residency. This was followed by a surgical oncology fellowship at Buffalo's Roswell Park Cancer Institute. Harlow joined Krag in 1994, just as the sentinel node's validation phase was getting under way.

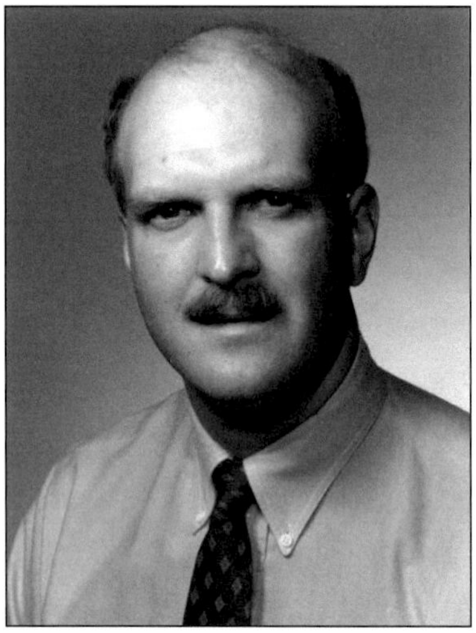

FIGURE 19-4. Seth Harlow arrived in 1994 to help Krag with the sentinel node trials, and to conduct his own research and clinical practice.

Harlow was a quick study, having already spent three years of dedicated research at Northwestern and Roswell Park. He shared Krag's enthusiasm for the sentinel node project, and threw himself completely into the effort. Harlow also took up the slack in endocrinology surgery, which had languished since Foster's departure. And he managed to attract some of the oddest general surgery cases during his call nights.

Under Krag's leadership, the NSABP conducted the 1999-2004 B-32 clinical trial in which sentinel node resection was compared to conventional axillary dissection in clinically node-negative breast cancer patients. Harlow was in charge of training surgeons, each of whom underwent surveillance of his or her performance. Ten trainers oversaw 270 surgeons at 76 institutions. Over 5,600 patients were eventually accrued making this one of the largest Phase III randomized surgical trials ever conducted.[8] Slides of all negative nodes were double-checked for occult metastases by three UVM pathologists. UVM's efforts during this study were truly heroic.

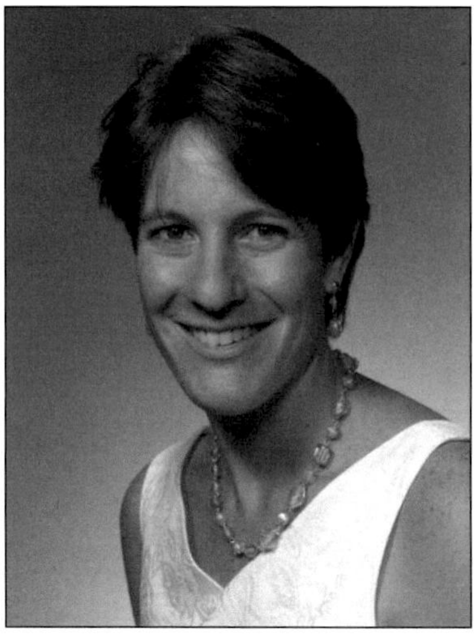

FIGURE 19-5. Mary Stanley bolstered the Breast Center following her 1998 arrival.

Krag and Harlow had realized that the B-32 study was going to consume a lot of their attention. As a result, new UVM hire Mary A. Stanley was assigned to the Breast Care Center. She had come to Vermont in 1998 with her husband, vascular surgeon Andrew Stanley. The pair had attended medical school at Dartmouth (which was still a two-year institution) and Brown, and then been residents at the UMass Medical Center. Mary Stanley had stayed on at UMass for a subsequent endosurgery fellowship.

Stanley, together with Harlow, amassed the largest number of patients for the B-32 trial. Unfortunately, the technology got ahead of the study. Consensus panels declared that sentinel node biopsy was the gold standard of care as of 2003, yet the NSABP trial was designed to continue until 2004. Stanley could no longer justify enrolling patients that might be randomized to "no sentinel node biopsy," so she dropped out. Stanley then turned her research energies to high-risk biomarkers, ductal lavage, and random peri-areolar fine needle aspiration.

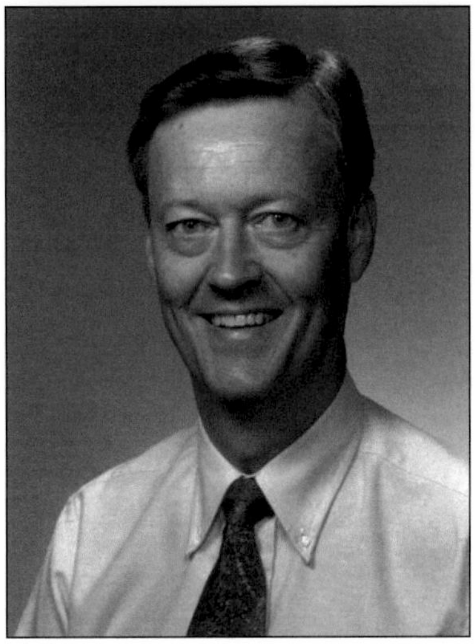

John David Beatty was brought on board in 1999 to take Krag's place as division chief and Breast Care Center director. Beatty had spent medical school and residency in Toronto prior to an oncology fellowship at the Medical College of Virginia. He had then been an attending at the Los Angeles-area City of Hope National Medical Center for seven years before moving to the National Cancer Institute of Canada in 1991. Beatty's role was strictly clinical, basically keeping the ship afloat while Krag and Harlow carried through with their B-32 commitments.

FIGURE 19-6. David Beatty led the UVM Breast Center and directed the Vermont Cancer Center.

Surgical Oncology Adopts Ultrasound

Krag's advances didn't stop with the sentinel node. He also followed the example set by UVM's vascular surgeons, and brought surgeon-controlled ultrasound to the office and operating room. The Department of Radiology was strongly opposed to letting surgeons perform any office-based imaging. The hospital refused to fund Krag's 1995 request, but donors came forth. With their help, the Breast Care Center purchased two ultrasound machines to use in its sixth floor DeGoesbriand office.

Ultrasound proved to be extremely useful in the outpatient setting. Cysts could be drained, benign masses could be followed, and unknown lesions could be biopsied. Intra-operative identification of non-palpable breast masses soon followed. This was far superior to needle localization with its inherent risk of wire dislodgement during transport from the radiographic suite to the O.R. UVM's oncology surgeons were among the first in the country to use ultrasound in this manner.[9]

Oncology Surgeons Tackle Liver Resections

More change and transition occurred at the turn of the 21st century. The Breast Care Center moved to larger space on the DeGoesbriand's first floor in 1998. Krag relinquished his Breast Care Center duties shortly thereafter in order to fully devote himself to research. The change was made possible by an extremely generous grant from one of Krag's grateful melanoma patients. Harlow, Stanley, and Beatty were keeping up with the increasing patient volume, but just barely.

Lawrence E. McCahill filled the staffing void in 2002. McCahill had attended Duke on a Navy scholarship. He took his residency at the University of Washington, where he learned

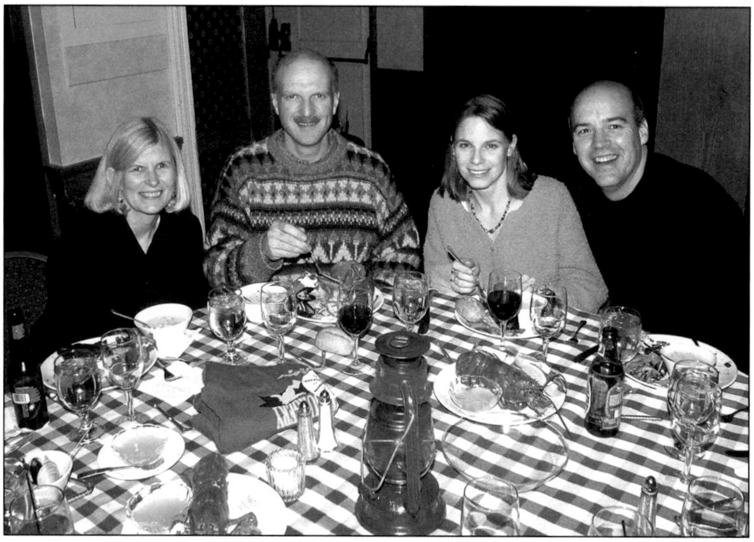

FIGURE 19-7. The Harlows and the McCahills enjoy a lobster supper during the annual Stowe winter surgery retreat.

excellent laparoscopic skills. McCahill considered a career in vascular surgery, but was torn apart when a peripheral bypass patient ended up with an amputation and later died, so he set his sights on oncology surgery. He liked the technical challenges of high-risk cancer operations, particularly those of major liver resections.

McCahill's four years of Navy payback were followed by an oncology fellowship at Beatty's former stomping ground, the City of Hope National Medical Center. McCahill chose this institution because it performed a large number of liver resections. He joined Beatty at UVM, and set his sights on performing major liver cases. This was an operation that had previously been done at UVM by the vascular surgeons, and later by the transplant surgeons.

Careful patient selection, low central volume technique, and a collaborative effort with dedicated anesthesiologist Mark Hamlin has led to a remarkable record: 50 major resections without a fatality. Moreover, only one in three cases have required a transfusion. Transplant surgeons do such cases at other institutions, but McCahill believes that an oncologic orientation makes for better cancer surgery. The new era seems to be paying dividends for the patients.

McCahill has teamed up with Edward Borrazzo to perform another cutting edge procedure, totally laparoscopic esophagectomy. The time constraints of this approach require that the pair work simultaneously. The technique results in smaller, less painful incisions, reductions in blood transfusions, and earlier discharge. Their sixteen cases compare favorably with the large series reported by other institutions.

McCahill has taken an interest in surgical approaches to palliative care. He is currently heading a Phase II clinical trial examining the utility of chemotherapy and monoclonal antibody treatment in certain patients with Stage IV colon cancer.[10] McCahill also studies breast cancer surgery quality outcomes and maintains the Breast Care Center's operative database.[11]

New Faculty and New Frontiers

Beatty left for a position with Seattle's Swedish Hospital in 2003. Harlow was promoted to chief of a division that found itself short a clinician once again, this time as the NSABP

B-32 trial was coming to a close. Stanley and McCahill stepped up, and a crisis was averted.

Ted A. James, who had attended the Medical College of Pennsylvania, and had completed a residency at North Shore University Hospital, was just finishing his Roswell Park fellowship. He joined the oncology division in 2005 after being suitably impressed during a Breast Care Center visit. His clinical interests include breast, thyroid, soft tissue sarcomas, and melanomas. James' research focuses on diagnostic melanoma markers and quality measures in breast cancer.[12]

James has been a Macy Scholar for Educators in the Health Professions at Harvard, and has been awarded a research fellowship by the Association for Surgical Education. As Director of the Surgery Clerkship for the College of Medicine, he is in the process of developing a "bridge" between the medical students' clinical core and their surgical rotations.

Krag's fertile mind continues to generate oncologic studies. He currently oversees eight grants with a total funding of over four million dollars. Most of this work centers on targeting cancer cells with peptides generated by bacteriophages. Krag and the division are also among the lead investigators for the NSABP's new BP-59 trial. This study aims to determine the predictive value of bone marrow micro-metastases in patients with early-stage breast cancer.

Stanley left for private practice in 2008, although she continues her affiliation with the Vermont Cancer Center. The division was bolstered around the same time, though, by the addition of David W. McFadden, the Department of Surgery's new chairman. McFadden, who has served as the primary investigator for over 30 different research projects, brings additional experience in cell signaling and tumor growth inhibition. UVM thus remains well poised in its efforts to overcome cancer through research, treatment, and education well into the future.

CHAPTER 20

Trauma and Critical Care Division

UVM's trauma tradition originated with John Davis. He oversaw burn and post-splenectomy sepsis research, edited the Journal of Trauma, and trained residents who became trauma care leaders.

UVM offered the first ATLS training courses to New England's practicing physicians and medical students. Davis and his successor, Steven Shackford, were presidents of the American Association for the Surgery of Trauma.

Shackford shaped the future of UVM's critical care. His head injury research had national impact, as did his promotion of surgeon-conducted trauma ultrasound through the American College of Surgeons.

Trauma Surgery Lags at UVM

People have been injuring themselves or each other accidentally or on purpose throughout recorded history. Since Vermont had largely avoided the battles of both the Revolutionary War and the War of 1812, UVM's earliest surgeons mostly dealt with wounds typical of life on the frontier. At that point in time the surgeon went to see the patient on foot or on horseback. Survivors obviously self-selected themselves while awaiting the arrival of help.

The Civil War, with its old-fashioned tactics and modern weapons, changed everything. Although many of UVM's medical faculty from this era served in one capacity or another, Henry Janes' methods not only stood out, they presaged those of modern trauma surgery. Janes oversaw logistically efficient U.S. Army hospitals at Gettysburg and Montpelier that employed non-operative treatments and comprehensive rehabilitation programs. He also maintained an inclusive outcomes database that documented his patients' progress by means of detailed notes and photographs. (see Chapter 4)

UVM's approach to trauma over the next hundred years was no different than that of any other mid-size teaching hospital. Most faculty members were the wrong age for World War I service. The staff that went overseas during World War II returned to practice either traditional general surgery or a sub-specialty. Vermont remained predominantly rural, and geographically isolated, since transportation was still an issue. It was thus left to Korean War veteran and innovator John Davis to bring contemporary trauma care to UVM.

The Division of Trauma and Critical Care

Davis was heavily involved with the prestigious American Association for the Surgery of Trauma (AAST). He served as president one year, and edited its Journal of Trauma for another 25. Davis did all of this from his Given Building corner office, Surgery's version of the White House Oval Office. He shared the space with departmental secretary Ruth Gilbert (whom he had brought from Cleveland) and editorial secretary Joan Young (whose husband had been the Department of Anatomy's chair). Joan remained a fixture there for years, even though others occasionally helped run the publication's editorial duties. The Journal was prepared to pay an editorial salary, but Davis never took the money!

Davis believed that general surgery was an all-inclusive specialty. Accordingly, he did not formally designate any sub-specialty divisions within the Department for years. This finally changed in 1980 with the arrival of emergency room physicians and the creation of the Division of Emergency Services. Around the same time, a few of the UVM surgeons took it upon themselves to form a trauma team, the purpose of which was to review trauma cases and improve trauma care.

Richard Gamelli ran the "Trauma Service" (which later became a true Division under Davis' successor Steven Shackford). A separate call schedule was put in place much to the relief of the more senior community surgeons. The service conducted daily X-ray rounds and had its own weekly Morbidity and Mortality conference. Special attention was paid to blunt trauma and burn care.

Burn Care at UVM

Topical burn treatment of the late 1950s was not dissimilar to that of the early 1900s, as described by former UVM chairman John Brooks Wheeler. It was performed:

> *"... in such a way to prevent the absorption of poisonous material, the result of germ infection, and to furnish a protective coating which would not need to be removed. This is done by spraying the burn with a 5% solution of tannic acid every two hours for twenty four hours and after that at longer intervals until the burned skin is actually tanned. This relieves pain, protects the burnt area and is not removed for two or three weeks, thus avoiding the painful daily change of dressing. When the tanned coating is removed a normal raw surface is left, which is treated like any other raw surface. In this treatment of extensive burns, there is almost no pain after the first few hours and the mortality rate is much lower and the raw surface smaller than in any of the older methods of treating burns. Further improvement has lately been made by using a 1% solution of gentian violet instead of tannic acid. It has the advantage of being antiseptic as well as absorbent and protective."* [1]

The revolution came during the early 1960s with the advent of antibiotic creams. The Army, thinking that there might not be enough doctors to go around in the wake of an atomic war, aggressively pursued potential uses for these compounds. Ischemic injuries were created in animal models by clamping arteries, and from inducing gunshot wounds; and were then treated with topical mafenide acetate (Sulfamylon®).[2] The cream, as expected,

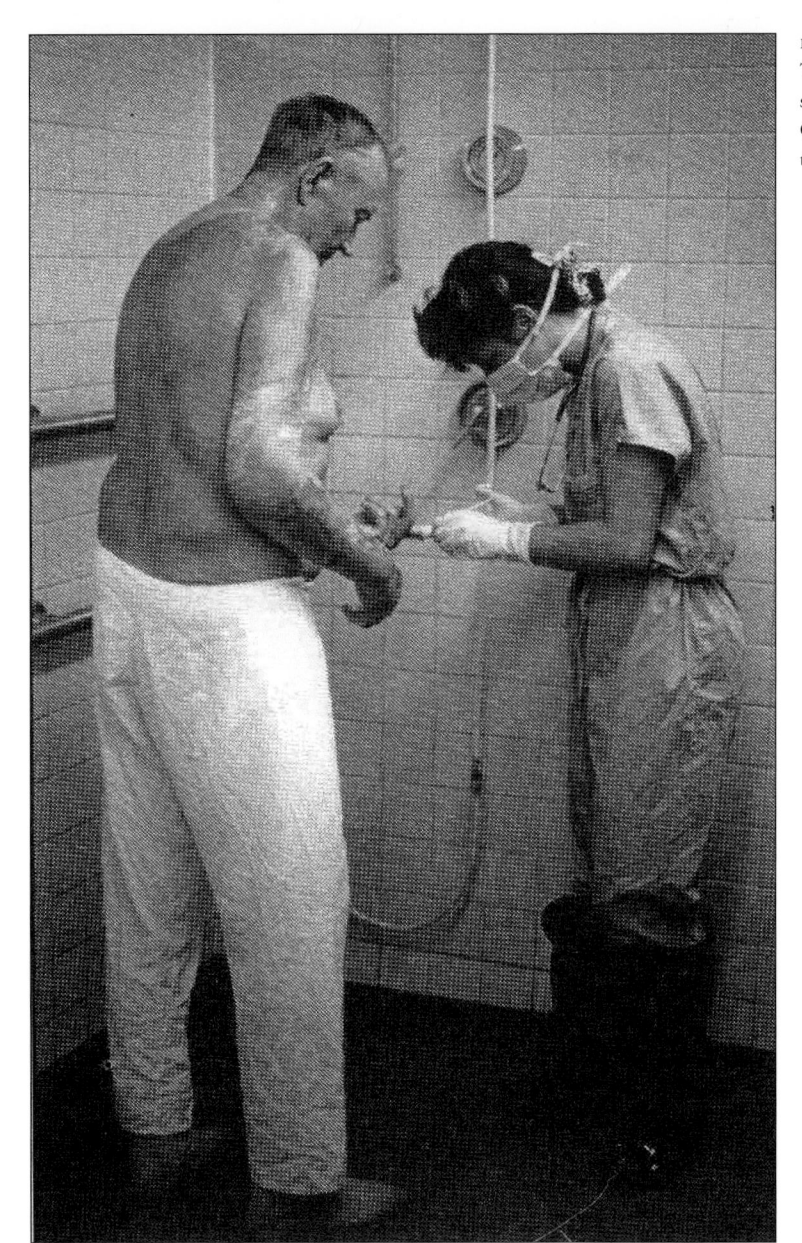

FIGURE 20-1. The Baird 3 burn shower was one of Gamelli's innovations.

decreased bacterial counts within the ischemic tissue and decreased deaths from sepsis. The Brooke Army team took the approach one step further by applying Sulfamylon® to burns. The substance was smeared over the affected site, washed off, and reapplied daily.[3] Burned soldiers came to call it "white lightning" because of the pain associated with its application.

Others used wet silver nitrate soaks, which were not nearly as painful. The initially clear soaks major drawback, however, was that upon exposure to light they invariably turned the patient's wounds, the room's furnishings, and the doctor's hands BLACK! A pH-balanced cream, silver sulfadiazine (Silvadene®), was eventually developed that proved to be more tolerable. Shortly before coming to UVM, Davis demonstrated that the new medication was just as effective as Sulfamylon against sepsis.[4,5] Silvadene still persists as the mainstay of burn treatment well into the 21st century.

Davis spearheaded UVM's major burn care until he turned the reins over to Gamelli in the early '80s. Gamelli carried on with credible results before going to Loyola in 1990. The field

FIGURE 20-2. Richard Gamelli treating a burn patient at UVM. Gamelli later became Chief of Surgery and Director of the Burn Center at Loyola University.

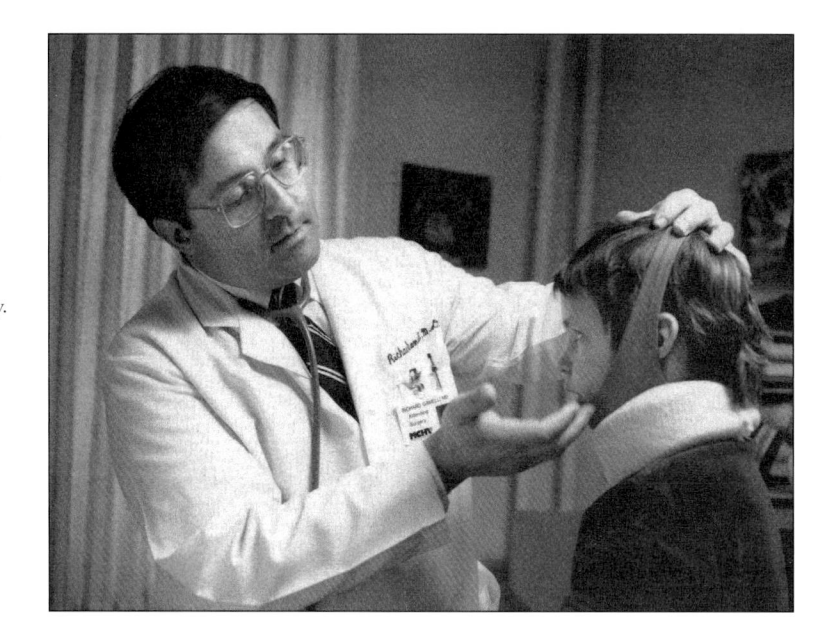

fell by the wayside for a few years, but was resurrected by Turner Osler in the mid-1990s. Although Osler has since left the clinical arena, UVM still treats severely burned patients in house rather than transferring them elsewhere.

Several of Davis and Gamelli's residents went on to become nationally recognized burn care leaders in their own right. Notable among these were Geoffrey Silver (who presently works alongside Gamelli) at Loyola, David Greenhalgh at the University of California Davis, and William Cioffi at Brown University.

Cioffi had followed Davis' example by serving at the Army Burn Center attached to San Antonio's Brooke Army Medical Center. He later led the Rhode Island Hospital response to the February 2003 fire that engulfed The Station Nightclub — the fourth worst such conflagration in U.S. history. Cioffi set-up a 24-bed burn ICU and a 34-bed acute burn ward on the hospital's fifth floor within minutes of receiving the alert. Every single one of the 64 burn patients admitted that night survived.

FIGURE 20-3. William Cioffi, pictured here as a UVM resident, directed burn care at Rhode Island Hospital following the 2003 Station Nightclub disaster.

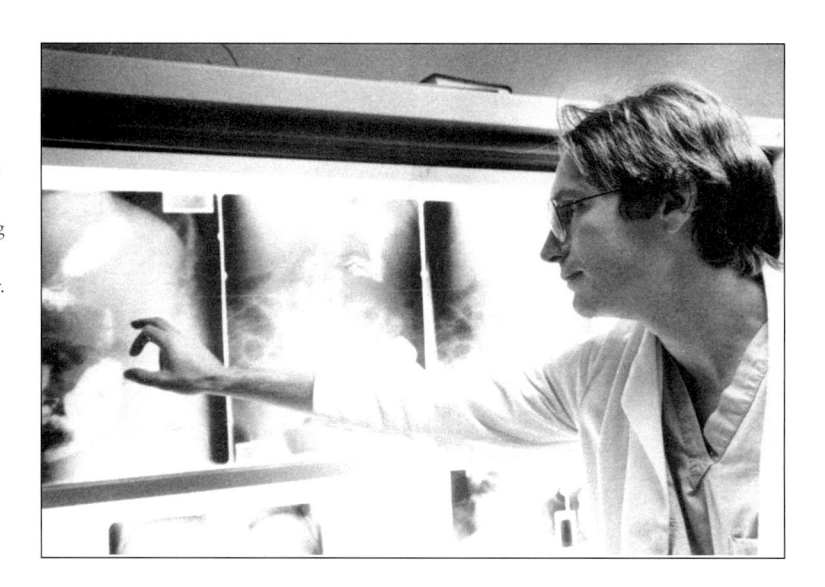

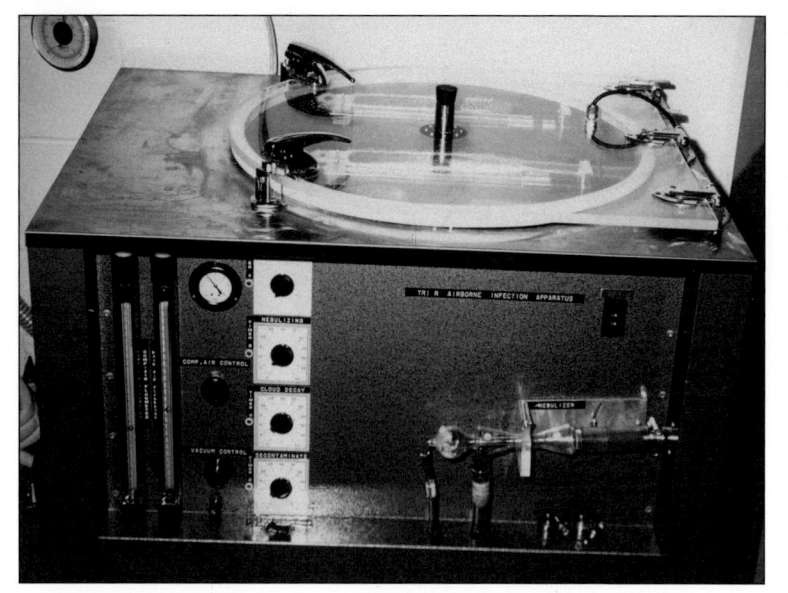

FIGURE 20-4. The centrifuge aerosol machine used by Coil, Dickerman, Davis, and Hebert still resides in the UVM surgical research laboratory.

Davis Promotes Trauma Research

Another of Davis' interests was post-splenectomy sepsis. Splenectomy was carried out during the 1970s for every type of splenic injury with the belief that there were no significant long-term consequences from asplenia. When late deaths from pneumococcus started to mount, Davis hired James Coil to investigate. Coil used a centrifuge to expose large numbers of mice to aerosolized pneumococcus. He then showed a significant increase in mortality among splenectomized mice.[6] James Hebert conducted further pneumococcal-related studies using this model following Coil's early '80s departure.

Hebert was one of several Davis-era residents to pursue trauma research. Some looked at the role of granulocyte colony stimulation factor in burns and abdominal sepsis, while others took a more clinical approach. Susan Pories, for example, studied the financial side of caring for the critically injured.[7] Her work was presented in 1987 at the first annual Resident Trauma Papers Competition, an event sponsored by the American College of Surgeons' Committee on Trauma. Pories won the New England region prize, a feat that has been matched by a number of other UVM residents through the years.

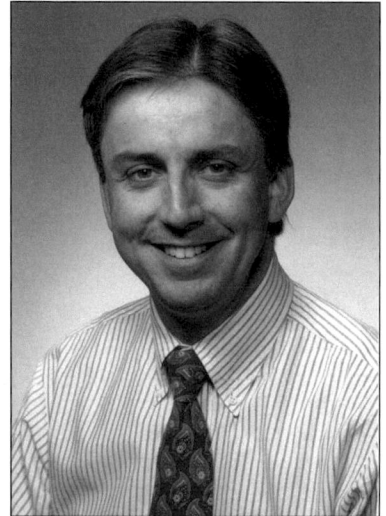

FIGURE 20-5. James Hebert continued his resident research after joining the staff in 1982, while simultaneously assuming huge academic and clinical loads. He never turned down a duty or an assignment.

UVM epidemiologist Julian Waller had published studies on preventable motor vehicle deaths during the early '70s. Shortly thereafter, an E.R. patient with a ruptured spleen bled to death while awaiting surgery. The two events motivated me (DBP) to review similar cases at MCHV. Not surprisingly, unrecognized hypovolemic shock monopolized the avoidable deaths in our series.[8] This foreshadowed work done by Shackford in Orange County California, who went on to produce the definitive studies on preventable trauma death.

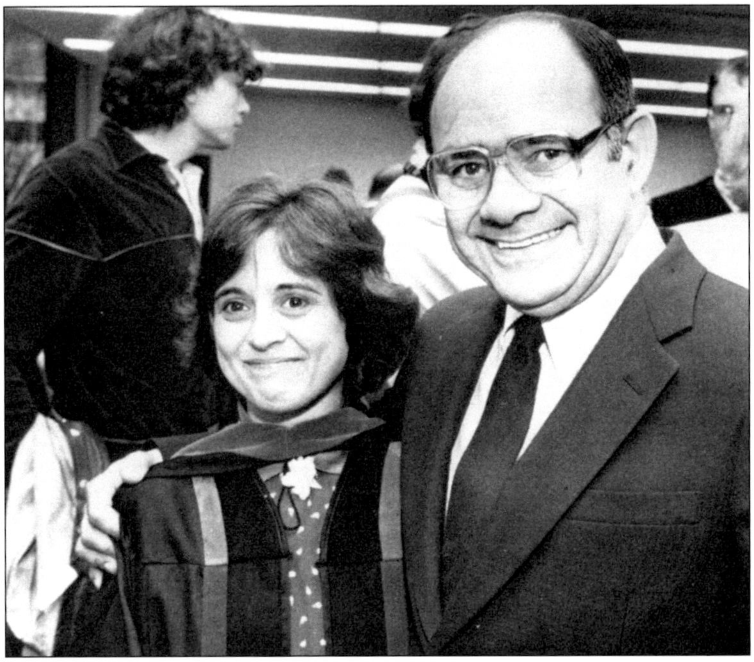

FIGURE 20-6. G-2 resident Susan Pories won the first New England Committee on Trauma resident competition in 1987. Here she is at her UVM COM graduation with her father, Walter J. Pories, the Chief of Surgery at East Carolina University from 1977-1996.

The Pilcher-Moore Shunt

One of the greatest difficulties that I had faced in Vietnam was the management of retro-hepatic vena caval injuries.[9] Clamping the cava too high had led to cardiac arrest in these hypovolemic patients. Theodore Schrock had described a shunt in 1968 that isolated the injury and thus facilitated its repair.[10] Schrock's shunt was inserted via the right atrium through a thoraco-abdominal incision. Although general surgeons received thoracic training, I felt that they would be uneasy with this approach.

It seemed to me that a shunt that incorporated a balloon catheter could be placed through the sapheno-femoral vein junction. Measuring flows in a canine model, G-4 resident Eugene Moore, medical student Kent Harman, and I proved the efficacy of this system in the lab.[11] The device was first commercially produced in 1977 as the "Pilcher-Moore Shunt." As time went by, it became known as the "Moore-Pilcher Shunt." Today it is simply referred to as a "Moore Shunt."

Moore was an exceptionally bright and hard working resident. His written consults frequently included references from the recent medical literature. It was odd then, that the perceptive Moore was not consulted about a litiginous trauma patient. He and his brother John had been assigned to the MCHV emergency room when an inebriated, paralyzed skier was brought in. The patient admitted that he had been skiing beyond his ability and had caused the accident. The insurance investigator dropped the ball, and the ski resort lost the lawsuit. Moore has gone on to have a prominent career as Chief of Surgery at Denver General Hospital, where he works alongside his brothers.

Advanced Trauma Life Support (ATLS) Courses Come to Vermont

Emergency trauma care was a mystery to most physicians prior to 1980. Our Emergency Medical Technicians (EMTs) frequently noted this distressing fact during MCHV emergency room case reviews. The EMTs justifiably complained that their carefully splinted patients were unwrapped and manipulated in the E.R. with little regard to the avoidance of further injury. The Department offered to address this issue by teaching the EMT course to first-year medical students, but the proposal found no support at the College of Medicine.

The American College of Surgeons (ACS), however, did appreciate the problem. In response, it adopted the Advanced Trauma Life Support (ATLS) course in emergency care. The course, taught through the ACS's Committee on Trauma (COT), emphasized treatment that had been advocated and endorsed by respected trauma surgeons. The system was organized and presented so that physicians with different levels of experience could execute it.

The ACS (on Davis' recommendation, no doubt) had appointed me Chair of the Vermont COT during the 1970s. Within a short while, I was named the COT Region I (New England) Chief. I accepted, provided that I could also remain Chair of Vermont! The regional Chiefs were among the first to obtain ATLS certification. This occurred at an expanded instructors' course held in Newark, New Jersey. The event was the prototype for today's courses. Fearing the streets of Newark more than I had feared the jungles of Vietnam, I stayed holed up in the hotel for two days. I studied the course book and took the open book pre-test, finding out later that the actual test was identical!

I had gone through high school, college, medical school, and surgical residency without learning how to give a proper speech. The ATLS course was the first to include professional instruction and videotaped sessions teaching communication skills. We all learned a lot about being effective teachers. One of the tips was that a red tie made one look more authoritative. I have watched television announcers and politicians ever since, and am surprised to note how many of them wear red ties!

Upon completion of the Newark seminar, we became "National Faculty." We were invited around the country to teach ATLS courses to both students and instructors. A cadre of teachers was created through the instructor courses that carried on the momentum. I was skeptical of the ATLS course's value at first, but turned into a convert. In the end, I was one of its greatest advocates. After the ATLS course was brought to UVM it soon became a requirement of the surgical residency program.

UVM hired an "educator" in February 1981 to help conduct the first New England instructor's course, which was only the 15th one conducted in the country thus far. The rest of our staff had yet to receive training, so we imported most of the other teachers. We charged non-UVM attendees so that we could teach our own faculty for nothing! We ended up training six Vermont instructors. The ACS limited each session to 16 students, so UVM gave eight more courses during the following year, and five more the next. We ended up teaching ATLS to 180 physicians in those first three years.

The ACS did not initially authorize the ATLS course for medical students. We believed that the students would be enthusiastic and would benefit from it, so we trained an

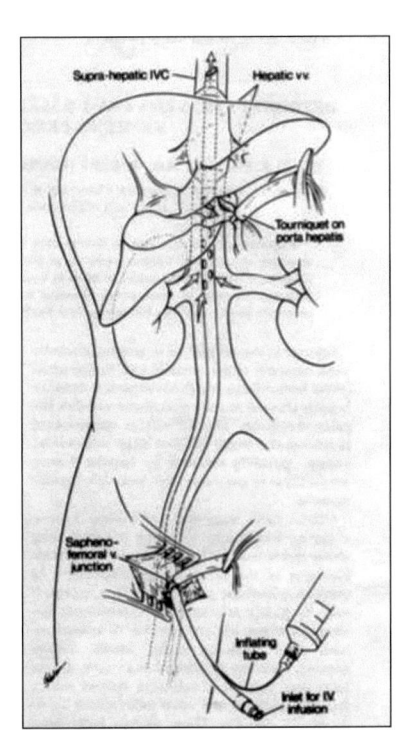

FIGURE 20-7. A Vena Caval shunt inserted via the Sapheno-femoral junction was developed at UVM by myself (DBP) and surgical resident E.E. Moore with medical student Kent Harman.

FIGURE 20-8. Richard Gamelli (upper left corner), Linda Sheehey, and Douglas McSweeney (Right) at a 1982 UVM ATLS course.

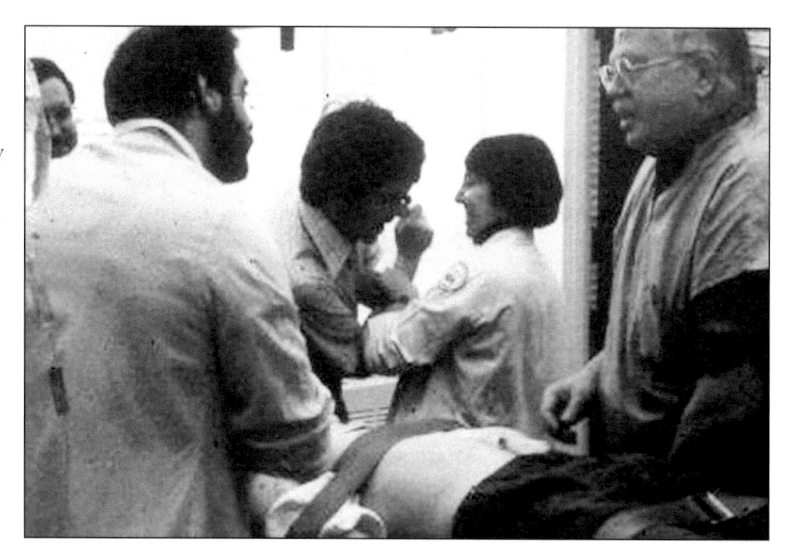

additional 43 of them during the first two years. We stuck to the rules by giving them their certificates after they got their MD degrees. We even traveled to Montreal in 1984 to give the first foreign ATLS course.

Gamelli and I shared the course directorship until pediatric surgeon Dennis Vane took over in 1989. Vane had been an ATLS instructor before coming to UVM, so he was a natural replacement. Linda Sheehey has been our one and only course coordinator since 1981. UVM still offers five ATLS courses a year.

ATLS instructor Eugene Grabowski of Bennington succeeded me as Chair of the Vermont COT. Vane, then Frederick Rogers and then Kennith Sartorelli, all of UVM, followed. Vane continued to spearhead the ATLS course during this time. He summed up this important undertaking thusly:

"It gives people a common language with which to deal with trauma patients. A trauma situation is a very stressful time. You have to be very methodical, so that you don't forget important things when treating the patient. Our course teaches you how to prepare, how to have the right people doing the right things, so that important things are never overlooked."[12]

Vermont ACS Chapter Meetings

Bishop McGill had preceded me as the Vermont Chairman for the COT. He convinced everyone that the Trauma Chair also served as the Program Chairman for the annual Vermont ACS Chapter meetings. Whether this had any basis in fact is unknown, but it left me as the Program Chair of the subsequent chapter meetings for more than ten years!

The best of these meetings was held one spring at the Mount Mansfield Trout Club in Stowe. Gordon Page commandeered the lodge for the meeting, along with a few other members of the exclusive organization. The restaurant's staff filleted and cooked the fish we caught from the Club's well-stocked pond and then served them for supper. Page, of course, caught the biggest trout!

We scheduled a screening of the movie "M*A*S*H". Richard Hornberger, author of the "M*A*S*H" book, agreed to come from Maine and give a presentation "provided he didn't

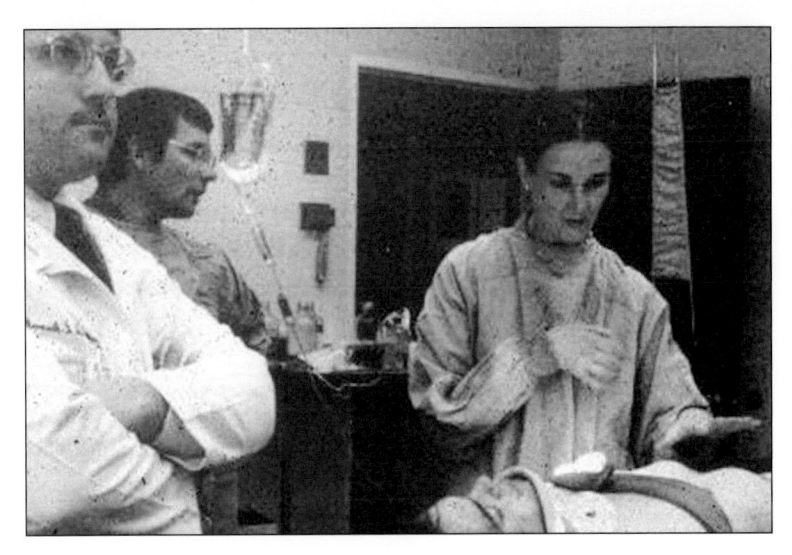

FIGURE 20-9. Gamelli (left), Fred Loy (Bennington surgeon), and Carrie Walters (UVM neurosurgery faculty) at the 1982 course.

have to watch the movie again." Hornberger cancelled at the last minute due to a "family emergency," but Davis filled in with his Korean War anecdotes. I completed the evening by showing movie footage that I had taken in Vietnam.

Most Vermont Chapter meetings were held at the Woodstock Inn. One year, we decided to put on a trauma symposium in emergency care. Our orthopaedic attendings staffed the femur and tibia and fibula fracture-splinting station. A surgeon from Brattleboro asked what should be done in order to get patients in better condition before transferring them to Burlington. Our UVM orthopaedist said: "Just get them to me as fast as you can, your treatment won't make any difference." This undid a lot of past good will towards UVM for years to come!

Critical Care Matures at UVM

Robert S. Deane (1933-1997) left his South African general practice in 1961 to become a UVM anesthesiology resident. During his voyage to the United States aboard a "tramp steamer," a passenger told Deane that great bargains were to be found at a certain east-coast car

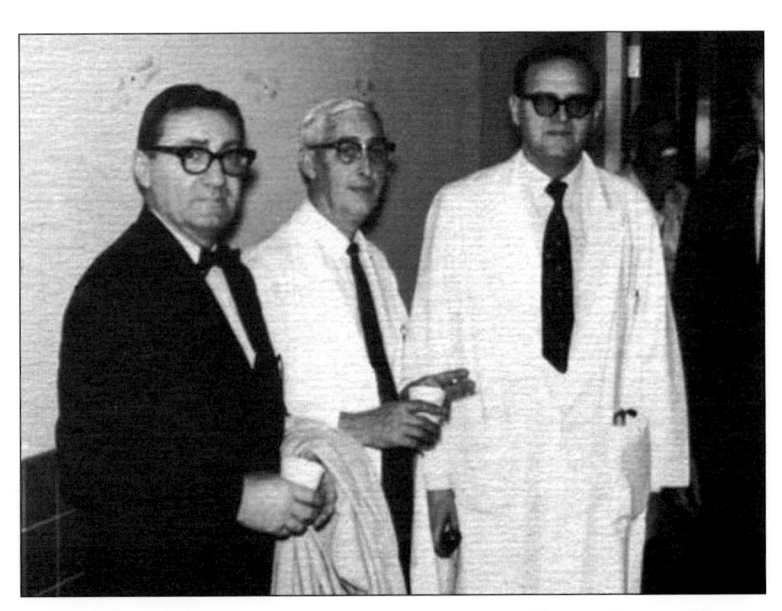

FIGURE 20-10. Ernie Mills (center) directed the ICU from 1961-65. Here he is meeting with Robert Deane (right), and Gino Dente (left).

Chapter Twenty: Trauma and Critical Care Division 295

FIGURE 20-11. Tamotsu (Tom) Shinozaki joined the ICU team in 1965.

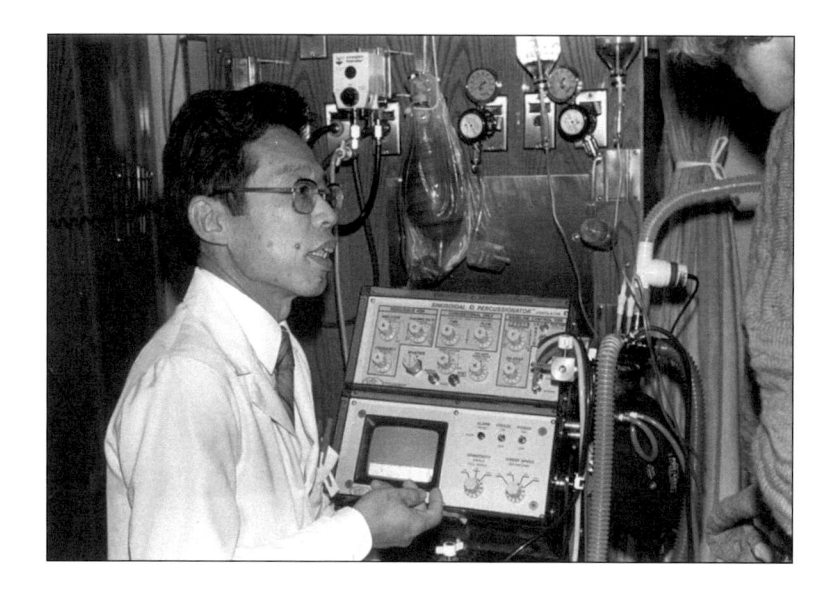

dealership. Deane arrived at said dealership, ready to pay cash for a new automobile. The salesman was so taken aback that he called John Mazuzan to vouch for Deane. After doing so, Mazuzan asked, "Where are you calling from?" The salesman replied, "Philadelphia." Mazuzan shot back, "Tell him he's going in the wrong direction."[13] Deane (who walked to work every day) ended up keeping his prized 1962 Plymouth convertible in showroom condition.

An Intensive Care Unit (ICU) had been started at the MFH shortly beforehand under the direction of Anesthesia's Ernest Mills. Deane, with his clinical background and newly acquired respiratory training, expressed an interest in critical care. Mills, meanwhile, was getting ready to step down. As Mazuzan tells it:

> *"When Mills retired in 1965, there were several anesthesiologists who could have been appointed to replace him, foremost being Eric Furman who had been at the MGH training in pediatric anesthesiology. The rumor of appointing Furman came to Deane's ears and ever the gentleman; he nevertheless let it be known that he was hurt by that idea, so Deane took over when Mills retired."*[14]

Deane was perfectly complemented by the engineering and mechanical skills of his fellow anesthesiologist Tamotsu "Tom" Shinozaki. The ICU, which treated medical and surgical

FIGURE 20-12. The 1962 ICU was an eleven-bed affair between Smith 2's operating suite and Patrick 2's patient wards.

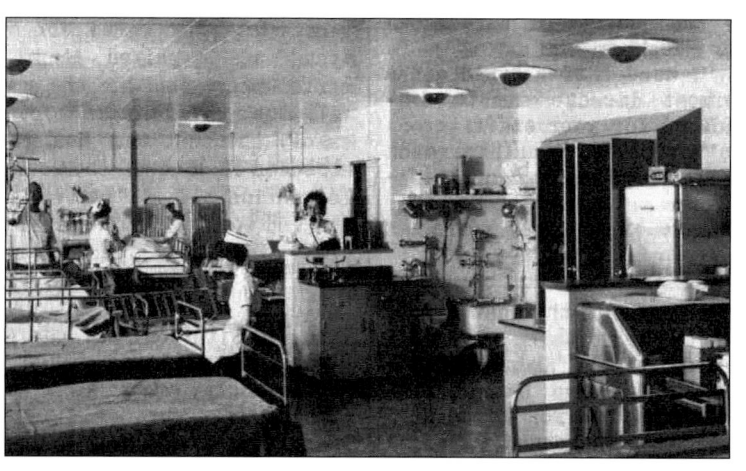

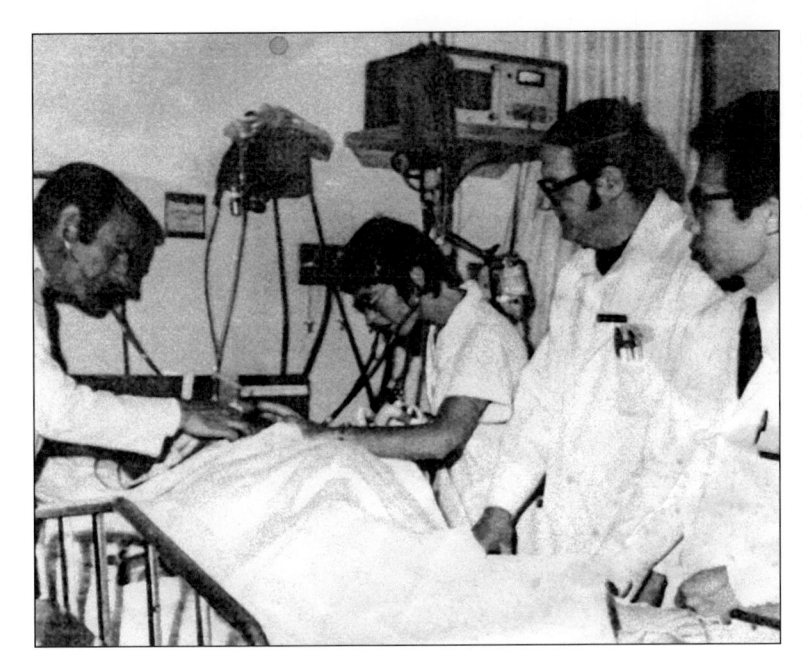

FIGURE 20-13. ICU rounds about 1972 (left to right): John Morgan, Wendy Marshall, Robert Deane, and Tom Shinozaki.

patients, grew increasingly busy over the next several years. This led to the recruitment of John Morgan in 1970. Deane, Shinozaki, and Morgan saw to the ventilators and respiratory care, although they also made other treatment suggestions. The surgeons were responsible for their own patients, but almost always followed the "suggestions" put forth by the ever-watchful anesthesiologists.

The medical service eventually established its own medical/pulmonary ICU one floor above the operating suites on Smith 3 in 1971. Deane hired Wendy Marshall, a physical therapist with respiratory experience, soon thereafter. Inspired by Deane and Morgan's example, Marshall went on to UVM medical school, and then pursued a career in critical care and trauma surgery at Loyola. She was one of many individuals who looked up to Deane and Shinozaki as role models.

The legendary pair had been synonymous with outstanding ICU care for almost 25 years at the time of Shackford's 1989 arrival. Shackford was board-certified in Critical Care, and felt that the surgeons should run the SICU. He and new vascular surgeon Ricci (who was also trained in critical care) shared call until full-time replacements were hired. Shackford had realized by then that a cooperative working relationship with anesthesia was appropriate. The two anesthesiologists' era came to an end a few years later. Deane was found to have end-stage pancreatic cancer — a condition that he stoically bore during his slow demise — while Shinozaki developed renal failure that necessitated a kidney transplant.

New Faculty Recruited for Trauma and Critical Care

Shackford brought Frederick B. Rogers in to head the Division of Trauma and Critical Care in 1990. Rogers had become interested in surgery and trauma while working as an EMT at Williams College. He was later intimately involved with the improvement of trauma care as a UVM medical student.[15] He went on to complete his residency and trauma fellowship at the University of Illinois' trauma rich Cook County Hospital. Rogers moved to the Chicago suburbs upon finishing his training where he organized a trauma center.

FIGURE 20-14. Frederick Rogers, Chief of the Division of Trauma and Critical Care, prepares a lecture using Kodachrome slides before the advent of PowerPoint.

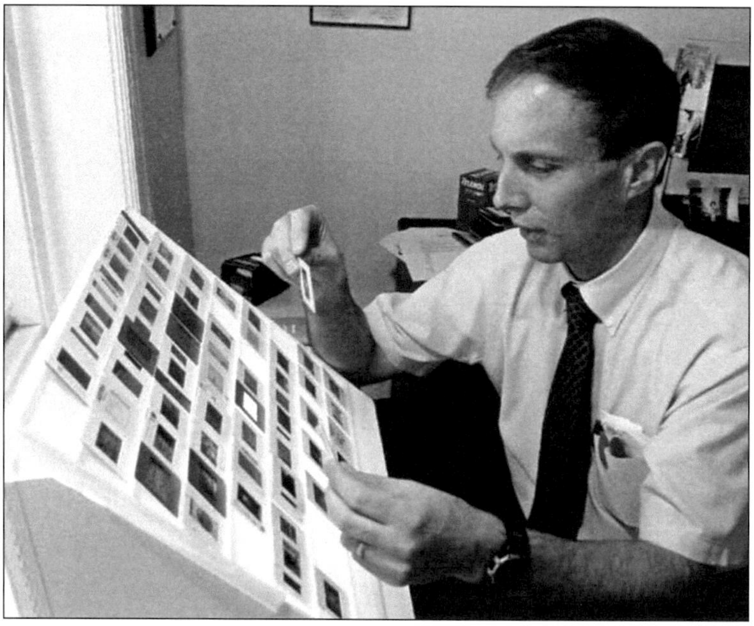

Rogers had always wanted to return to Vermont. When he heard that Gamelli was leaving for Loyola, he called Shackford at once. UVM cardiac surgeon Bruce Leavitt put in a good word for his former medical school classmate. Rogers was definitely in the right place at the right time; he came back to Burlington the same day that Gamelli left.

Krista L. Kaups, fresh out of her UMass critical care fellowship, was hired around the same time. She was technically assigned to the SICU side of the division, while Rogers was designated the head of trauma. In reality, the pair split Burn/Shock/Trauma (BST) team duties, trauma call coverage, and weekly SICU rotations, the latter of which were always conducted alongside either Deane or Shinozaki. The arrangement lasted five years until Kaups took a similar position at the University of California at Fresno.

Turner M. Osler replaced Kaups in 1995. Osler's background and interests were wide-ranging, to say the least. He had started out as a neurosurgery resident but switched to general practice and then general surgery with the Alaska Native Health Service. This was followed by a burn surgery fellowship in Galveston, Texas. Osler moved on to the University of New

FIGURE 20-15. The ICU team in 1998 (left to right): G-1 resident Patrick Forgione, unidentified medical student, Steven Shackford, Todd Havener G-3 orthopaedic resident, G-1 resident Lawrence Novak, Frederick Rogers, and Turner Osler.

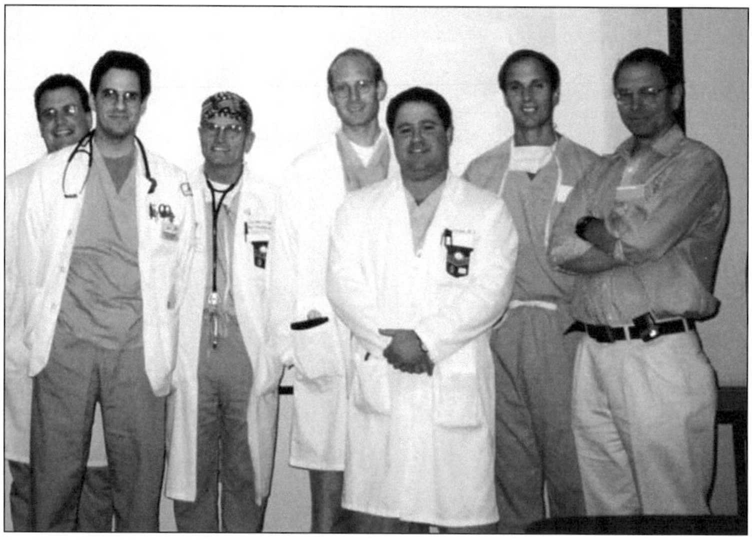

Mexico for an eight year run directing the SICU, the burns and trauma service, and the burn unit.

Osler immediately upgraded UVM's burn care upon his arrival. Fascination with probabilities and predictions led to the study of advanced statistics. Osler was allowed to take a half-time sabbatical in order to get a master's degree in the subject. Conflicts arose, however, when the trauma and SICU services grew busier than anticipated. Osler, having been called back into service one too many times, finally resigned from the clinical staff in 2000. He has continued to assist the Department with its statistical research needs ever since.

Research Strengthens Under Shackford

Once the new critical care team was set, Shackford started a new basic science research program. Building on his background and an NIH grant, he conducted a number of studies of traumatic brain injury using a swine model. Initial projects focused on resuscitation. A number of permutations soon evolved. Among these was resuscitation with isotonic versus hypertonic saline, and immediate versus delayed resuscitation. Later studies looked at variables affecting oxygen delivery and secondary brain injury.

A few clinical resuscitation trials followed, but were hampered by the small numbers of eligible patients. Shackford later examined the more global realms of trauma care delivery in a rural setting, the epidemiology of traumatic deaths, injury severity scoring, and critical care quality assurance. He somehow found time to promote the Focused Abdominal Sonogram for Trauma (FAST) exam through the ACS alongside national leaders Edward Staren and Grace Rozycki. Shackford, like Davis, also served a term as AAST president.

Rogers, in the meantime, was an early adopter when it came to placing vena cava filters in critically injured patients. UVM's blunt trauma victims, with their head injuries and broken bones, were perfectly suited for this non-coagulopathic method of deep vein thrombo-embolic prophylaxis. A number of papers outlining short and long-term ICU filter deployment outcomes were subsequently compiled. Rogers also worked in tandem with Shackford on population-based trauma care delivery studies.

UVM Achieves a Level I Trauma Center First

Trauma centers, such as the one in which Rogers trained at Cook County, had sprouted up across the country during the '70s and '80s. In order to ensure national standards, the American College of Surgeons developed a trauma center ranking system. Among the criteria were hospital volume, staffing, and sub-specialty coverage. Some services had to have staff surgeons on hand 24 hours a day, while others merely had to provide availability within certain time constraints. Levels ranged from I to III, with I being the highest. All Level I trauma centers were located in large, urban tertiary referral hospitals that were dedicated to injury research, education, and prevention programs.

In 1991 Shackford charged Rogers with attaining Level I trauma status verification for UVM. This turned out to be a huge undertaking. UVM's physicians were entrenched in their routines, many of which were not in compliance with ACS Level I trauma center standards.

There had been fifteen or so surgeons taking trauma call. This number was reduced to a core of five that were willing to arrive within minutes of a "trauma alert." Rogers also worked with the rescue squad, the E.R., and the Departments of Anesthesia, Radiology, and Orthopaedics in order to meet the ACS guidelines.

The verification went through with flying colors in 1994. Vane had assisted Rogers throughout the endeavor. Building on UVM's model land transport system for premature infants, Vane obtained separate pediatric verification in the process. This made UVM the first rural hospital to achieve both adult and pediatric Level I trauma status. The hospital has been successfully re-verified every three years since then.

Today's Critical Care Staff

Osler's place was filled on a temporary, yet unsustainable basis. Rogers covered the SICU by himself again, although Vane pitched in and took a few call nights each month. Word spread through the trauma network that UVM was looking for a critical care leader. Help finally came in July of 2003 when William E. Charash was appointed SICU director, giving Rogers some much-needed relief.

Charash had gone to medical school at Cornell, and then trained at Albany. This was followed by a trauma and critical care fellowship at Tennessee under Timothy Fabian. Charash practiced in Lexington, Kentucky for the next few years, before being sidetracked by private enterprise. Putting his inventiveness and PhD in physiology to good use (in conjunction with a million-dollar NIH Small Business Innovative Research program grant) he helped develop a novel near-infrared spectroscopy catheter. The device has since been used to detect vulnerable coronary artery plaques and to measure the inflammatory response following resuscitation from hemorrhagic shock.[16]

Charash has collaborated with vascular surgery's Ricci to expand the trauma side of telemedicine. He has also tried to conduct more clinical critical care research, but has been limited by the ACS-based national registry system currently in place. In that system, outcomes from a representative proportion of trauma cases can be compared with other hospitals nationwide, but physicians cannot alter data entry points in order to customize the data. Charash is also interested in bringing more protocols and evidence-based medicine to the SICU.

Bruce A. Crookes joined Charash within five months. Crookes had been at Mt. Sinai for medical school and Abington Memorial Hospital for residency. He then completed fellowships in critical care and trauma at the University of Miami. Crookes has carried on Shackford's swine research model of traumatic brain injury. He was named director of the trauma division following Rogers' 2008 departure to set up a trauma center at Pennsylvania's Lancaster General Hospital.

The division continues to uphold Davis and Shackford's legacies. It does so clinically by caring for over 1000 critically injured patients a year and providing on-line consultations 24/7 through telemedicine links with the region's community hospitals. And it does so educationally by conducting research at the basic science and clinical levels, in addition to teaching students and the next generation of physicians ATLS and emergency care.

CHAPTER 21

Neurosurgery Division

The Division of Neurosurgery achieved international prominence under R.M.P. Donaghy's watchful eye. His developments of microneurosurgery and the innovative extra-cranial to intra-cranial (EC/IC) bypass are landmarks in modern medicine.

His successor, Henry Schmidek, edited a wildly successful textbook that is still considered the gold standard for neurosurgical education. More academician than administrator, he was supplanted by dynamic clinician and scientist Cordell Gross.

Gross brought the Division back from the brink, but was struck down by cancer before he could fully implement his ideas. The revival of neurosurgery at UVM continues as a work in progress under Bruce Tranmer.

Diseases of the Mind and Nervous System

While it is true that John Pomeroy and Nathan Smith performed trephinations and elevated depressed skull fractures, surgical treatment of the nervous system at UVM was largely unknown for most of the 19th century. The first Special Professors in the "diseases of the mind and nervous system" arrived during the chairmanship of James L. Little. Among these were former Civil War Surgeon General William Alexander Hamilton and William James Morton, the son of William T.G. Morton — the Boston dentist who "discovered" anesthesia.[1]

If a surgeon in Burlington of this early era did attempt a neurosurgical operation, it was usually done under the supervision of a visiting New York or Montreal neurologist. Spinal procedures fell under the domain of UVM's orthopaedists during the 1910s — about the same time that Harvey Cushing was establishing neurosurgery as its own distinct discipline. Former UVM chief Lyman Allen took an interest in the subject, but was hardly a specialist. Patients with serious head injuries or brain tumors were sent to either Boston or Montreal for treatment well into the 1940s. This all changed with the arrival of UVM's first dedicated neurosurgeon in 1946.[2]

R.M.P. Donaghy: In the Beginning

Canadian-born Raymond Madiford Peardon "Pete" Donaghy (1911-1991) had grown up in Plainfield, Vermont living near the poverty line. Luckily, his grades earned him a full UVM scholarship right as the Great Depression hit the state. He underwrote his housing costs with a proctorship and obtained free milk from the dairy school. Donaghy enrolled at the College of Medicine in 1933. He soon became fascinated with the intricate procedures and rapid decision-making presented by the burgeoning field of neurosurgery.

Donaghy did a preceptorship with Leon Sample of St. Albans, Vermont. One of Sample's patients was a woman with a complex neurological condition. Donaghy studied her problem extensively and then presented her case to a visiting Montreal neurologist. The neurologist was so impressed that he offered Donaghy an internship and a neurology residency at Montreal General Hospital. Donaghy accepted instantly, since this gave him a chance to return to his native Quebec and put his bilingual skills to good use.

Donaghy stayed at Montreal General for another year, and then did a year in surgery at Montreal Children's Hospital at Winfield Penfield's urging. The outbreak of World War II put an end to research plans at London's National Hospital for Neurology and Neurosurgery, so he completed a neurosurgery fellowship at the Lahey Clinic. A neurosurgery residency followed at the Massachusetts General Hospital under chief neurosurgeon William Jason Mixter and neuropathologist Charles Kubic.[3]

In 1942, Donaghy, by now a trained neurosurgeon, enlisted in the Army. He was sent to Fort Sam Houston and then to England with the other specialists of the First Auxiliary Surgical Group. After conducting basic research on nerve injuries and frostbite, he was mobilized for the Normandy Invasion. Donaghy's Neurosurgical Unit consisted of two neurosurgeons, one anesthesiologist, one operating room nurse, and several technologists.

The other "surgeon" was Lester J. Wallman (1912-2007), a Yale medical graduate with just a single year of neurosurgery training. The pair treated head and peripheral nerve injuries on the front lines in France and later, Germany. The Unit went back to the United States in preparation for a deployment to Japan. Donaghy, still suffering from pneumonia he had acquired in Europe, remained stateside.[4]

Donaghy was faced with two job options upon his 1946 discharge from the service, the neurosurgery position at UVM and a similar opportunity in Richmond, Virginia. Donaghy chose UVM since he was familiar with Burlington from his college days and wanted to be in a small town with a medical school. He later jokingly claimed that he had really come back because the skiing was poor in Virginia.

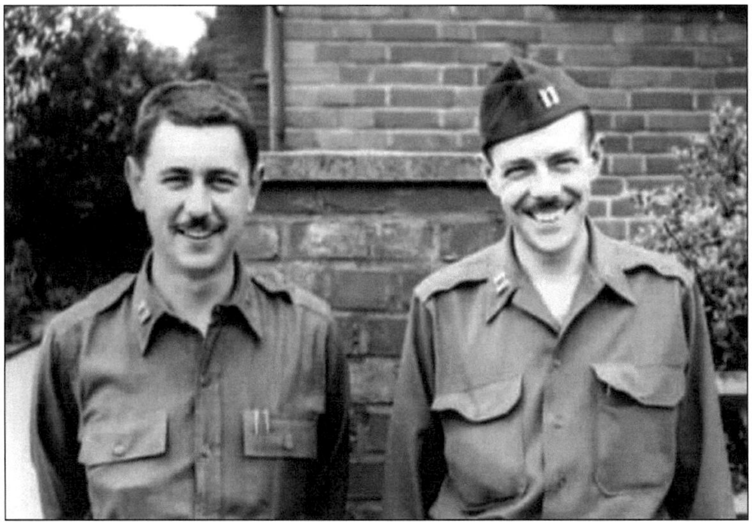

FIGURE 21-1. R.M.P. Donaghy (right) was joined by Lester Wallman (left) during World War II. The two campaigned as a special neurosurgical team throughout Europe.

The dean asked Donaghy to head a new Department of Neuroscience consisting of neurology, neurosurgery, and psychiatry. Donaghy had observed this combination before and felt that it did not work well. It was his opinion that the chairman's own field usually took precedence under this arrangement, so the other disciplines were seldom of first-rate quality. Donaghy's concerns led to the creation of the stand-alone Division of Neurosurgery within the Department of Surgery in 1946.

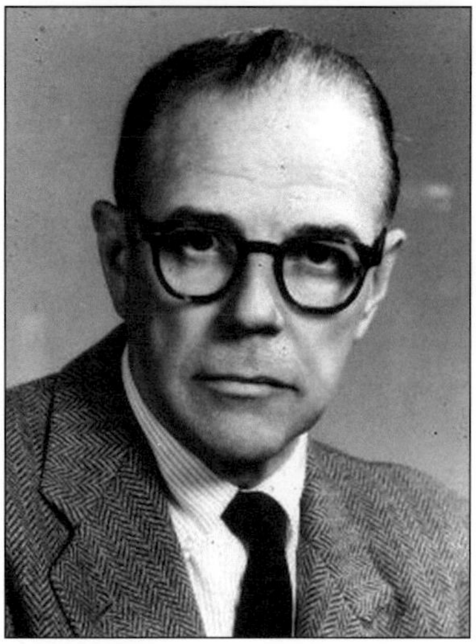

Donaghy wrote to Wallman and invited him to come to UVM as a fellow. His former Army colleague could complete his neurosurgical training and help run the service. Money for Wallman's salary was a problem, but the G.I. Bill contributed $100 a month, and the dean found additional funding. The compensation package even included farm vegetables obtained through a deal with the School of Agriculture. Donaghy himself was only paid $5,000 a year as a "part-time" faculty member, a sum that UVM expected to recoup through his clinical practice.

FIGURE 21-2. Donaghy came to UVM as Chief of Neurosurgery after the war and recruited Wallman to join him.

Research on a Shoestring Budget

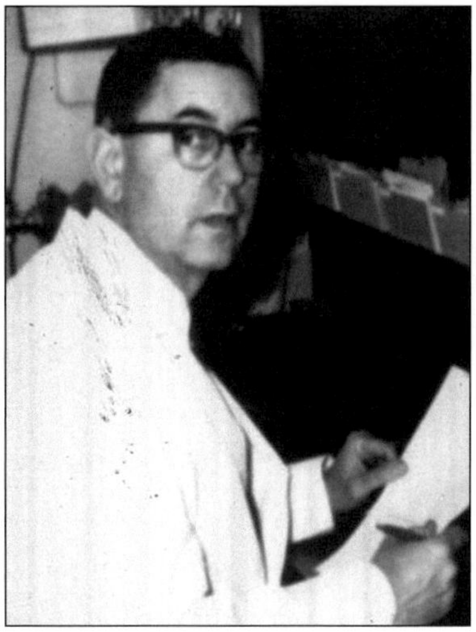

Donaghy started a neurosurgery research program in 1948. Funding, of course, remained an issue. The first year's budget was set at $25. The dean suggested that if Donaghy personally supplemented this meager amount, his donations could be tax deductible. The dean also donated a corner of the Physiology Department's Quonset hut and the use of the animal operating room. Discarded suture material and instruments were scrounged from the operating room, and experimental rats were somehow acquired.

Early experiments focused on peripheral nerve repair. Transected sciatic nerves were reattached either with or without systemic corticosteroids. The slides were saved and catalogued for year-end interpretation. Unfortunately, the identification "key" was lost along the way. As a result, the experimental slides could not be distinguished from the controls.[5] Donaghy later turned to stroke research that was funded by the Hartford Foundation and the Shattuck family.

Donaghy met pioneering microvascular surgeon Julius Jacobson soon after the latter's arrival at UVM. Jacobson's Medical Alumni Building basement research facility seemed to have an inexhaustible supply of funding and equipment. Donaghy knew that Jacobson's microscopic techniques could be applied to the repair of peripheral nerves and small, previously inaccessible intracerebral blood vessels. Donaghy spent hours in Jacobson's laboratory and soon became a superb microvascular surgeon.

He teamed with Jacobson in 1960 to clear an embolic occlusion from a middle cerebral artery. The procedure was partially successful, so it was followed by another such operation for thrombosis secondary to plaque.[6] Their work was presented at the Harvey Cushing

FIGURE 21-3. Wallman was accredited as a fellow under Donaghy in order to gain board certification. An excellent neurosurgeon, he spent his entire career at UVM.

FIGURE 21-4. Donaghy brought micro-vascular and micro-neurosurgery into the clinical operating room. Former Mary Fletcher head O.R. nurse Esther (Jackie) Roberts usually scrubbed with him.

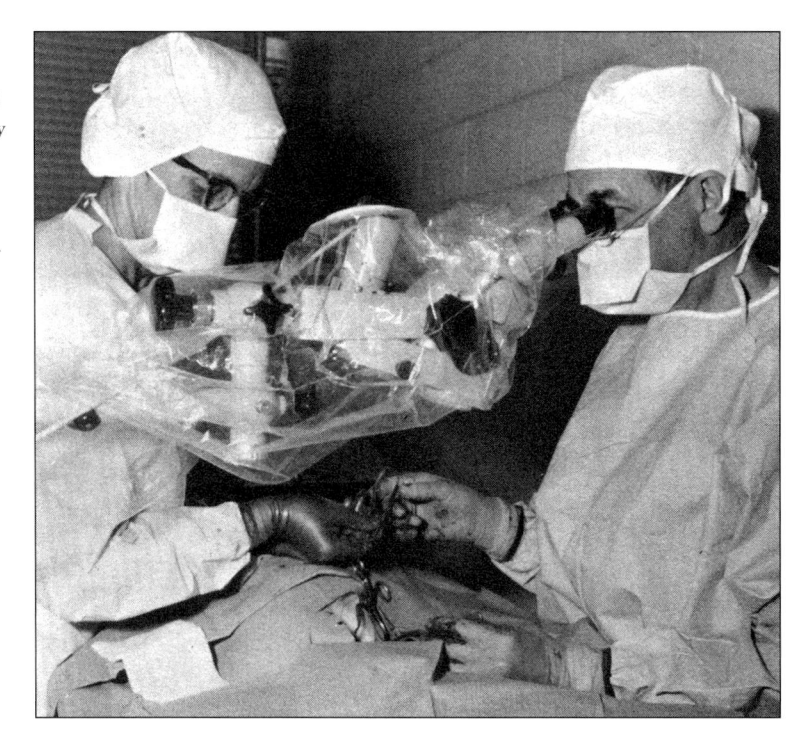

Society meeting on April 17, 1961 in Mexico City — the same day as the "Bay of Pigs" invasion. Jacobson still remembers the signs and chants of "Yanqui, go home" as he walked to the hotel to present the paper.[7] Two of nine middle cerebral endarterectomies were still patent as of 1962. Improved Zeiss microscopes, smaller sutures, and more delicate instruments soon improved the quality of their work.

Mitsuo Numoto joined the division in 1962. Numoto had been trained in biomechanics as well as neurosurgery. Working in the lab alongside Donaghy, he developed an intracranial pressure (ICP) monitor switch, which ultimately led to the development of the Ladd fiberoptic ICP monitor. Numoto also created a device to measure evoked potentials following spinal cord injuries. The pair also studied the cause and mechanism of fat emboli arising from long bone fractures. They came up with some interesting observations over the years, but no earthshaking breakthroughs. Numoto worked in Donaghy's lab until 1974, before moving on to Okayama, Japan.

FIGURE 21-5. Gazi Yasargil studied with Donaghy at UVM before widely disseminating such micro-vascular techniques as the extra-cranial-to-intra-cranial (ECIC) bypass.

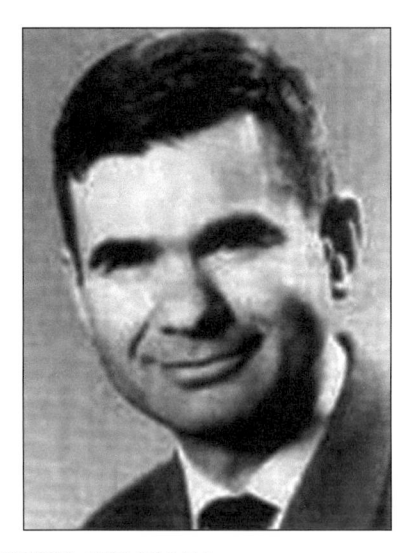

The Yasargil Connection and EC/IC

M. Gazi Yasargil left the University of Zurich in November 1965 to work with Jacobson, who had since taken a position at Mount Sinai. Yasargil started in New York, but was sent to UVM shortly thereafter at Jacobson's suggestion to spend a year with Donaghy. Yasargil's studies were funded with a $2000 Hartford Foundation grant.

Yasargil was brilliant and dynamic, but often provoked his peers. Donaghy was brilliant too, but reserved and beloved by his peers. Yasargil promoted and expanded Donaghy's ideas. He gave Donaghy his due, but overshad-

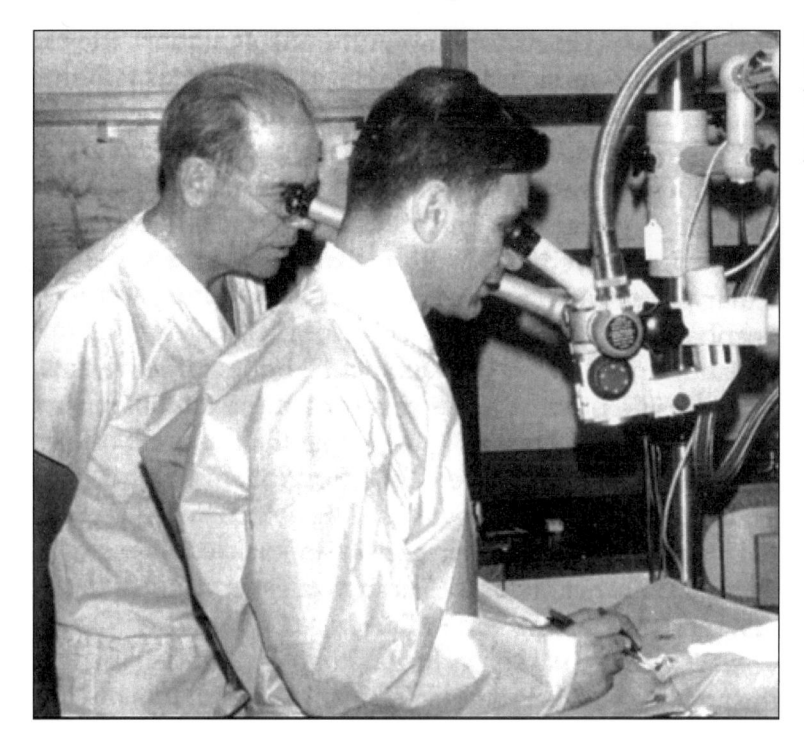

FIGURE 21-6. Donaghy and Yasargil working under the diploscope as a team.

owed him with his energy, huge caseload, and numerous publications. Yasargil returned to Zurich where he gained fame as the father of microneurovascular surgery. It can be argued that the title was more deserving of Yasargil's teacher, Donaghy.

Yasargil, however, did come up with the idea for the superficial temporal artery to middle cerebral artery anastomosis for occlusive cerebrovascular disease. Yasargil and Donaghy developed the operation, also known as the extra-cranial to intra-cranial (EC/IC) bypass, in tandem. The first procedure on a human was performed in Zurich on Oct 30, 1967. The second was done in Burlington one day later. The Burlington bypass remained patent until the patient's death in 1978.[8] Yasargil's publications, including a book on the subject, led to his designation as a pioneer. The quiet, more modest Donaghy's recognition came later.

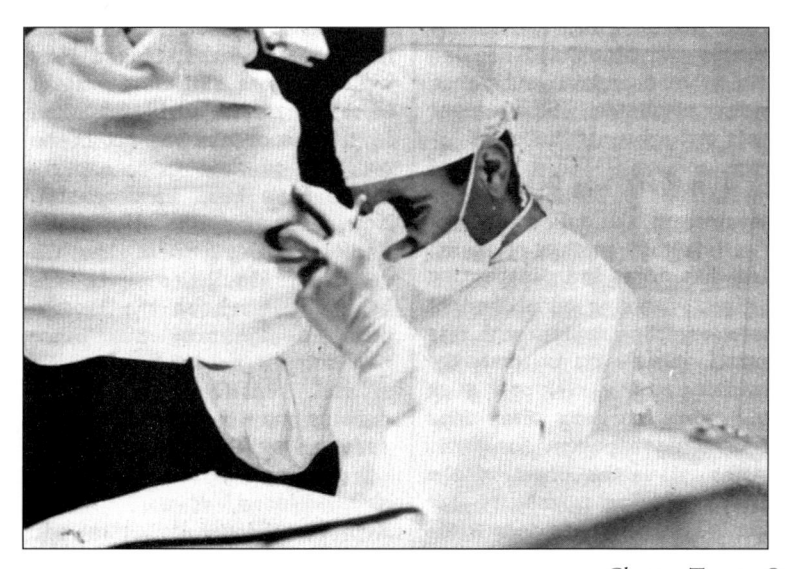

FIGURE 21-7. Yasargil working at the UVM Surgical Research Lab in 1960.

EC/IC lost favor in 1985 after a controlled study failed to demonstrate its efficacy. Although the post-op patency rate was 96%, the 30-day mortality stroke rate was 2.5% versus only 0.6% in the control group.[9] The study's operative indications were somewhat broad, however. EC/IC has regained some of its popularity recently, as there are some situations in which it is both indicated and beneficial. UVM's two most recent chairs, Gross and Tranmer, have each performed successful procedures in Burlington.

International microneurovascular surgery conferences were held in Burlington in 1966 and 1969. Donaghy also ran a hands-on practical laboratory course for visiting neurosurgeons. Grafting and microsuturing were taught using rat carotid arteries and rabbit superficial epigastric arteries (a branch of the femoral artery in the leg). Course attendees returned to their communities ready to perform EC/IC bypasses.

Donaghy enticed Esther (Jackie) Roberts RN to leave the O.R. in order to lead the microvascular lab course. Jackie was technically accomplished in her own right. Self-important visiting surgeons sometimes had a hard time accepting instructions from a nurse — until they realized that their success hinged on Jackie's expertise. Yasargil actually credited her as "my main teacher in microtechniques."[10] Jackie taught her successor, Elaine Lavigne, who kept the course going for many years.

Plastic and hand surgeons continued to come to Burlington throughout the 1970s for microvascular training. As late as 1979, the course was still taught by Donaghy with help from orthopedic hand surgeon Philip Davis, general surgeon Richard Gamelli, and ENT surgeon Robert Sofferman. Plastic surgeons Peter Linton and David Leitner, and I (DBP) occasionally chipped in. The UVM microvascular lab continued long after Donaghy's retirement and subsequent death. As Wallman later put it:

"He [Donaghy], more than anyone else, is responsible for having introduced the microscope into neurosurgery. His efforts have made possible surgical accomplishments with acoustic neuromas, aneurysms, arteriovenous malformations, and intramedullary tumors of the spinal cord which were not previously possible. It would be difficult to over-rate what he has done." [11]

FIGURE 21-8.
In 1980, Donaghy continued to work in the micro-surgical laboratory after his retirement where he served as an inspiration to all.

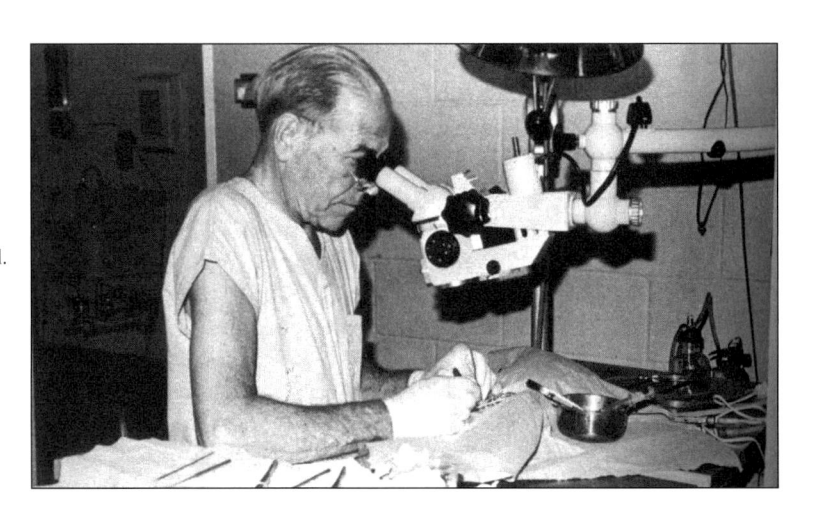

Beyond Microvascular Neurosurgery

Donaghy's inquiring mind was always active. He was convinced that clamping the carotid artery during an endarterectomy, even momentarily, deprived the brain of oxygen. His solution was to cannulate the femoral artery and send circulating blood to the brain via a roller pump and a needle placed in the internal carotid artery above the level of the stenosis. Donaghy's system eliminated any chance of temporary cerebral ischemia, but it was complex and time consuming. Meanwhile, his fellow surgeons were obtaining superb results with internal shunts and other methods of cerebral protection. In the end, Donaghy's idea was a blind end, and won no converts.[12]

Carotid endarterectomies were (and still are) done to reduce the risk of stroke. Donaghy's concern about the effects of cerebral ischemia led him to wonder if correcting a stenotic carotid artery might also lead to improved brain function. He performed psychometric testing both pre- and post- operatively, but was unable to prove any benefit from revascularization.[13]

Donaghy retired in 1976 at the age of 65 after a nearly 30 year run at UVM. Wallman succeeded him as chief, presiding over the division for the next one and a half years. Wallman, however, was also nearing retirement age. He thought that the ensuing chief should be younger, and not at the end of his career.

Henry Schmidek Builds a Department and Then Leaves

Donaghy, who had maintained his ties to the Massachusetts General Hospital (MGH), called chief neurosurgeon William Sweet, and asked for a recommendation. Sweet suggested one of his recent graduates, Henry H. Schmidek (1937-2008). Schmidek had trained in Ontario and Montreal before going to the MGH. He then became the chief of neurosurgery at Philadelphia's Hahnemann University, the youngest person to hold such a position at that time. Schmidek was approached in 1978, and subsequently decided to move to Vermont even though he had only been at Hahnemann for two years. He thought it would be a good place to raise his children and build a neurosurgical program.

Somehow forgetting that he had given Schmidek's name to Donaghy in the first place, Sweet told his former resident not to take the position! Sweet posed some valid concerns. The first was that neurosurgery was a division of surgery, and not an independent department. The second was that Donaghy and Wallman were essentially retired, leaving the division with one clinical neurosurgeon, Martin Flanagan. Finally, the staffing void had led to a reduction in cases, which in turn had led to probation for the UVM neurosurgery residency program.

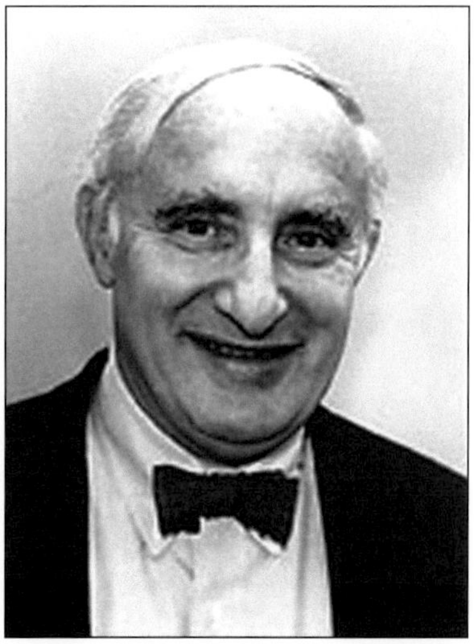

Schmidek had taught himself to use the operating microscope before coming to UVM. Nevertheless, he still took Jackie Roberts's lab class upon his arrival. He became the titular head of the microvascular course. Schmidek set

FIGURE 21-9. Henry Schmidek came to UVM during a period of turmoil. Martin Flanagan was the only active faculty member in a Division on probation.

about reassembling the division. He contacted Yasargil, who had since become the Director of Neurosurgery at Zurich's University Hospital. Yasargil loved Vermont, but never seriously considered the offer for obvious reasons.

Help soon came in a different manner, when Schmidek went with youth over experience. Low starting salaries may have played a role, though Schmidek (who was still only 43) may not have wanted to be outnumbered by more senior partners. Carol L. (Carrie) Walters thus arrived in 1980 fresh out of a fellowship with the Public Health Service. The Northwestern University medical school alumna and University of Chicago residency graduate was considered such a novelty in the male-dominated discipline, that she garnered a feature story in People magazine![14]

Walters was brought onboard to do vascular neurosurgery, such as aneurysm clippings. The clippings however fell to Schmidek. Walters often had to do complex back cases. These were sometimes performed with Martin Krag of orthopaedics. Flanagan, in the meantime, was excising herniated discs using the microscope. Schmidek recalled that 60% of the division's cases during this era were spinal in nature.

Another young hire was pediatric neurosurgeon Steven Wald. The University of Cincinnati neurosurgery resident was about to finish his pediatric training at Toronto's Hospital for Sick Children. He had expected to join a practice group in Cincinnati, but political upheaval eliminated the job. Wald was then offered a spot in Toronto, but would have had to renounce his U.S. citizenship in order to accept it! After talking to Schmidek, Wald decided to remain on this side of the border. His July 1981 arrival coincided with the return of cardiac surgeon Frank Ittleman.

Schmidek was in the process of writing a textbook in conjunction with his old chief, Sweet. Wald was asked to contribute four chapters. Linton, Leitner, Sofferman, Walters, and neurosurgery resident John Duckworth also wrote chapters. Schmidek was characterized as an outstanding editor by his peers with great insight and productivity. "Schmidek and Sweet's Operative Neurosurgical Techniques" was exceedingly successful, and is currently in its 5th edition.[15]

The book's popularity led to greater national prominence for Schmidek. He was frequently unavailable due to his increasing out-of-town obligations. Flanagan, now approaching his 60s, did not relish taking extra call. Walters, meanwhile, was not being used to her full potential, so she went to Arizona. This left Wald feeling overwhelmed covering both general and pediatric neurosurgery alone. When Walters called about an opportunity at a new Phoenix Children's Hospital, Wald went west too. The division's volume dwindled to around 200 cases a year and the residency program remained in jeopardy.

Sweet's warnings about neurosurgery's divisional status had come true as well. Schmidek, the chief of the Division, came into constant conflict with Davis, the chief of the Department. Schmidek, perceiving his loss of control of the staff and the division, left in 1985 to become Chief of Neurosurgery at the New England Deaconess Hospital, Consultant Neurosurgeon to the Dana Farber Cancer Institute, and a molecular genetics researcher at Harvard/MIT. After later stops at Henry Ford Hospital and Dartmouth, he retired to a farm in A.G. Mackay's hometown of Peacham, Vermont.

Cordell Gross Becomes Chief of a Phantom Division

Martin E. Flanagan (1930-2002) once again found himself as the only member of the division at the time of Schmidek and Wald's departures. Flanagan had been with the division almost from the beginning, first as a 1950s-era College of Medicine student and then as UVM's first neurosurgery resident. He had joined the staff in 1962, focusing primarily on spinal procedures. Flanagan was very supportive of the residents, but did not conduct much in the way of basic or clinical research. As such, he knew that he was to remain chief only on an interim basis.

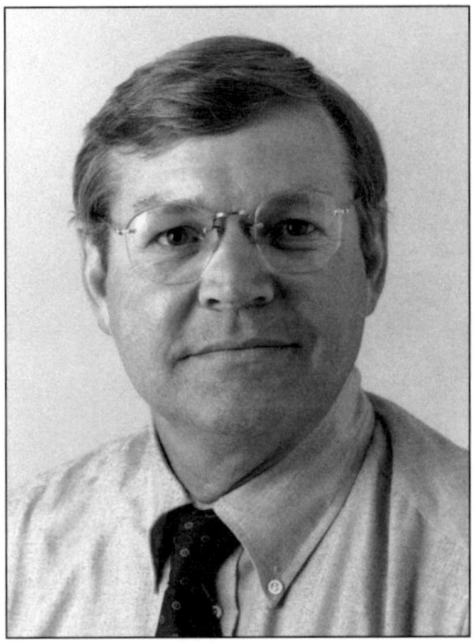

A search committee was convened and appropriate candidates were screened. The selection, Cordell E. Gross (1942-2000), proved ably suited to continue Donaghy's legacy. Gross had New England roots, but grew up in Florida. After attending the University of Florida for both college and medical school, he took an internship at Yale. A neurosurgery residency at SUNY Syracuse under Robert King followed this. Gross obtained an academic appointment at the University of Iowa in 1977. He became Iowa's EC/IC specialist, and played a part in the previously mentioned landmark study of that procedure. Gross moved on to the University of Colorado in 1982, before becoming chief of neurosurgery at Loma Linda in 1986.

FIGURE 21-10. Cordell Gross arrived in time to right a still foundering neurosurgical ship.

Gross arrived at UVM in 1987 to find a tired, overworked Flanagan manning the fort. Graduating UVM neurosurgery resident Nancy Binter had decided to stay in Burlington, and she had a strong interest in spinal cases. Gross and Flanagan were already entrenched in that practice. Binter went into private practice. Another recent graduate, Paul Penar, was recruited instead. Penar had attended medical school at the University of Michigan and then trained at Yale. His keen interest in neurological oncology complemented the rest of the division's strengths. Wald, meanwhile, had realized that the "Children's Center" position was not going to work out after all, so he came back to UVM in 1988.

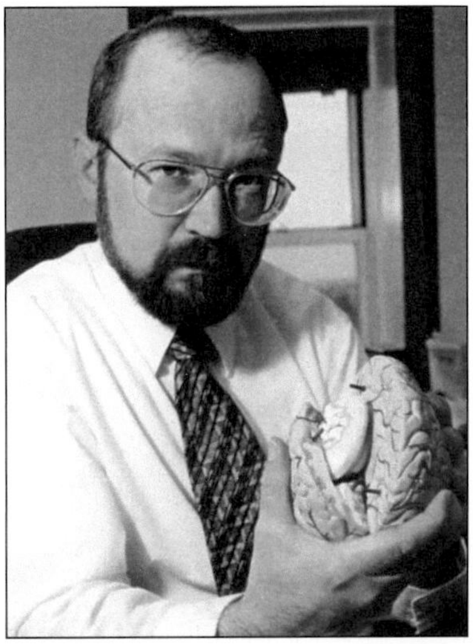

Gross was clinically superb and rapidly restored the operative volume. He was an outstanding hands-on teacher who inspired loyalty among the staff. Demanding high standards of the residents, he successfully rebuilt the training program. Gross championed the underdog, and usually saw the good side of colleagues and residents that others failed to appreciate. An excellent experimental neurophysiologist, he succeeded Richard Gamelli as the Department of Surgery's director of research in 1990. He also served as Vice Chair of the Department of Surgery.

FIGURE 21-11. Clinical and research productivity took off once Paul Penar (pictured), Steven Wald, and Martin Bednar joined the Gross team.

Gross was an idea man who recruited staff that could write grants, implement plans, and bring projects to fruition. Gross studied cerebral ischemia in a rabbit model and human electrical muscle stimulation in an attempt to help paralyzed patients walk. The procedure was tried on Davis following his paralysis, but it did not work. Gross asked UVM neurosurgery resident Martin Bednar to join the faculty and to work in the research lab in 1992. Their collaboration was successful and yielded prolific publications.

Angiography-guided coiling and balloon occlusion of intracranial aneurysms was developed in Europe during the 1990s. The technique was safer and less invasive than the traditional method of open clipping. When Gross was unable to find someone to bring the procedure to UVM, he characteristically said, "I'll do it myself." A three-month sabbatical at the University of Vienna followed in 1996. Gross returned with the requisite skills, but was impeded by the lack of regular access to the radiology suite. The idea was timely, but an aggressive colon cancer was discovered in the fall of 1996. Gross went on sick leave and the attending staff rallied and pulled together. Gross continued to work in the laboratory and on research projects at Woods Hole.

In under two years metastatic disease incapacitated him further and he participated in the search for a new chief, while Wald directed the department.

Tranmer Resuscitates the Division

A new chief was selected. The candidate, however, turned down the position at the last minute. Another search began. Wald threw his hat into the ring this time. The search committee chose external candidate Bruce I. Tranmer. Wald decided that another move was in order, so he took a job in Dayton, Ohio at the end of 1999. Bednar left shortly thereafter for a non-clinical position with a pharmaceutical firm. Flanagan had finally retired in 1994, so it was now Penar's turn to help keep the division afloat. Binter, still in private practice, graciously helped with the call schedule.

Tranmer, like Donaghy, was born in Canada. He had gone to medical school at Queen's University and trained in neurosurgery at the University of Toronto. Tranmer worked with Gross at the University of Colorado in the mid-80s, before going to Europe on a nine-month traveling fellowship. While there, he had the opportunity to study with Yasargil in Zurich. Then it was on to the University of Calgary, where he helped duplicate the cerebral blood flow machine that he had developed in Colorado. Tranmer then became chief of neurosurgery at New York's Albany Medical College in 1995.

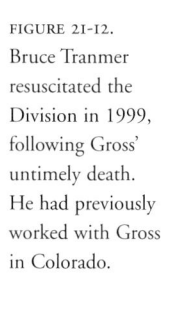

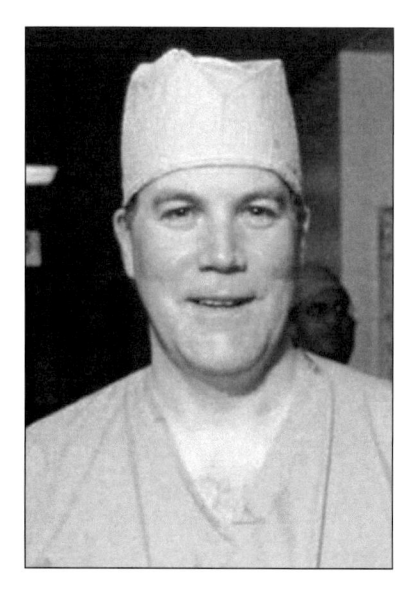

FIGURE 21-12. Bruce Tranmer resuscitated the Division in 1999, following Gross' untimely death. He had previously worked with Gross in Colorado.

One of Tranmer's first UVM recruits was Michael Horgan in 2000. Horgan was finishing a skull base and cerebrovascular fellowship in Portland, Oregon. A neurosurgery residency preceded this in the same city, so he was glad to return to his native New England. In addition to his fellowship skills, Horgan brought minimally invasive discectomies and spine fusions to UVM. He is currently initiating a study comparing transnasal versus transoral odontoid excision.

Horgan required a skull base lab, which Tranmer guaranteed even though he didn't have the funds. In an inspired move, the pair asked the Zeiss Company to support a lab dedicated to Donaghy, the father of microneurosurgery. Zeiss agreed and donated five operating microscopes. The lab was initially housed in UVM's remote pig facility, but returned to its former Given Building home in 2003. It is believed to be the only microneurosurgery lab in New England. Every New England neurosurgery resident attends a four-day course each year of their residency held at this lab with a visiting professor.

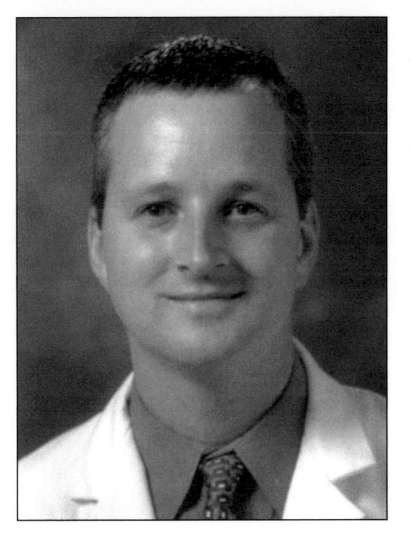

FIGURE 21-13. Michael Horgan's arrival buoyed the Department at a critical time.

Todd Maugans rounded out the division in 2000, filling the pediatric neurosurgery position vacated by Wald. Maugans had been in the Family Practice program at UVM before completing a neurosurgery residency at Dartmouth. He stayed until 2003, when he decided to take a similar job at Cincinnati Children's Hospital. The division's remaining members have shared straightforward pediatric cases since then.

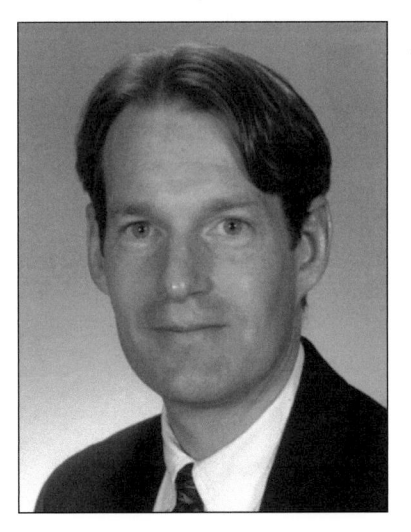

FIGURE 21-14. Todd Maugans filled the pediatric neurosurgery void created when Wald left.

Tranmer worked in collaboration with the Pharmacology Department to establish the Totman Center for Cerebrovascular Research. The lab studies the physiology of human arteries and the vascular consequences of established risk factors. One such investigation is looking at the incidence of late vasospasm-related stroke after subarachnoid hemorrhage or aneurysm rupture. Understanding the role that smooth muscle calcium channels play in this phenomenon may lead to improved outcomes.[16]

A regional outreach program coupled with Tranmer's upstate New York connections from his time in Albany helped restore the clinical volume lost in the wake of Gross' illness. As the referrals began to accumulate, it became clear that a spinal specialist was needed. The division hadn't offered much in the way of this service since Flanagan's retirement. The focus of spine surgery had been elsewhere. Luckily, Tranmer didn't have to look far for his next hire, Ryan Jewell.

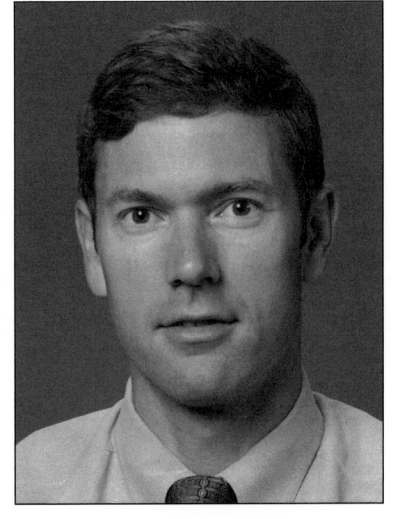

FIGURE 21-15. Ryan Jewell seemed destined for "anything but neurosurgery." Luckily for UVM, he embraced the discipline, sub-specializing in spinal surgery.

Jewell had been born at MCHV while his father was a medical student. The youngster was later taught by his vascular surgeon father (in jest) that neurosurgeons stole carotid endarterectomies from vascular surgeons and spinal cases from orthopods. Jewell, as a College of Medicine student, decided on an operative career in anything but neurosurgery. His attitude changed after he rotated through

Chapter Twenty-One: Neurosurgery Division

the discipline during his UVM internship. A month at Boston's Brigham and Women's Hospital was enough to convince Jewell that he needed to stay in Vermont, though. An opening occurred and he transferred directly into UVM's neurosurgery residency program.

Jewell joined the division in 2007 after completing a spine fellowship at the University of Alabama at Birmingham. As a known quantity, he has been able to work with the orthopaedic group on spinal cord trauma. Neurosurgery now receives unassigned spinal cord injury patients one fourth of the time. Jewell has also become the principal investigator for the division's first randomized, controlled trial. The Phase III study is evaluating a medication called Cethrin®, which blocks an axonal growth inhibitor. The thought is that the compound will promote spinal cord nerve repair when applied at the injury site during decompression surgery.[17] Perhaps a revival of an interdisciplinary spinal injury center is coming in the future.

Today's Division embodies Donaghy's innovation, Schmidek's academics, Flanagan and Wald's loyal service, and Gross' expertise and enthusiasm. It is well positioned to provide comprehensive clinical care and cutting-edge research.[18]

CHAPTER 22

Ophthalmology Division

Ophthalmology was tied to ENT until the 1950s. Research and a residency program were transient under part-time faculty members.

A full-time group was established during the Davis years and stationed at UHC. Division member Geoffrey Tabin organized and led an attack on blindness in the third world during the 1990s.

The division continues to provide excellent patient care and student instruction as a growing faculty in new facilities greets the 21st century.

Ophthalmology is Originally Combined with ENT

John Pomeroy, Nathan Smith, and Edward Phelps performed the ancient art of "couching the cataract" during their UVM tenures. The trio restored vision by pushing patients' opacified lenses to the sides of their eyes, out of the line of sight. They had access to Benjamin Bell's "A System of Surgery", which also demonstrated cataract removal as an alternative operation to couching the cataract. Bell advocated the liberal use of opium. Following either couching or cataract extraction, Bell recommended postoperatively:

> "For several days after the operation, no light should be admitted to the patient's apartment. A very low diet is absolutely necessary, and the eye being very apt to inflame, repeated blood lettings are frequently requisite from the jugular vein or the temporal artery."[1]

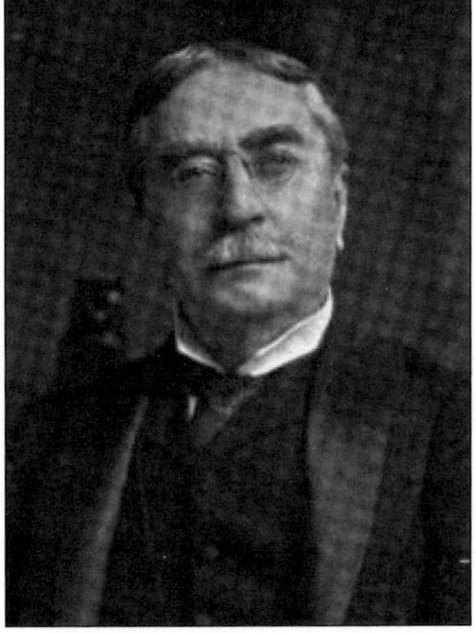

Smith lectured on "Dropsy of the Eye" and "Coagulated Substances on the Cornea" and operated on drooping eyelids, tumors of the eyelids, and cancerous eyes. He considered that the latter procedure, "On the whole [was] a simple operation".[2]

Daniel Bennett St. John Roosa (1838-1908) served as UVM's first Special Professor of "Diseases of the Eye and Ear" in 1875, and again during 1879-1883. The close friend of UVM chairman James L. Little and President Chester A. Arthur had conducted a special study of ophthalmology in

FIGURE 22-1. D.B. St. John Roosa was UVM's first Professor of Diseases of the Eye and Ear in 1875.

FIGURE 22-2. Benjamin Bell's, A System of Surgery, 1796 edition shows the following plate depicting cataract surgery. Figure 1: A needle is inserted into the anterior chamber to push or "couch" the cataract out of the line of vision. Figure 2: A scalpel is inserted through the cornea, and then either sliced up (Figure 3) or down (Figure 4) to allow the removal of the cataract. The text does not describe how this could be done without anesthesia!

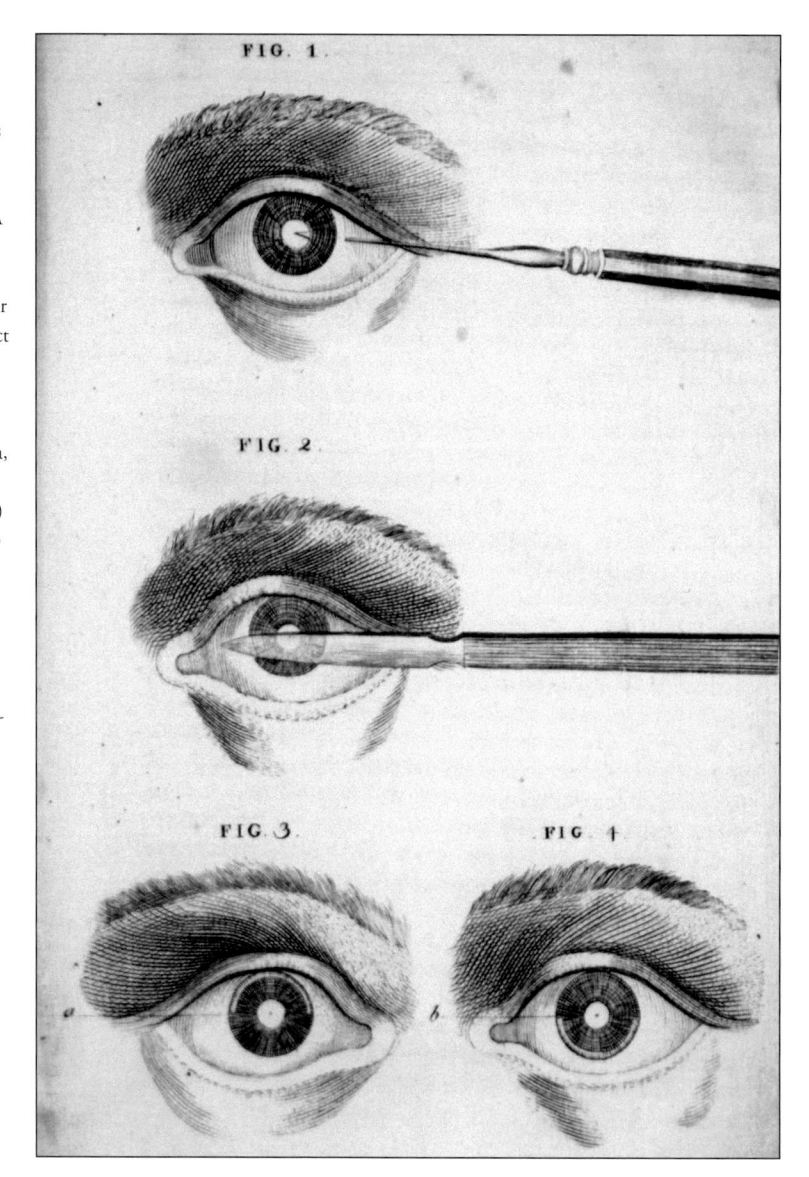

Vienna and Berlin during the 1860s. Roosa established the Manhattan Eye and Ear Hospital in 1869 and even gave the main address at the Mary Fletcher Hospital's 1879 dedication. He left UVM to found and preside over the New York Post-Graduate Medical School and Hospital.[3]

William O. Moore (1841-1930), one of Roosa's associates at the Post-Graduate, lectured at UVM from 1885-89. Moore had made headlines in 1884 by reporting the local anesthetic properties of Cocaine. Moore noted that, "the mydriatic [papillary dilatation] effect of cocaine is well marked and will make it a valuable contribution to our list, as ophthalmoscopic examinations can be made, and the inconvenience of atropine not be felt."[4]

Julius H. Woodward (1858-1916), the grandson of Benjamin Lincoln's old Castleton Medical School nemesis Theodore Woodward, was next. Woodward was a skilled ophthalmologist who also served as UVM's special professor of "Diseases of the Throat" during his 1889-1898 term. This cemented the relationship between Ophthalmology and ENT at UVM for the next 50 years. Woodward moved to New York City in 1897, where he eventually took Roosa's place as professor of ophthalmology at the Post-Graduate in 1908.[5]

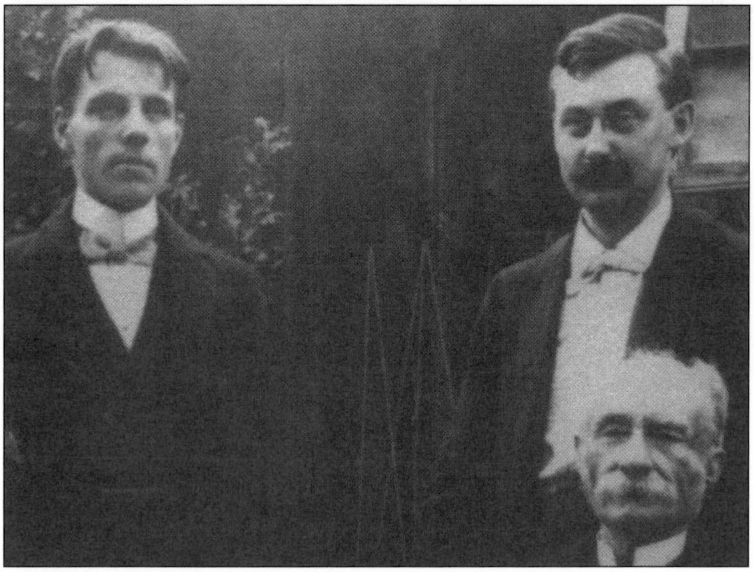

FIGURE 22-3. Emmus George Twitchell (top L) (younger stepbrother of MCT), Marshall Coleman Twitchell (top R) first Professor of EENT at UVM), and Marshall Harvey Twitchell (Bottom R).

The Twitchells of UVM

Marshall Coleman Twitchell (1871-1949) was Special Professor of "Diseases of Eye, Ear, and *Throat*" from 1899 to 1909, branching out into "Eye, Ear, *Nose*, and Throat" until 1917. He was succeeded by Edmund T. Brown (1871-1944), who in turn was followed by Twitchell's stepbrother, Emmus George Twitchell (1881-1963), in 1928. The younger Twitchell became the first chair of the formal Department of Ophthalmology, Otology, and Rhinology in 1938 as part of the College of Medicine's grand reorganization.

The Twitchells were the sons of Marshall H. Twitchell, a Union soldier from Vermont turned Reconstruction carpetbagger. The Elder Twitchell amassed cotton lands and political power in Louisiana while working for the Freedman's Bureau. He made a considerable number of enemies in the process, and was viciously attacked by a gang of white supremacists in 1876. The assassination attempt failed, but gunshot wounds to both arms necessitated double upper extremity amputation. Twitchell became a northern hero of sorts, and was named Consul to Canada in 1878 by President Rutherford B. Hayes.[6]

The Twitchell boys grew up in Kingston, Ontario as the sons of a famous, yet handicapped father. M.C. graduated from the College of Medicine in 1893, and then studied at the New York Ophthalmological and Aural Institute, the New York Eye and Ear Infirmary, and the Post-Graduate before coming to UVM. E.G. went to Queen's University in Kingston for medical school and, like M.C., attended the New York Eye and Ear Infirmary. He then came to UVM in 1914 to work with his stepbrother, joining the faculty in the process as an instructor.

M.C. was reportedly very difficult to work with in the O.R. According to past chairman A.G. Mackay, former attending Walford Rees learned this the hard way during his 1924 internship:

"As was Dr. Twitchell's habit when he was irritated with his assistant, he rapped Dr. Rees on the knuckles. Dr. Rees pulled back from the operating table and pulled off his gloves, and Dr. Twitchell said, 'Where are you going, Doctor?' Dr. Rees said, 'I am going to leave this operating suite until I can be treated as a professional gentleman.' Dr. Twitchell said, 'Good

for you boy! Come back here, and I will be glad to have you assist me, and I will treat you as a gentleman.' Their relations were always good from that time on."[7]

Although M.C. had deferred the special professorship to Edmund Brown in 1909, he remained on staff, serving well into the mid-1940s under his stepbrother E.G. Twitchell. Mackay had this to say about M.C. when he was a junior medical student in 1930-31:

"M.C. Twitchell, Sr., was the professor of ophthalmology and highly respected, a power in the town and on the faculty, and a very dignified man who some held in great awe. It was thought that he was hyper-critical, but I always found him to be absolutely charming if he was well served and you were accurate and punctilious in performing the duties that he assigned for you to do."[8]

Marshall Twitchell, Jr. (1912-1987) joined his father and uncle shortly after World War II. He had gone to Harvard for medical school, and the Massachusetts Eye and Ear Infirmary for subspecialty training. He favored ophthalmology, and had little to do with otolaryngology. His 1977 retirement marked an end to more than three quarters of a century of Twitchells at UVM in Ophthalmology and ENT.

A New Department Looks Into Research

John C. Cunningham (1910-1971) was named chief in 1946 upon E.G. Twitchell's retirement. Cunningham, who had trained at the Eye Institute of the Columbia-Presbyterian Medical Center in New York, was fresh out of the Air Corps service. His partner, Twitchell, Jr., made all of the lesson plans and directed medical student instruction. Cunningham didn't relish being chief of "Otology and Rhinology", as those subjects were beyond his area of expertise. He was greatly relieved when Ophthalmology and ENT were separated in 1951.

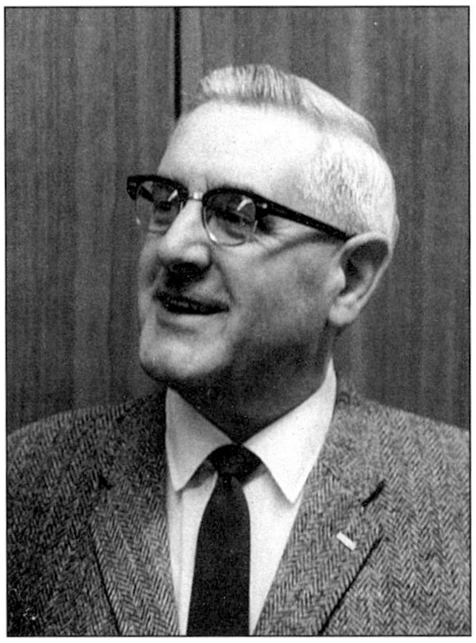

FIGURE 22-4. Edward Irwin started an ophthalmology practice at UVM in 1958 and became Chief of the Division in 1972. (1971 photo)

Edward S. Irwin and Thomas R. Kleh eventually joined Cunningham and Twitchell. Irwin had graduated from UVM in 1940 and the College of Medicine in 1955. The delay stemmed from a WW II Army deployment and a short-lived career as an optometrist. Irwin then completed an ophthalmology residency at the University of Rochester before coming back to UVM. Kleh had left the University of Maryland in 1949 for medical school at George Washington University. Ophthalmology training at Stanford followed this. Although the four "oculists" held UVM faculty appointments and taught medical students, they maintained separate but collegial private clinical practices.

Irwin teamed up with a group of UVM pharmacologists in 1958 to study ocular reaction to embedded foreign material. The project employed a rabbit model, and was a precursor to intraocular lens implantation. It had arisen following reports about WW II pilots who had tolerated similarly embedded pieces of Perspex® (polymethyl methacrylate) from shattered airplane windshields remarkably well.[9] Irwin spent one afternoon a week at the Quonset hut research lab placing such particles in the anterior eye chambers of his animal models. Ophthalmology research efforts came to a halt when funding dried up and the pharmacologists left UVM.

Ophthalmology Briefly Attempts a Residency Program

The department, in an attempt to start a residency program, hired its first resident in 1960. Each of the four faculty devoted an afternoon a week to the hospital's largely indigent clinic patients. The attendings spent the rest of their time seeing private patients in their offices. The resident was only allowed to operate on clinic patients. It became clear before the year was up that the department didn't have enough patients to satisfy the requirements of a residency program. The one (and only) UVM resident transferred to Boston where he completed his residency, and the UVM program was abandoned.

Cunningham pretty much worked right up until he died. Twitchell, Jr. was reaching retirement age as well, so Irwin became chief from 1972-77. Robert C. Guiduli, the UVM medical student that I (DBP) had worked with in Julius Jacobson's lab, had joined the staff in 1966 after completing residencies in ophthalmology and neuro-ophthalmology at New York University Medical Center. The remaining practitioners thus consisted of Irwin, Kleh, and Guiduli. They continued in separate private practices, yet still shared common clinical duties.

Chairman John Davis convinced virtually all of UVM's part-time general surgeons to become full-time faculty under the mantle of Surgical Associates and the University Health Center (UHC). Irwin, Kleh and Guiduli, however, chose to remain in their independent practices. Davis felt that UVM needed a full-time ophthalmology staff, so he started the recruitment process.

UVM Recruits Full-time Ophthalmologists

Philip A. Aitken had worked with charismatic virologist Alan Phillips as a student at the Baylor College of Medicine. After Phillips and his wife Carol, a pediatric resident, took positions in infectious disease and pediatrics respectively at UVM, Philips talked Aitken into considering UVM for his internship. Aitken finished a rotating internship at MCHV and then stayed on for a neurology residency. He subsequently trained in ophthalmology and neuro-ophthalmology at George Washington University and in England. After briefly practicing in Rutland, Vermont and back at George Washington, he became UVM's first full-time Chief of the Division of Ophthalmology in 1977.

Alan E. Irwin was following in his father Ed's footsteps. Alan had graduated from UVM medical school and gone to Richmond, Virginia for residency. He was drafted into the Air Force in 1972 where he performed induction physicals for the next two years. The assignment gave him a chance to be with his family, something that had been hard

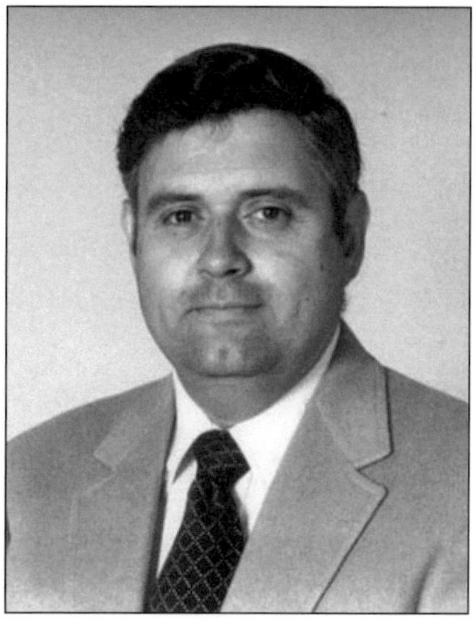

FIGURE 22-5. Alan Irwin joined his father on the UVM faculty as a partner with new Division Chief Phil Aitken.

to do in Virginia. Irwin left the military for training at Philadelphia's Wills Eye Hospital, the largest institution of its kind in the western hemisphere. Irwin then asked Davis about returning to UVM. When Davis put his après ski boot-clad feet on his desk during his interview, Irwin realized that it was really nice to be home.

Irwin had another interview with Aitken in Washington, DC. The pair agreed to establish two separate practices, but otherwise function as partners. They came to UVM together, and were the first physicians to practice in the newly renovated DeGoesbriand space that had become UHC. In fact, Irwin occupied the Bishop's old suite. Aitken and Irwin held full-time appointments. Although Ophthalmology had been termed a "department" before, it was now clearly a division of general surgery, in contrast to the situation at most other medical schools.

Cataract Surgery Evolves to Intraocular Lenses

Cataract extraction dated back to the time of the ancient Egyptians. The removal of opaque lenses improved vision by allowing light to get into the eye. Imperfectly focused vision was partially restored with thick glasses. These techniques placed objects at different depths, however, at best. Adjustments in elderly patients were difficult and cataract extraction was restricted to those who were virtually blind.

The United States' first intraocular lens implant was done by Turgot Hamdi in 1949 at the Wills Eye Hospital. Alan Irwin had trained with Hamdi during his time at Wills, and had learned the technique. Irwin, in turn, then did the first intraocular lens placement in Vermont in 1977 following a cataract extraction.

The first lenses that Hamdi and Irwin placed within anterior chambers were rigid. Post-op courses were occasionally complicated by severe iritis, and focus was far from normal since the lenses were placed at different distances from the retina. Lenses soon became more flexible, and some were placed closer to the retina on the iris itself. The real breakthrough came during the mid-80s in the form of extracapsular lens extraction. Under this method, the opaque lens was removed but the transparent avascular lens capsule was left behind. An implant lens was then placed within the capsule, the lens' normal anatomic location. Complications dramatically decreased, and remarkably excellent vision resulted.[10]

Cataract surgery became a routine procedure in Burlington following Irwin's lead. The local ophthalmologists picked up the new procedure, while the division's future additions learned how to perform lens implants during their residencies.

1980: Happy Times and Harmony

Kathleen J. Maguire (1950-2007) joined the full-time UHC group in 1980. Maguire had graduated from UVM medical school, and trained in ophthalmology at Boston University and the Massachusetts Eye and Ear Infirmary. She then did an extra year in advanced retinal surgery with Boston's Retina Associates. Thomas J. Cavin came on board in 1985. He had gone to medical school at Harvard, finished his ophthalmology residency at the University of Iowa, and then done extra work in corneal surgery.

The division of ophthalmology seemed to be a congenial and secure group from 1980 to 1987 that provided excellent care throughout the community. The emergency call schedule was evenly spread between the full and part-time staff so that each physician took call once a week. Aitken arranged the medical student teaching schedule with active input from the other faculty members. Happy times seemed to prevail.

Davis did not exactly approve of sabbaticals, a benefit that every UVM faculty member was supposedly entitled to. His frequently quoted words were: "If I can do without you for a year, I can do without you." Aitken, however, managed to arrange a four-month sojourn in England with full pay in order to learn oculoplastic and orbital surgery. How this trip did not become common knowledge is one of the Department of Surgery's mysteries. The repercussions among the rest of the faculty from knowledge of such a breach in the Davis doctrine are hard to imagine!

1987: The First Exodus

McGuire and Cavin decided to leave UHC in 1987 for Burlington-based private practice. Aitken and Irwin held down the full-time sector for the next two years. UHC eventually replaced Maguire with retinal specialist Robert Millay and Cavin with corneal surgeon Michael Vrabec.[11] Vrabec was a graduate of the University of Wisconsin's medical school, where he had remained for his ophthalmology residency. This was followed by a corneal transplant fellowship at the University of Iowa.

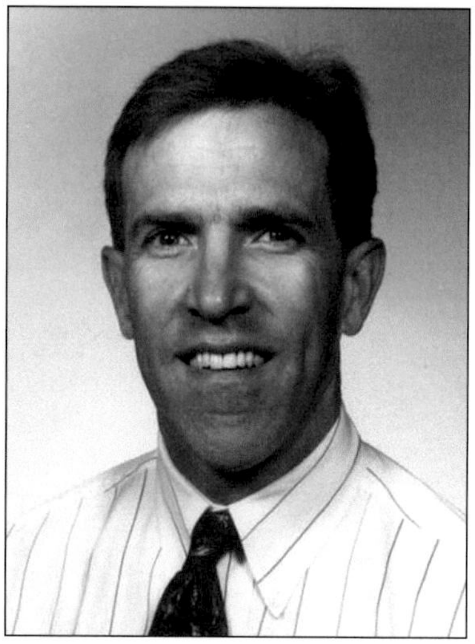

Millay had enrolled at the UVM College of Medicine, but had to complete his studies at the Medical School of Virginia for family reasons. He finished ophthalmology training and a retinal fellowship at Oregon Health and Science University Hospital, and then practiced in Seattle. He joined the full-time UHC group alongside Vrabec in 1989, taking a 40% salary cut in the process. His wife Donna was simultaneously hired to fill dual surgical needs in ENT and plastic surgery. The couple were the last additions to the staff under the Davis regime.[12]

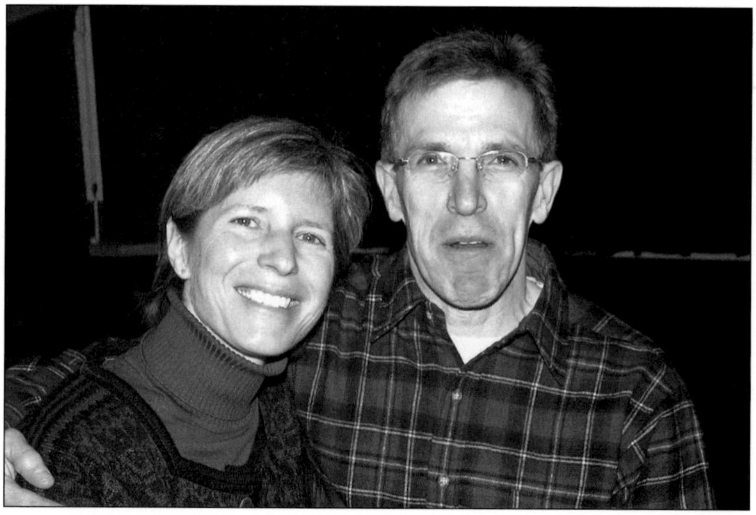

FIGURE 22-6. Robert Millay, hired as a retinal surgeon, later was asked to be the Chief of the Division.

FIGURE 22-7. Robert and Donna Millay relaxing at the Stowe winter surgery retreat.

1994: The Second Exodus

Aitken stepped down as chief in 1994, after having served for seventeen years, in order to take a position at Baylor University. Vrabec returned to his native Wisconsin at the same time, leaving Irwin and Millay alone at UHC. Their workload was heavy, and they often saw more than 50 office patients a day! Millay assumed the duties of Division Chief in 1995. Aitken returned to Burlington after a couple of years, but went into private practice instead of rejoining UHC.

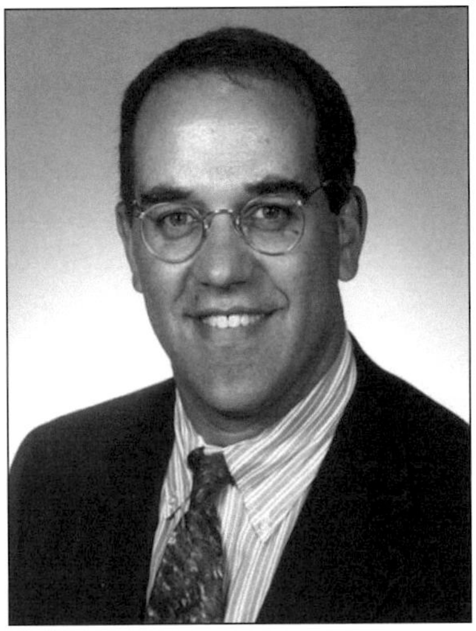

FIGURE 22-8. David Weissgold supplemented the full-time group alongside David Weinberg and David Lawlor.

David J. Weissgold took Vrabec's place as UHC's corneal expert. Weissgold had graduated from SUNY Syracuse and done an ophthalmology residency at Philadelphia's Scheie Eye Institute before finishing his retina fellowship at the Massachusetts Eye and Ear Infirmary. UHC hired David P. Lawlor in 1999 to cover glaucoma problems. Lawlor (whose grandfather had been a UVM ENT surgeon, and whose father was a Burlington opthalmologist) had attended the College of Medicine and trained at the University of Washington before assuming a glaucoma opthalmology fellowship at the University of Nebraska.

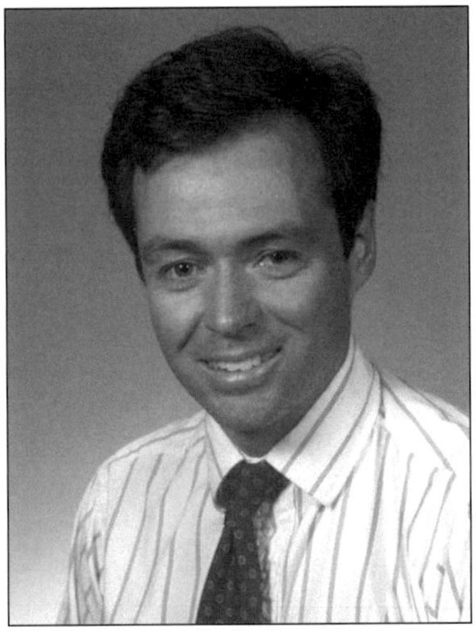

FIGURE 22-9. David Lawlor arrived in 1998.

Another new face at this time was David A. Weinberg, who was arguably UVM's most academically oriented ophthalmologist. He had gone through a six-year bio-medical program at Rensselaer Polytechnic Institute and Albany Medical College, been an ophthalmology resident at the University of Cincinnati, and done a neuro-ophthalmology fellowship at Michigan State University. Weinberg then completed a second neuro-ophthalmology fellowship at Wills Eye Hospital, and an oculofacial-plastic surgery fellowship at UCLA's Jules Stein Eye Institute. Weinberg was knowledgeable, energetic, and outgoing. Residents rotating on the SICU service always appreciated his friendly and scholarly input. Weinberg was an excellent teacher, who subsequently ran an oculofacial plastic surgery fellowship at UVM for five years.[13]

An Unlikely Ophthalmologist Prepares to Come to Vermont

Geoffrey C. Tabin was the remaining hire during this era. Tabin had dropped out of Harvard medical school not once, but twice in order to go mountain climbing. He had gotten back into Harvard the second time by stating that he had been doing "high altitude retinopathy" research on Mount Everest. Seven years from start to finish at Harvard Medical School was followed by an internship at the University of Colorado under former UVM resident Eugene Moore. After two years of orthopaedic surgery at Chicago's Michael Reese

Hospital, Tabin dropped out again to go mountain climbing. Here's what he was up to on October 2, 1988:

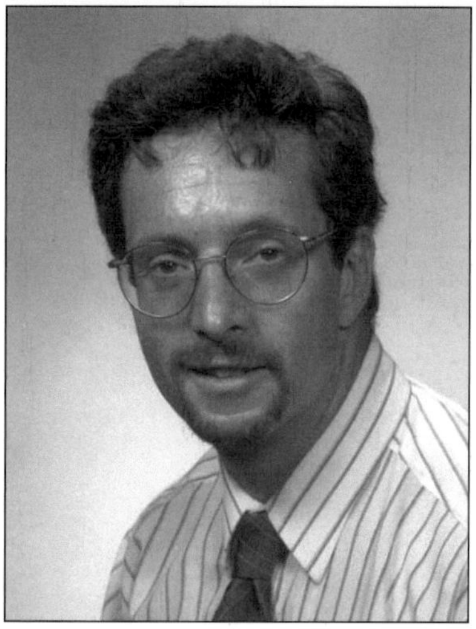

> "The ridge I am climbing is barely two feet wide. To the east is a sheer drop of twelve thousand feet into Tibet. Westward it is eight thousand feet down to the next landing in Nepal. The angle increased from seventy degrees to vertical at the Hillary Step. Climbing un-roped, I delicately balance the crampon points on my right foot on an edge of rock. I swing my left foot, with all my remaining strength, into the adjoining ice. Precariously balanced on quarter-inch ice spikes attached to my boots, I gasp for breath. Forty feet higher the angle eases. Adrenaline mixed with joy surges through me. After eight hours of intense concentration, I know I will make it. The seventy mile-an-hour wind threatens to blow me off the ridge; the ambient temperature is far below zero. Yet I feel flushed with warmth. Ahead stretches a five-foot-wide walkway angled upward at less than ten degrees. Thirty minutes later, just after ten o'clock in the morning, the path ends in a platform of ice the size of a small desk. Everything is below me. I am the 209th person to stand on the summit of Mount Everest.
>
> "The sky is deep blue and cloudless. The cliché is true, the vistas do seem to stretch infinitely in all directions. ... The Tibetan plateau on the other side extends to the horizon, where I can see the curve of the world dropping away. For fifteen minutes I savor the view as the highest person on earth."[14]

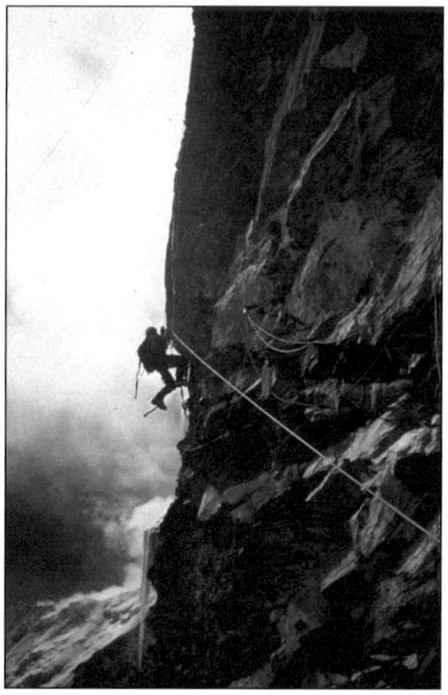

FIGURE 22-10. Geoffrey Tabin came to UVM in 1995. His third-world adventures as a corneal specialist complimented his teaching expertise.

FIGURE 22-11. Tabin clings to the rock headwall on the East Face of Mt. Everest.

Tabin, who had worked as a general practioner in Nepal during this time, was transformed after watching a Dutch team restore sight to a totally blind woman by means of an intraocular lens implant. Knowing that the Himalayas were home to over 300,000 people blinded by cataracts, Tabin took an ophthalmology residency and comprehensive fellowship at Brown University's Rhode Island Hospital. He then set off for Melbourne, Australia's Royal Victoria Eye and Ear Hospital for a corneal surgery fellowship. Tabin described his international eye career in his book "Blind Corners" as follows:

> "I completed my training in America and faced the difficult question of how I could make a dent in the blinding diseases of mountainous Asia. It seemed like a bigger obstacle than any mountain I had faced. Serendipity led me to Professor Hugh Taylor in Melbourne Australia [who] sent me to Nepal to work at a high volume cataract surgery camp with Dr. Sanduk Ruit as part of my fellowship year. Ruit is a master surgeon who spent a year perfecting his microsurgical technique. He took modern state-of-the-art cataract surgery with a lens implant and adapted it to Nepal. Ruit was performing perfect cataract surgery in seven min-

FIGURE 22-12. Tabin visits with Nepalese post-op patients as part of his ongoing battle against blindness in the Himalayas.

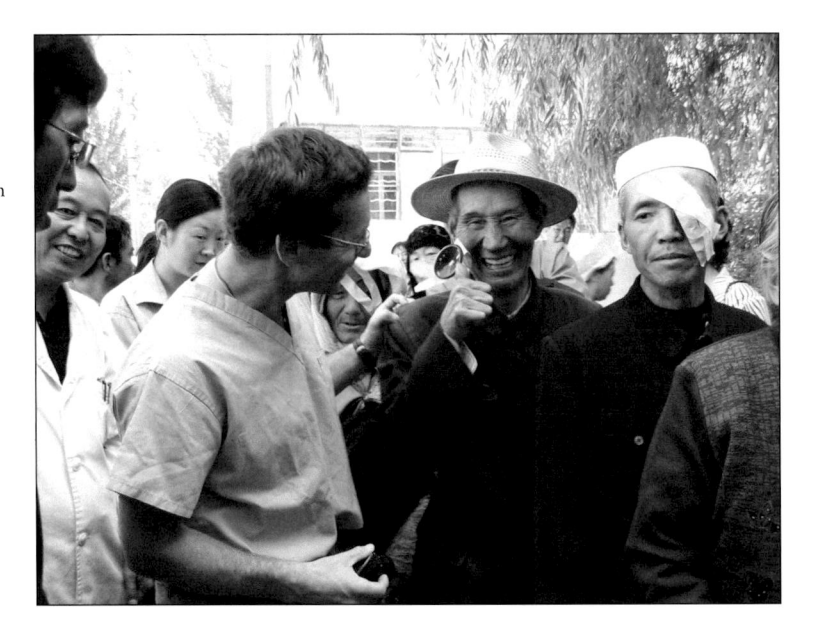

utes at a cost of twenty dollars. I was an instant convert to his methods and stayed in Nepal after my fellowship to work with him for a year. Before I left Nepal Ruit and I vowed to work to overcome needless blindness in the Himalayan regions in our lifetime. We formed the Himalayan Cataract Project to teach other doctors in the region modern surgical techniques."[15]

The following 1994 episode at a Tibetan eye camp was typical of Tabin's many Himalayan experiences:

"When we arrived, hundreds of elderly Tibetans and their families had already gathered. Some had traveled sixty miles or more by tractor or on the backs of family members. Some had been waiting for months. For the next three days, twelve hours a day, Dr. Ruit and I performed surgery side by side in a makeshift operating room without any high tech equipment beyond a microscope. When the generator failed we continued working through the microscope on eyes illuminated by flashlights. Technicians injected local anesthetics to numb the eyes and prepare the patients for surgery. When an operation finished, the patient was rolled off one side of the table and the next patient was rolled on from the other. The new

FIGURE 22-13. Himalayan post-op patients with intraocular lenses can do much more than count fingers, giving obvious satisfaction to Tabin.

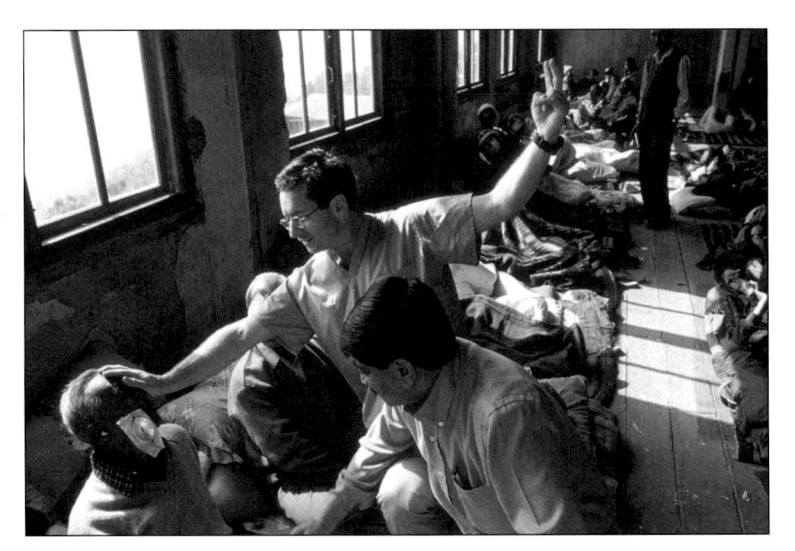

patient's face was painted with antiseptic and surgery continued. The turnover time between patients was less than one minute."

"Dr. Ruit had no trouble sustaining a rate of seven perfect surgeries per hour for a twelve hour operating day." ... "There is a new sky for my eye." ... "I am free from the hell of blindness." ... In three days Dr. Ruit and I performed two hundred such "miracles."[16]

Tabin had already climbed the highest mountains on each of the seven continents at the time of his 1995 UVM arrival. Hired to replace Vrabec as the UHC corneal specialist, Tabin continued to travel to Nepal and attend meetings where he presented lectures about his adventures and raised funds for his Himalayan Cataract Project organization. Tabin kept a picture of himself with the Dalai Llama on his office wall, along with one of himself climbing a rock wall on Mount Everest. National Geographic magazine even sent a photographic team to FAHC to record Tabin's operative skills.

UVM happily basked in the celebrity of Tabin's accomplishments, especially with regards to his Himalayan outreach programs. Tabin gained widespread national acclaim, however his share of the workload at UVM often fell on his partners' shoulders. His independent and adventuresome nature also occasionally went against UVM protocols. The one-minute gaps between patients in Nepal were a far cry from the traditional FAHC operating room turnover times.

2005: The Third Exodus

Tabin took an offer that he couldn't refuse, leaving UVM in 2004 for an endowed professorship at the University of Utah. The rest of the recent additions to the UHC group followed suit. Weinberg followed Tabin to Utah, before relocating to Portland, Maine in 2007. Lawlor went into private practice in Newport, VT, and Weissgold made a similar move locally.

Millay stepped down as Chief of the Division in 2005, but remained with UHC as a full-time faculty member. The division was short-handed once again after a relatively stable

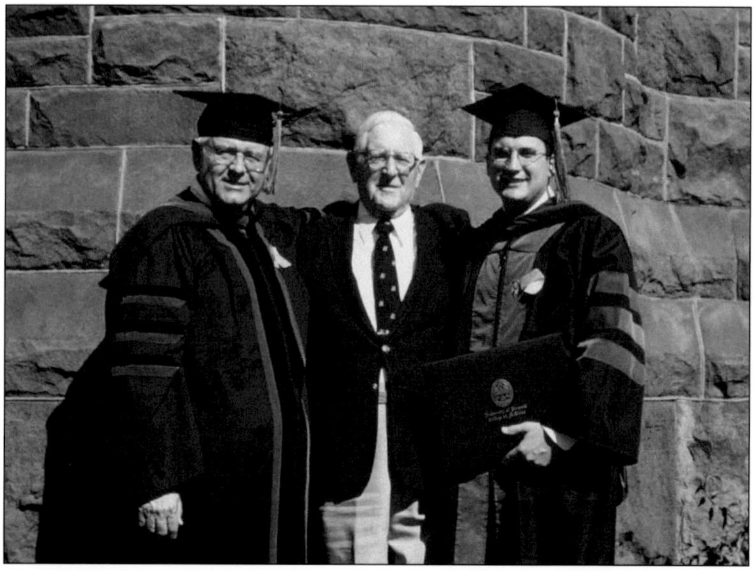

FIGURE 22-14. Three generations of Irwins have studied at the COM and joined UVM's surgical faculty. Left to right: Alan and Edward at Brian Irwin's 2001 graduation.

decade. Irwin remained as a loyal practitioner and stalwart teacher, but didn't want to be chair. Shackford had to step into the resulting vacuum and run the division.

A New Division at UVM

Neuro-ophthalmologist Terry D. Wood arrived in 2005 and served as interim chair before leaving for Washington State in 2008. Stephen M. Pecsenyicki has since taken Wood's position as interim chief. The Medical College of Wisconsin alumnus and former University of Colorado/Rocky Mountain Lions Eye Institute resident, like Tabin, traveled "down under" to do a cornea fellowship at the Royal Victorian Eye and Ear Hospital. The fellowship included time in Nepal, so it is perhaps fitting that Pecsenyicki succeeded Tabin as UVM's corneal specialist.

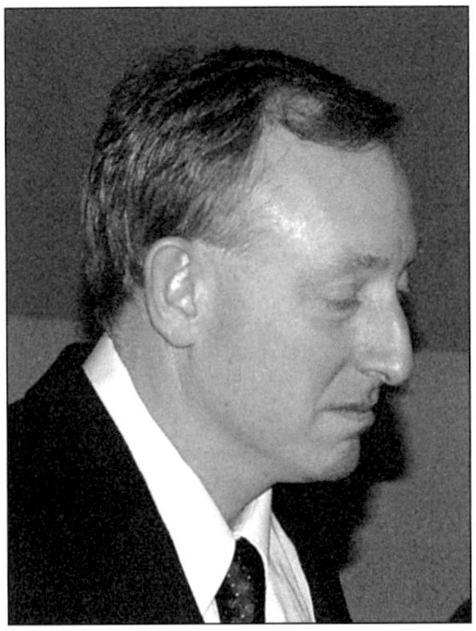

FIGURE 22-15. Terry Woods became the Chief of Ophthalmology in 2005 and rebuilt the Division.

Millay moved to the Courthouse Plaza FAHC retinal center where he was joined by Michelle L. Young in 2004 and Brian Y. Kim in 2005. Young had attended medical school in Nova Scotia at Dalhousie University and completed her ophthalmology residency at McGill before a vitreoretinal fellowship at the Cleveland Clinic's Cole Eye Institute. Kim had graduated from St. Louis University and then done both residency and a vitreoretinal fellowship, like Young, in Cleveland.

Irwin remains busy at UHC's successor, the new FAHC Ambulatory Care Center. The full-time group also maintains a presence at satellite clinics in Rutland, Barre, Stowe, and Middlebury. Kleh retired in 1993, but Aitken, Cavin and Guiduli are active and adding younger talent to their private practices at their South Burlington locations.

Although a few positions remain vacant, the division's future looks bright. The faculty members continue to teach medical students at the preclinical and clinical level, as well as Family Practice, Neurology, and ENT residents. The division treats a wide array of clinical conditions, and leads the way when it comes to complex procedures. Just as cumbersome rigid lenses gave way to flexible intraocular lens implants, and radial keratotomy was supplanted by LASIK surgery (laser-assisted in situ keratomileusis), new advances will undoubtedly be forthcoming.[17]

CHAPTER 23

Otolaryngology Division

Otolaryngology was initially divided between visiting professors of the "Eye and Ear" and the "Throat" before being linked with ophthalmology. This changed with the creation of a separate division in 1951.

The first few chairmen were idealistic, but often on their own and constrained by limited resources. Development of a competitive, high quality residency therefore fell squarely upon the shoulders of Robert Sofferman, who was just out of his fellowship.

With this accomplished, UVM went on to lead the country in optic nerve decompression surgery, parathyroid surgery, and ultrasound training for the ENT surgeon.

Horace Green: Vermont ENT Pioneer

Vermonter Horace Green (1802-1866) was the first American physician to specialize in diseases of the throat. The Chittenden native had obtained a degree from Castleton Medical School in 1824, and then studied in Philadelphia and Europe. While in London, he was told that laryngeal disease was untreatable because the means to apply medication to the organ's membranous lining did not exist. Green's solution was to attach a sponge to the tip of a specialized probe ("proban") made out of curved whalebone. He then used the device to put silver nitrate on affected laryngeal tissue.[1]

When Green reported his successful outcomes in 1840, he was promptly accused of fraud. Most physicians did not think that the larynx could withstand the presence of any foreign substance. Green's results spoke for themselves however, and his practice increased as people came from all over the world to receive treatment. Green performed a tonsillectomy on "Miss R." at his Rutland home in 1850. She related the circumstances of her operation in the following letter:

> "Dr. Green sent for me to go to the office a few days after I came and looked at my throat. "Bad enough", was his exclamation. "There is a deep ulceration out of sight, your physicians have not discovered it." Said he, "What would you say Miss R. if I should be obliged to cut away some of that bad flesh that is in your way there?" I replied, "Whatever you think best to do I will endeavor to submit to patiently" — "Well then the sooner it is over the better, do you not say so?" I answered, "Yes by all means."

FIGURE 23-1.
Horace Green's instruments with the "Proban" from whalebone on the right. The sponge tip can be used to apply medications to the larynx, or remove obstructions.

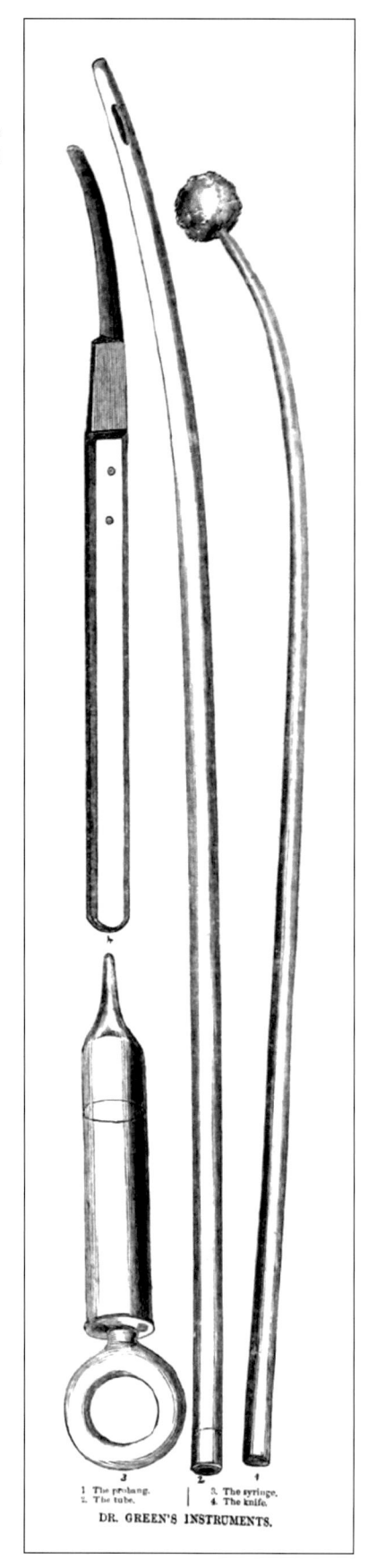

I sat perfectly still, and the Dr. cut off my left tonsil. The blood streamed from my mouth for about half an hour, and then I sat down and had the right one cut off, — after it stopped a little, a sponge application of nitrate of silver was applied and almost strangled me. The bleeding began again and continued until two o'clock — and for a few days I suffered a great deal of pain, but I had kind nursing and "French fixins" to get well on." [2]

Green, by then a professor at Castleton, left Rutland in 1850. Unable to find another academic position in Vermont (UVM's College of Medicine did not reopen until 1854), he became professor of materia medica at New York Medical College. While there, Green popularized the use of the newly invented laryngoscope. He engaged in "the employment of local treatment of the air passages" until his death.[3] A bust of Green was donated to the New York Academy of Medicine by his family in 1901 at a ceremony presided over by D.B. St. John Roosa.[4]

UVM's Early Otolaryngologists

Roosa from New York, had been UVM's first Special Professor in "Diseases of the Eye and Ear" in 1875 and again from 1879-1883. He was one of the many specialists brought to Vermont by chair James L. Little, who himself was facile with the ophthalmoscope and laryngoscope. Little had, after all, trained in New York during Green's heyday.

Roosa's associate in New York, Clinton Wagner (1837-1914), was UVM's first Special Professor in "Diseases of the Throat" from 1879-1882. Wagner had founded the New York Laryngological Society in 1873 and the American Laryngological Society in 1878. He "devised many new instruments and surgical methods. His rare skill enabled him to attempt with success operations upon the throat and neck which few specialists were in the habit of undertaking." Wagner, like Roosa, left UVM to devote his full energies to the creation of the New York Post-Graduate Medical School.[5]

George B. Hope (1847-1926), another Post-Graduate veteran, filled in from 1886-1893. William C. Jarvis (1855-1895) followed Hope in 1894. The special professorship was then combined with that of "Eye and Ear" under the charge of Julius H. Woodward from 1895-1898. Thus, Marshall C. Twitchell (1871-1949) became Special Professor of "Eye, Ear, and

Throat" in 1899 when Woodward moved to New York City. Twitchell, in keeping with the terminology of the day, formally became professor of "Eye, Ear, Nose, and Throat" in 1910. Edmund T. Brown (1871-1944) succeeded Twitchell from 1917-28, before being replaced by Emmus George Twitchell, Marshall's stepbrother.

The younger Twitchell favored otolaryngology over ophthalmology, as former chairman A.G. Mackay well remembered. When Mackay was a junior medical student in 1930-31, "There were 32 hours of lecture in ear, nose, and throat given very kindly and pompously by Dr. E.G. Twitchell." And during Mackay's time as a rotating intern at the Mary Fletcher Hospital, "Fridays brought fish to the table and tonsils to the clinic, and we used to think of 'fish and tonsils' on Friday, with another tonsil clinic on Tuesday."[6]

E.G. Twitchell became the chair of the newly created Department of Ophthalmology, Otology, and Rhinology in 1938. Additional staff members were hired as the needs of the clinic and classroom dictated. Karl C. "Mickey" McMahon (1897-1955) came on board in 1926, Arthur L. Larner (1881-1950) joined in 1936, and Peter P. Lawlor (1890-1969) arrived in 1939. Twitchell subsequently presided over the Department until his 1946 retirement.

The First Chief of ENT

Twitchell's successor, John C. Cunningham (1910-1971), was primarily an ophthalmologist, as were McMahon and later recruit Marshall C. Twitchell, Jr. (1912-1987). Larner, Lawlor, and subsequent hire Elmer M. Reed (1911-1993), on the other hand, were otolaryngologists. Neither group was particularly well trained in the field of the other. The specialties were therefore sub-divided under mutual agreement, on the condition that ENT was to be run by a board-certified otolaryngologist. Rufus C. Morrow (1913-1987) was chosen for the position in 1951.

Morrow, the son of a Presbyterian missionary, had grown up just outside Mexico City. Mexican revolutionaries, in fact, had jailed his father at time of Rufus' birth. The family left the country for Virginia upon his release, but returned when peace resumed. The younger Morrow did a little missionary work himself as an undergraduate before attending Yale medical school. He completed ENT training in New York City, and then joined the Army during World War II. Fluent in Spanish, Morrow was assigned to the American Friends Service and sent to the tropics where he worked on malaria control.

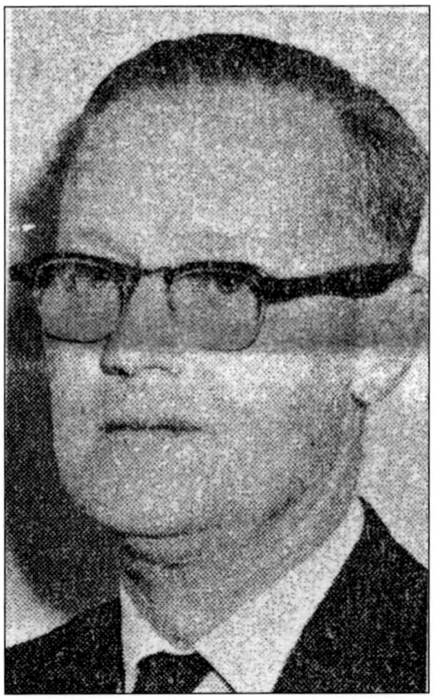

After the War, Morrow practiced in New York City before coming to Vermont in 1951. He conducted very thorough examinations and allowed generous time for patient discussions, so his Burlington office was always full of waiting patients. Morrow at one point shared space with John W. Heisse, Jr., who was an efficient and technically superb otolaryngologist interested in microsurgery. Rumor has it that Heisse's side of the waiting room was frequently empty, even though he saw many more patients than Morrow did.[7]

FIGURE 23-2. Rufus Morrow became UVM's Chief of ENT in 1951. He started the residency program, and traveled frequently to third-world countries aboard the ship "SS Hope."

There were no real guidelines for setting up an ENT residency back then, other than a desire to act as a preceptor and the ability to provide enough operative cases. Morrow started the residency program in 1959 with one resident per year.[8] A similar program was begun by UVM's ophthalmologists, but failed due to a smaller clinical load. The ENT group's wasn't much larger, but the residency managed to survive.

The SS HOPE (Health Opportunities for People Everywhere), the world's first peacetime Hospital Ship, had also been launched around the same time. Project HOPE worked to bring modern medicine and education to the under-served areas of the world. Morrow, with his missionary and malaria control background, was still excited about third world medicine. He was also committed to teaching, so the HOPE's mission piqued his interest. Morrow and his pediatrician wife signed up, and took their first trip aboard the ship in 1961.[9]

Morrow took medical students on later excursions. As he described it:

"Teaching on the Project Hope occurs at many levels simultaneously. There is extensive training for nurses and paramedical personnel and health education for teachers and even the general public. Hope's mission to medical students is to involve them in clinical experience and free discussion."[10]

Morrow's trips aboard the HOPE became more frequent as time went by. A 1965 lawsuit dampened his enthusiasm for traditional medical care (Morrow was acquitted, but the MFH had to pay a hefty fine after a young girl received burns from exposure to a sterilized, piping hot oral retractor). Morrow finally requested an extended leave of absence and embarked on a long tour of duty with the HOPE in 1969. He never returned to private practice.

Charles F. Tschopp replaced Morrow as chief when it became clear that the "leave of absence" was really a resignation. Tschopp had gone to the University of Kansas for medical school, and then trained under Morrow at UVM. After the completion of his ENT residency, he had worked at the Alaska Native Hospital. Tschopp returned to UVM shortly thereafter to join Morrow and Reed on the staff. Larner and Lawlor (whose son and grandson later became Burlington ophthalmologists) had both retired during the 1950s.

FIGURE 23-3. Charles Tschopp was UVM's first ENT residency graduate. He became chief when Morrow left for third-world endeavors.

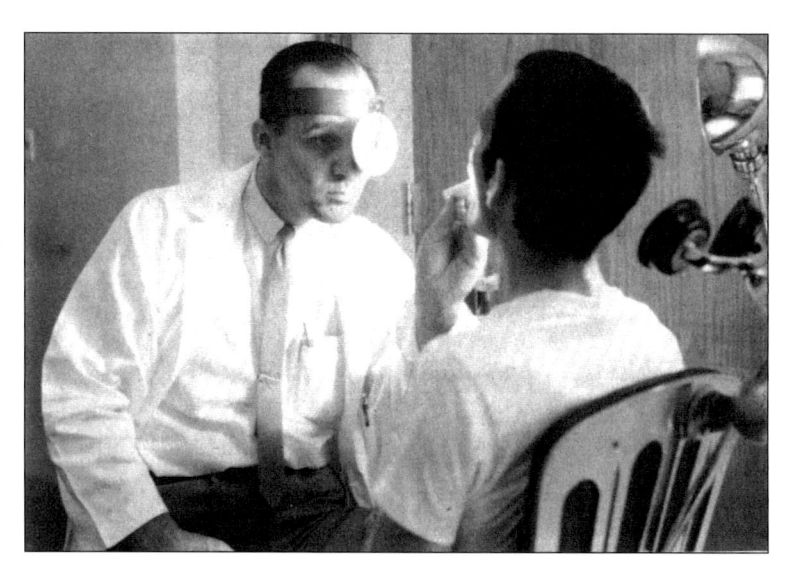

An "Un-needed" Surgeon is Put in Charge

John M. "Jack" McGinnis, Jr. had graduated from the College of Medicine and then studied ENT at the University of Michigan. He had always wanted to come back to Vermont, but was told that there were already enough otolaryngologists in town. After successfully petitioning the hospital for staff privileges, he set up private practice in Burlington. Within a few months, Morrow had set sail on the HOPE and Reed had moved to Pennsylvania. McGinnis was subsequently offered an instructorship in ENT by UVM despite being told that he was not needed. According to McGinnis, there was "No salary, a $500 a year expression of appreciation from UVM, and a $50 a year deduction from tuition for any children."[11]

Tschopp decided to leave UVM in 1974 to permanently relocate in Anchorage, Alaska. This left McGinnis, the "unneeded" surgeon of just five years earlier, as UVM's chief of ENT. McGinnis worked quickly to rebuild the faculty, recruiting Hans W. Behrens from the University of Minnesota, and Robert A. Sofferman from the Massachusetts Eye and Ear Infirmary. The day that Behrens and Sofferman arrived in Burlington was the same day that Tschopp left for Alaska. McGinnis was thus faced with two new partners that were fresh out of training.

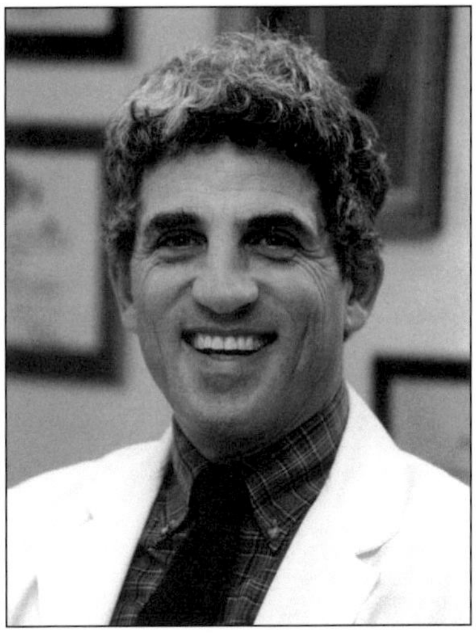

Sofferman's professor at Massachusetts Eye and Ear had trained at the College of Medicine, so when the UVM job notice arrived, he suggested that Sofferman talk to Dr. Frank Lathrop about the opportunity. Lathrop, who had retired from the Lahey Clinic to a Pittsford, Vermont farm, gave Sofferman a favorable recommendation. When Sofferman came to UVM, however, he found that "the place was a dump."[12] The remodeled UHC office space at the DeGoesbriand was poor and the equipment that it contained was outdated. Nevertheless, Sofferman knew that UVM had potential and he felt equal to the challenge ahead.

FIGURE 23-4. Robert Sofferman became the Chief of ENT three years out from his fellowship.

The residency program, in the meantime, was not attracting enough qualified candidates. The dean sought to suspend training, but was opposed by McGinnis and Sofferman. McGinnis grew frustrated over the situation. He was the chief of the division, but did not feel he had any independence or power. He was also concerned that a large multi-specialty group such as UHC might swallow ENT, an outcome that seemed inevitable. McGinnis, who was always very prim and proper in his bow tie and crew cut, left for a one-month vacation. He returned to UVM a different man, with no tie, a beard, and sandals. Reassessing his goals while camping in Vermont, McGinnis decided that he would be happier practicing at Central Vermont Hospital instead.

Sofferman Assumes Control Three Years Out of Fellowship

Behrens moved to Michigan in 1977 in order to care for his ailing father. This left Sofferman by himself at UVM, although both Heisse and Richard H. Goldsborough were across town in private practice. Davis asked Sofferman to assume the chief's role in 1978.

The division desperately needed new faculty. Sofferman hired Moshe Ziv from Ohio State University, and Howard L. Delozier from Syracuse University. ENT then became sub-specialized. Sofferman focused on major head and neck oncology and reconstructive surgery. He was at the forefront of the cochlear implant revolution and developed a team that achieved maximum benefit performing this new procedure. Ziv was responsible for general otology, while Delozier was a master at functional endoscopic sinus surgery and with laryngeal/tracheal problems. The private practitioners emphasized allergy.

Davis and Sofferman agreed there was a need for a pediatric otolaryngologist, the only service that the group did not offer. Sofferman told ENT resident Richard N. Hubbell that if he took a pediatric fellowship at Cincinnati Children's Hospital, there would be a job waiting for him in Burlington when he got back. Hubbell was a true Vermonter whose family had been in residence since 1740! He went to UVM for college and medical school, and started as a UVM surgical resident before transferring to ENT in 1981. His inspiration for the change had been the division's charismatic chief, Sofferman.

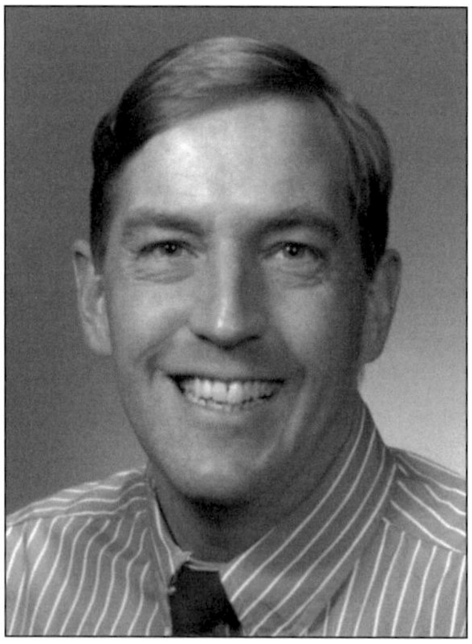

FIGURE 23-5. Richard Hubbell was UVM's first specialist in pediatric otolaryngology.

About 50 sets of pediatric pressure equalization tubes (PE tubes) had been placed at UVM in the four years preceding Hubbell's fellowship. The devices, developed during the 1970s, radically improved childhood otitis media by giving the smaller Eustachian tubes a channel through which to drain. Since Hubbell's 1986 return, each resident in the program has done over 500 such operations! Hubbell also pursued clinical research to prove the hypothesis that routine administration of antibiotics after PE tubes was only necessary in those with mucoid drainage.[13]

Sofferman remembers the day that John Davis became paralyzed in late 1986, not long after Hubbell's arrival. Sofferman had been referred an 11 year-old oral surgery patient with persistent bleeding around a tooth. He planned to extract the tooth and sew in a pack in order to control the hemorrhage. When he got to the O.R., however, he found a hemangioma within the mandible. After an eight-liter blood loss, the patient was transferred to the ICU as coagulopathy set in. Embolization of an artery to decrease bleeding from a hypervascular site was without precedent at this time. Sofferman successfully embolized the feeding vessels and then went back to the operating room where he packed the hemangioma-filled medullary canal with cancellous bone and fat. Innovation always needs to be entertained, even in a rural medical center.[14]

Donna J. Millay was a welcome addition in 1989, having come to UVM as part of a double hire with her husband Robert Millay, Davis' hire as retinal specialist for ophthalmology. She had graduated from the Medical College of Virginia and been an ENT resident at Oregon Health Sciences University Hospital. She had then trained in facial, plastic, and reconstructive surgery at Seattle's Virginia Mason Clinic. She was hired jointly by ENT and plastic surgery. Millay concentrated on rhinology and obstructive sleep apnea, leaving Sofferman, Ziv, Delozier, and Hubbell to tend to their chosen subspecialties.

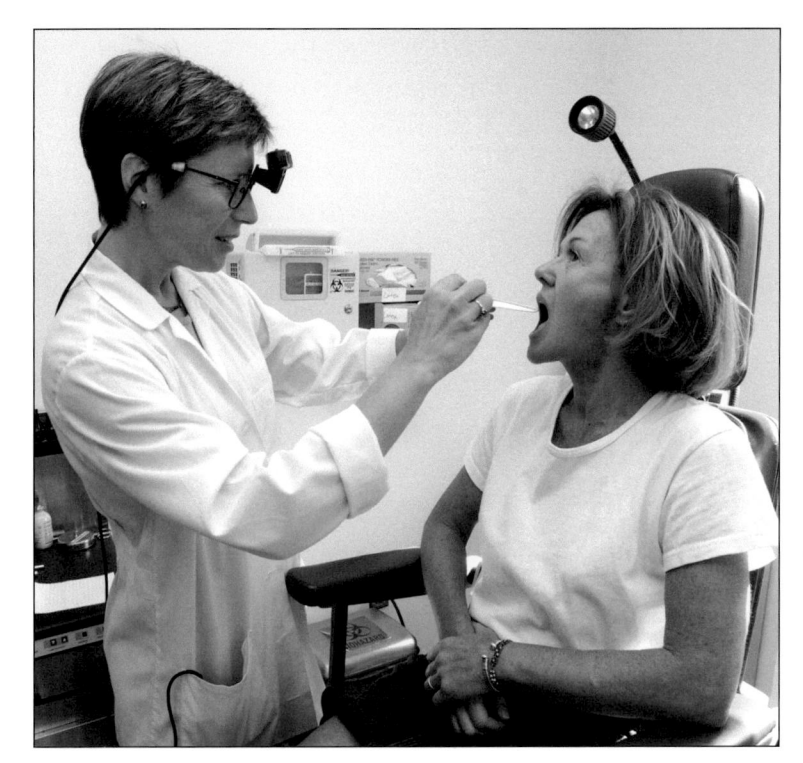

FIGURE 23-6. Donna Millay complemented the other members of the ENT group with her additional training in facial plastic surgery and sleep apnea.

Challenges Arise During the 1990s

Ziv went back to Columbus, Ohio in 1992, and was replaced by recent UVM ENT graduate Paula B. Pyle. Delozier's 1994 departure, however, came as a great blow to the division. Delozier had recovered from a serious spine injury suffered during an automobile accident, but then left medicine entirely. His considerable skills and excellent teaching were sorely missed. Fortunately, Heisse's partner in private practice, Gary P. Landrigan was available. Landrigan had trained at Nova Scotia's Dalhousie University before coming to Burlington. Heisse retired within two years of his arrival, so Landrigan joined Sofferman's group. Landrigan picked up Delozier's endoscopic sinus work, and developed his own niche in allergy control.

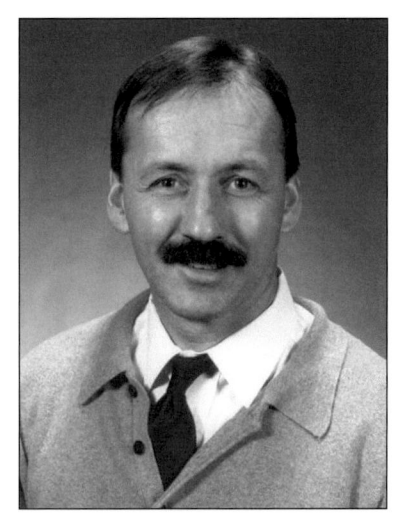

FIGURE 23-7. Gary Landrigan left private practice to join UVM full-time.

Meanwhile, ENT residency programs were undergoing increasing scrutiny nationwide. There were only five programs in the entire country like UVM's with just one resident per level. Each was in danger of being shut down by the Residency Review Committee. As Sofferman put it:

> *"We didn't seem to have enough big cases for the residents, so I approached Dartmouth where there were five ENT attendings and no residents. We sent one resident per year to Dartmouth, and our residents doubled their case numbers."*[15]

The program was still in danger two years later because it lacked a research component. Sofferman followed Shackford's lead in general surgery by adding twelve months to the ENT

Chapter Twenty-Three: Otolaryngology Division   331

residency between the first and second years. Half of the time was devoted to research, and the other half was spent on specialties such as oral surgery, oculoplastic surgery, Mohs chemosurgery, allergies, and a month at the Armed Forces Institute of Pathology in Washington, D.C. learning surgical pathology. The added year brought new depth to the program, which became a highly sought after residency.

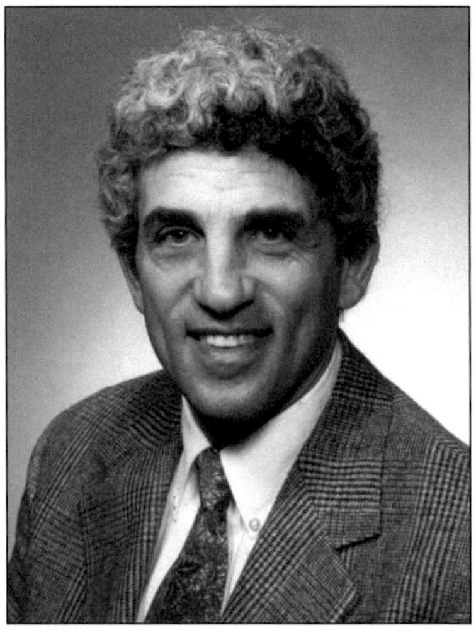

FIGURE 23-8. Sofferman finished his 33 years of practice as a leader in thyroid and parathyroid surgery, as well as ultrasound for ENT surgeons.

Having solved the problems of staffing and residency training, Sofferman got back to business. His early research had been on extra-cranial microsurgical approaches to the optic nerve, but shifted to the blood supply to the parathyroid glands.[16] The change of focus came when ENT started to dominate thyroid and parathyroid surgery following Roger Foster's 1991 departure. UVM was soon recognized nationally as a leader in endocrine surgery of the head and neck.[17]

UVM, through the efforts of Shackford and myself (DBP), also became known as a pioneer in the application of surgeon-directed ultrasound both in the office and the operating room. Because of this influence and the applicability of ultrasound to disorders of the thyroid and parathyroid, Sofferman rapidly embraced its use. He subsequently helped integrate ultrasound training into residency programs. Sofferman also developed a course for practicing ENT surgeons that is still given throughout the country. He currently serves as the chair of the American College of Surgeons National Ultrasound Faculty Executive Committee and is the Module Director for Head and Neck training.[18]

A New Era Unfolds

William J. Brundage decided to trade big city life for the country after living through a particularly bad Philadelphia garbage collectors' strike. The Jefferson Medical College graduate finished his UVM ENT residency, and then joined the Indian Health service. Brundage returned to UVM in 1998 after a six-year stint in Anchorage, Alaska, where he worked alongside Tschopp. He was then sent on a mini-fellowship in voice and laryngology in order to fill that slot and to help with head and neck oncology. Brundage founded the Vermont Voice Center, which was staffed with physicians and speech language pathologists who worked as an organized team. This was at the cutting edge of patient care and unique for a rural program.

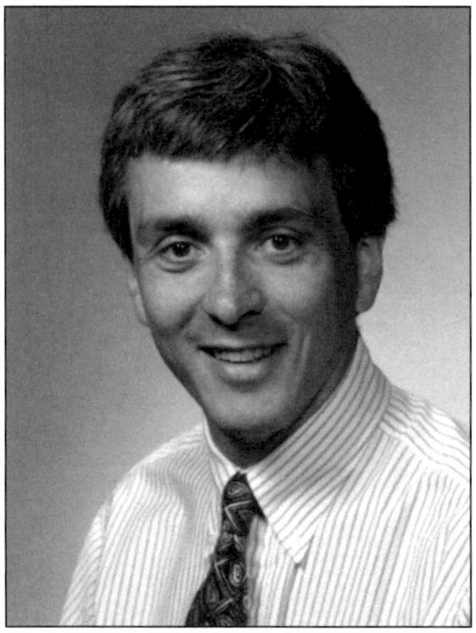

FIGURE 23-9. William Brundage added the Chief's role to his huge clinical load following Sofferman's retirement.

Meanwhile, Damon A. Silverman was training in ENT at the Cleveland Clinic. Silverman had attended Middlebury College, and had set his sights on joining the UVM faculty. His skills were legendary at Cleveland, and his persistence in seeking a position at UVM when an opening did not exist was reminiscent of McGinnis' plight 37 years earlier. After learning that UVM needed someone with laryngology and voice surgery expertise, he completed a fellowship at Vanderbilt's prestigious voice program.

Silverman was subsequently hired in 2005. Brundage was more than happy to let Silverman take over voice surgery so that he could concentrate on head and neck oncology. ENT gained another attending and the Vermont Voice Center has since thrived under its new director.

The most recent addition to the division's staff was Mark E. Whitaker in 2008. Whitaker has brought additional skills in otology and neurotology that were gained during his training at Geisinger and his fellowship at the University of Pittsburgh.

Sofferman stepped down as chief in 2007. Brundage has since been named chair of the division. Hubbell remains in his niche of pediatric otolaryngology as Millay pursues facial plastic surgery. Landrigan concentrates on sinus surgery and sleep apnea, while Silverman and Whitaker tackle voice and skull base disease, respectively. Active satellite clinics in Barre and St. Albans extend the division's reach. Research and resident education continue to flourish, as does the division's outpatient clinic under its cohesive staff. Not bad for a place that was once considered "a dump" by its former boss.[19]

CHAPTER 24

Pediatric Surgery Division

R.W. Paul Mellish established a one-man pediatric surgery division that endured for twenty years. When his successor did not match his tenure, a general surgeon took up the slack and kept the program going.

Dennis Vane's clinical experience and business acumen revived the division. His interest in trauma strengthened the ATLS program and led to Level I Pediatric Trauma Center verification by the American College of Surgeons for UVM's main hospital.

The addition of Kennith Sartorelli brought minimally invasive skills and urological expertise. Although Vane has since moved on, the division continues to provide a broad array of services under Sartorelli's able leadership.

Mackay Builds UVM's Program with a Pediatric Surgeon

UVM's general surgeons performed routine pediatric operations for decades. If the case was complicated enough, the patient was shipped to Boston Children's Hospital. As advances were made in anesthesia and medicine, it became apparent that children's surgical needs differed from those of adults. An aging A.G. Mackay, meanwhile, was trying to improve the Department by recruiting academically oriented specialists, rather than searching for a new Chief. Acquiring a pediatric surgeon was therefore high on his priority list.

Mackay lured Richard Wallace Paul Mellish (1923-2008) away from future U.S. Surgeon General C. Everett Koop's staff in 1962. Mellish, a minister's son, had been born and raised in London, England. He trained at St. Mary's Medical School at the University of London during the early years of the Second World War. As in the United States, medical students were deferred from armed forces duty. Mellish graduated at war's end in 1945, so he felt that he owed his country some military service. He joined the Royal Air Force (RAF) and was deployed to India and Pakistan for two years.

Mellish did not regard England's National Health Service as an inviting place to practice, so he set off for the United States upon his discharge from the RAF. An internship at Seton Hospital in the West Bronx was succeeded by surgical residency at Bellevue from 1950-1953. The Korean War was in full swing by then, and doctors were needed. Mellish, who had become a U.S. citizen in the meantime, was drafted into the U.S. Air Force. His previous RAF stint was disregarded, and he was sent to an air base in England![1,2]

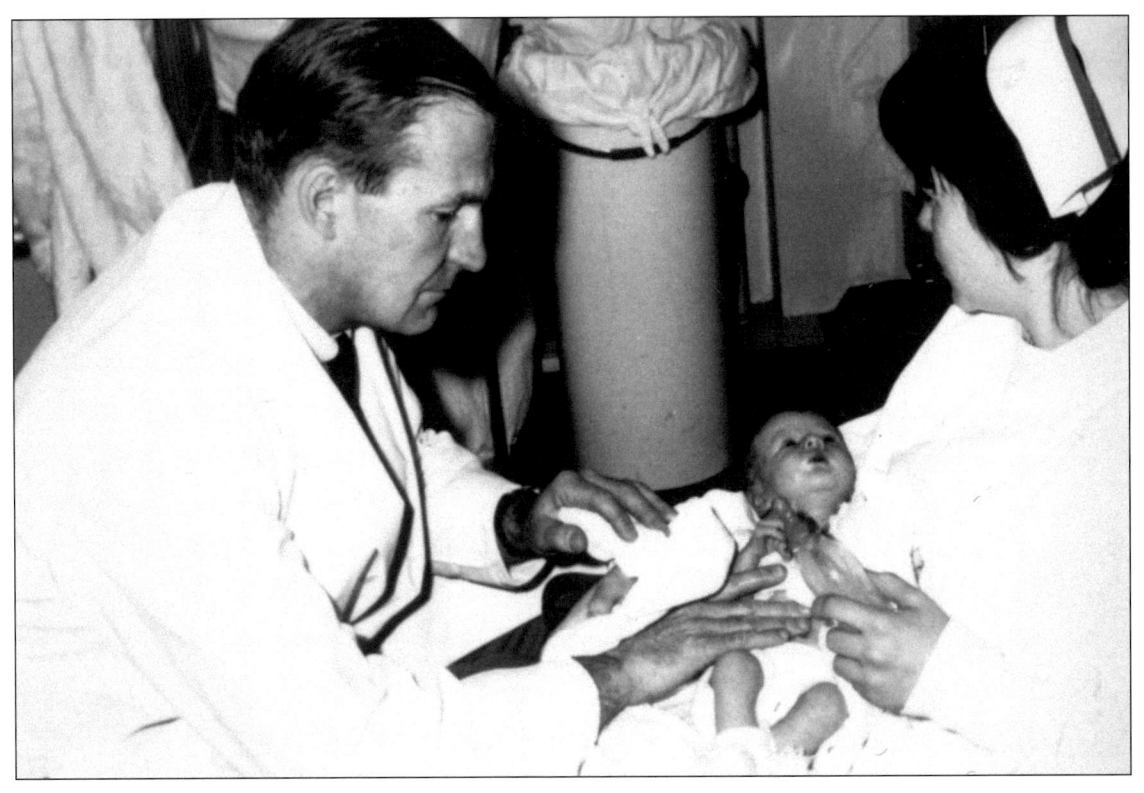

FIGURE 24-1.
R.W. Paul Mellish, UVM's first pediatric surgeon, trained under C. Everett Koop in Philadelphia.

After another two years of military service, Mellish took a position at the Children's Hospital of Philadelphia, one of the few pediatric surgery-training programs of that era. While there, he completed a fellowship under Koop. Although he and Koop published a couple of papers on small bowel duplication and pediatric nutrition, Mellish felt that he did not have much of a future as Koop's junior associate.[3, 4] UVM provided Mellish with his long-sought opportunity to practice as he saw fit.

According to Mellish, UVM's pediatricians were divided between the Mary Fletcher Hospital and the nearby DeGoesbriand. The Mary Fletcher's staff did not enter the Catholic hospital and those associated with the DeGoesbriand did not go to "the hospital on the hill." Like their brethren in internal medicine, the two groups would barely associate with each other. The Department of Surgery, however, covered both institutions. Mellish worked closely with each of the pediatric groups, as neither hospital was willing to give him operative time without a fight. Oddly, neither he nor the pediatricians traveled the three miles to Colchester's smaller Fanny Allen Hospital.

Mellish was the sole pediatric surgeon in not only Burlington, but also the entire State of Vermont for twenty years. He was on call 24 hours a day, almost seven days a week except for two or three years when Anthony Ty, an associate in general surgery at UVM, provided some temporary relief. The general surgeons otherwise covered Mellish if he went on vacation. This duty usually fell to Mackay or Page during Mellish's early years, and then either Gerald Howe or Cemaletin Topuzlu later.

Mellish remembers approaching Mackay when one of the other surgeons, in his opinion, was not performing very well. Mellish said that Mackay refused to take action and that he said, "If you feel that way, why don't you leave?" Mackay ended up freezing Mellish's salary, which Mellish already felt was quite low. Nevertheless, Mellish stayed on and strengthened all aspects of pediatric surgery at UVM.

Mellish took a comprehensive approach to the pre- and post-op aspects of pediatric surgery. He wrote a seminal paper about preparing young patients for surgery and hospitalization.[5] He also worked with UVM's pediatric anesthesiologist, J. Christian Abajian, to develop pioneering spinal anesthetic techniques for routine and high-risk pediatric patients.[6]

Mellish finally departed in 1982 to join the Aramco Medical Center in Dhahran Saudi Arabia. While the perceived low salary wasn't the only reason he left UVM, there were huge financial rewards waiting in Saudi Arabia along with a reasonable call schedule. Mellish retired from practice in 1992 to Charleston, SC, and later Hanover, NH.[7]

UVM's Second Pediatric Surgeon

Allen F. Browne had gone to medical school at George Washington University (GWU) and then finished a general surgery residency at the Maine Medical Center. He had decided to become a pediatric surgeon while at GWU upon attending an inspiring lecture given by Judson G. Randolph. The accomplished Randolph was, among other things, Surgeon-in-Chief at Children's National Medical Center, Professor of Surgery at GWU, and consultant to a number of military and government institutions. The charismatic leader was also at the forefront of surgical education. Browne subsequently completed two separate pediatric fellowships at the University of Cincinnati's Children's Hospital and the Ohio State University's Nationwide Children's Hospital.

Browne, who was fresh out of training at that point, wanted to return to New England. Openings, however, were hard to find, so he pursued a position at Johns Hopkins. Just before he signed on the dotted line, he called John Davis again to see if anything had changed at UVM. As it turned out, Mellish had announced that he was leaving the day before. Davis invited Browne to come for an interview, and subsequently offered him Mellish's position. Davis, careful with his budget, set the starting salary at $40,000. Browne hesitantly asked for $50,000, to which Davis agreed.[8]

Browne came to UVM in 1982 and did approximately 200-250 cases a year for the next several years. He still remembers battling the pediatricians so that he could care for his own surgical patients in the intensive care unit. Browne eventually moved on to the Maine Medical Center. His salary was doubled once he got to Portland, and additional partners shared his workload. Browne later spent time at the University of Illinois Chicago, before recently relocating to Nationwide Children's Hospital.[9]

Dennis Vane Fills the Pediatric Surgery Void

Browne's departure left UVM without a pediatric surgery specialist. General surgeon Hebert provided coverage for routine cases and shared night call with some of the other staff members. But the patient pipeline to Boston, which had been inactive for many years, soon resumed its flow. When Shackford assumed the chair from Davis in 1989, filling the vacancy in pediatric surgery became one of his priorities.

FIGURE 24-2. Dennis Vane, one of Shackford's first recruits, arrived in 1990. He later assumed several major administrative roles.

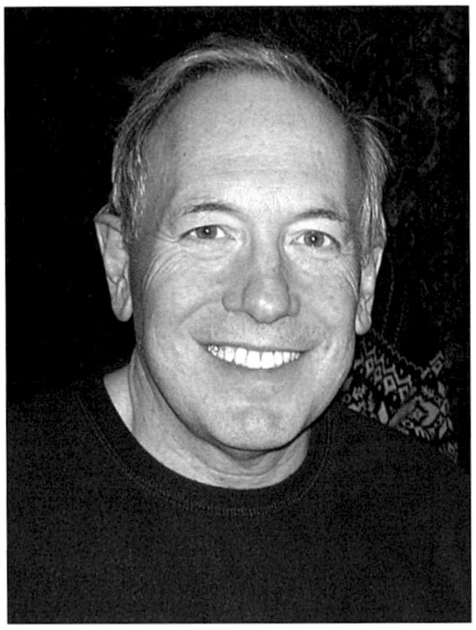

Shackford hired New York City native Dennis W. Vane within a year. Vane had gone to medical school at the Faculté de Médecine, Université Libre de Bruxelles, a French-speaking school in Brussels, Belgium. While there, he did an "away" rotation in pediatric surgery at George Washington University, the home of Browne's surgical hero Judson Randolph. The experience working with Randolph, inspired Vane to become a pediatric surgeon as well. Upon graduating, he completed a surgery residency at Indiana University, followed by a pediatric fellowship at the Ohio State University, finishing three years behind Browne.

Vane became a junior staff member of Indiana University's Pediatric Surgery Section in 1985. While there, he worked with Chairman Jay Grosfeld to start a residency program in pediatric surgery and develop the Kiwanis-Riley Regional Pediatric Trauma Center in Indianapolis. Although Vane was not actively looking for another job, he was convinced to investigate the opportunity that UVM offered. Shackford and Vane developed an immediate bond during their first meeting. Vane's wife was enamored with Vermont after she accompanied him on his second visit. That clinched the deal.

Vane's appointment came with the condition that UVM develop a pediatric Intensive Care Unit (ICU) and an Intensive Care Nursery (ICN). While an ICU and ICN were of benefit to the surgeons, Vane knew that they were essential for the continuation of the pediatric residency program. The units were established in record time. Although the pediatricians were not accustomed to such direction by surgeons, they enthusiastically embraced Vane's energy and expertise.[10]

Richard Gamelli and I (DBP) had been teaching the Advanced Trauma Life Support (ATLS) course at UVM since its inception, but Gamelli had just left for Loyola. Vane, formerly, had been teaching ATLS at Indiana. Vane filled the staffing void without missing a beat, and directed UVM's ATLS training courses for the next 18 years. He was later appointed the Vermont chairman for the American College of Surgeons Committee on Trauma. Vane also helped UVM obtain Level I Pediatric Trauma Center verification.

Research had never been one of Mellish or Browne's priorities (each had published a half dozen or so articles during their UVM tenures). Vane, however, was different. He had either authored or collaborated on nearly 50 papers before coming to Vermont. Vane continued Mellish's spinal anesthetic work with Chris Abajian, but his real interest lay in the epidemiology, imaging, and non-operative management of pediatric trauma. Much of this work was carried out in conjunction with either Shackford or one of the surgery residents.

UVM Needs Two Pediatric Surgeons

Andrew R. Hong had been a UVM general surgery resident during the period after Browne's departure but before Vane's arrival. The University of Wisconsin Medical School graduate had already decided upon a career in pediatric surgery, so he went north to Montreal

Children's Hospital in order to complete a fellowship. Hong then returned to UVM in 1992 to help with pediatric surgery. Things, however, did not quite work out, so he left in 1994 for a position with the North Shore-Long Island Jewish Health System. Vane was thus left to cover pediatric surgery by himself once again.

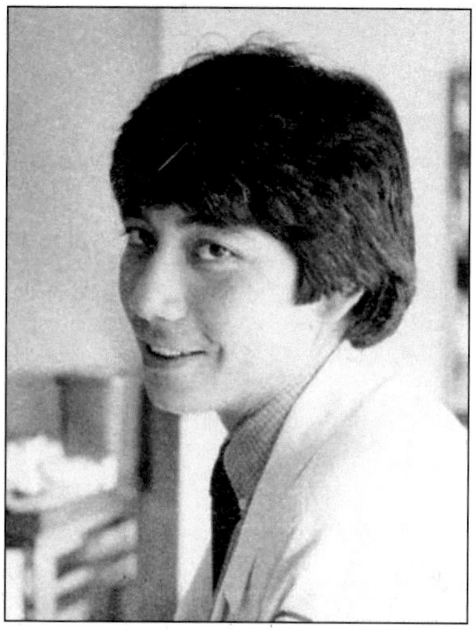

UVM's pediatric surgery load had increased from 400 to 750 cases a year during Hong's two and a half year stay. Vane knew that he could not perform every operation by himself and take call each night. At the same time, he did not want to start sending patients to Boston again. It was clear that UVM needed a second full-time pediatric surgeon.

Vermonter Kennith H. Sartorelli was another UVM general surgery resident during the late Browne/early Vane years. He had followed his residency with a pediatric fellowship, and then a pediatric urology fellowship at the University of Colorado. Sartorelli was a fitting candidate to replace Hong due to his additional training and his tremendous interest in teaching. Performing major pediatric cases alongside Sartorelli was, and continues to be, one of the UVM surgical residency program's highlights.[11]

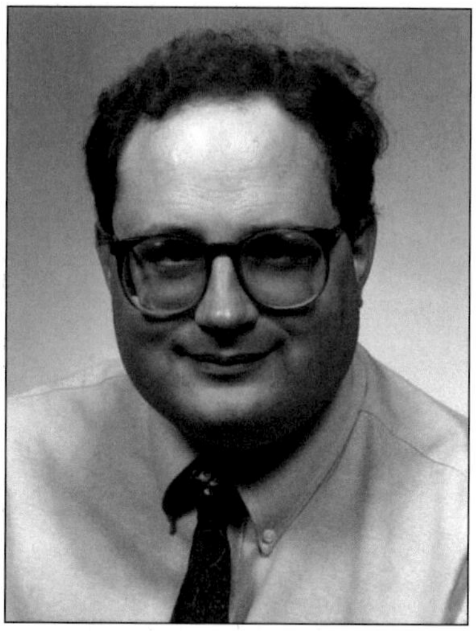

FIGURE 24-3. Andrew Hong came to assist Vane in 1992, but left for Long Island, NY after only two years.

FIGURE 24-4. Kennith Sartorelli returned to UVM in 1995 after completing pediatric training in Colorado. The superb and stalwart surgeon is also the current Residency Program Director.

Pediatric Trauma: How Old is Too Old?

The need for continuous specialty coverage demanded that UVM employ two pediatric surgeons. Unfortunately, Vermont's rural environment did not guarantee a steady stream of patients. The situation was partially solved by entrusting Vane and Sartorelli with a number of administrative positions. Vane, as Vice Chair of Clinical Affairs, oversaw the hospital side of the Department's clinical practice. He also found time, somehow, to earn a UVM MBA during his off-hours. Sartorelli, meanwhile, assumed the important role of Director of Residency Programs from Hebert.

Clinically, the pediatric trauma age limit was redefined to include those 16 or under, so that the teenagers previously treated as adults were cared for by the pediatric surgeons. Knowing that Vane and Sartorelli laid claim to any underage trauma patient, I (DBP) decided to have a little fun one day. I was down the hall from the Pediatric Surgery office at the UHC Vascular Clinic, and had just seen a man with a slowly growing, pulsatile, golf-ball sized mass in his groin. The lesion, located at the site of an earlier injury, was consistent with a pseudoaneurysm. I injected it with thrombin under ultrasound guidance, which successfully thrombosed the pseudoaneurysm. The technique was relatively new, but it worked beautifully. I then set off for the pediatric surgery clinic.

Finding Sartorelli at his desk, I said, "Ken I have a patient that fell onto the tip of a ski pole when he was sixteen. How far out do you see patients from their injuries?" Sartorelli sat back. "Does he have a hernia?" "No," I replied, "a pseudoaneurysm." His brow furrowed. Although Sartorelli didn't do much vascular surgery, he remained undeterred. "I could take a look at him. He'd have to go to the O.R. and have it resected. It's been a while since I've done one." I shook my head and said, "That's unnecessary. I just fixed it with the ultrasound machine." As I walked away, it finally dawned on Sartorelli to ask the truly pertinent question. "By the way, how old is he now?" I turned around, and with a big smile answered, "Sixty-five!"[12]

Back to Basics

Vane's national prominence steadily grew during his stay at UVM. He had by this time written another 50 manuscripts, and was involved with at least twenty professional organizations. His sons were fully grown, and he was ready for a change. Accordingly, when the opportunity to become the Chair of Pediatric Surgery at Saint Louis University arose, Vane took it. He settled in as Surgeon-in-Chief at Cardinal Glennon Children's Medical Center in 2008, where he oversees a team of three additional pediatric surgeons and works alongside a wide array of pediatric sub-specialists.

Sartorelli, like Mellish, Browne, and at times, Vane, now manages the division without additional help. He continues to offer a full complement of services, and remains an expert in minimally invasive procedures. The Department of Surgery's other divisions provide complementary pediatric coverage. Ittleman even ligates the occasional patent ductus arteriosus, although patients with more complex congenital abnormalities still travel to Boston.

And just as C. Everett Koop, Judson Randolph, and Jay Grosfeld influenced the division's first three pediatric surgeons, Vane and Sartorelli have inspired 7 of the past 57 UVM surgical residents to pursue careers in pediatric surgery. It is a very high percentage for such a small program, and a reflection of the difference that good teachers can make.

CHAPTER 25

Plastic Surgery Division

Plastic surgery has evolved from the domain of a solitary part-time physician into a full-time four-person division. UVM's plastic surgeons have donated their services to underserved third world patients for decades.

The staff built on groundbreaking microvascular surgery innovations learned from Jacobson, R.M.P. Donaghy, Harry Bunke, and Stephen Mathes. UVM remains a notable center of excellence for these techniques.

The division is at the leading edge of cleft lip pre-surgical molding and early one stage reconstruction. UVM is also one of the few centers that perform intricate rectosigmoid neo-vaginal reconstruction for gender reassignment surgery.

Early Plastic Surgery at UVM

UVM's early general surgeons performed a wide variety of "plastic" operations. Nathan Smith, as usual, led the way. Listed within his account ledger of 1800 were two instances of

FIGURE 25-1.
Cleft lip repairs performed by J.L. Little on patients older than in present day practice.

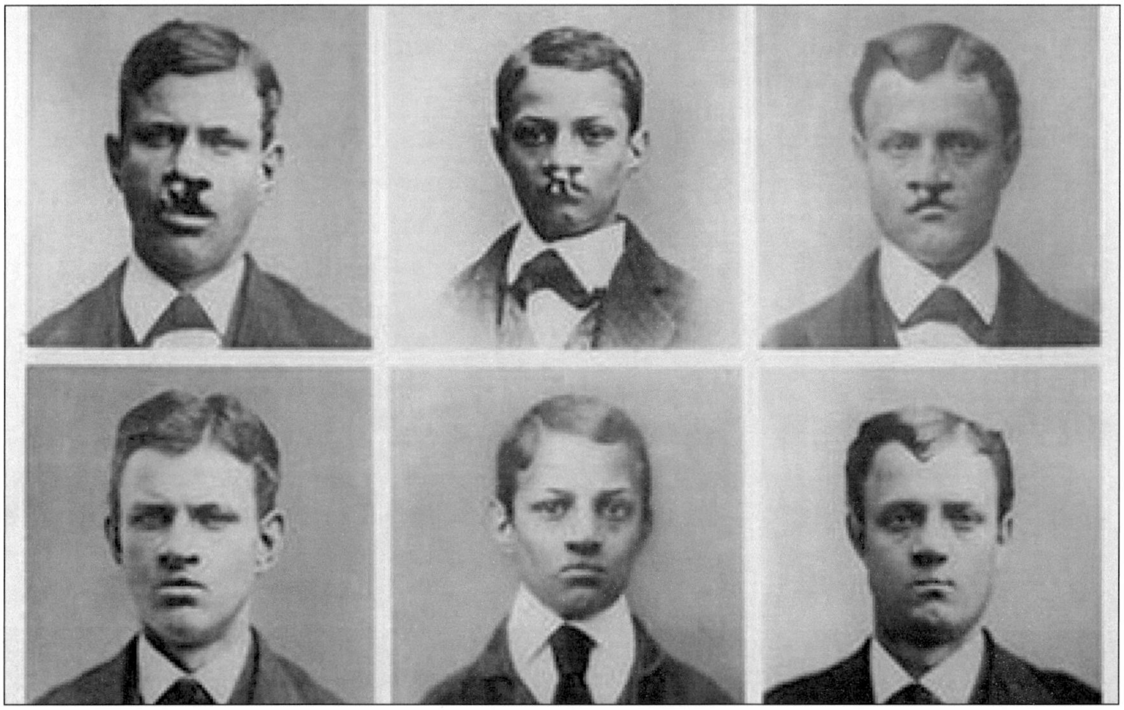

"Operation for a harelip."[1] James L. Little, another of UVM's multitalented surgeons, was also extremely adept at repairing cleft lips. The techniques unique to the discipline, however, evolved from the terrible injuries and incredible reconstructions of World War I. The year 1921 saw the formation of the American Association of Oral and Plastic Surgery. Members were required to have both medical and dental degrees. The American Board of Plastic Surgery was finally recognized in 1937, although the Society of Plastic and Reconstructive Surgery had to wait until 1941 for its debut.

Plastic Surgery Comes to Vermont in 1955

Another type of debut occurred in 1941. That was the year that Bernard B. Barney (1914-2003) enrolled at UVM's College of Medicine. The industrious young man had worked as a merchant marine engineer for seven years before starting college, having saved enough to pay his way through UVM as an undergraduate. Barney also supported himself by working each summer as an engineer on a number of different ships, or as a janitor.

At the outbreak of World War II, UVM's medical school training was accelerated and its students were enrolled in the Army Reserves. As the cash-strapped Barney later put it, "Things were a cinch. We were studying now on Uncle Sam's payroll." Three years of military service were followed by an internship and general surgical residency at Bellevue. Barney then studied head and neck tumor surgery at the Kingsbridge Veterans Administration Hospital in New York. This was succeeded by plastic surgery at the Royal Victoria Hospital in Montreal and the University of Pennsylvania.[2] He ended up being board certified in general, ENT, and plastic surgery.

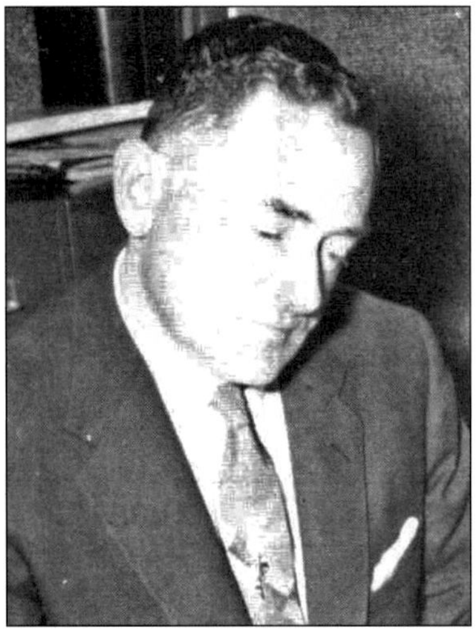

FIGURE 25-2. Bernard Barney, pictured here in 1955, was UVM's first plastic surgeon.

Barney returned to Vermont in 1955 and went into private practice, joining the UVM faculty part-time in 1961. He used his home office/studio to photograph his plastic surgery patients' pre-op conditions and post-op results. Visiting UVM medical students were shown many of the before and after pictures as part of their training. Modesty draping was not Barney's forte. Patients came from distant places as his fame spread. More than one famous face made the trip to Burlington to acquire a new look away from the glare of the paparazzi.

While it was true that Barney did excellent work, it was also true that he was a bit of a character. I (DBP) had the chance to experience this firsthand in 1974. Barney had done a breast augmentation on a young lady who developed an intestinal obstruction the day after surgery. I subsequently took her back to the operating room for an emergency laparotomy and lysis of adhesions from a prior appendectomy. As she lay anesthetized on the O.R. table, the dressings covering her breast augmentation were removed. There, in two-inch high black magic marker was the artist's signature, "BREASTS BY BARNEY."

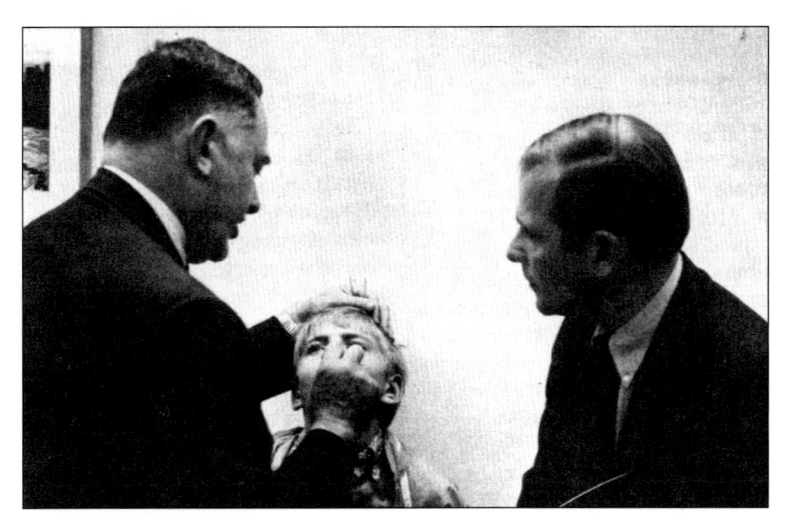

FIGURE 25-3.
Peter Linton and Barney confer about an operative case in 1969.

Linton Arrives in Burlington

Peter C. Linton (1930-2004) was finishing medical school at Albany Medical College just as Barney was settling into his Burlington office. The Brooklyn native completed a plastic surgery residency in Albany, and then moved across the lake to Vermont in 1965. Linton established his own private practice on Colchester Avenue in one of the many Victorian houses that had been turned into doctor's clinics.

Linton became fascinated with Julius Jacobson's and R.M.P. Donaghy's pioneering work in microvascular surgery. Linton spent half a day each week practicing under the microscope, even though his clinical opportunities were limited. He ended up staffing the microvascular teaching lab alongside Donaghy, which was ably run by former operating room nurses Jackie Roberts and Elaine Lavigne. Hand surgeons and neurosurgeons from across the country attended the UVM microvascular courses. Donaghy and Linton reinforced the value of listening to instruction from the nurses, an innovative approach for that time.

Linton also saw post-op patients that had been to Boston Children's Hospital for cleft lip and palate repair. He became convinced early on that he could do a better job than the Boston surgeons. Linton founded the Vermont Cleft Palate Clinic in 1968; and within a few years he was treating nearly every case of cleft lip and palate in the entire state. Later associate David Leitner (and indeed all who saw Linton's work) marveled at his "ability to visualize and create balance and proportion of the human face where before there had been none." Leitner added that he had never seen anyone repair a cleft lip as well as Linton.[3]

Barney and Linton also took facial trauma call. In 1969, a Copley Hospital O.R. nurse crashed her car after hitting a patch of black ice. She was taken to Copley by the hearse/ambulance, but was referred to Linton by community surgeon Philip Goddard. Linton performed a miraculous reconstructive repair. He liked the results (and the patient) so much that he turned her office visits into ski dates. Linton traveled to India for three months in 1973 where he donated his skills to the needy. Returning rejuvenated and

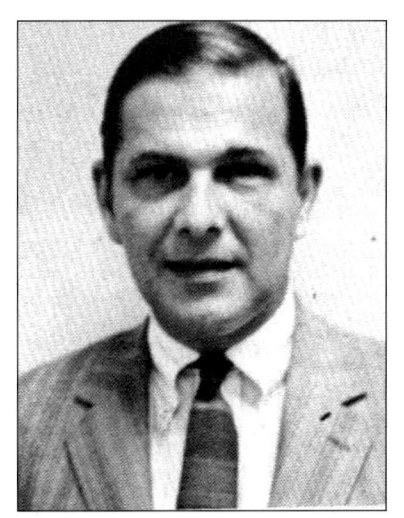

FIGURE 25-4.
Linton did such a superb job repairing facial injuries on a Copley Hospital nurse that he ended up marrying her.

Chapter Twenty-Five: Plastic Surgery Division

inspired, he married his Copley patient, who was now a UVM surgical nurse. Linton joined Surgical Associates as a full-time member, and became chief of the Department's new Division of Plastic Surgery shortly thereafter.[4]

A Unique Search Committee Hires a Plastic Surgeon

Barney was aging and operating less frequently by the early 1980s, although he did not retire until the end of the decade. Linton, meanwhile, was doing more and more of the division's work. After a bit of grumbling, Chairman John Davis finally allowed Linton to look for another plastic surgeon. Coincidentally, there was also a need for a hand surgeon. This came at a time when general surgeons, orthopaedic surgeons, and plastic surgeons were battling over which specialty was responsible for hand surgery. Davis' search "committee" consisted solely of Dr. and Mrs. Linton.

Their selection of David W. Leitner proved to be excellent. Leitner had graduated from Wayne State University, done a general surgery residency at Berkshire Medical Center, and trained in plastic surgery in Phoenix. He had then gone to the University of California at San Francisco (UCSF) for a hand fellowship under Harry J. Bunke, the father of replantation microsurgery. Bunke had developed his microsurgical methods apart from, but in parallel with Jacobson, and had later attended UVM's 1966 international microvascular conference. Bunke, like neurosurgeon Gazi Yasargil, then embarked on his own spectacular career.

Leitner was hired without a contract and without having met the chairman. He was also unaware of the turf battle over hand surgery. Upon arriving at UVM, Leitner discovered that he did not have a Vermont medical license and therefore couldn't work for several weeks. This happened to many a new faculty member before and after Leitner! It was an inevitable consequence of the Department's informal hiring process.

Leitner attended a surgical course in Las Vegas as he awaited his Vermont license. While there, he came across a fully loaded silver Saab. Leitner had been in the market for a car, but

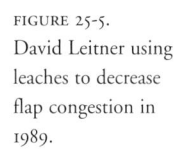

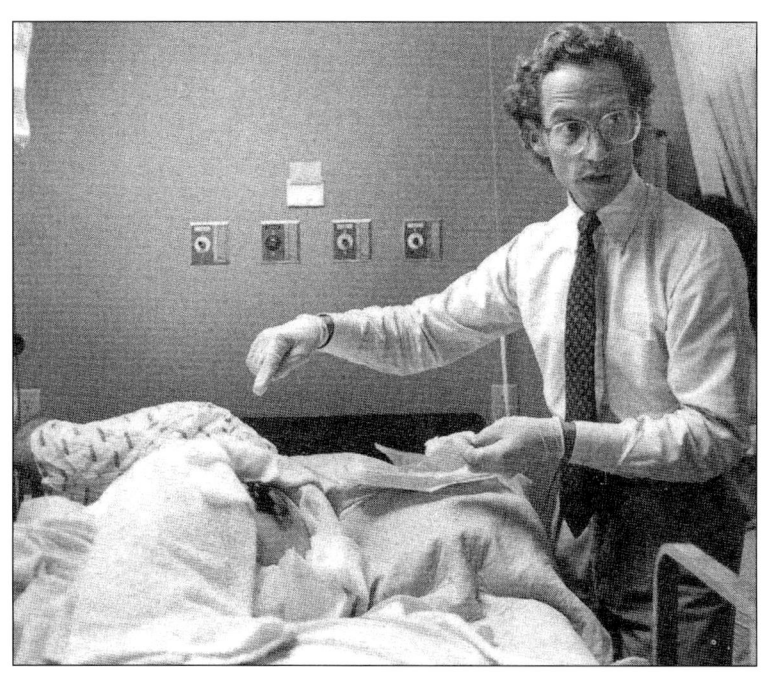

FIGURE 25-5. David Leitner using leaches to decrease flap congestion in 1989.

had not yet found one to his liking. Having recently discovered that the surgeons received a leased car as part of their employment package, Leitner called the Department's business manager and asked if Surgical Associates would buy the car for him. After being given the OK, Leitner had his wife Linda drive the Saab back to Vermont while he flew on ahead to start work.

Leitner organized a replantation service shortly after his 1984 arrival. He subsequently took replantation call every night until others joined the service in 1990. Microvascular skills were employed for nerve and vessel re-anastomoses. Digits were the most commonly replanted structures, although several scalps and an arm have also been reattached. One of Leitner's most gratifying experiences as a doctor came when he saw a young woman with a well functioning replanted arm many years out from her injury.[5]

The Plastic Surgeons Engage in Outreach Programs

Leitner, like Linton, had an interest in helping the underserved. While doing his hand fellowship in San Francisco, Leitner learned about an organization called Interplast® that was dedicated to providing free reconstructive plastic surgery for poor people in developing countries. Donald Laub, Sr., the chief of plastic surgery at Stanford and an associate of Leitner's fellowship director Harry Bunke had founded the group in 1969. Leitner took the first of his five trips to Peru with Interplast upon the completion of his fellowship.

Vermont medical doctors Arthur and Renee Bergner, meanwhile, were regularly volunteering at Hôpital Albert Schweitzer, Haiti during the 1980s. William Larimer Mellon, Jr., the hospital's founder and the grandson of financier Andrew Mellon, happened to be at their Burlington office one day. The Bergner's noticed some skin cancers on Mellon's face, so they called Leitner to remove them. Afterwards, Mellon wrote and asked Leitner if he would like to perform surgery in Haiti. When Linton saw the opened letter on Leitner's desk, he volunteered to "take care of this for you."[6] The opportunity was clearly ideal for each of UVM's plastic surgeons.

Linton and Leitner started going to Haiti on an alternating basis once or twice a year. Each trip lasted one or two weeks, and was conducted on the surgeon's own time without any compensation. During one visit, Linton discovered that Haitian children could not attend school unless they had shoes. He gathered all of his family's used sneakers before his next trip to Haiti, so that he had something to give the island's disadvantaged youngsters. Linton's kids subsequently had to hide all of their shoes so that they would not end up shoeless themselves![7]

Trabulsy Walks into Plastic Surgery

Philip P. Trabulsy grew up in New York City during the 1970s idolizing diver and respected scientist Jacques Cousteau. He chose Old Dominion University for college so that he could get a good education, play college football, and be near the Cousteau Society for the Protection of Ocean Life. Trabulsy, however, could not put his marine biology degree to good use after graduating, so he worked as a hospital orderly for the next year at Eastern Virginia Medical School (EVMS) hospital.

FIGURE 25-6. Philip and Mario Trabulsy preparing to join Linton on an outreach trip to Haiti.

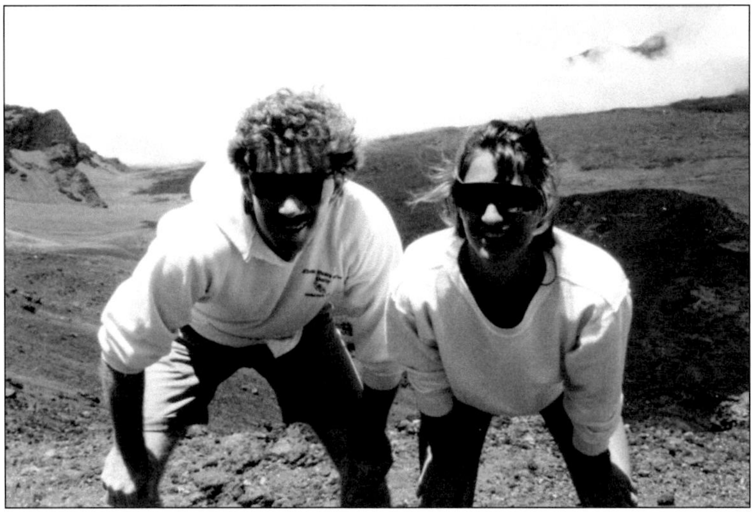

Luck was with him when he walked into the EVMS research laboratory of plastic surgeon Julia K. Terzis. He asked if they needed any help, and was told, "We have just moved here and need someone to set the lab up." Terzis was yet another microvascular pioneer and had just come to EVMS from Montreal. When Trabulsy mentioned that he was familiar with operating rooms, he found himself hired as a laboratory assistant right on the spot. The exciting research lab experience prompted Trabulsy to apply to EVMS with the goal of becoming a plastic surgeon.

Having now spent the better part of a decade in Virginia, Trabulsy thought that he should take his surgical residency elsewhere. He was urged to look at John Davis' UVM program. After matching at his number one choice, he started residency in 1985. Those were the days when the surgical residents spent 24 hours on and 24 hours off during their emergency room rotations. One of the emergency room volunteers plied Trabulsy with chocolate chip cookies. The gesture led to romance and eventual marriage.

During Trabulsy's chief year, he and his new wife Mario (by then a UVM medical student) accompanied Linton to the Schweitzer Hospital. Several young male patients had been scarred on one side of the body from burns sustained at Voodoo "cleansing" ceremonies. The operation to release the resultant axillary contractures was tedious and particularly bloody. Trabulsy remembers tearing his glove and injuring his hand during one such case. He bled significantly, and came into contact with the patient's blood in the process. Trabulsy put on another glove, and continued with the procedure. It was nearly impossible, after all, to follow universal precautions under such conditions.

Two weeks after returning to Burlington, Trabulsy noticed that he was tiring easily and that his eyes were yellow. He saw his physician and blood samples were drawn. The results showed abnormal liver function. When the antibody tests were negative for blood-borne hepatitis B, Trabulsy was reassured that it was probably atypical food-related hepatitis A. The other possibility was "non-A non-B hepatitis", an entity that could not be further investigated in 1989. The symptoms remitted, and Trabulsy put the problem out of his mind.

A plastic surgery fellowship at UCSF followed, under Bunke's successor Stephen J. Mathes, whom Trabulsy had met while Mathes was a visiting professor at Terzis' EVMS lab. Mathes was a world leader in musculocutaneous flaps and had authored the major text in the field.[8]

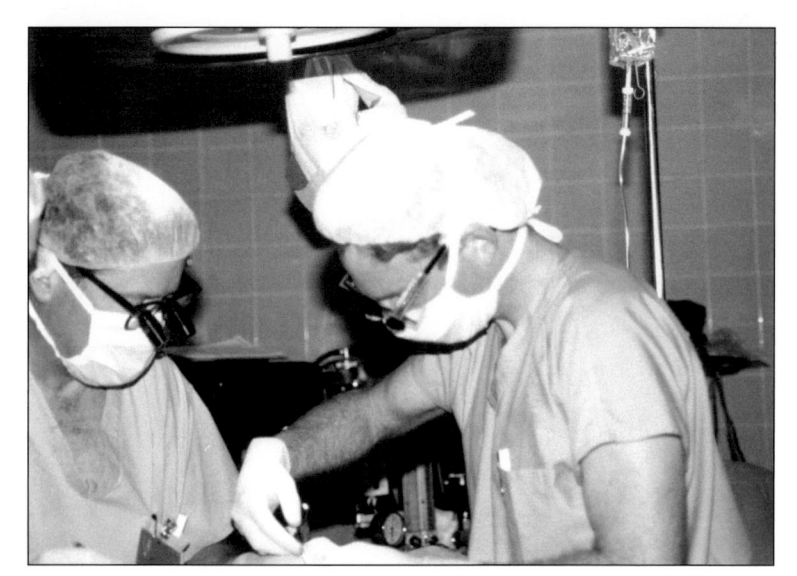

FIGURE 25-7. Trabulsy performs minor surgery in the old UHC 6th floor suite.

Trabulsy stayed on after his training, and became the Chief of Plastic Surgery, Hand Surgery, and Burn Surgery at San Francisco General Hospital for the next four years.

Mario Trabulsy was invited back to UVM in 1996 to practice as an emergency department physician. Her family lived in Vermont, which the young couple considered a wonderful place to raise a family. Linton, by this time, was ready to retire. When Leitner and Shackford offered Trabulsy a position at UVM in plastic surgery, the move was made. He accepted a dual appointment with orthopaedics that focused on hand surgery.

Vignettes of Microvascular Plastic Surgery in Three Decades

UVM's plastic surgeons put the microvascular techniques learned at the hands of Donaghy, Bunke, and Mathes to good use over the years. Here are a few examples:

1973

A motorcyclist lost a significant amount of soft tissue from his leg after a high-speed crash. Linton transplanted a latissimus dorsi free flap to the affected portion of the patient's lower extremity. The pioneering operation, which was essentially done with two medical students as assistants, took fifteen hours. Exhausted, Linton returned home to relax and listen to his beloved opera music. He was awakened several hours later by a report of a dusky flap. Linton dragged himself back to the operating room, revised the vascular graft, and performed a thrombectomy. The maneuvers rescued the flap, which in turn saved the patient's limb.[9]

1984

The surgeon and the style were different, but the wound and the outcome were the same. Leitner, having recently arrived at UVM, performed a similar latissimus dorsi free flap procedure on yet another injured motorcycle rider. The flap flourished without further incident, and the leg was salvaged.[10]

1996

A seven year-old girl sustained massive tissue loss below and behind her knee from a high-powered rifle bullet. Trabulsy was not on call, but had been visiting his wife in the E.R. when the alert came in. He and I (DBP) debrided the girl's leg and bypassed the damaged artery

FIGURE 25-8. Philip Trabulsy examines the patient described in the text with a below-knee salvage amputation from a major gunshot wound.

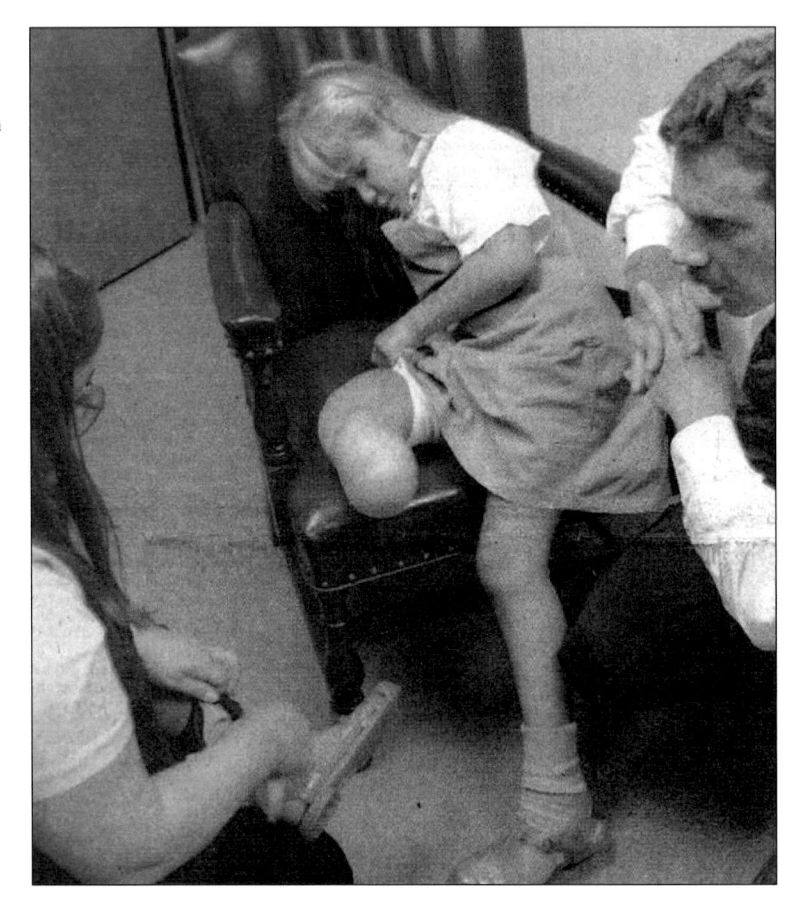

and vein. Unfortunately, the anterior compartment muscles did not survive. The tibia and fibula were intact, but completely exposed. An amputation was unavoidable; the only choice left was whether to amputate through or above-the-knee. Neither option was likely to provide a satisfactory result.

Trabulsy, inspired by work Mathes had done, suggested protecting the bones with a musculocutaneous flap.[11] The medial ankle tissue remained well vascularized from the vein graft, and provided sufficient coverage for a below-the-knee amputation. The procedure, although viewed with skepticism by dozens of well-meaning "consultants" was successfully carried out.

FIGURE 25-9. A below-knee amputation is much more functional than an above-knee amputation, as described in this 1996 example.

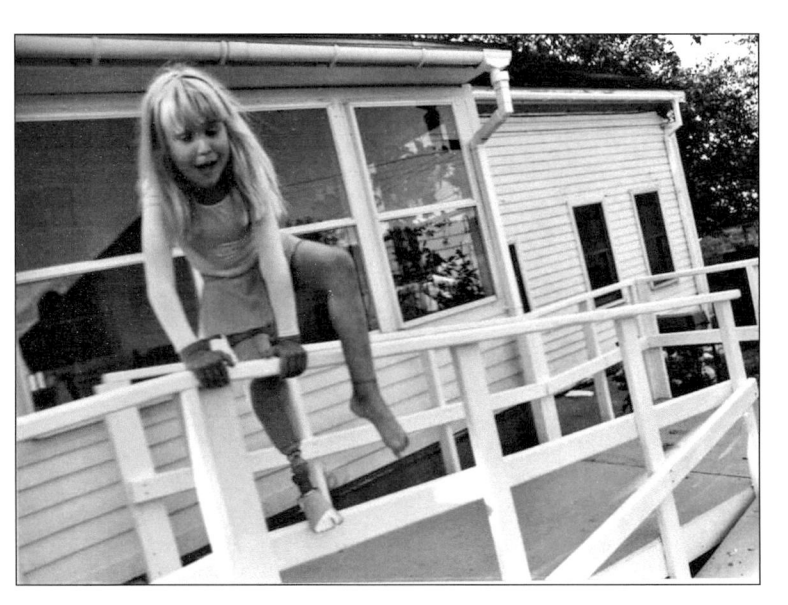

The patient ended up with a remarkably well-shaped and functional amputation on which she can run and play soccer.[12]

What Would You Do if You Contracted Hepatitis C?

Ten months and 350 operative cases into his UVM career, Trabulsy had another episode of fatigue and jaundice. He returned to the physician that he had seen six years earlier when he had "atypical hepatitis A". Routine lab tests showed poor liver function and anemia. The physician decided to recheck hepatitis titers. As Trabulsy put it, "I remember it like yesterday when Dr. S. called at 7 pm on a Tuesday to tell me I had hepatitis C. I asked him what that meant, and he said I had a virus affecting my liver."

Trabulsy met with an infectious disease doctor the next day. The two found three or four published reports of a surgeon transferring hepatitis C to a patient during an operative procedure. The infectious disease doctor suggested that Trabulsy put his surgical cases on hold, and perhaps take a medical leave. Trabulsy postponed his scheduled cases, saying that he was ill. Four days later, he told Leitner the bad news.

Many people thought Trabulsy should continue to operate despite the problem. But at this point, the hospital got a call from a patient. "I hear I was operated upon by a surgeon who has hepatitis. Am I at risk?" Alarmed, the hospital prompted Trabulsy to go public. A statement was sent to each of Trabulsy's UVM patients that read: "The surgeon has decided to curtail his surgical practice and undergo treatment for his condition." Trabulsy was eventually advised that he could officially return to the O.R. since the risk of transmission was so low; however he took the high road. He did not want to take even the slightest chance of passing hepatitis C virus on to a patient during a procedure.

Trabulsy's depression over his situation was compounded by the medication that he was receiving as part of his treatment. Sitting at home was not helping, so he returned to one of his favorite pastimes, golf. While on the links, he met William Allen, the chairman of the local Make-A-Wish Foundation® chapter. Allen befriended Trabulsy and invited him to join the Foundation's board. After a while, Allen suggested that he and Trabulsy build a tree house in order "to keep you occupied." A magical three-room structure was built in the canopy next to Trabulsy's home. It was a far cry from the shacks we all remember from our childhoods.

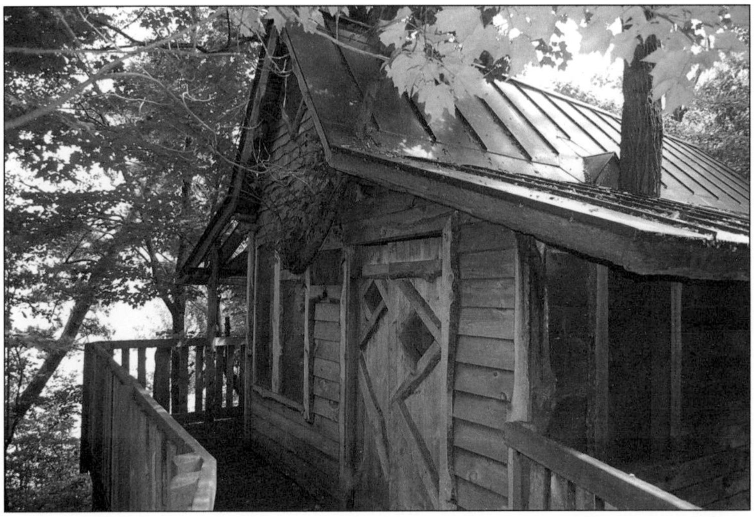

FIGURE 25-10. Trabulsy's first handicapped accessible tree house at Camp-Ta-Kum-Ta.

FIGURE 25-11. Trabulsy is leaning on a live tree that has sprouted leaves inside the Camp Ta-Kum-Ta tree house.

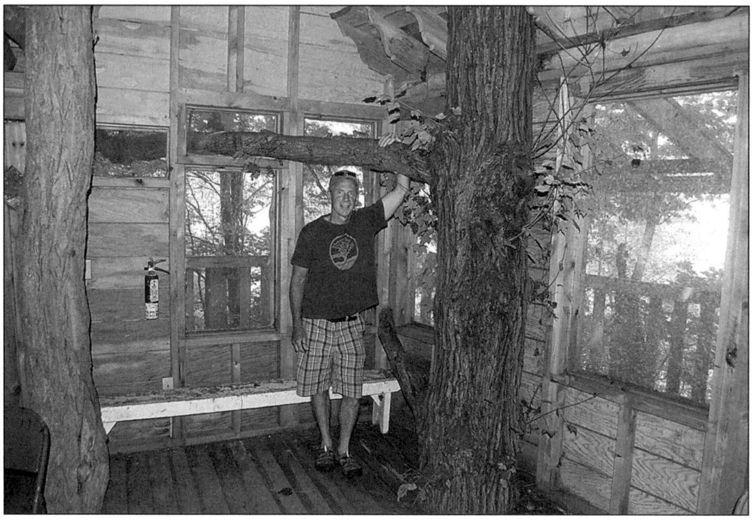

Trabulsy and Allen came up with the idea of building a wheelchair-accessible tree house at a Make-A-Wish board meeting, even though none of the kids had ever asked for one. In fact, no one had ever attempted such a project before. The pair offered the idea to Camp Ta-Kum-Ta, a Vermont retreat for children with cancer. They were told, "Show us you can build a handicapped-accessible tree house first." Trabulsy and Allen approached Vermont's "Yestermorrow Design/Build School®," for help and developed a prototype. Camp Ta-Kum-Ta approved the prototype, and the tree house was built on the site of the camp's Colchester Point location.

FIGURE 25-12. The ramp leading to the handicapped accessible tree house built by Forever Green Treehouses® for Paul Newman's Hole in the Wall Gang Camp.

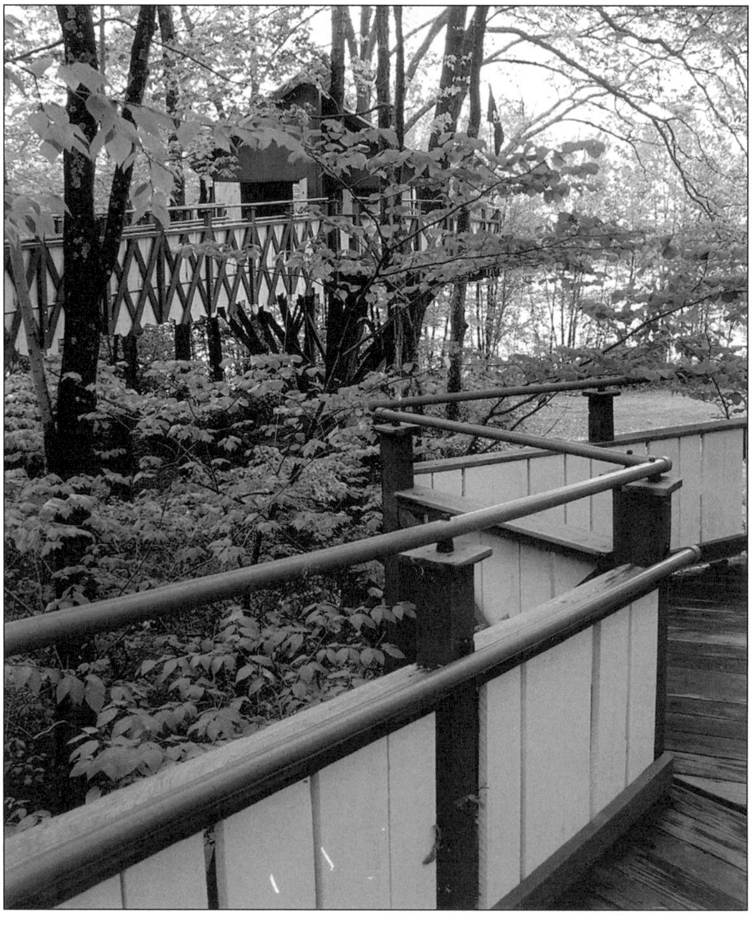

Paul Newman heard about the tree house, and had one built for his "Hole in the Wall Gang Camp®" in Ashford, Connecticut. Trabulsy and Allen's firm, "Forever Young Tree Houses®," has built nearly two-dozen universally accessible tree houses in the past decade. One of their most recent projects is a glorious Los Angeles structure costing over $500,000.[13]

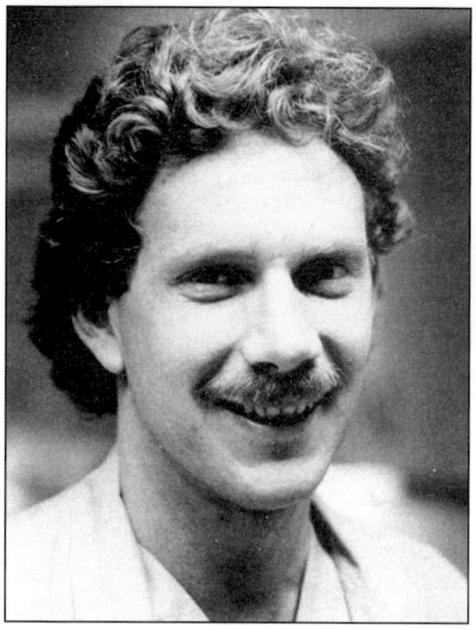

Trabulsy continues to see hand patients at UVM's orthopedic clinic, but does not operate. There isn't a minute of the day that he doesn't dream of doing surgery again! For the past year he has been exploring complementary and alternative medical practices.[14] Trabulsy's integrity and perseverance are an inspiration for medical students, residents, and other doctors. Hopefully, their paths will not be strewn with such thorns.

FIGURE 25-13. There isn't a minute of the day that Trabulsy (pictured in 1998) doesn't dream of doing surgery again.

Another New Plastic Surgeon is Hired

Leitner was one-man division of plastic surgery following Linton's 1996 retirement and Trabulsy's 1997 leave of absence. It did not seem like there was enough plastic surgery at UVM for more than one and one half surgeons. As such, the dual plastics and orthopaedic appointment was continued, so that Trabulsy's replacement could also help with hand surgery. No one foresaw that UVM was going to be home to four busy plastic surgeons within ten years.

Donald R. Laub, Jr. knew that he was not going into medicine after watching his plastic surgeon father work so hard at Stanford. The younger Laub graduated from U.C. Berkeley, but could not find a job. As a result, he became a research assistant at his father's lab in 1983. While there, he crossed paths with Leitner and future Dartmouth plastic surgeon Joseph Rosen. Laub also accompanied his father on several Interplast sponsored trips to Ecuador and Honduras. The exposure to third world plastic surgery inspired Laub to pursue medicine after all and become a plastic surgeon.

Laub graduated from the Medical College of Wisconsin and did part of a general surgery residency at Oregon Health Sciences University and Hospital. Then it was on to a plastic surgery fellowship at Dartmouth with Rosen, followed by a hand fellowship at Stanford. Laub finished at the right time with the right credentials. Leitner remembered Laub from his San Francisco lab assistant days and recruited him to UVM.

Linton's tradition of excellent cleft lip and palate repair has continued in the Vermont Craniofacial and Cleft Lip Clinic. Laub, oral surgeon Thomas Connolly, and orthodontist Richard Reed have developed innovative improvements to cleft lip and palate surgery. Laub brought the pioneering work to UVM from NYU following a brief mini-sabbatical. The trio starts their patients' naso-alveolar molding at three weeks of age with a retainer plate that brings the alveolar ridges into alignment. Single stage corrective surgery is subsequently performed at three months of age.

FIGURE 25-14. Donald Laub during a trip to Honduras with Interplast® with a young patient and his parents following a cleft lip repair.

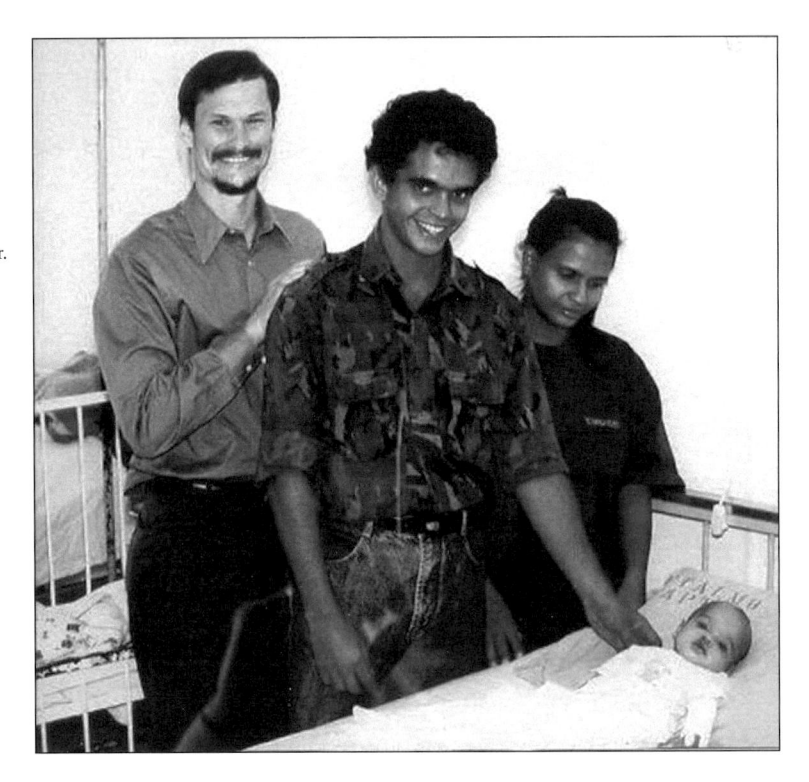

Laub has also followed in his father's footsteps by taking on gender reassignment surgery. As a result, UVM is now one center in the country capable of constructing a vagina for male-to-female patients using sigmoid colon. The process uses a relocated piece of sigmoid colon and is done in collaboration with a colorectal surgeon.[15] The operation is not frequently done elsewhere because of its technical difficulty, and the requirement for low anal anterior colon resection and re-anastomosis. A radial forearm flap is employed for urethral/penile construction in female-to-male patients. This operation is performed elsewhere, but not frequently as it may take multiple stages to achieve a suitable result.[16]

The Division's Approach to Breast Reconstruction

Leitner and Laub were soon overwhelmed by their workloads, especially with respect to breast surgery. Susan E. MacLennan joined the practice in 2000 after the case for hiring a third surgeon had been made. She had been a Dartmouth medical student when Laub was a resident. MacLennan scrubbed in on a breast reduction procedure the first day of her plastic surgery rotation. By the time the case was done, she knew that she wanted to be a plastic surgeon. MacLennan completed an integrated general and plastic surgery residency at the University of Cincinnati, and then came to UVM with a special interest in breast reconstruction.

Breast augmentation was still in its infancy prior to 1960. Ivalon® (polyvinyl alcohol-formaldehyde) sponges were often deployed, but became quite firm after implantation. The first silicone gel implants were placed in 1962, largely without prior FDA safety monitoring.[17] UVM's surgeons used silicone implants until their dangers were exposed to the public on the 1990 TV show "Face to face with Connie Chung."[18] Concerns included autoimmune reaction and cancer. The FDA effectively banned silicone implants in 1992, requiring that their use be considered investigational. Saline-filled implants were introduced around the same time. Replacement of silicone implants with their saline counterparts increased many a plastic surgeon's caseload.

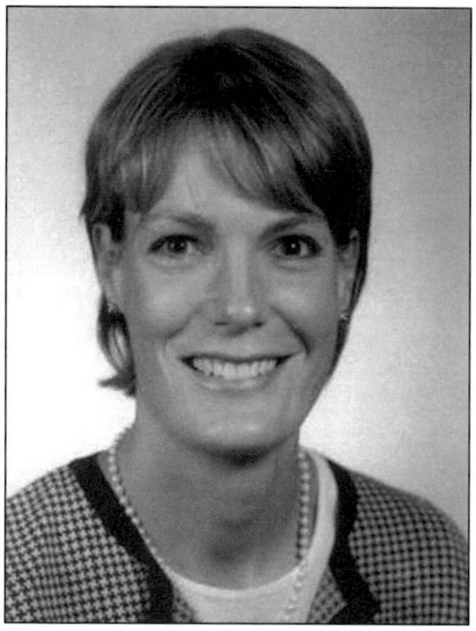

A National Academy of Science report later determined that "Evidence suggests diseases or conditions such as connective tissue diseases, cancer, neurological diseases or other systemic complaints or conditions are no more common in women with breast implants than in women without implants."[19] The FDA approved silicone implants in 2002 under stricter guidelines for patients requiring reconstruction or revision. The devices were released four years later for elective augmentation in women over 22 years of age. The worries over autoimmune reaction and cancer were dismissed.

FIGURE 25-15. Susan MacLennan joined the practice in 2000, having previously trained at Dartmouth with Laub.

MacLennan was mainly interested in post cancer surgery reconstruction. With this in mind, she started attending UVM's weekly Multidisciplinary Breast Conference. This collaborative effort among oncologists, pathologists, and radiologists has led to many more autologous tissue reconstructions. An example is the pedicled transverse rectus abdominus myocutaneous (TRAM) flap. First described in 1982, it requires the use of an entire rectus abdominus muscle. The drawback is that it weakens the abdominal wall and produces a bulge as it passes over the rib cage toward the breast. A free TRAM flap only sacrifices part of the rectus muscle, but it requires microvascular anastamoses.

The latest tissue reconstruction technique involves deep inferior epigastric perforator (DIEP) flap transfers. This uses abdominal skin and fat to reconstruct the breast mound in place of the rectus muscle. The approach is similar to a free TRAM flap in that it requires microvascular anastamoses. Such autologous tissue reconstructions usually yield superior results when compared to implants, but involve more extensive surgeries and have more potential complications. Although DIEP flaps are not yet done at UVM, the division continues to offer a wide range of breast reconstruction options.

The Future

Demand for plastic and reconstructive surgery continued to grow. This led to the hiring of Robert D. Nesbit in 2006. The Medical College of Georgia graduate finished his general surgery residency at the University of Tennessee before undergoing additional plastics training in Charlotte, North Carolina. Laub's dual appointment with orthopaedics was technically dissolved the same year so that he could devote himself to plastic surgery full time. He has since succeeded Leitner as chief of the four-person division.

"Giving Back" surgery thrives under Leitner, Laub, and MacLennan. Leitner has traveled abroad more times than he can count, and continues to find it a satisfying aspect of his career. Laub has temporarily foregone overseas surgery in order to maximize time with his young family, having already taken nine trips as a plastic surgeon with Interplast to Ecuador, Honduras, Vietnam, Brazil, and Guatemala. MacLennan has been to Peru twice. Their work has been facilitated by the Department of Surgery's policy of allowing three weeks with pay for such efforts. In most practices, volunteer services are charged up to vacation/meeting time.

The division's focus, understandably, has not been as research oriented as some other divisions over the years however the future looks bright. Nevertheless, UVM's plastic surgeons have ably served as excellent clinicians and role models for medical students and surgical residents, many of whom have pursued similar careers themselves. This is the true mark of the division's educational impact.

CHAPTER 26

Transplant and Immunology Division

The task of starting UVM's kidney transplant service fell to surgical oncologist Roger Foster. His superb operative skills and knowledge of immunology sustained the program for nearly 15 years.

More and more transplants were done as anti-rejection medications improved. The service steadily grew under Foster's successors, each of whom had received fellowship training in transplantation.

The carefully regulated discipline remains restricted to centers that generate enough volume and have satisfactory outcomes. Despite its small referral base, UVM continues to meet these criteria under the leadership of a new generation of surgeons.

The Recent Rise of Transplantation

Organ transplantation remained the stuff of science fiction until well into the 1960s. Although vascular surgeon Alexis Carrel had the expertise and audacity to move kidneys, hearts, spleens, and legs between dogs as early as 1908, his experiments were thwarted by rejection. Peter Medawar advanced the cause in 1951 with the discovery that tissue intolerance could be suppressed with medication. Cortisone was initially employed for this purpose before being augmented by azothioprine at the end of the decade.

Joseph Murray, meanwhile, had successfully performed a kidney transplant between a set of identical twins in 1954. He then carried out the world's first cadaveric renal transplant in 1962 thanks to azothioprine. James Hardy transplanted a lung in 1963, and Thomas Starzl started his liver transplantation work the same year. Starzl achieved success in 1967, but the accomplishment was overshadowed by Christiaan Barnard's human heart transplant a few months later. Long-term outcomes remained mixed, however, in spite of the increasing popularity of these procedures.

Kidney Transplantation Arrives at UVM in 1971

Chairman John Davis decided that UVM needed a transplant service if it were to remain competitive with other New England medical centers. After some consideration, he assigned the job to Roger Foster in 1971. Although Foster's clinical field was surgical oncology, his research interest was immunology. The choice made sense, since the most challenging part of a kidney transplant was the management of post-operative immunity, suppression, and rejection. Davis didn't exactly explain it to Foster that way, though. As he recalls, he asked Foster into his office and said: "We need a transplant program and you can do it."[1]

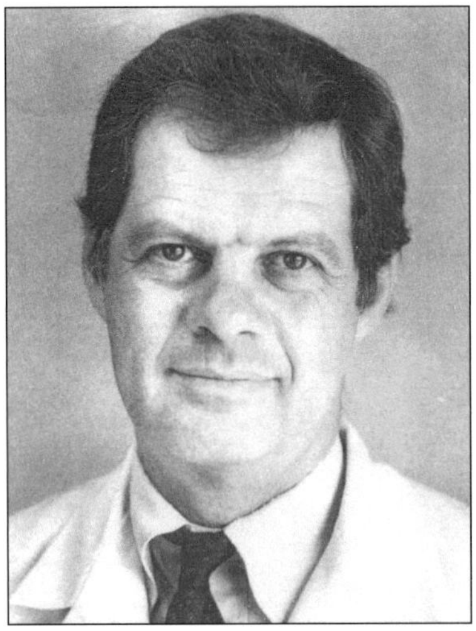

FIGURE 26-1. Roger Foster performed the first kidney transplant at UVM in 1971.

Foster agreed to the assignment, but asked me (DBP) to share the load when it came to arteriovenous hemodialysis shunt placement. Nephrologist Carl Runge came to the operating room and showed us how to properly implant a Ramirez shunt. The device differed from the classic Scribner shunt in that each limb of its silastic tubing had a "wing" that was tunneled under the skin. These kept the Teflon tips (which were tied to the interrupted yet undivided artery and vein) from rotating. Learning how to perform an operation from an internist was a unique experience, to say the least.

Davis was on call one weekend covering vascular surgery. He had been involved with dialysis while in Korea and at Fort Sam Houston. Davis was facile with dialysis needles and temporary access catheters, so he felt qualified to place a Ramirez shunt even though he had never seen one. When Davis asked the third year resident if he had done one of these before, the resident (incorrectly) assured him that he had. Davis and the resident placed the shunt in the radial artery and vein, but failed to bury the wings.

When Runge examined the pair's work on rounds the next morning, he exploded in my presence: "Who the hell put this shunt in this way?" He complained so vociferously that the

FIGURE 26-2. Artificial kidney used at UVM in 1959 for eight-hour long dialysis sessions.

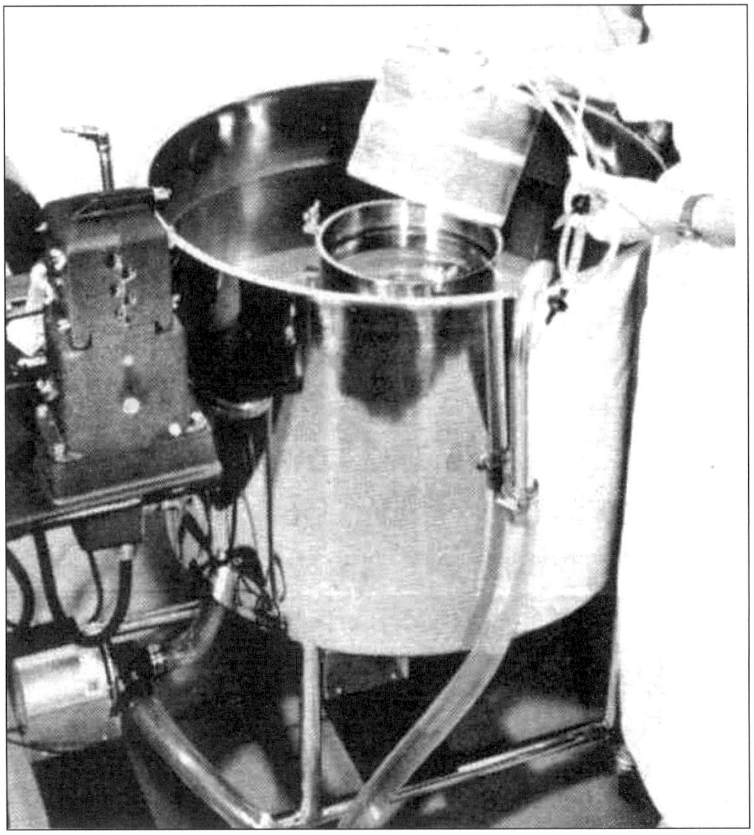

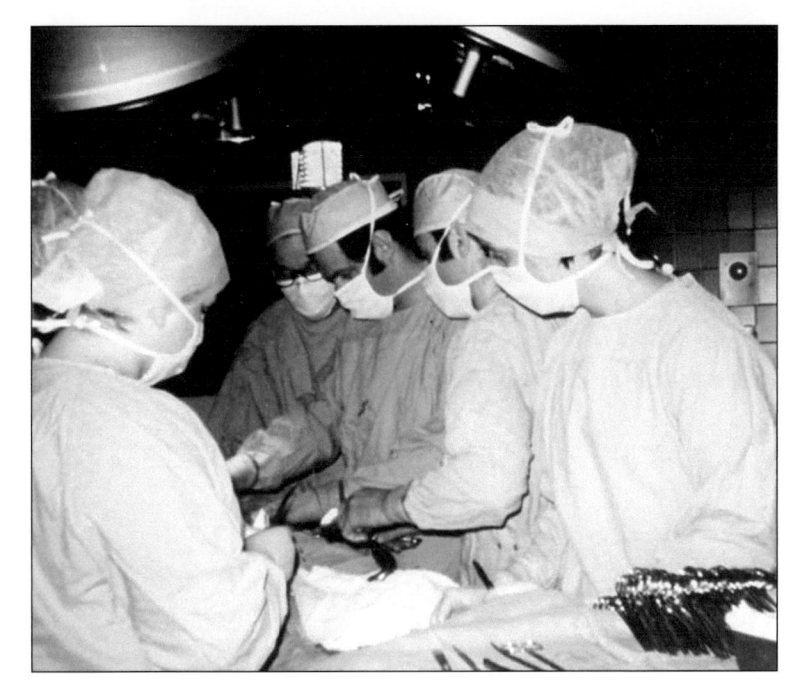

FIGURE 26-3. John Davis (4th from R) assisted Foster (3rd from R) during UVM's first kidney transplant. Young surgeons such as Foster didn't need eyeglasses, and the concept of universal precautions had yet to be mandated. Davis never scrubbed again for a kidney transplant.

surgical team took the patient back to the O.R. and revised the shunt according to Runge's protocol. Davis never discussed the event again, nor did he ever place another dialysis shunt or fistula!

Foster learned how to do the various steps required in a kidney transplant at a variety of surgical programs. He picked up a technique in which the ureters were tunneled through the bladder prior to their attachment during a visit to San Francisco. This led to less leakage than the standard method for ureteral implantation. UVM's urologists originally wanted to be involved with the transplants, specifically with the ureter-to-bladder anastomosis. Scheduling was a problem, as was the nature of the procedure itself. The urologists stood around during the first transplant operation and watched Foster do the vascular anastomoses while they waited for their fifteen minutes of surgery. Once the case was done, they decided that Foster could do the entire procedure himself. The urologists seemed happy to stay out of this arena from that point on.[2]

Operating room technician turned chief open-heart pump perfusionist Clement Comeau transported the procured kidneys. These were placed in a chilled solution that prevented cellular structures from swelling. Comeau also ran the perfusion pump that kept the kidneys preserved for up to 48 hours following removal.

The hemodialysis access surgery fell to the vascular surgeons as arteriovenous fistulas replaced silastic shunts. Foster performed the kidney transplants without backup from the other attending surgeons, although the nephrologists helped with post-operative medical management. Foster called the hospital several times a day whenever he was out-of-town to adjust his patients' anti-rejection medications. He basically took call for the service 365 days a year.

Organ Procurement Then and Now

Most transplanted organs came from cadavers during the '70s. Policy dictated that patients thought to be brain dead were to be taken to the operating room and then removed from the ventilator. If spontaneous respiration and a palpable aortic pulse were clinically absent, the patient was formally declared dead. The kidneys and/or other organs were then removed. Foster, as the transplant surgeon, was not allowed to perform the harvest or even be present in the O.R.

This was in sharp contrast to 21st century protocols. Patients are declared brain dead at the bedside via cerebral flow scans. Organs are harvested in the O.R. while perfusion continues, and a transplant surgeon usually does the procedure. Donation after cardiac death (DCD) can be carried out when support is withdrawn before checking for brain death. Such a scenario often plays out after failed emergency room trauma resuscitation.[3] The United Network for Organ Sharing (UNOS) stipulates that transplant surgeons cannot be involved with the consent process in any way. The surgeon is not allowed to proceed with procurement until five minutes have passed from the time that the patient was declared dead by the E.R. or ICU team.[4]

The Legionnaire's Epidemic of 1977

Transplants were performed in Room 7, the largest of Smith 2's operative suites. Unfortunately, the air conditioner intake was immediately adjacent to Room 7. As a result, the space routinely filled with external odors. For example, when a rescue helicopter landed outside, one could immediately smell the exhaust fumes in the room. The phenomenon was largely regarded as a nuisance by the hospital, despite repeated protests by the O.R. staff.

The Vermont Legionnaire's disease epidemic of 1977 struck the hospital with a vengeance. A total of 69 patients and staff came down with the abrupt onset of headache and diarrhea, followed by fever, rigors, and a cough that produced minimally purulent sputum. The infection could not be identified at first, and did not respond to standard antibiotic therapy. Respiratory failure, hypotension, and septic shock led to fourteen deaths during the May to December outbreak.[5]

The transplant service was hit especially hard. Fourteen of UVM's 101 transplant patients contracted the disease. The causative organism, Legionella pneumophila, did not take Gram's stain and was not easily cultured. Suspicions were raised and then finally confirmed through antibody testing. Seven of the transplant patients were successfully treated once the disease was identified, although it was later found within two infected hemodialysis fistulas.[6]

A second, less severe outbreak occurred at UVM in 1980. Epidemiologic and environmental studies pinpointed a Legionella breeding ground within the cooling tower atop the Given Building. The Room 7 air intake was just 500 feet downwind from the tower. Clusters of the disease have sporadically appeared throughout the State since then, but the hospital has been spared following appropriate decontamination and rerouting of its ventilation equipment.[7]

Low Urine Output Isn't Always Rejection

Foster had transplanted a second living-related kidney into a 13 year-old girl with chronic renal failure. The transplant was technically "successful," but functioned poorly. There were no signs of rejection. The patient was in severe congestive heart failure, so she continued to undergo dialysis through a huge saphenous vein arteriovenous fistula in her left thigh. Foster and I (DBP) postulated that this enormous fistula was causing high-output congestive heart

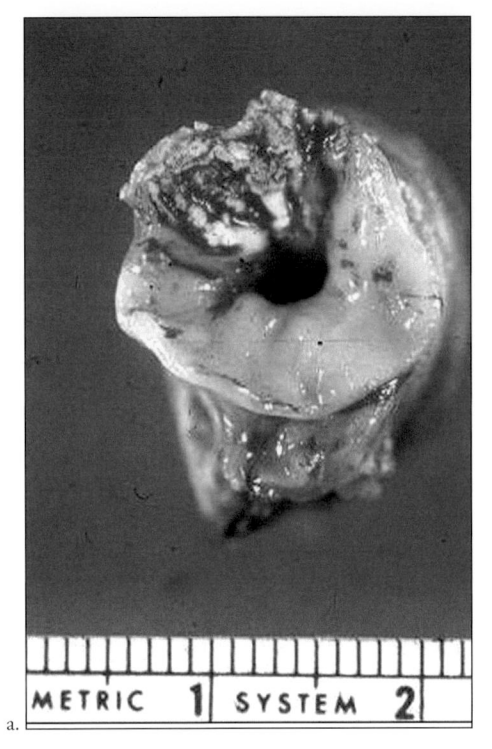

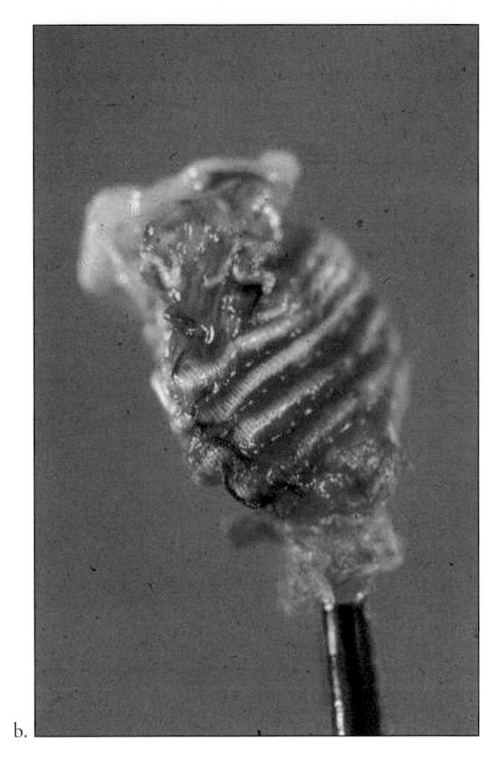

FIGURE 26-4.
After removal of the no longer needed saphenous loop arterio-venous loop fistula, the specimen shows the Dacron® band in place. Proximal luminal view (a) and side view (b).

failure, which in turn was leading to hypoperfusion of the transplanted kidney. Digital compression of the fistula produced a Branham's sign (bradycardia seen with obstruction of a high flow fistula) and confirmed the diagnosis.

I exposed the fistula's arterial origin in the operating room and found its flow rate to be 5.2 liters a minute. This was more than twice what this small girl's normal cardiac output should have been, and it was all short-circuiting through the fistula. In fact, this fistula's flow was greater than any that had ever been reported in the surgical literature. Her overworked heart was enlarged and failing. I reduced the fistula's inflow to 1.5 liters a minute with a constrictive Dacron band. Within hours, her congestive heart failure was gone. The transplanted kidney made supernormal amounts of urine, and relieved the fluid overload from her congestive failure. The patient never needed dialysis again. The fistula was subsequently ligated and removed, and the kidney remains functional 30 years later.

UVM Recruits Fellowship Trained Transplant Surgeons

Foster performed all of UVM's transplants until 1984. A change in leadership was undertaken at that juncture for several reasons. The most obvious was that Foster's obligations to surgical oncology in general and the Vermont Cancer Center in particular were consuming much of his time. The second was the appearance of cyclosporine on the market in 1983. The safer and more powerful immunosuppressive agent facilitated transplants in previously unsuitable candidates, which led to a greater number of cases.

Carl E. Haisch was fresh out of a clinical transplantation fellowship at Albany Medical College when he assumed the transplant service mantle from Foster. The University of

Washington medical school graduate had completed four years of research over the course of his general surgery residency, two of which were in transplant and vascular surgery at East Carolina University. Haisch did all of the dialysis access surgery, much to the relief of the busy vascular surgeons. He subsequently achieved excellent fistula patency and renal transplant survival rates. Haisch also helped increase organ procurement for the New England Organ Bank.

Haisch returned to East Carolina University for a similar position in 1992, and was replaced by Jeffrey C. Reese the following year. Reese had trained in general surgery at St. Louis University and had taken transplant fellowships in St. Louis and Pittsburg with Thomas Starzl. Reese, like Haisch, wanted to perform all of the access surgery. He also wanted to do elective liver cases, such as metastatic tumor resections and portocaval shunts, since he had been exposed to a lot of liver surgery under Starzl.

Reese considered establishing a liver transplant program at UVM, but the plans withered. Nevertheless, the kidney transplant service flourished. Some of the increase in volume came from Dartmouth, which had lost its transplant surgeon. Reese worked to raise UVM's stature within the New England and Albany programs. This ensured that Vermont's transplant patients received their fair share of the region's donated organs.

The Montreal Transplant Connection

Reese left for the greener pastures of Kansas City, Missouri in 2001. UVM was suddenly left without a kidney transplant program. The hospital scrambled to give two McGill transplant surgeons, Jean Tchervenkov and Peter Metrakos, surgical privileges to do a few transplants in Burlington. UVM nephrologist Mark Weidner helped out by coordinating post-op immunosuppressive therapy. Abrar Khan was brought in as UVM's attending transplant surgeon in 2002. With the assistance of the Montreal group, UVM continued to perform about 30 total organ transplants per year. This included 6 combined kidney-pancreas transplants.[8]

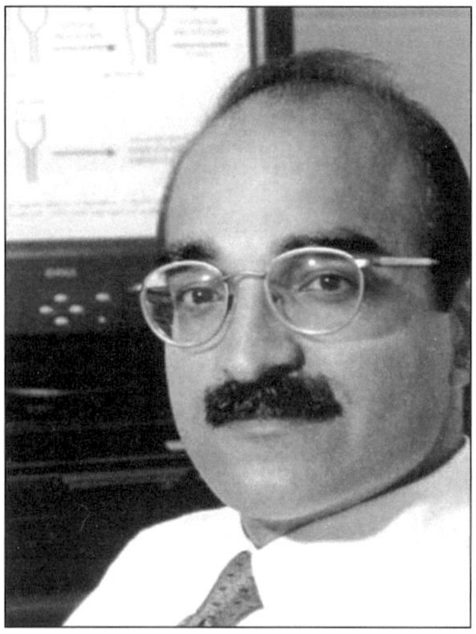

FIGURE 26-5. Abrar Kahn proved a productive researcher at UVM.

UVM hired McGill alumnus Anthony Di Carlo upon Khan's 2005 departure. Di Carlo had also trained in surgery at McGill before doing a multivisceral transplantation fellowship at the University of Wisconsin. He has continued to work with the Montreal group in order to maintain his liver transplant skills with the goal of eventually bringing hepatic transplantation to UVM. Di Carlo initiated a total laparoscopic approach for living related kidney donors, which attracted new patients to UVM. This technique is associated with decreased morbidity and improved cosmesis. Other nearby transplant programs do not routinely offer this option in 2008.

Jon S. Yamaguchi is the latest transplant team addition, having joined UVM in 2007. Medical school at Temple was followed by surgery residency at the University of Maryland and a multi-organ transplant fellowship at Emory. Yamaguchi waited until his chief resident year to embrace transplant surgery. By then, what had previously seemed to him like monotonous operations on incredibly sick patients turned out to be technically demanding procedures with tremendously gratifying outcomes. Yamaguchi was subsequently attracted to UVM for its lifestyle, and the chance to be a full partner from day one in a small, young division that was attempting to start a liver transplant service.

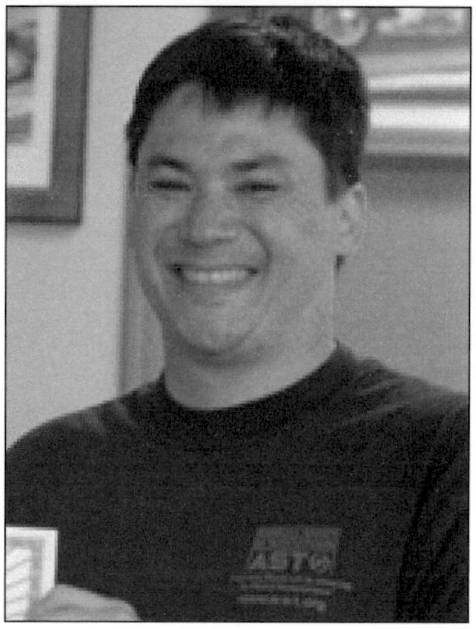

Widespread transplantation remains limited by the supply of organs. The deceased donor rate has increased 23% since 2003 nationwide. Implementing donation after cardiac death (DCD) has also expanded the number of available organs. Di Carlo and the Wisconsin group have demonstrated that this is a successful strategy.[9] The UVM team is also exploring whether organs from less-than-ideal donors can still benefit recipients in an era of improving anti-rejection agents. The outlook is encouraging as UVM embarks on its fourth decade of performing highly successful renal transplants.[10]

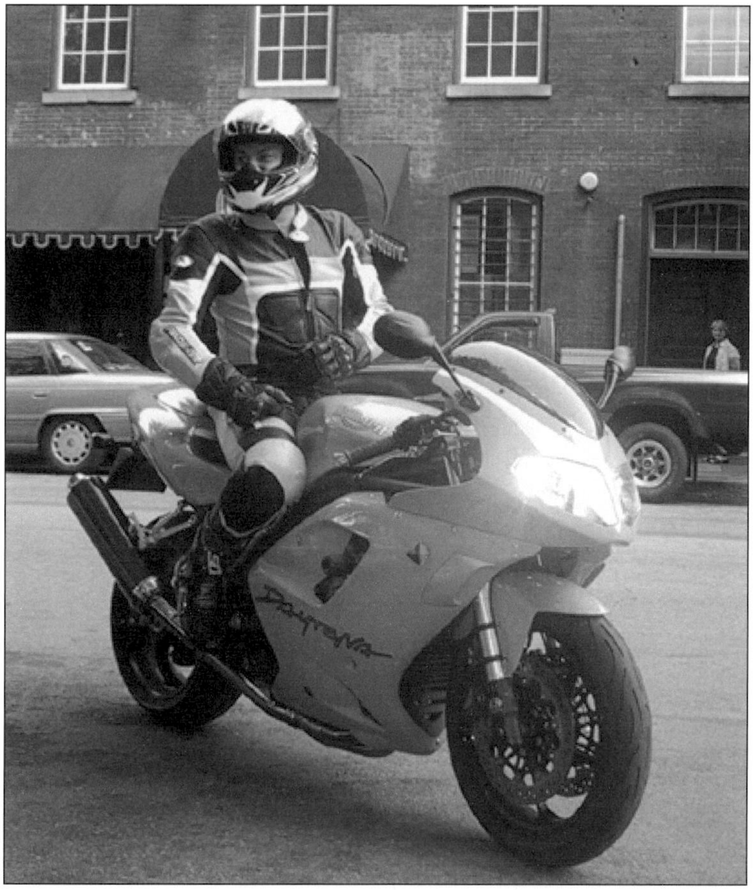

FIGURE 26-6. Jon Yamaguchi in his transplant society t-shirt accepting his certificate of completion for his motorcycle racing course.

FIGURE 26-7. Yamaguchi here has just completed an eight hour ride!

CHAPTER 27

Urology Division

Visiting professors gave way to part-time faculty at UVM as the field of urology evolved. An already excellent clinical program was enhanced with new blood and skills in 1967. The group remained independent during the Davis regime even though other divisions joined the UHC fold. When the chief retired in 1992, the urologists fell on hard times and lost their residency program.

The division gradually rebuilt itself by joining UVM full-time and increasing its academic pursuits. Stable, proven leaders currently oversee a full spectrum of cutting-edge services.

Stone Crushers Become Skilled Specialists

Bladder stones were, until recently, one of most commonly treated surgical conditions in all of western civilization. Poor diet, chronic infection, and urinary stasis led to the formation of incredibly painful calculi. Dramatic relief came with rapid perineal incisions that either removed the stones or crushed them so that they could pass through the urethra. Described as early as 50 A.D., such procedures were the domain of practitioners known as "stone crushers" or "lithotomists." These itinerant "specialists" usually did not deliver any other surgical or medical treatments.

By the early 1800s, most respected surgeons "cut for the stone." Nathan Smith was especially skilled in this operation. As he told his students:

> *A large stone is the most frequent cause of unfortunate operations. It is not the frequent introduction of the forceps that causes the death of the patient. In one case I operated successfully where there were 40 stones in the bladder but they were small. The forceps were introduced a great number of times ... After the operation the bladder should be examined with the finger and after all the stones that can be found are removed, the bladder should be washed out with a syringe of warm water.[1]*

The procedure, while straightforward, remained dangerous in the era before anesthesia and asepsis. Further advances came with Maximilian Nitze's development of the modern cystoscope in 1877. The device had magnifying lenses like a telescope, and an incandescent filament. Alexander Brenner modified the design in 1887 to include a curved tip and a channel for ureteral cannulation.[2] Diagnostic and therapeutic measures, such as superficial tumor removal and prostatic channel enlargement, were advanced through the additions of miniature light bulbs, cautery, and improved optics. Traditional surgical training, however, did not incorporate the specialized skills required of the new cystoscopes.

Open procedures evolved along the same lines. William Belfield performed a prostate resection at Cook County Hospital in 1886.[3] Hugh Young conducted the first radical perineal prostatectomy for cancer in 1904 at Johns Hopkins. Young, the father of American Urology, initially had no interest in what was still a new field. When told by William Halsted that he was to "take charge of the Department of Genito-Urinary Surgery" in 1897, Young replied, "This is a great surprise. I know nothing about genitourinary surgery." Halsted replied, "Dean Welch and I said you didn't know anything about it, but we believe you could learn."[4]

Visiting Professors Become Part-Time Staff

Young's experience at Johns Hopkins was typical, as UVM too was without a qualified urologist at the turn of the century. The College of Medicine filled its teaching gap, as it had done in other sub-specialties, with special professors of "Genito-Urinary and Venereal Diseases" from elsewhere. The first person to hold the position was James R. Hayden (1862-1921) of Columbia University's College of Physicians and Surgeons. Hayden, whose preceptor at Columbia was none other than William Halsted, lectured at UVM from 1892-1898. Eugene Fuller (1858-1930) of the New York Post-Graduate School succeeded him from 1899-1901. Fuller, like Belfield, had been one of the first surgeons to resect the prostate.

Frank R. England (1862-1942) of McGill followed from 1903-04. The suffragette work of his more famous wife, Octavia Grace Ritchie (the first woman in Quebec to receive a medical degree), soon drew him back to Montreal. James E. Pedersen (1864-1947), yet another Post-Graduate staffer, was next in 1905-07. Walter S. Reynolds (1864-1919) of the College of Physicians and Surgeons succeeded him from 1909-10.[5]

The revolving door of specialists stopped turning after the College of Medicine's 1911 reorganization. New Jersey native William Warren Townsend (1870-1928) was brought in from Rutland to be Special Professor of Genito-Urinary Disease later that year, a position that he held until his death. Townsend had graduated from the College of Medicine in 1893, and had obtained his urologic training in New York. He was quite academic for a rural practitioner, having published numerous articles prior to his UVM appointment. Among these were treatises on renal efficiency, chronic anterior urethritis, and one with the squirm-inducing title "Bicycle-riding upon improperly fitting saddles as an aetiological factor in prostatitis and stricture of the urethra."

Townsend's son, William Graves Townsend (1896-1944), joined UVM's staff as an instructor in 1926. Tod, as he was known, was another College of Medicine product. The younger Townsend had learned urology in New York and at the feet of his father, whom he eventually succeeded as the first full-time Professor of Urology. Former chairman A.G. Mackay had been a medical student and intern under Townsend, and remembered him as, "a fine man, much beloved by his confreres."[6]

Winthrop M. Flagg (1910-1955) joined Tod Townsend in 1938. Flagg had also received his MD from UVM before taking a urology residency at Morrisania Hospital in the Bronx.

Townsend and Flagg learned how to use the cystoscope during the late 1930s. The pair then started to perform trans-urethral resection of the prostate (TURP), a procedure first described in 1932. In order to prevent anyone (particularly the general surgeons) from stealing their secret technique, patients were wheeled on a half-stretcher into a little-used room in which the two performed the surgery.[7]

Urology Residency Starts After World War II

Flagg was appointed Chief of Urology upon Townsend's death and his own return from WWII military service. Urology formally became a division within the Department of Surgery in 1945. Shortly thereafter, Flagg received approval to start a urology training program. His first resident, Platt R. Powell, had been brought up in Milton, Vermont, where his father ran a grocery store. Powell was an engineering student while an undergraduate at UVM, but went on to the College of Medicine. He interned at Bryn Mawr Hospital in Philadelphia and then returned to Burlington for a pathology year. Powell's urology residency at the University of Pennsylvania was interrupted, however, when he was called up into the Army at the start of the Second World War.

Powell served two years as a general surgeon with Boston's harbor defenses. He was then sent to England where he worked with Boris Petroff, a trained urologist from New York City. During this time, Powell frequently saw buzz bombs traveling overhead en route to London. He was subsequently transferred to East Anglia to help care for the Third Division of the Eighth Air Force. Powell managed to acquire two years of urology credit in the process. Following his 1946 discharge, he resumed his urology residency at Morrisania Hospital. One year later, he became the first urology resident at UVM.[8] Powell then spent six months studying prostate surgery in Brooklyn prior to joining Flagg as an attending urologist in 1949.[9]

William T. Fagan, Jr. became the fifth resident to complete the UVM program in 1952. He had chosen a medical career while he was still a teenager after helping a doctor operate on a child with an infected eardrum. Fagan subsequently attended UVM for both undergraduate and medical school before embarking on a Mary Fletcher internship. Fagan remained in

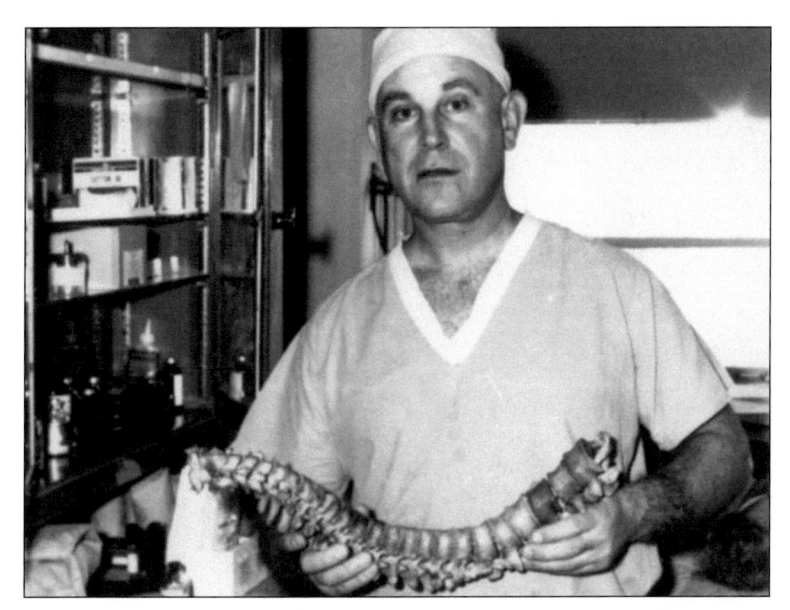

FIGURE 27-1. Platt Powell, UVM's first urology residency graduate, later became the Chief of Urology.

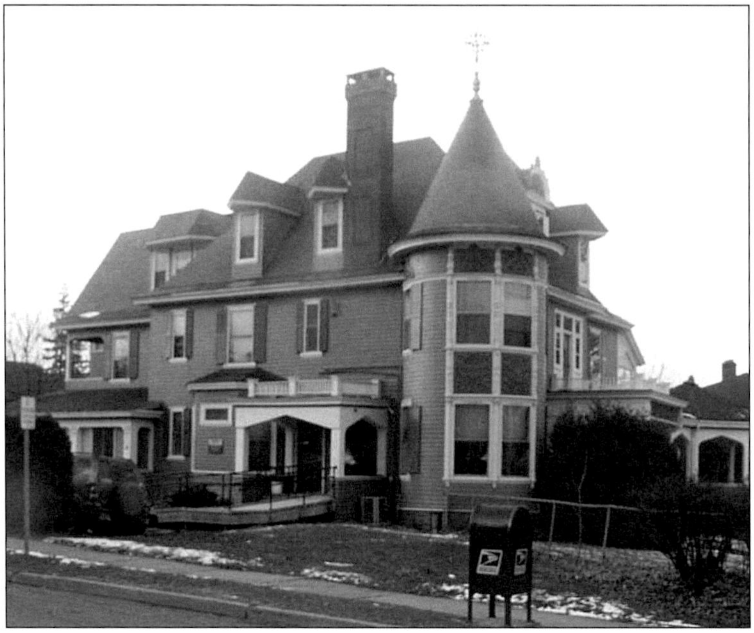

FIGURE 27-2. The Pearl Street Urology office originally belonged to William Fagan, and more recently to the UVM Department of Family Practice.

Burlington after finishing his training. Within a few years, Flagg died and Powell became chief of the division of urology.

The division moved into Fagan's Pearl Street office. Powell and Fagan did endoscopies, TURPs, and open prostatectomies through suprapubic or retropubic approaches. In addition, the duo performed radical cystectomy with urinary diversion, radical nephrectomy, and some pediatric urologic procedures. General surgeons assisted with the intestinal portions of these operations, and rendered assistance when the chest was open. Powell also conducted urological procedures at such institutions as the Vermont State Hospital in Waterbury, often taking a resident with him to assist.

Powell and Fagan's unique partnership steadily added more members over time. Income was pooled and divided equally among all of the partners regardless of their productivity. Fagan remembers that he and Powell approached Dean Edward Andrews about the part-time urologists joining the faculty full-time. Andrews said that he could not afford to match the group's salaries. He asked that they remain part-time, but continue to teach and provide cases for the College of Medicine.[10]

A New Chief of Urology is Recruited From the MGH

Powell decided that the division of urology needed new leadership if it was to keep offering the latest procedures. This was despite the fact that his retirement date was still more than ten years away. Powell planned to continue practicing; he just felt that it was time to step down as Chief. Both Powell and Fagan were acquainted with the chair of urology at the Massachusetts General Hospital (MGH), Wyland F. Leadbetter. They also knew that Wyland's younger cousin Guy W. Leadbetter, Jr. was a urologist. Guy had hoped to inherit the MGH chair from Wyland, but decided to leave Boston when that seemed unlikely. Powell and Fagan took advantage of the situation and hired the younger Leadbetter as the division's chief in 1967 to improve teaching and surgery.

Guy Leadbetter had followed his orthopedic surgeon father into medicine and his cousin Wyland into urology. He had attended Johns Hopkins, regarded by many as the home of American urology, for medical school. This had been followed by three years of general surgery and three years of urology training at the MGH. Leadbetter then joined the MGH urology staff upon the completion of his residency in 1959.

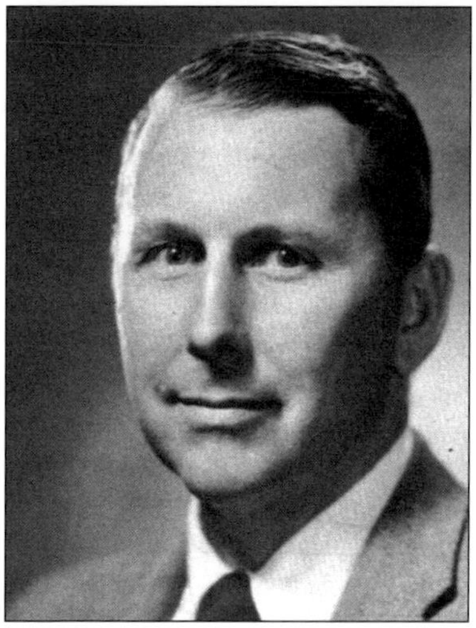

Leadbetter pioneered research in hypertension due to renal artery stenosis while at the MGH, performing the angiograms himself. This was done by puncturing the aorta of a prone patient with an extra long 16-gauge spinal needle. Intravenous bolus angiograms were carried out occasionally as well. Leadbetter followed the Cleveland Clinic's lead and performed the first renal artery bypass for hypertension control at the MGH. Although vascular surgery giants Robert Linton and Clement Darling were at the same institution, they had little interest in the procedure. As a result, Leadbetter did all of the MGH's renal artery bypasses until his departure for UVM.

FIGURE 27-3. Guy Leadbetter brought new urological skills to UVM, and built a new division when Powell stepped down.

While at the MGH, Leadbetter developed a procedure to rectify total urinary incontinence in children. He also came up with a technique for fixing megaureter, and a two-stage perineal correction for urethral strictures. After coming to UVM, Leadbetter performed major oncologic and pediatric urologic operations on patients that had previously been sent to Boston. Well trained in general surgery, he constructed the ileal loops required of urinary diversion procedures himself. This displaced UVM's general surgeons from their accustomed roles in these operations.[11]

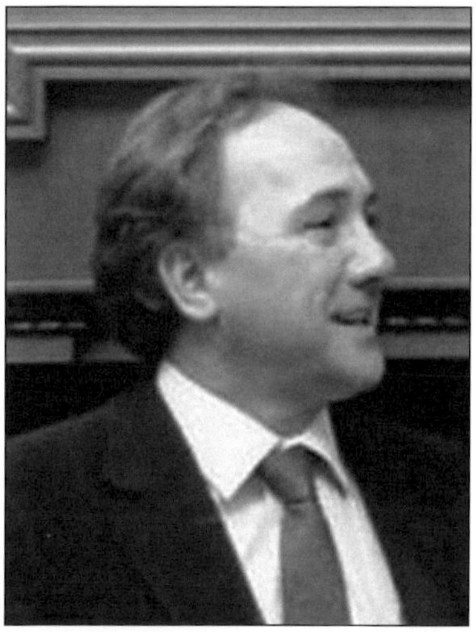

Paul M. Morrisseau was brought on board in 1969. The Burlington native and College of Medicine graduate had completed an internship and a year of general surgery while in the Army. Morrisseau's father died, however, just as he started his Army urology residency. He left the program and returned to Burlington to run his father's restaurant. Powell and Fagan offered him a position in UVM's urology residency program, which he completed in 1969. Morrisseau was planning to go elsewhere, but was convinced to stay by Leadbetter. Nevertheless, he cleverly obtained a Florida license after he finished his residency. This allowed him to move his practice to Florida later and semi-retire at a young age.

FIGURE 27-4. Burlington native Paul Morriseau was recruited by Leadbetter.

Morrisseau remembers that his salary was $25,000 when he became a partner in Urology Associates. He felt that this was much less than what others in New England were making. The group contacted all former UVM urology residents practicing in New England and had them submit records of their charges and reimbursements from Blue Cross/Blue Shield. It turned out that almost everyone else was paid twice as much as Urology Associates! As Morrisseau put it, "We just hadn't increased our fees with the times and inflation!" The group

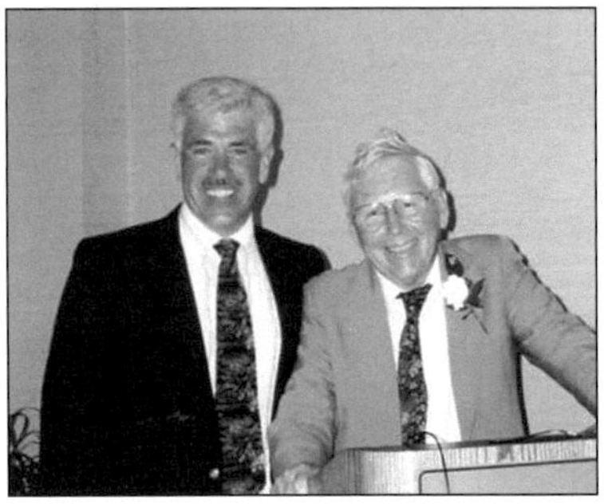

FIGURE 27-5.
Robert Vinson and Leadbetter happily share a podium.

submitted the data to their insurance companies, and asked that their rates be doubled. After their initial outrage, the insurers realized that this was fair after all and granted fee increases across the board![12]

Robert K. Vinson joined Urology Associates in 1977. He had gone to Harvard for medical school and then finished a urology residency at the University of Michigan. Vinson and Leadbetter bought Fagan's office building from Fagan together. This was then used as the Urology Associates clinic. "Vinson had a Midas touch. He managed to buy the building with no money down and pay it off with the rents."[13]

The Calm Before the Storm

Powell stuck to his plan to retire in 1978 at age 65, even though he was still in good health. Leadbetter continued as chief of the division, performing oncologic and reconstructive procedures. Morrisseau kept busy with general urology and outreach at North Country Hospital in Newport, Vermont. Vinson took over most of the pediatric urology. The urology residency was flourishing, and the urologists were doing well financially — at least in the eyes of some general surgeons. When Fagan stepped down in 1984, it was determined that he could be replaced with two or even three new partners.

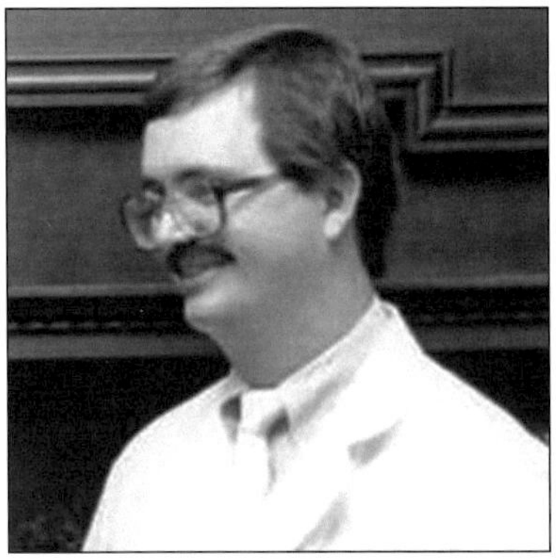

FIGURE 27-6.
Sam Trotter's first taste of Vermont came when he started his UVM urology residency.

Samuel J. Trotter had gone to medical school at the University of Illinois and had done two years of general surgery residency at Chicago's Rush University. Nevertheless, he was actively looking for a urology position somewhere else. Most urology residencies, including the one at UVM, recruited residents from their own general surgery training programs. UVM, however, had an opening because one of its residents had switched to anesthesia. Morrisseau interviewed Trotter at a meeting in Chicago and hired him on the spot, even though he really didn't have the authority to do so. Trotter had never been to Vermont before, but came without hesitation. He became a staff member upon finishing his residency in 1986 and has grown deep roots since.[14]

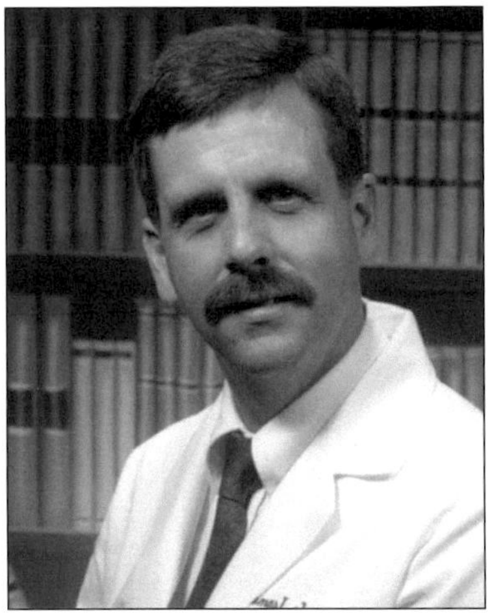

FIGURE 27-7.
Tom Jackson was a UVM urology resident three years behind Trotter, and then joined him on the faculty.

Thomas L. Jackson was the next to join the faculty in 1989. He had attended medical school and completed two years of general surgery at nearby Dartmouth before crossing the Connecticut River upon accepting a urology residency at UVM. Christopher S. Fukuda was brought into the group in 1992. Fukuda, whose father had been one of John Abajian's early anesthesiology residents, had long-standing UVM ties. He had obtained an M.D. from the College of Medicine before going to the University of Washington for his urology training. With a vibrant new staff in place, prosperity seemed assured.

The Perfect Storm

A turning point arrived during 1992, however. Leadbetter retired, as he had intended, at age 65. According to Morrisseau and Trotter, Vinson felt that he should replace Leadbetter as Chief of the Division of Urology. Leadbetter had indeed wanted to leave Vinson in charge, but had not discussed his succession plan with the rest of the group. Morrisseau, Trotter, Jackson, and Fukuda all objected. Morrisseau became the acting Chief.[15]

In the meantime, the Department of Surgery had recently hired a new chairman and the College of Medicine had appointed a new Dean. The Dean wanted all of the town's urologists to join UVM and UHC as a full-time group. The urologists felt that they were better off on their own, happy with their fee schedules and reimbursements. However dissatisfaction within the group over perceived workload inequities that were rewarded with equal pay arose. Some of the partners essentially felt they were working more than the others, but were not being paid appropriately.

The pressure to join the full-time faculty was accompanied by trouble with the residency program. During a site visit, the ACGME found that a couple of long-term problems had worsened since its last visit. The first was that the residents spent too much time operating and not enough time in clinic. This was an understandable issue at a chronically understaffed hospital. The second more troublesome concern was that the residents were not receiving adequate didactic training. The needed changes fell by the wayside during the disagreements that arose following Leadbetter's retirement, and the program lost its accreditation. The final UVM trainee, Richard Phelps, graduated in 1995.

Morrisseau planned to retire around the same time, so the furthest thing from his mind was staying on as the division's leader. Vinson, after failing to be appointed chief, took a three-month sabbatical at 80% pay and never came back. Fukuda left the group for a Burlington-based private practice. Urology Associates and its residency program, in place since the late 1940s, were both extinct by 1996.[16]

After the Storm

Making the most out of the opportunity, the Dean turned the Division of Urology into a full-time practice group. Shackford appointed Trotter as Chief of the reconstituted division. Jackson signed on, thereby forming a two-person group. The pair picked up the pieces of Urology Associates, winning back most of the group's former patients. The fact that they continued to be located in Fagan's old 371 Pearl Street office may have helped. Jackson was eventually given the task of revising, refining, and running the general surgery clinical core training program for the medical students.

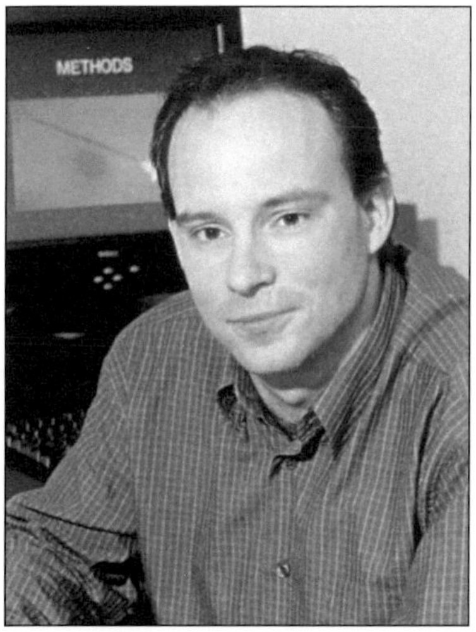

Volume was sufficient enough to hire additional urologists that same year. Mark K. Plante had attended McGill for medical school, and general surgery and urology residencies. He had also engaged in laser-guided minimally invasive prostatic therapy during his time in Montreal,

FIGURE 27-8. Mark Plante engaged in active research at UVM upon his arrival in 1996.

something that was not offered in Burlington. He met Trotter and Jackson during an elective month at UVM during his chief year, and liked what he saw. Plante consequently joined the division of urology upon the completion of his residency in 1996.

A. Cengiz Esenler arrived around the same time. The Medical College of Toledo graduate had gone through general surgery and urology training alongside Plante at McGill. After taking up some of the slack at UVM's hospital, he additionally set up an outreach clinic in nearby St. Albans.

Urology Research Shifts Into High Gear

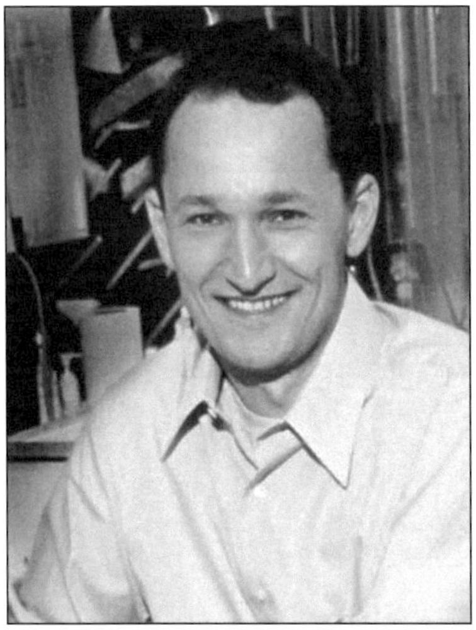

FIGURE 27-9. Peter Zvara was brought on board in 1999 to expand urology's research.

Plante's minimally invasive skills were accompanied by academic endeavors. In 1997, he joined a clinical trial that investigated the new drug Flomax®. He also engaged in a trial that examined radiofrequency needle ablation of enlarged prostates. Plante encouraged his former McGill associate Peter Zvara to join UVM's research lab. The two then initiated prostate ablation experiments using alcohol placed through the hollow needles that had been employed for radiofrequency ablation. Their initial work was funded and published in 1999.[17] This led to a phase I/II trial with Plante as lead investigator.[18]

Zvara and Plante switched their focus when prostate ablation funding was no longer available. They turned to studying the correlation between sensory innervation and function of the bladder, reasoning that suppression of sensory input could benefit bladder hyperactivity. Their experimental mouse model, which employs microsurgery and uses homemade electrodes, is unique to UVM. Zvara has since left to form a clinical testing company. Nevertheless, project funding for Plante's bladder research remains secure through an NIH grant.

New Horizons

The division made enough progress under Trotter, Jackson, and Plante to warrant further expansion within a decade of its formation. Its newest members have brought additional expertise in a variety of urologic sub-specialties. Richard T. Kershen arrived in 2004 to establish and manage the Fletcher Allen Continence Center. Kershen built on his urology training at Boston University with fellowships at the Baylor College of Medicine in female urology and voiding dysfunction, and neurourology and urodynamics.

The staff assumed its current form following the hiring of Scott D. Perrapato and Gerald C. Mingin, Jr. in 2007. Both graduated from the University of Medicine and Dentistry of New Jersey (UMDNJ), but they each bring a different skill set to UVM. Perrapato completed an oncology fellowship at Roswell Park Cancer Institute after taking a urology residency at Metropolitan Hospital of Grand Rapids, Michigan, so he focuses on major cancer cases. Mingin, on the other hand, went to the University of California at San Francisco for a pediatric urology fellowship following his UMDNJ urology training. He thus became the first full-time pediatric urologist in UVM's history.

The division's members continue to offer cutting-edge approaches to prostate disease, incontinence, erectile dysfunction, infertility, and kidney disease. All have become proficient at robotic-assisted surgery, the latest in minimally invasive urologic surgery. The division also provides excellent clinical instruction to medical students and the occasional general surgery resident on an elective rotation. Re-establishment of its own residency program remains a goal, although it may prove to be challenging. Nonetheless, the foundations upon which to accomplish such a task have been properly laid.[19]

CHAPTER 28

Vascular Surgery Division

UVM's first vascular procedures were performed during an age of operative innovation by self-taught general surgeons. Later staff members completed formal training programs as the field rapidly changed and expanded.

Aneurysm growth suppression by using beta-blockers was a clinical and laboratory focus until a randomized trial failed to demonstrate significant benefit. UVM missed an opportunity in non-invasive segmental artery testing, but capitalized on vascular ultrasound.

UVM has since become a nationally recognized leader in ultrasound training for physicians and technicians. Vascular surgery currently finds itself at the forefront of the nationwide trend toward endovascular repair.

Vascular Surgery has a Long Legacy

More often than not, a concept or procedure thought to be new has actually been around for years. Such has often been the case in vascular surgery. Historically, arterial injuries were treated with ligation or amputation. But in 1759, Samuel Hallowell of Newcastle, England fixed a leaking brachial artery aneurysm by performing a lateral arteriorrhaphy.[1] No one took this route again until Chicago's John Murphy reported the successful end-to-end repair of a lacerated femoral artery in 1897.[2] The father of modern vascular surgery, Alexis Carrel, published a paper on vascular anastamoses in 1904 that outlined many of the principles and practices still in use today.[3]

A venous autograft was done in Madrid, Spain in 1906, but the procedure did not catch on. During all of WW II, there were 2,471 reported arterial injuries, yet only 40 vein graft repairs. It was left to French surgeon Jean Kunlin to revive interest in this technique with his 1951 report.[4] Even then, his outcomes were hard to duplicate. As a result, many surgeons used arterial homografts taken from cadavers as conduits.

Aneurysms were another matter. Former UVM surgery chair James Kent Platt had stood by as Sir Astley Cooper ligated an abdominal aortic aneurysm with disastrous results in 1818. John Brooks Wheeler, chairman from 1900-1923, recounted another harrowing story that occurred during his 1880 residency at the Massachusetts General Hospital under Professor of Surgery Henry Bigelow:

"He was dealing with a left subclavian aneurysm, about four inches in diameter. Dr.

> *Bigelow wanted to cure this aneurysm by clotting the blood in it, in the hope that the clot would become transformed into a solid lump of fibrous tissue and thus avert the danger of bursting and prevent any further pressure. Blood tends to clot around any foreign substance that is put into it, and his plan was to stick a trocar (a pointed steel rod surrounded by a metallic tube) into the aneurysm, withdraw the rod, leaving the tube in position and stuff catgut into the aneurysm through the tube which could then be withdrawn, after which it was expected that clotting would take place. Some strands of catgut being ready at hand, he plunged the trocar into the aneurysm and withdrew the rod, leaving the tube in position. The blood spurted from the tube several feet into the air, with such force that he could not push the catgut into the tube. For a moment or two he was fairly "stumped" and fumbled among his instruments, catching up and dropping one after another. Suddenly he stopped fumbling, pulled the tube out, pressed his thumb on the wound controlling the hemorrhage, and remarking as he did so, "Well, I suppose I shall have the pleasure of holding onto this damned thing for the next 24 hours!" His anticipations were not realized, however, for in ten or fifteen minutes he very cautiously took his thumb away and there was no bleeding. A gauze compress was fastened firmly over the wound with sticking-plaster and the patient was very carefully put to bed. He was not under my care and I don't remember what became of him. He could not have lived long, but I think he went home and died there."[5]

The literature recounts that Arthur Blakemore revived Bigelow's packing technique in the early 1950s. Blakemore put strands of 30-gauge stainless steel wire into the lumens of abdominal aortic aneurysms through 18-gauge needles. He applied an electric current to the wires, thinking that they would generate heat in the aneurysm's stagnant outer layers. This would induce gradual aneurysm thrombosis, which in turn would lead to collateral formation. The aneurysm would then eventually thrombose, thereby forestalling rupture.[6] In the end, Blakemore's results were not much better than Bigelow's.

Vascular Surgery Comes to UVM in the 1950s

Burlington's first modern vascular procedure occurred during the early 1950s when Jay Keller, using leg compression and suction catheters, extracted a popliteal artery embolus. This technique was successfully employed for years until the Fogarty® balloon catheter came on the market in 1963. The ingenious little device facilitated clot extraction with more ease and completeness in a shorter amount of time.[7]

H. Gordon Page was stationed at Boston's Fort Devens after finishing his Korean Conflict tour of duty. He frequently went to the Massachusetts General Hospital during this period to watch pioneering vascular surgeon Robert Linton operate with resident Stanley Crawford. When Page started his Burlington practice in 1953, one of his friends was found to have a contained but leaking abdominal aortic aneurysm. Page urged him to transfer to Boston, but the patient insisted on staying in Burlington. No one could offer him appropriate surgery and he died.

Determined to avoid another such episode, Page visited Crawford in 1955 to learn the latest vascular procedures. Crawford had relocated to Houston, Texas, where Michael DeBakey was also holding demonstrations. Page ended up completing a weeklong mini-fellowship under these vascular giants. Upon returning to Vermont, he set up a homograft tissue bank containing harvested cadaver aortas and arteries frozen at -10°F. Homografts, however, were limited by their availability and durability. Arthur Voorhees introduced vascular grafts made from vinyon-N parachute fabric in 1953, which worked well but unraveled along their cut edges unless heat-sealed with cautery.[8] DeBakey and others introduced Dacron® grafts in 1957, eliminating the need for Burlington's tissue bank.

One of Page's initial cases was an urgent aortic embolectomy for severe bilateral leg ischemia. The clots were successfully extracted with suction, resulting in pink lower extremities and palpable pedal pulses. Page then did his first elective aortic case, which turned out to be "a matter of poor selection." An endarterectomy was attempted on an individual with severe aortic stenosis, but the tissues fell apart and the patient died.

Page repaired a traumatic popliteal arterial injury shortly thereafter. The patient hailed from New York City and wanted to return there, but was advised that the severity of his ischemia contraindicated the time-consuming transfer. The family then asked the MGH's Linton to fly up in order to save the leg. He refused, but reassured them that Page would do a good job. The crushed artery required resection of a short segment prior to its reanastamosis. Page kept the patient's leg flexed almost 90 degrees in a long-leg cast to avoid tension on the fresh suture line. The patient was subsequently sent back to New York City, where he presumably regained leg extension.

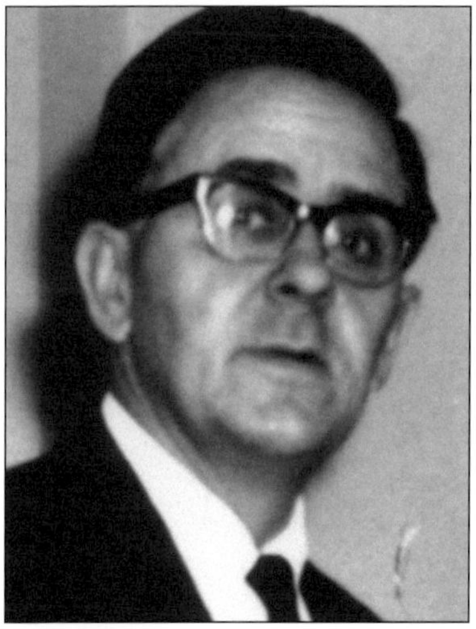

FIGURE 28-1. H. Gordon Page started practice in Burlington in 1953, and went on to establish himself as UVM's leading vascular surgeon.

Page also encountered aneurysms that he felt were not safe to resect and graft. He treated these technically inoperable lesions by coiling large amounts of wire inside them as Blakemore had done, but did not apply electric current. Some of the wire doubled up on itself and extended into the thoracic aorta. The efficacy of this maneuver was unknown, but patients were reassured because something had been done. Page recalls more than a few long-term survivors. Their X-rays, were remarkable.[9]

Knitted or woven Dacron grafts were placed around other "inoperable" aneurysms and tacked down posteriorly. The lumbar arteries were not dissected or divided, so there was no protection against posterior rupture, but at least patients could sleep easier since once again, something had been done. Other centers wrapped aneurysms with cellophane to induce perianeurysmal fibrosis. This technique, with dissection and division of the lumbars, was later championed by Francis Robicsek but never widely adopted.[10]

Other Burlington general surgeons learned how to do these procedures on the job. Nonetheless, Page performed the bulk of the vascular cases. Chairman A.G. Mackay actually told Keller that Page should do every such operation.[11] Page was ALWAYS available, and fearlessly took on all vascular cases.

UVM's First Fellowship Trained Vascular Surgeons

In an attempt to bolster UVM's academic reputation, Mackay appointed Julius H. Jacobson, II director of surgical research in 1960. Jacobson had been trained in thoracic and

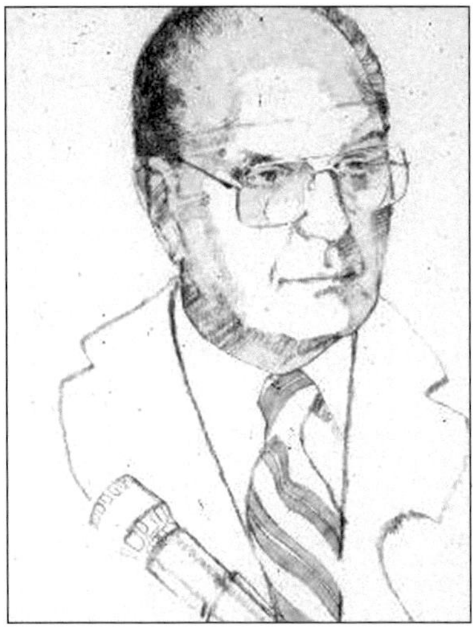

FIGURE 28-2. Julius H. Jacobson II was hired as UVM's director of surgical research shortly after completing his Columbia cardiothoracic fellowship. Jacobson did peripheral vascular and cardiothoracic procedures whenever he wasn't innovating with the operating microscope.

peripheral vascular procedures during his residency and fellowship at Columbia's New York-Presbyterian Hospital. While he and neurosurgeon R.M.P. Donaghy are mostly remembered today for their pioneering cerebrovascular developments, Jacobson's microvascular work also included a number of peripheral vascular applications.

Jacobson remembers operating on an 86-year-old man with a leaking abdominal aortic aneurysm during his stay at UVM. Pleased that the patient survived the surgery, Jacobson presented the case at a morbidity and mortality conference. Instead of being praised, he was severely criticized for taking the individual to the O.R. This prompted Jacobson to check actuarial statistics for elderly patients. He was gratified to learn that his aneurysm patient had survived far beyond the statistical prediction, and was now ensured a few more functional years. Jacobson's ensuing article was widely quoted for its actuarial data, rather than the technical success of the operation![12]

Jacobson continued his microvascular and adjunctive hyperbaric work at Mt. Sinai after migrating back to New York City. William Stahl, who had trained in vascular surgery and performed arterial procedures in his Connecticut private practice, succeeded Jacobson in 1962. Stahl was a superb technician and an excellent vascular surgeon. UVM faculty members augmented their incomes during this time by conducting their own private practices. A few cases came Stahl's way under this policy, even though Page still had the busiest practice and did the most vascular procedures. Stahl left to pursue a trauma career in the late 1960s, eventually becoming the Chief of Surgery at the Lincoln Medical and Mental Health Center in the Bronx.

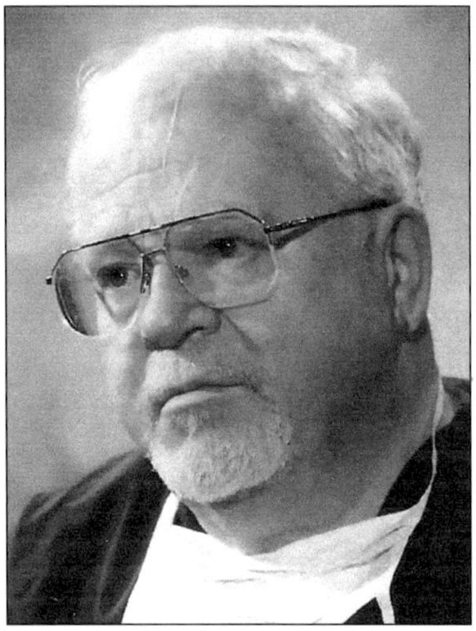

FIGURE 28-3. E. Douglas McSweeney completed vascular training at McGill and in San Francisco.

E. Douglas McSweeney was a true Burlingtonian. His father Edward was a UVM gynecologist, his aunt Katherine practiced internal medicine, and his grandfather Patrick had been a gynecologist and general surgeon. In fact, three generations of McSweeneys were members of the American College of Surgeons. Douglas returned to UVM in 1964 fresh from vascular surgery training at McGill and the University of Oregon. He joined the full-time group hoping to continue the research that he had conducted during his fellowship, but claimed he was stymied by Mackay and not supported by the Department.

Disillusioned, McSweeney left the UVM full-time group for private practice in July 1965, setting up shop on lower Pearl Street in his aunt's old office building. Practice patterns dictated that established community surgeons accrued and kept their own patients. The hometown Catholic boy was therefore busy from the start, thanks in part to referrals from his relatives' old associates.

"Quite a Piece of Surgery"

Like many others of his era, John Davis was a self-taught vascular surgeon. He had done capillary-centered research, which had always fascinated him, and had performed some venous procedures and arterial embolectomies during residency, but had never witnessed arterial or aneurismal repairs. Aortic grafting was just coming into its own when Davis started working at Cleveland's Metropolitan General Hospital in 1956. The Cleveland Clinic's Alfred Humphries (who had trained as an orthopedic surgeon) was the only other person in town doing vascular surgery.[13, 14]

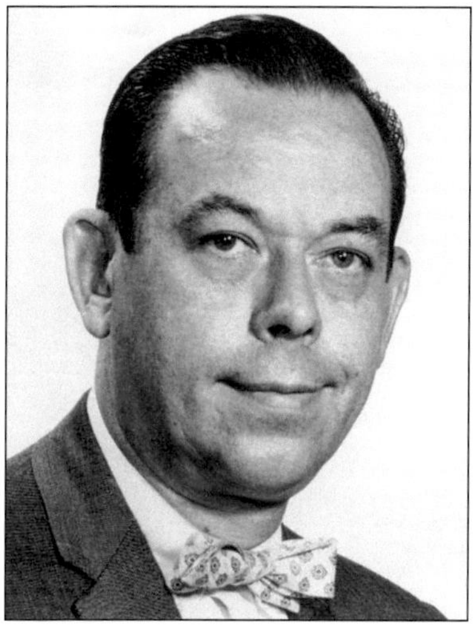

FIGURE 28-4. John H. Davis was a technically masterful self-taught vascular surgeon. He believed that vascular surgery should not become an independent specialty, a view opposed by many of his peers.

Davis tells of a patient from 1957 that presented with a dissecting thoraco-abdominal aneurysm that involved the mesenteric and renal vessels. Davis broke scrub and went to the morgue for a homograft. The only available cadaveric aorta was far too calcified to use, so Davis returned to the O.R. with a vinyon tube graft instead. He burned side holes for the celiac, superior mesenteric and renal arteries. He then attached freeze-dried iliac artery homografts (which were serendipitously available from the research laboratory) as branches. Davis finally sewed a second tube graft above and below the aortic clamp sites to be used as a shunt during the aneurysm resection.

Davis implanted the improvised graft during a thirteen-hour marathon case that encompassed a total of ten anastamoses. The left kidney was without flow for 53 minutes, and the right was ischemic for 70. The patient was essentially anuric for 6 days, but regained renal function without dialysis, which was not clinically available anyway. Intestinal function took more than a week to return, but re-operation was never considered. Davis submitted the case to the Archives of Surgery once the patient had fully recovered. This was only the fourth report of a successful thoraco-abdominal aorta repair (Etheredge 1954, Rob 1955, and DeBakey 1956) and the first with a synthetic graft.[15] The Archives' acceptance letter read: "That's quite a piece of surgery. Keep up the good work." This left Davis "walking on air" for quite some time thereafter.[16]

Davis Brings Vascular Specialists and Innovation to UVM

I (DBP) first met Davis in 1969. He was still in Cleveland, but had already been tapped to succeed Mackay at UVM. I was completing my vascular fellowship at UCLA, having returned from my tour of duty in Vietnam six months previously. I was now looking for a full-time a job, preferably at UVM. Davis, fortunately, was in the process of assembling a versatile staff. During the course of my interview, I asked Davis if I could be a vascular surgeon as well as a general surgeon. Davis said, "Okay, but you have had great trauma experience, so you will ALSO be a trauma surgeon and chief of the emergency room!"

We were summoned to the recovery room in the midst of our interview session to see a patient that had undergone an aneurysm repair. Adhesive straps had been attached to each of his flanks, to which Q-tips had been taped and then rubber-banded together anteriorly. Davis noted that the Q-tips were two inches beyond the mark applied an hour earlier. This indicated that the abdomen had massively expanded and that the patient required an immediate re-operation to control bleeding! End of interview. The "Cleveland straps" eventually became a UVM tradition. Of course, an experienced surgeon should realize the importance of a tense, distended post-op abdomen without relying on straps.

Davis brought other excellent vascular skills and experience from Cleveland, introducing UVM to portosystemic shunts soon after his arrival. Although Nikolai Eck had described a canine porta-caval shunt in 1877, and Blakemore had reported a similar operation on humans in 1948, the treatment of esophageal varices was still in its infancy during the 1970s.[17] As a result, the vascular surgeons frequently performed these "Eck fistulas" on incredibly sick patients. Therefore we were soon entrusted with all forms of liver surgery. Endoscopic and endovascular therapy has evolved since then, as have liver transplants, largely making portosystemic shunts a thing of the past.

Page sent me an obese, alcoholic patient in 1974 who should have had esophageal varices. His vascular problem, however, was a large abdominal aortic aneurysm that involved the mesenteric and renal arteries. I took him to the O.R. and sewed a 20 mm Dacron tube graft

FIGURE 28-5. The author (DBP) performing aortic aneurysm surgery at UVM. I covered Davis' cases during his increasingly frequent out-of-town commitments.

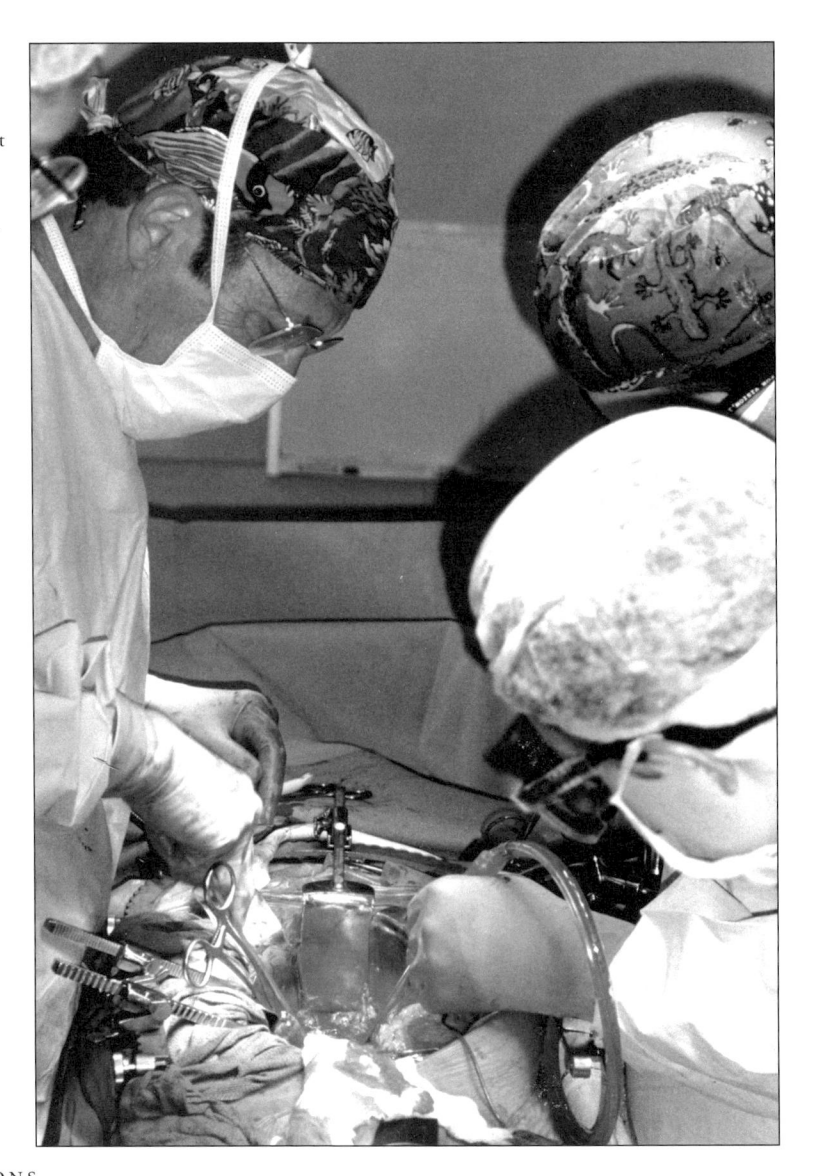

to the lower thoracic aorta in an end-to-side fashion through a thoraco-abdominal approach. A series of 8 mm Dacron grafts were utilized for mesenteric and renal vessel side branches. Upon finishing the end-to-end anastomosis to the celiac artery, the aortic clamp was re-positioned on the next graft, thus restoring perfusion to the proximal intestine. The ensuing branch was sewn to the superior mesenteric artery in a similar manner before moving the clamp distally again. The process was repeated for the renals.

The ischemic time for each vascular anastamosis was limited to 15 minutes or less. The distal end-to-end aortic anastomosis was done last. There was no renal failure. The patient not only lived for 22 more happy years, but also overcame his alcoholism to become a leader of the local AA chapter and rehab center. I do not know why Page felt that I was capable of doing this case, but I appreciated his confidence. I had neither seen nor done a thoraco-abdominal procedure before this one! My colleague apparently felt that I could do anything, having completed a vascular fellowship.

It's a Vascular Team, Not a Division

UVM's on-call surgeons were overwhelmed by emergent vascular problems every now and then. As such, the overnight coverage system was modified in 1970 to include a "vascular call schedule." Davis didn't dissuade the general surgeons from performing vascular procedures if they were comfortable doing so; he just ensured that a vascular specialist was always available to take care of difficult cases. Davis, McSweeney, and I rotated on the original vascular call schedule. Although none of us restricted our practice to vascular disease, a natural shift occurred so that the majority of elective vascular and "unassigned emergent cases" were directed to the three of us.

Carl Haisch succeeded Roger Foster as transplant surgeon in 1984. Upon arriving, he announced that he wanted to do all of the arteriovenous access procedures for dialysis patients AND do vascular procedures. Seeking to expand his vascular involvement, he requested that I help him with clinical decisions and more intricate cases. His vascular skills markedly improved. McSweeney developed angina shortly thereafter. The condition limited his ability to tolerate operative stress, so he gave up vascular call. This left Davis, Haisch and me as the vascular team.

The Non-Invasive Vascular Laboratory

The Massachusetts General Hospital developed a pioneering device during the early 1970s that measured segmental extremity arterial supply. This was packaged and promoted as the Pulse Volume Recording (PVR) machine.[18] The innovation swept the nation. It enabled surgeons everywhere to quantitate the arterial supply to the extremities and apply objective data to subsequent vascular procedures.

One of Davis' Cleveland acquaintances, electrical engineer Marvin Buffington, visited UVM in 1972. Buffington had invented another novel "PVR" machine that was simpler and less expensive than the MGH system, yet still gave the same information. He donated the equipment to UVM, which we tested and successfully used for many years. As with many other innovations, promotion, advertising, and marketing were everything. The "Buffington

PVR System©" never left UVM despite its validation in the surgical literature.[19] We were on the right road, but forgot to put up a road sign!

A non-invasive vascular laboratory was established, although it lacked a dedicated office. Initially run by an EKG technician, the lab performed PVRs, indirect carotid stenosis testing, and non-invasive venous thrombosis analysis. The Department had originally purchased the venous testing equipment with money from a DVT prophylaxis study grant. The hospital later took over machine maintenance and supplied an office in exchange for equipment ownership. The hospital paid the technicians and billed for their services, while the Department billed for the physicians' interpretive skills. This model was based on the existing Radiology system. Our initial technician, Vicki Gonyeau, ran the laboratory for more than fifteen years.

Making Movies and Teaching Residents

Suture manufacturer Davis and Geck® produced a number of educational medical movies and maintained a film library for the American College of Surgeons (ACS). John Davis had a strong relationship with the firm, therefore he was the natural choice to be featured in a movie about abdominal aortic aneurysm repair. The Davis and Geck team came to UVM and filmed Davis as he performed an operative procedure. A couple of lumbar artery orifices bled into the aneurismal sac as the cameras rolled, so Davis covered them with a laparotomy pad. He commented that these arteries (which were indeed merely oozing) did not need to be ligated since they stopped bleeding spontaneously by the time the graft was placed and the sac was closed over the repair.

The operation continued without complication, and seemed to be the ideal case for a teaching film. As the patient's blood pressure increased post-op, however, the previously quiescent lumbar arteries started to bleed. By 10 pm, it was obvious that the patient needed to go back to the O.R. Davis had taken an afternoon flight to the West Coast to attend a meeting, so I ended up ligating the offending lumbar orifices during the wee hours of the night. Luckily, the film crew had already left town as well.

Davis wrote the narrative and the movie was edited at Davis and Geck's Danbury, Connecticut production facilities. It was then shown during the "Cine Clinic" program of the annual ACS meeting in 1971 with Davis providing live narration. A sound track was later added and a copy was placed in the ACS film library. All movies were available to any surgeon free of charge as part of the ACS' educational outreach. The 16 mm films were converted to VHS tapes during the '80s, but the film library itself was disbanded within the next decade. All films and tapes were subsequently returned to their original authors. The video reveals that even in the 21st century, open repair of AAAs has changed little.

David Finley, who became a fellowship trained vascular surgeon after his UVM surgical residency, recalled an episode from 1977 that illustrated Davis' teaching abilities:

> *"Our own attending Nolan Cain presented with an aortic aneurysm which involved the renal artery. I was the Chief Resident on vascular that month. I did not particularly want to operate on Dr. Cain, and so I asked Dr. Davis how he was planning to handle the revascularization of the kidney. He said since I was the Chief Resident on the service that he want-*

ed to know how I thought the revascularization should be handled. I spent the next three days on and off in the library, analyzing the various ways to revascularize, and chose jump graft of Goretex from the aortic graft. That worked fine. I learned a lot about many things from that experience."[20]

Vascular Surgery at UVM's Referral Hospitals

UVM remained without a designated vascular service or division, since Davis felt that Vascular was integral to general surgery. Many established vascular surgeons disagreed. They stipulated that Vascular should be a separate division of surgery with its own requirements and certifying board, modeled after cardiothoracic surgery. Davis supported the group opposed to further sub-specialization. When a special American Board of Surgery vascular certificate finally became available, none of UVM's surgeons were allowed to obtain it per Davis' instructions. Ironically, younger board-certified vascular surgeons ended up working at the area's community hospitals, but not in Burlington!

In due time, more and more vascular procedures were performed at UVM's referral hospitals. DeBakey, however, had publicly proposed funneling aneurysm surgery to large-volume centers in order to improve results. Smaller hospitals argued that their outcomes were just as good, and that they needed to perform elective cases if they were expected to handle emergencies. This sounded remarkably similar to UVM's initial justification for treating vascular (and cardiac and pediatric) patients rather than sending them to Boston. Davis and I conducted a statewide study in 1980 that showed some of the smaller hospitals did indeed have excellent results when it came to aneurysm repair.[20]

The pendulum had completely swung the other way by the 1990's. Surgeons certified by the Vascular Surgery Board of the American Board of Surgery did all of UVM's vascular procedures. Most community surgeons, meanwhile, stopped performing vascular operations. The advent of interventional radiology and endovascular repairs had a lot to do with this, as did the modern phenomena of escalating vascular surgery malpractice premiums.

Davis Hires a New Vascular Surgeon but Forgets to Tell the Dean

When Davis became paralyzed in 1987, Haisch and I were faced with an increasingly busy service. Despite his opposition to sub-specialization, Davis finally relented and allowed me to become board-certified. Later, upon realizing that his paralysis was permanent, Davis began to look for another vascular surgeon. Michael A. Ricci, meanwhile, was ensconced in a vascular fellowship at McGill. His father had lost a leg during World War II, a circumstance that may have steered him toward the sub-specialty.

Ricci had been a four-year letter winner in football at Hamilton College before training at Syracuse and the Guthrie Clinic. He had decided to supplement his income while in Montreal as a vascular fellow, by working in the Emergency Rooms at Plattsburgh and St. Albans. Ricci needed a Vermont license in order to do this, which necessitated an interview with Page at UHC as part of the approval process. Page mentioned that UVM needed a good vascular surgeon. The UHC facility looked excellent to Ricci, and Page was convincing.

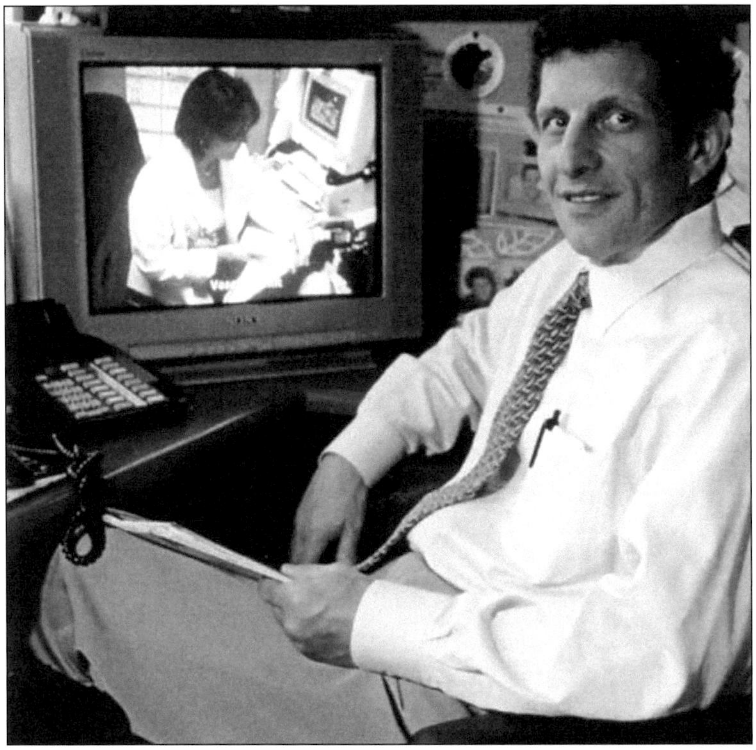

FIGURE 28-6. Michael Ricci was the first UVM vascular surgeon to complete a two-year fellowship. Trained in ultrasound, his arrival coincided with that of the new ultrasound machine that no one else knew how to use.

Ricci arrived in March of 1989 to make practice and housing arrangements. Davis had assured him that he was hired, so Ricci declined his other job offers. It was thus a shock to discover that Davis had failed to create a spot for him within the College of Medicine. Ricci called Dean Luginbuhl, defended his agreement to come to UVM, and fought for his position. The Dean thought that Davis, as the outgoing chairman, should not have made any appointments. A compromise was finally reached in the form of a one-year contract. Ricci hit it off with new chair Shackford, so there were no further appointment issues.

Ricci was UVM's first two-year, fellowship-trained vascular surgeon. His vascular ultrasound and computer skills, as well as his excellent technical abilities enhanced UVM's vascular service. Ricci had also done research at McGill on compartment syndrome, and to a lesser extent, a procedure termed "arterio-venous reversal." This was employed for ischemic limbs without adequate revascularization targets. Arterial inflow was anastamosed to the proximal end of a large distal vein, in essence arterializing the vein.[21] Publications were in press at the time Ricci journeyed south. He subsequently spent two days a week in the lab investigating arterio-venous reversal at UVM. One of Ricci's first clinical cases was a miraculous success. His enthusiasm waned when neither he nor the rest of the vascular world were able to match this result.

Ricci then joined forces with me (DBP) to study the clinical effects of beta-blockers on aneurysm growth. One of his old McGill associates was working on an experimental rat aneurysm model at Loyola. This seemed to fit well with our clinical study, so Ricci focused on the laboratory work. General surgery resident Jeffrey Slaiby assisted during his research year, and several publications followed.[22, 23] It seemed that UVM was about to become a leader in an exciting, new area of medical treatment for aortic aneurysms. Randomized studies did not support this approach, however, and dashed our hopes.

Shackford Takes Over Thoracic Outlet Syndrome Care

Steven Shackford succeeded Davis as chair shortly after Ricci's arrival. He was board-certified in general, vascular, and critical care, and brought a tremendous amount of trauma surgery know-how with him from San Diego. Shackford formally codified many of the Department's current divisions following his arrival. Vascular Surgery had been functioning as a division with me as its head, but Shackford finally separated vascular from general surgery, formally establishing a Division of Vascular Surgery.

Shackford seemed to have no end of energy or endurance. He administered the Department of Surgery and was at the same time an innovative and productive vascular surgeon. He carried his fair share of the clinical workload and took call on a regular basis. Shackford was also a huge clinical presence in the Surgical Intensive Care Unit, a domain previously controlled by the Anesthesiologists. Both he and Ricci (who was also board-certified in critical care) provided overnight SICU coverage for nearly a year, until new hires made this unnecessary.

I was at the peak of my productivity, but had reservations about performing first rib resections for thoracic outlet syndrome after experiencing a couple of less than optimal outcomes. I had already decided that the residents could no longer actively assist, since only one person could see the nerve and artery through the transaxillary route. Shackford, though, felt that he could carry out this demanding procedure and still teach the residents. He took on the entire caseload, eventually treating a large number of people with thoracic outlet and other upper extremity vascular issues. His results were admirable, and I was gratified to know that the procedure was of benefit after all.

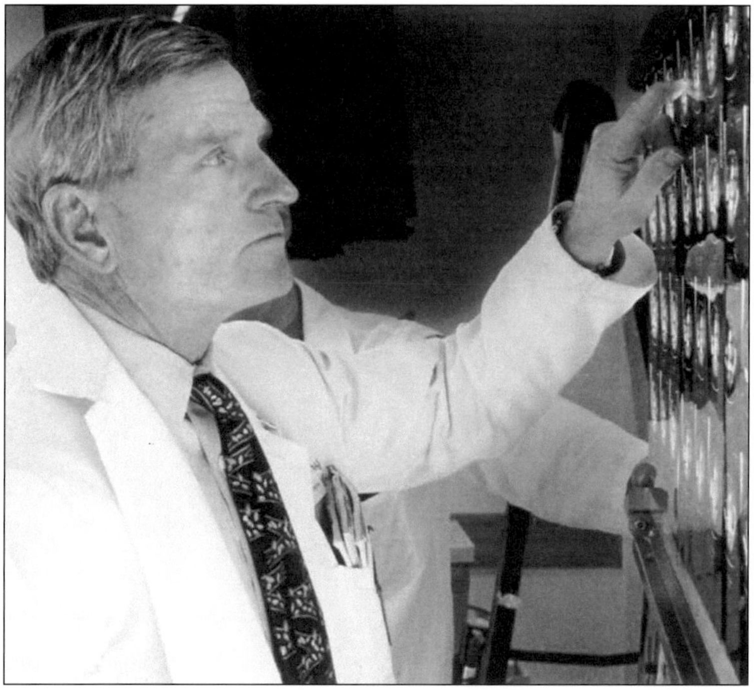

FIGURE 28-7. Steven Shackford was board-certified in general surgery, vascular surgery, and critical care. The majority of his UVM clinical practice was devoted to vascular surgery.

Ultrasound Comes to Vascular Surgery via the Caribbean

I had attended a vascular ultrasound course in the fall of 1988 at Frenchman's Reef Hotel on St. Thomas. The event — which was all business of course — left me evangelistically enthusiastic about using ultrasound for non-invasive vascular testing. Davis, in one of his last major acts as chairman, purchased a duplex ultrasound machine at my request. This original machine, a Quantum Medical Systems QAD-1, was outdated the day it arrived. I had gone to Seattle for an ultrasound physics course put on by Quantum, and had toured their nearby factory. The newer Q-2000 was ready for marketing, but it was not on display. The company never mentioned it at the time they sold us the obsolete model!

Shackford was none too pleased when he found out that the device was to be paid for on his watch. He was also skeptical as to whether the expense could be recouped. The machine, however, paid for itself many times over in the long run, and was a wonderful adjunct to patient care!

The non-invasive laboratory was relocated to the DeGoesbriand Unit, just down the hall from the vascular surgery outpatient clinic. Registered vascular technologist (RVT) Donna Wallace was hired at the time of Ricci's July 1989 arrival. Ricci, meanwhile, had already been trained in vascular ultrasound interpretation during his vascular fellowship at McGill. Working together, the pair initiated the Department's vascular ultrasound endeavors. They tutored me and helped me develop my ultrasound skills on the job. Ricci helped me manage and direct the now expanded Vascular Laboratory. When I became Chief of the Division of Vascular Surgery, I turned the directorship of the Vascular Non-invasive Laboratory over to him.

Ricci took the initiative to study for, and pass, the RVT exam. I successfully achieved the same RVT certification the next year. This entailed learning a lot of ultrasound physics. It imparted knowledge that put us in good stead later, but was far beyond what we needed to interpret an ultrasound image. Laura Merchant came to the vascular lab from the Department of Radiology shortly thereafter. She improved our productivity with her knowledge, reliability, and work ethic. With her help, and that of Steven Knight, we achieved certification in many areas set forth by the International Certifying Authority for Vascular Laboratories (ICAVL).

FIGURE 28-8. Laura Merchant's ultrasound skills complemented UVM's vascular laboratory. She was instrumental in obtaining the lab's ICAVL credentialing.

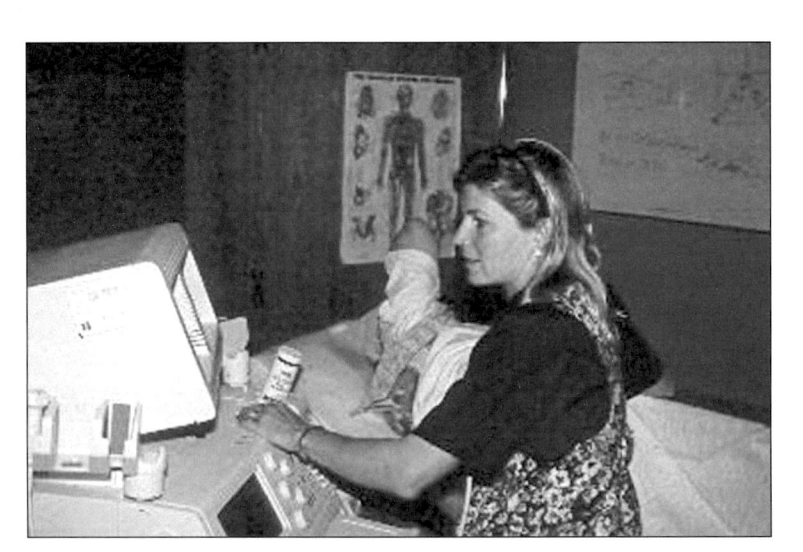

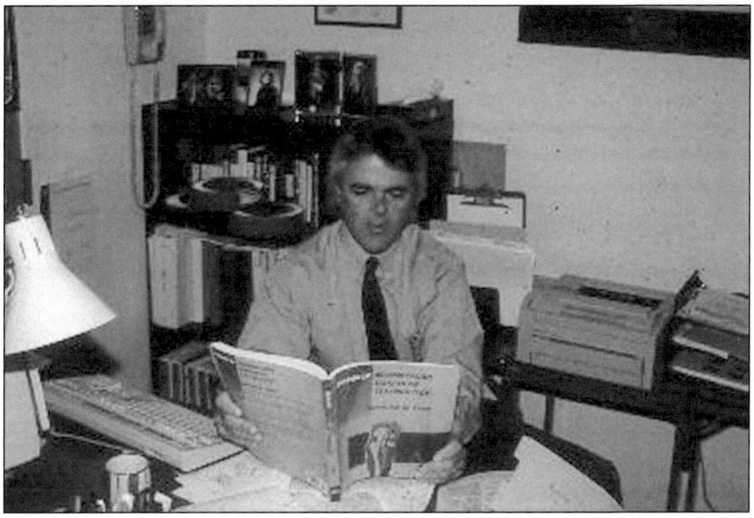

FIGURE 28-9. Terrence Case helped UVM introduce vascular ultrasound into the national arena. The annual non-invasive laboratory seminar was highly popular amongst those seeking credentialing and certification.

Terrence Case came to UVM in 1992 to become the non-invasive vascular lab's chief technician. He had been doing similar non-invasive testing in Brattleboro, Vermont, but had family ties to Burlington. Case was an academically minded RVT who, with the help of Ricci and me, started an annual preparatory course for the RVT exam. All vascular labs had to employ technicians possessing the RVT credential in order to be accredited by the ICAVL. Our course, given in the fall just before the exam, was popular and well attended during its 1992-98 run. This program helped establish UVM's national reputation for being at the forefront of non-invasive vascular testing.

Case went on to publish a text for RVTs while he was in our vascular lab and produced a nationally distributed movie on the many facets of ultrasound. We also began accepting trainees for a one-year preceptorship during his time at UVM. Case left for other endeavors in industry and teaching. Nevertheless, the vascular lab grew by leaps and bounds under the leadership of his successor, Mary Anne Waters, who had been working at Dartmouth. By 2006, the lab employed five technologists, ran five duplex ultrasound machines, and generated one-fifth of vascular surgery's gross billings!

Academically, Ricci has authored the non-invasive carotid testing chapter for the most recent editions of Rutherford's "Vascular Surgery" and has taught national courses on intravascular ultrasound.[24, 25] I have directed the American College of Surgeons' postgraduate course "Ultrasound for Vascular Surgery" for the past eight years and have written several treatises on vascular ultrasound for national audiences.[26] My most recent focus has been on intra-operative completion duplex ultrasound exams.

The Dawn of the Endograft Era

I visited Brooklyn's SUNY Downstate Medical Center in 1988 as a Visiting Professor at the request of surgery chief and former UVM resident Richard Wait. One of Downstate's new vascular surgeons was Thomas Panetta. He had recently worked with Frank Veith, the first American surgeon to perform an endovascular aneurysm repair. The Brooklyn group gave a yearly postgraduate course on advanced vascular subjects, one of which was endovascular grafting. Ricci wanted to learn the approach, so I introduced him to Panetta the next year. The two rapidly established a working relationship.

FIGURE 28-10. General surgery resident Whitney McBride performs a completion duplex ultrasound after carotid endarterectomy. UVM has become nationally prominent in this area.

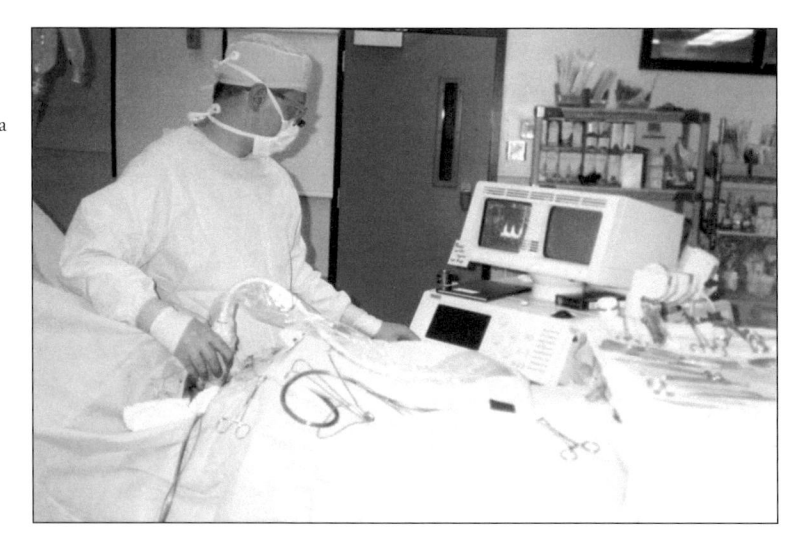

UVM already had *intravascular* ultrasound equipment. Ricci, as one of the few in the region with experience in this field, taught intravascular ultrasound and angioscopy at the annual Brooklyn course. Ultrasound's ability to penetrate blood vessels and measure the flow within was widely known. The intravascular equipment was costly, though, and the disposable probe that it utilized was prohibitively expensive. Angioscopy allowed for direct internal arterial or graft visualization, but only worked if large volumes of clear fluid were pumped into the structure of interest. This was not only time-consuming, but also potentially dangerous if a plaque or thrombus was dislodged. Although the two modalities were intriguing, neither one proved to be practical.

The Brooklyn course and the connection to Panetta, however, did introduce Ricci to endografting. General surgeons had already embraced laparoscopy, whereas orthopaedists had adopted arthroscopy. For vascular surgeons, the minimally invasive revolution originated with endografts. The devices were placed under fluoroscopy, usually during the course of a diagnostic angiogram since a guide-wire was already in place. Vascular surgeons therefore started doing diagnostic studies to determine whether endografting was indicated.

Some surgeons performed the procedure independently, while others collaborated with radiologists or cardiologists. Proficient surgeons mentored their colleagues and credentialing

FIGURE 28-11. The surgeon usually does a completion carotid duplex in conjunction with an ultrasound technician from the vascular laboratory.

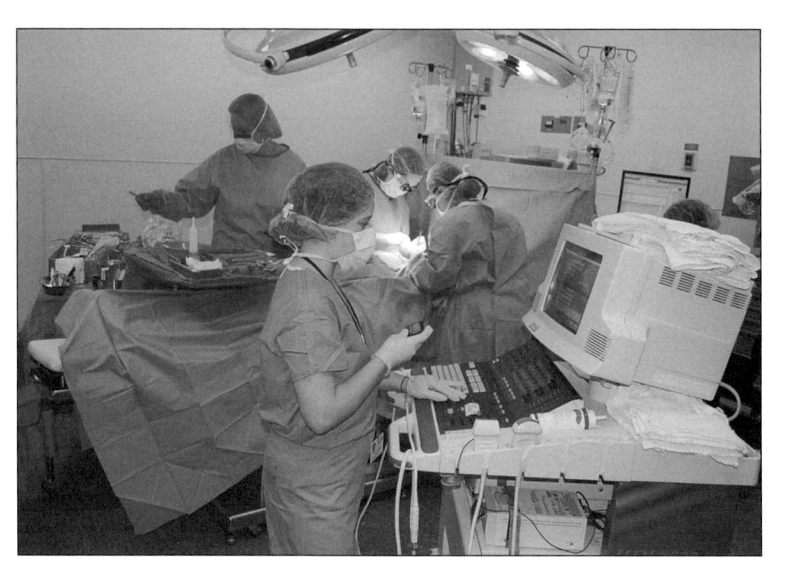

criteria were created. Pharmaceutical companies and device manufacturers pitched in by developing training courses based on animal models. UVM's most recent vascular surgeons learned endovascular grafting during their fellowships.

As percutaneous technology advanced, radiologists and cardiologists began to deploy endografts without surgical assistance. Many institutions permitted this even though such "interventionalists" did not usually admit patients, provide follow-up, or deal with complications. We chose to team up with our interventional radiologists to maximize our collective strengths and avoid a turf war. Panetta himself came up from Brooklyn to help Ricci place UVM's first endovascular graft in 1993.

UVM participated in a clinical trial that evaluated iliac endografts, which led to further funded research. The study was also of great personal benefit to Ricci, who ended up marrying the research coordinator! UVM did not participate in any aortic aneurysm endografting trials, but followed other ongoing studies. These endografts were originally intended for high-risk patients that could not tolerate an open repair. Demand grew when patients realized they could trade a large, painful abdominal wound for a small groin incision. The fact that the early grafts were not proven and required frequent surveillance CT scans to rule out leakage did little to dampen the public's enthusiasm.

The same situation occurred with peripheral lesions. More than 90% of all critical iliac stenoses are currently managed with percutaneous angioplasties and endografts. Now that it is easier to treat these blockages, it is tempting to lower the criteria to include less severe and less threatening lesions. Most vascular surgeons are still hard pressed to find any benefit in treating early, minimally symptomatic arterial disease.

Although UVM did not pioneer these endografts, we did get in on the ground floor. Our surgeons worked with our radiologists in a cooperative manner, stayed current with the technology, and matched the rest of the surgical world's outcomes.

Vascular Surgery Partners With a Podiatrist

Deaconess Hospital vascular surgeon David Campbell came to UVM as a visiting professor in 1993. The Deaconess worked closely with Boston's Joslin Diabetes Center, and was renowned for its diabetic limb salvage results. When the question of neuropathic diabetic ulceration was broached during vascular rounds, Campbell's response was brief: "We let our podiatrist manage those issues." This was news to those of us in attendance, as Vermont's podiatrists traditionally provided outpatient foot care. Several practiced in Burlington, but each had limited hospital privileges for minor foot procedures.

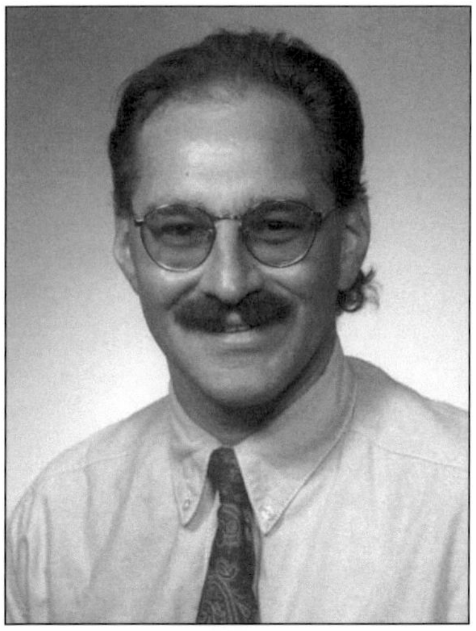

Podiatrist Marc Sarnow moved back to Plattsburgh, NY (a town in which his podiatrist father had practiced for over 40 years). Sarnow had just completed a residency in podiatric surgery at New York College of Podiatric Medicine and a fellowship in diabetes/foot and ankle surgery at the Deaconess. He was interested in continuing his

FIGURE 28-12. Marc Sarnow, an extremely well trained podiatrist, brought advances in the field of diabetic foot management to vascular surgery.

research, and wanted to practice at an academic institution.

UVM's podiatric privileges were granted by the Department of Orthopaedics at that time. Sarnow approached the general and orthopaedic surgical staffs in 1994 seeking an affiliation and practice opportunity. The full-time orthopaedic group rejected his overture, but the vascular surgeons were thrilled to have a skilled podiatrist available to help with diabetic foot management. Another benefit of this eventual partnership was Sarnow's participation in student and resident teaching.

Vermont statutes were changed in 1999 so that podiatrists could perform major surgery below the ankle. Hospital privileges then became the sticking point, since such cases required access to inpatient facilities. Sarnow overcame Fletcher Allen's original restrictions by operating in the presence of a vascular surgeon; however this often presented logistical problems. Stephan LaPointe brought impeccable podiatry credentials and experience in ankle surgery to UVM when he joined Sarnow in 2000, but returned to Georgia a short time later after tiring of the hospital's credentialing process.

Sarnow's association with the Division of Vascular Surgery ended under similar circumstances a few years later. He continues to run busy private practices in Plattsburgh and Colchester, but feels he has not reached parity with other medical staff members despite board certifications in foot surgery and reconstructive rear foot and ankle surgery.[27]

New Blood Arrives at UVM as Communities do Fewer Vascular Cases

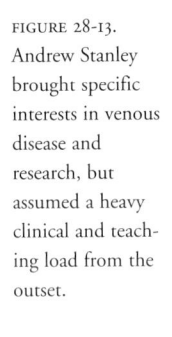

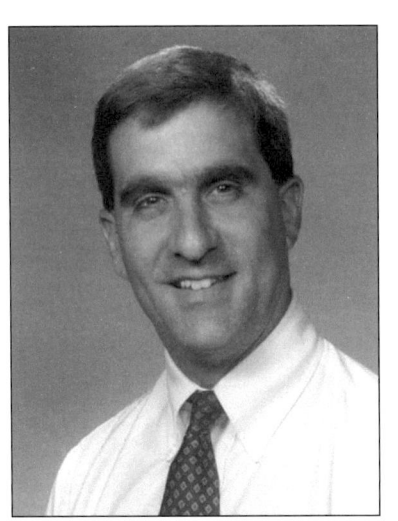

FIGURE 28-13. Andrew Stanley brought specific interests in venous disease and research, but assumed a heavy clinical and teaching load from the outset.

Rhode Island native Andrew C. Stanley spent his first two years of medical school at Dartmouth and his last two at Brown under the Brown-Dartmouth program. UMass surgical residency was then followed by a vascular fellowship at Boston University. Stanley presented a paper in 1997 on critical pathways and lower extremity vascular disease at the New England Society for Vascular Surgery (NESVS) annual meeting. Impressed by his performance, Ricci and I recruited him to UVM. Stanley and his wife surgeon Mary Stanley were ready to get out of Boston. After giving an equally engaging Grand Rounds at UVM in the spring of 1998 on venous disease, Stanley was in.

Stanley brought a new, less invasive varicose vein "closure" treatment to UVM. In this method, a probe is placed in the saphenous vein at knee-level and threaded toward the groin via ultrasound guidance. A radiofrequency signal or laser heated probe then occludes the vein as the probe is slowly withdrawn. The procedure's efficacy is similar to traditional vein avulsion or "stripping," but is much less morbid and painful. Stanley's leadership in this area was recognized with an invitation to teach the technique at a NESVS postgraduate course.

Shackford gladly relinquished varicose vein surgery and vein injections to his new partner. Stanley also pursued venous disease research in the laboratory, concentrating on the widespread problem of venous stasis ulcers. The non-medical UVM faculty held the medical fac-

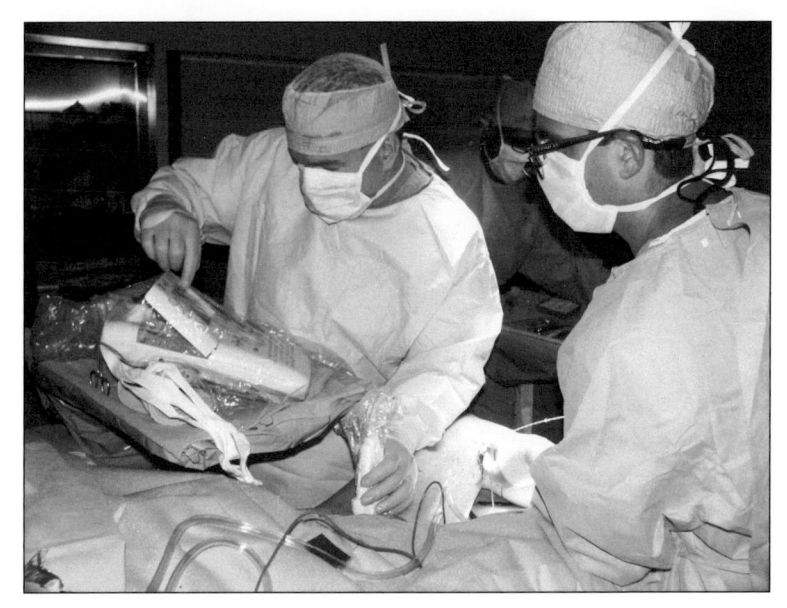

FIGURE 28-14. Stanley performs a "Vein Closure®" procedure using intraoperative ultrasound at the Fanny Allen Hospital.

ulty to their own rigorous criteria of research standards. As such, it became increasingly difficult for many of the surgeons to accomplish enough basic research to satisfy UVM's eligibility requirements for tenure. Stanley, faced with decreasing funding and an increasing clinical practice, switched from the tenure track to the clinical track in 2005.

The caseload grew as community surgeons stopped performing vascular procedures. At the same time, Shackford and Ricci were devoting more and more time to administration and telemedicine, respectively. Wallace C. Tarry filled the ensuing void in 2000. Tarry had gone to Duke for medical school, the Medical College of Virginia for residency, and Dartmouth for a vascular fellowship. While still a fellow, he presented a paper on "The fate of the contra-lateral leg following infra-inguinal bypass" at the same NESVS meeting where Stanley had given his critical pathways presentation, thus bringing him to our attention.[28]

Tarry had the unusual habit of rounding on his patients each morning well before the residents made their way to the hospital. He checked the wounds, wrote the day's orders, and then returned home. By that time, Tarry's wife and children had arisen and were ready for breakfast with dad. The patients, students, and residents loved him, voting Tarry Teacher of the Year at the end of his first year on staff. Tarry's southern roots drew him back to North Carolina in 2002 after a brief, but happy stay at UVM.

Paramedical personnel have since taken on much of the Division's day-to-day activities. Nurses Beth Nutter-Gamache and Deborah Soter are a constant presence, while secretaries and other support staff have come and gone over the years. Patients and doctors alike appreciate their dedication and expertise. Nurse practitioner Janet Stiles-McSorley performs most of the pre-admission history and physical exams in the wake of resident work-hour restrictions, and collects and correlates the division's outcomes data. Such angels smooth the way for UVM's vascular patients and staff.

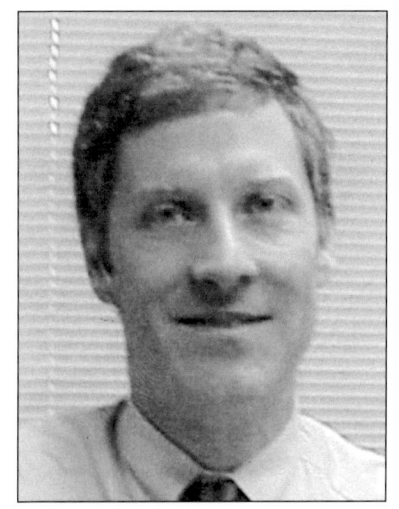

FIGURE 28-15. Wallace Tarry complemented the vascular staff, uniquely rounding on his patients before the house staff awoke before going back home to have breakfast with his family.

The Vascular Study Group of Northern New England

The Division was intimately acquainted with telemedicine thanks to Ricci's interest and involvement. Our existing relationship with the Maine Medical Center's vascular surgeons was enhanced through a monthly telemedicine conference. The MMC group, however, thought that the sessions lacked a certain bit of educational emphasis. After some discussion, we decided to invite Dartmouth's vascular surgeons to join us in a three-way conference. When the idea was presented to Dartmouth's Jack Cronenwett, he instead suggested that we form a consortium similar to the highly successful Northern New England Cardiovascular Disease Study Group to track and improve clinical outcomes.

The Vascular Study Group of Northern New England (VSGNNE) was founded in 2001 under Cronenwett's guidance, and Stanley's input. The Group has since created a regional registry that prospectively logs data associated with carotid endarterectomies, lower extremity bypasses, and both open and endovascular abdominal aortic aneurysm repairs.[29] A report is then generated on a biannual basis that includes procedure volume, process characteristics, and trends over time. This information is used to "improve the quality, safety, effectiveness, and cost of caring for patients with vascular disease."[30] It has already helped standardize pre-op beta-blocker usage across the region.

The Present Faculty Comes Together

Georg Steinthorsson replaced Tarry in December of 2002. Steinthorsson had graduated from the University of Iceland's medical school, a tuition-free institution with a huge attrition rate. Only 36 of more than 200 students advanced to the second year of school during Steinthorsson's time. There were no surgery training programs in Iceland, so Steinthorsson went to Dartmouth for residency, and then Yale for a vascular fellowship. He took an endovascular course at SUNY Downstate, where he met Ricci. Steinthorsson gained further endovascular experience during a three-month away rotation in Belgium. He settled into private practice in Iceland, but came back to New England at the behest of his homesick wife, physician Susan Dunning, MD, who was also hired by UVM.

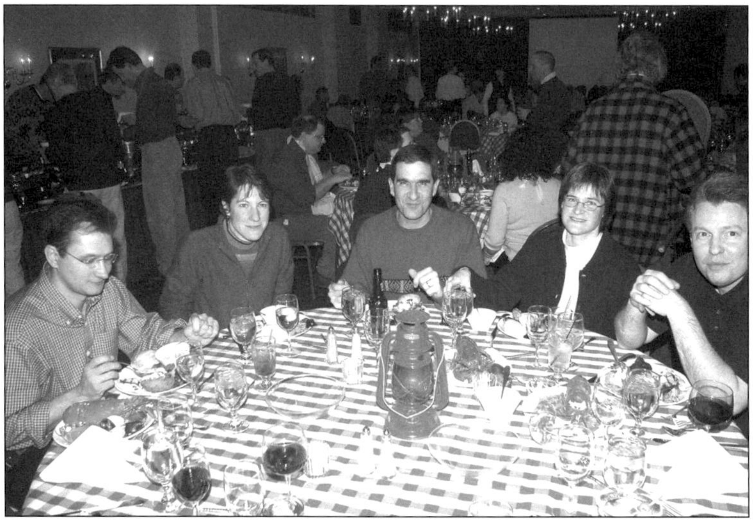

FIGURE 28-16. Enjoying a lobster supper at the Stowe winter retreat (left to right): Daniel Bertges, Mary Stanley, Andrew Stanley, Susan Dunning (Steinthorsson), and Georg Steinthorsson.

The Division hired Daniel J. Bertges upon my retirement in 2003. He was followed by former UVM resident Julie E. Adams two years later. Both were well trained in minimally invasive vascular procedures during their respective fellowships at the University of Pittsburg and the Cleveland Clinic. Each has been assigned interventional radiology suite block time in which to perform atherectomies, angioplasties, and endografting.

The Division remains at the forefront of medical education as well. It has compiled an online textbook that is available to students and residents alike as part of the College of Medicine's new computerized curriculum.

A genuine concern exists among residency programs that general surgery graduates do not perform enough vascular index cases. Volume has already fallen at programs with vascular fellowships and/or endovascular centers that no longer carry out routine "open" procedures. UVM's general surgery residents remain uniquely prepared, though, since they do not compete with fellows for our ample supply of major open cases. In fact, most of our housestaff graduate with enough cases to satisfy vascular board requirements!

CHAPTER 29

UVM Frontline Surgeons and the Evolution of Forward Surgical Hospitals

Wartime medical care evolved over the centuries as combat required and technology permitted. Even so, a certain structural hierarchy remained constant.

Those within the fighting units rendered immediate assistance, whereas frontline facilities delivered stabilizing treatment. Definitive procedures and recovery were the purview of general hospitals.

UVM surgeons played a part in this evolution from World War II onward, especially with regard to forward military hospitals. Their global experiences led to improved care for the citizens of Vermont.

The Evolution of Frontline Surgical Hospitals

Surgeons have been treating battlefield wounds for as long as armies have been fighting battles. But until the 1690s, it was largely up to the injured soldier to find his way to the regimental surgeon. This changed during the War of the English Succession (1688-1697) with the establishment of 300-bed "marching" hospitals that traveled with the army. Each had its own tents, wagons, and supplies, and was staffed by a physician, a surgeon, an apothecary, and eleven mates. These units were augmented by larger "fixed" hospitals, which were situated within the commandeered buildings of adjacent towns.[1]

The hospitals were renamed "flying" and "general" hospitals by the time of the French and Indian War (1754-63), but the three-tiered division of responsibility remained intact. The Continental Army emulated the British model during the Revolutionary War. John Pomeroy, after all, got his start as a surgeon's mate with the 9th Massachusetts Regiment. Likewise, Nathan Smith's teacher John Warren was chief surgeon of a general hospital at Cambridge, and "flying" hospitals on Long Island and in New Jersey.

Despite their designation, "flying" hospitals were situated several miles from the action. This was not an inconsequential matter, as it often took more than 24 hours to cover such a distance by litter bearer or cart. Realizing that soldiers were dying from their injuries during transport, French military surgeon Dominique Larrey decided to deliver lifesaving care at the front. Inspired by highly mobile horse drawn artillery wagons ("flying artillery"), he outfitted similar carriages with medical supplies and trained corpsmen. Larrey's *ambulance volante* was successfully deployed as a mobile frontline hospital in 1792. Hundreds of "flying ambulances" eventually accompanied Napoleon's forces across Africa and Europe over the next 25 years. Larrey usually manned one himself.[2]

Lack of a standing army, combined with the far-flung nature of the conflict, precluded the use of "flying hospitals" during the War of 1812. All the same, Pomeroy, William Beaumont, and Henry S. Waterhouse tended to the injured at three of the four general hospitals on the northern front in Burlington, Plattsburg, and Malone. Similarly, poor direction and distant supply lines plagued U.S. forces throughout the Mexican War. Medical personnel were on their own when it came time to set up "regimental" and "divisional" hospitals in captured towns.

Union and Confederate military surgeons were at a distinct organizational disadvantage when the Civil War erupted. Soldiers wounded at the Battle of Bull Run, for example, lay on the field of battle for up to three days. Later UVM professor of neurology William Hammond was appointed Surgeon General in the wake of the fiasco. Hammond, in turn, ordered Jonathan Letterman to overhaul the Army's medical corp. Letterman, as medical director of the Army of the Potomac, had the skill and authority to make sweeping changes.

Letterman started by implementing an efficient ambulance system. He also introduced another of Larrey's innovations — triage. Letterman's lasting legacy, though, was the establishment of the Army's echelons of care. The first level consisted of field dressing stations close to the battlefield. The second were the home and barn-based "field" hospitals. Large "general" city hospitals comprised the third level. The system saved lives through rapid transport, especially by railcar. UVM's Henry Janes oversaw Gettysburg's ultimate field hospital, the 1,600-bed tent facility dubbed Camp Letterman.

"Clearing" and "convalescent" hospitals were in place by the Spanish American War, only to be replaced by the "clearing" and "rest station" hospitals of World War I. These were serviced by railways, and for the first time, mechanized ground ambulances. A literal "flying hospital" called the *Aeorchir* was later deployed during the French Colonial wars of the 1920s.[3] The stage was thus set for the innovative front line surgical care of World War II and beyond, care that was delivered by several surgeons with ties to UVM.

William I. Shea: 30th Portable Surgical Hospital: Pacific Theater, 1944-45

Knowing that it would be waging an extended island-hopping war against the Japanese, the U.S. military aligned its specialized South Pacific forces into lean, nimble units. Colonel Percy J. Carroll, Chief Surgeon of U.S. Army Supply of Services under Douglas MacArthur, had this in mind when he conceived the Portable Surgical Hospital (PSH) in mid-1942. Three surgeons, one anesthetist, thirteen technicians, and twenty support staff manned the 25-bed facilities. Each contained enough supplies to perform 45 major operations. At war's end, 103 outfits were in service across the Theater.

Shea, meanwhile, had spent 1942-43 completing a UVM internship and a St. Vincent's residency in medicine and anesthesiology. By March 1944, though, he was in command of a medical clearing company caught up in the Battle of Los Negros. The 30th PSH was also on Los Negros Island, having supported the 1st Cavalry Brigade's assault during the early days of the Admiralty Islands campaign. Shea learned that the 30th's anesthesiologist was debilitated by a morphine addiction, thereby preventing the group's lone surgeon from operating. Shea stepped up and volunteered to give anesthesia. This led to a permanent transfer to the 30th PSH shortly thereafter.

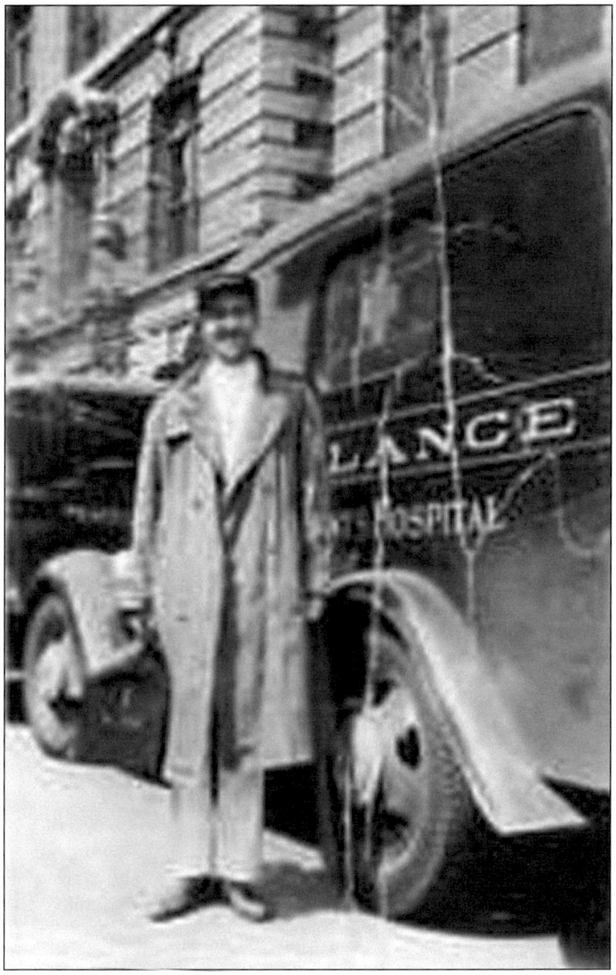

FIGURE 29-1. William Shea as a resident in NYC just before his military service.

The unit was sent to eastern New Guinea that June to regroup after completing its duties on Los Negros. While there, the surgeon was replaced with a green recruit whose only prior training had been a six-month surgical internship. Shea, as the senior officer, was given command. When the 30th PSH was redeployed in October for the invasion of the Philippines, Shea begged for competent help. His appeal was "filled" by two doctors without any surgical experience! Shea read a surgical atlas and practiced sewing intestinal anastamoses on his socks during the three-day naval transport to Leyte Island.

The 30th PSH accompanied the assault waves during the early stages of the Battle of Leyte. The four untrained surgeons and their crew set up shop on the beachhead until the Seabees dug them in under the coral and palms. Shea's first patient was a soldier that had placed his helmet over an incoming grenade and then sat on it. As can be imagined, the soldier's buttocks and rectum were destroyed. Shea performed his first colostomy and rectal resection during the ensuing four-hour operation. The soldier survived, and Shea's surgical career was launched.[4]

In addition to such emergency laparotomies, Shea and his comrades set compound fractures, carried out débridements, and performed amputations. Plasma and whole blood were widely available and frequently used. Surgery was considered "only when it was thought that the wounded soldier could not stand the arduous trip to the rear or when his condition would not permit the delay necessary for evacuation."[5] The 30th PSH went to Japan in 1945, where it remained in service until its October inactivation. It later received the Presidential Unit Citation for its work at Los Negros, and the Philippine Presidential Unit Citation for its performance on Leyte.

The PSHs functioned as designed overall, but were a dead-end as far as forward hospitals went. Supplies were limited to those that could be manually carried by the Hospital's complement of 37 men. The lines of command, communication, and supply with the larger, more remote field hospitals were either inconsistent or non-existent. As a result, severely injured soldiers often lingered, taking up much needed bed space. These deficiencies were overcome by the slightly larger, self-sustaining successor to the PSH, the Mobile Army Surgical Hospital (MASH).

Albert J. Crandall: 1st American Airborne Surgical Team: European Theater, 1944

The Army took a different approach when it came to the surgical support of its European forces. Acting on recommendations by Michael DeBakey and other advisors to the Surgeon General, the military created five Auxiliary Surgery Groups (ASGs). Each ASG consisted of twenty general surgery teams and twelve specialized thoracic, neurosurgery, orthopedic, plastic, and maxillofacial teams. Every team was attached to a medical company or field hospital and staffed by a chief surgeon, an assistant surgeon, an anesthesiologist, a nurse, and two technicians.[6] Neurosurgical Team Number 4, 1st Auxiliary Surgical Group, for example, was manned by future UVM neurosurgeons R.M.P. Donaghy and Lester Wallman.[7]

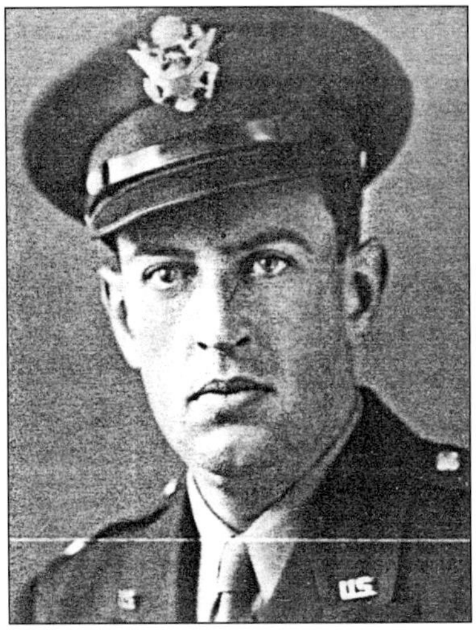

FIGURE 29-2. Albert Crandall enlisted in 1942 to later precede the allied invasion in France, June 5, 1944.

Unlike Shea, Fanny Allen surgeon Albert Crandall already had several years of surgical practice under his belt when he volunteered for duty in June of 1942. Initially assigned to Augusta, GA, Crandall petitioned the Surgeon General for overseas duty. The request was granted and he was transferred to the 3rd Auxiliary Surgery Group in England. Crandall worked and took courses throughout Britain before being given command of his own general surgery team in January of 1944.[8]

D-Day planning was well underway by this point.

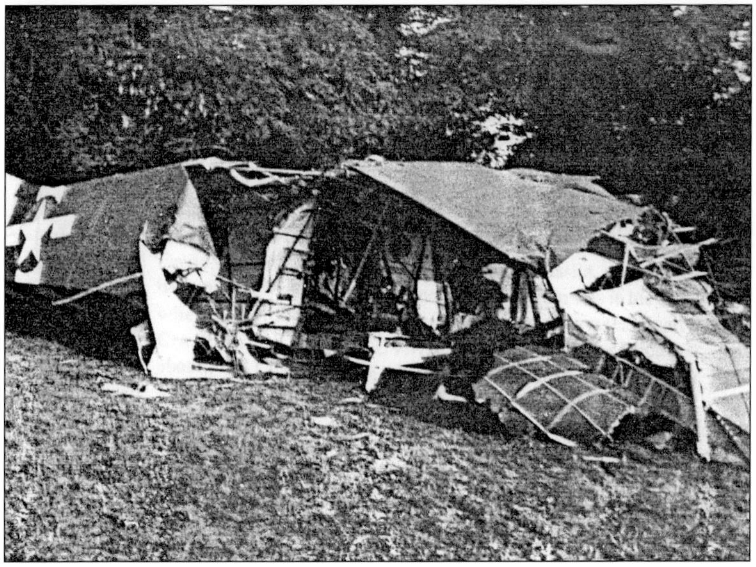

FIGURE 29-3. Crandalls gliders' crash landing in France, destroyed their jeep but not their medical supplies.

Appreciating the need for frontline surgeons, Crandall volunteered to lead a ten-member airborne surgical support team. Attached to the 326th Medical Company and the 101st Airborne Division, the group underwent intensive airborne and parachute training. Crandall later remarked that,

"Our men trained with the Division — qualified as paratroopers and gliderists and took part in the spring maneuvers. On March 23, 1944, the division was inspected while on maneuvers by Prime Minister Winston Churchill and General Eisenhower. Both were very interested in our field set up, examined it carefully and discussed it. Upon leaving, the Prime Minister commented 'It is a great idea — if you can get it in there.' General Eisenhower was all for it." [9]

Crandall's Team is Operational in France Before the D-Day Invasion

The first American Airborne Medical Team headed across the English Channel the night of June 5, 1944 in a series of gliders packed with medical equipment.

"About 11:00 pm on the night of June 5, 1944, we left England — Operation Overlord — the invasion of France. Our destination was to be a large field near Hiesville and St. Mère Église, Normandy. We were there to set up in a large 52 room Chateau. Every member of the team was injured." [10]

Crandall's son-in-law recounts:

"The sound of machine guns roar with the wind through antiaircraft flak holes in Doc's crippled glider. He crash lands on the Cotentin Peninsula, more than a mile off target. Blood oozes from a gash between his eyes when the fragmented craft hits the ground. He runs from the wreckage, crouched, trying to stay down. Nazi soldiers are everywhere. Enemy fire is heavy ... Ahead near a line of tanks is invasion leader Michael Murphy's glider. "I saw the form of a glider at the edge of a field" Crandall says, "Inside I found Gen. Donald Pratt,

FIGURE 29-4. None of the dead were members of Crandalls' surgical team, but the 101st Airborne took casualties.

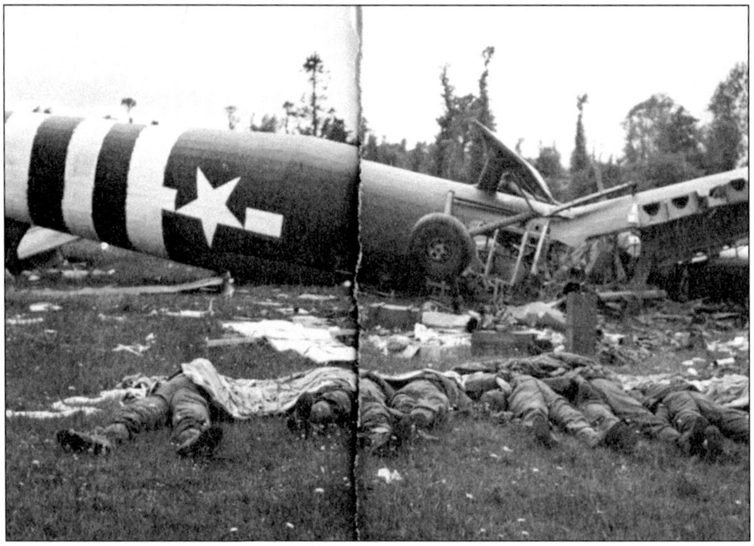

killed during the landing. I could hear other gliders crashing, gunfire increasing ..."

"Murphy, a barnstormer before the war and one of the world's best known pilots, is on the ground, watching Crandall, "one of the bravest men I ever saw" come toward him. He'd run a few feet, the Germans would let him have it, and he'd flop on his belly. Then he'd get up and repeat his action ... Crandall pulled the wounded Murphy to a hedgerow, put a splint on his broken leg, and he and his medics gathered there with other wounded, whom Murphy guarded with his .45 caliber pistol."

"The doctor ... leads another paratrooper to the nearby Chateau Colombieres in Hiesville, which they commandeered to be the first Allied hospital in France. Murphy makes history as the first patient. D-Day is hours away."

"By 9 am the (Utah beach) landing force has broken through German lines. Casualties are coming into the 326th Airborne Medical Company's hospital by cart, captured vehicle, litter and on foot. Surgical officer Crandall commands the United States' first fully qualified and equipped surgical company to accompany vanguard troops into battle."[11]

Crandall continues:

"The unit operated in the chateau for a little over four days and nights — 104 hours — we received two direct hits by enemy bombers that night. 250-300 men were treated at the surgical station. Immediately following the bombing, a company of German paratroopers were dropped in the area. Before daylight they were neutralized by our own troops."

"Fortunately, our patients had been moved into an adjoining building after treatment and the losses were small. However, we did suffer losses in personnel of the medical company."

"Within a few hours after daylight, we received supplies of equipment by air drop from England and were soon back in operation at a new location."

"We operated at the chateau until 2345 on 9 June. At that time we were attacked by dive bombers and the entire station [chateau] was destroyed ... I was performing an operation at the time the first bomb struck. Fortunately, we had evacuated most of our patients that after-

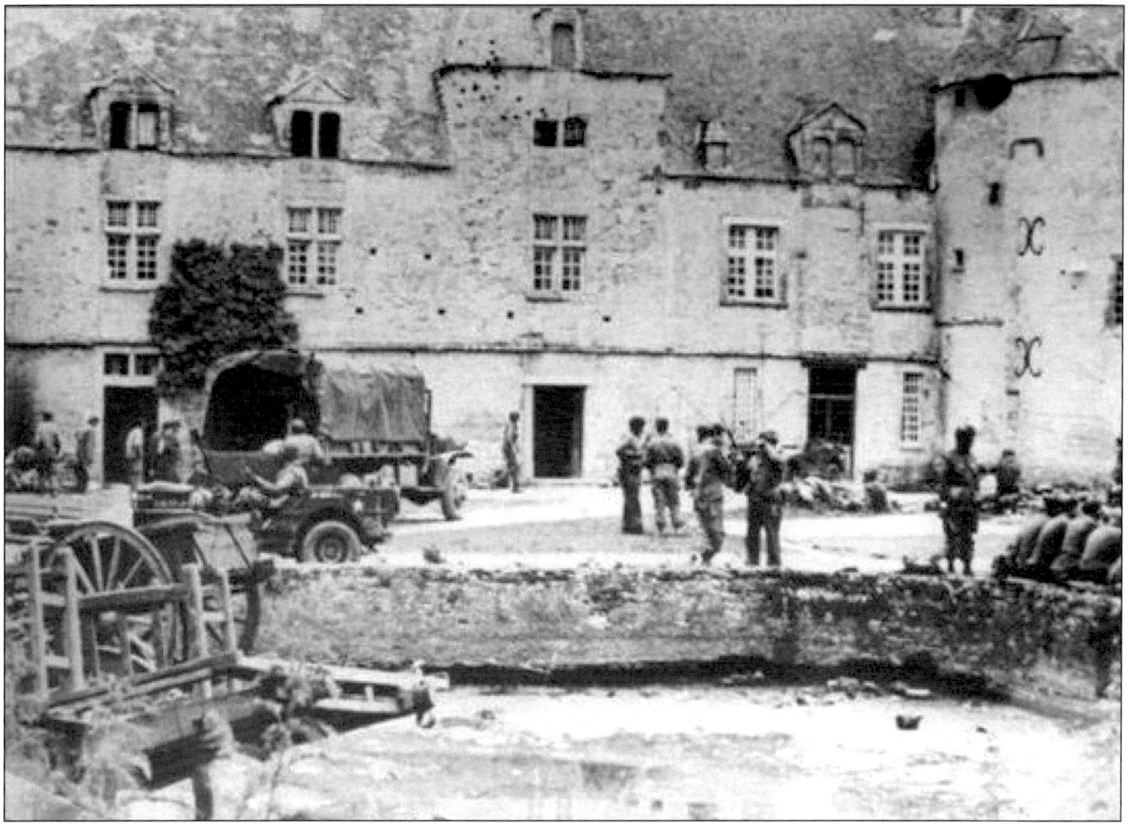

FIGURE 29-5.
The courtyard of Chateau Colombieres where Crandall's team operated for four days before the Chateau was totally destroyed.

noon, so there were very few patients left in the hospital. However we lost a lot of equipment and also some personnel. None of the surgical team were killed, although three were injured. The following day we moved to another site, borrowed some tentage from other units and set up again."[12]

"*The unit continued operation in Normandy for 37 days. By that time, large troop forces with accompanying field and evacuation hospitals were well established and the 101st was ordered back to England."*[13]

The unit was again deployed in "The invasion of Holland, Sept 17, 1944 ... the unit was much larger in this campaign. A field hospital was added — all airborne, but in late waves after the position was secured."

The original team event was on the first assault wave and we set up in a Dutch hospital in Zon and were in operation before the main wave of paratroopers and gliderists arrived. We were entirely encircled by German forces, but well protected by the 101st forces." [This battle was immortalized by the book "A Bridge too Far."]

"*We were able to use positive pressure anesthesia, which permitted us to do exploratories on chests, to go into the thoracic cavity in order to take care of the injury. We had a very low mortality on this type of case. There were only two or three of these thoracic cases that reached surgery that didn't survive. ... Almost all the cases that reached surgery survived and were evacuated ..."*[14] "*The surgery, in both Normandy and Holland, ran fourteen to sixteen percent head cases, twelve to fourteen percent chests, four to six percent abdomens, and the rest extremities. These percentages are similar to those in other operations. We had more fractures from jump casualties than usual; for instance, there were more leg, back, and ankle injuries than would occur in an infantry outfit. Aside from those, the injuries were typical of those seen on any war front.*[15]

"The surgical unit worked 87 days in Holland with combat conditions throughout the period. There was a small evacuation channel open at times during the latter part — "Hell's Highway" — alternately taken by the enemy or the airborne which helped in removal of post-op cases."[16]

"... On December 16, 1944 ... the division was ordered up to Bastogne (Belgium) ... About one half of the surgical unit was committed including our original team. The unit set up and operated on the outskirts of Bastogne — this time under tents and we did have a small channel for evacuation. The whole front was a bedlam and there were casualties from about every division on the front. We operated around the clock and evacuated as many as possible, until about 10 pm on December 19, 1944, at which time we received the full onslaught of Hitler's crack 2nd Panzer division. There was about a two hour warning and many of our men were able to get out as well as some of the wounded. However the rest of the original team was overrun by the German tanks and crack troops. Thus we became prisoners of war."[17]

When Crandall was finally liberated by the Russians the following February, he was told to head east for Moscow.[18] Left to fend for himself, Crandall hitchhiked to Warsaw during the dead of winter. He stowed away on a train headed for Odessa, and then secured passage to France on a British troop ship. Upon disembarking, he reported to the local command center and asked to resume active duty. Ex-POWs did not just return to normal service, however. Crandall, fifty pounds lighter and suffering from beriberi, was sent back to Washington, D.C. for interrogation and rehabilitation.[19]

The private and humble Crandall resumed his low-key role as a surgical instructor at war's end. Few beyond his immediate family ever knew the details of his war experiences. Even fewer knew that he had received the Legion of Merit, the Bronze Star with cluster, and the Purple Heart with cluster. Or that under his leadership the world's first airborne surgical team had been awarded multiple American, French, Dutch, and Belgian citations.[20]

John H. Davis: 8209th Mobile Army Surgical Hospital: Korea, 1951

The ASGs were reorganized into Mobile Auxiliary Surgical Hospitals in August of 1945. The outfits combined the portability of a PSH with the staffing and the equipment of a field hospital. Fourteen medical officers, twelve nurses, three non-medical officers, and 93 enlisted men ran each 60-bed unit. Facilities could be broken down and loaded onto trucks in six hours, and then reassembled within four hours of reaching their next destination. Japan's unconditional surrender weeks later, though, precluded any further MASH development.

The Army therefore had to scramble to get three of the newly renamed Mobile Army Surgical Hospitals to Korea in June of 1950 following the North's incursion across the 38th parallel. Four more were soon added to meet the goal of one unit per division. Casualties were stabilized at Battalion Aid Stations and then immediately routed to MASHs, usually by helicopter. Overland travel occurred, but was hampered by poor roads and railways, rugged ter-

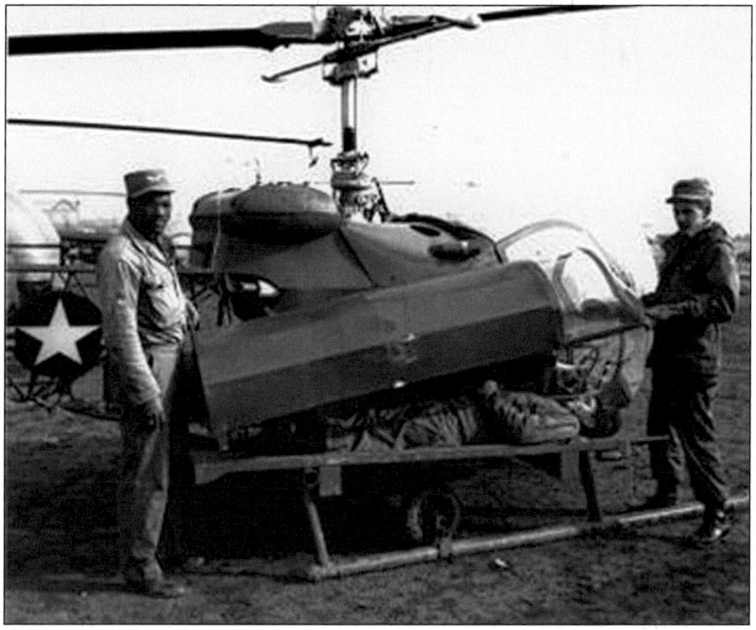

FIGURE 29-6. The injured were first evacuated by helicopter in Korea, but exposed to the elements.

ritory, and rapidly shifting battle lines. Conditions were just as Spartan for patients strapped to the exposed stretchers atop the helicopter's skids.

The MASHs moved repeatedly during the first year of fighting, staying within twenty miles of the action at all times. The only units closer were the Battalion Aid Stations and non-surgical clearing companies. Enemy shells occasionally landed within hospital compounds due to their proximity. The front lines stagnated after 1952, so the MASHs stayed put unless presented with the prospect of invasion. Their original 60-bed capacity grew to 150, and then 200 beds as casualties mounted.

John Davis was six months into a Brooke Army Hospital research project when the Korean War started, having entered the lab as a private citizen following his second year of surgical residency. Davis thus knew of the observational group led by his former professor Fiorindo Simeone that had been sent to the front lines "to observe the outstanding problems confronting the military surgeons." Curtis Artz, Davis' research director at Brooke, had assisted Simeone. The pair found that soldiers were surviving their initial injuries, but dying days later of infection and what the Surgeon General's Office called "irreversible shock." A closer look, however, revealed that renal failure brought on by inadequate fluid resuscitation was the real culprit.[21, 22]

A Surgical Research Team focused on "wound infections, dehydration, post-traumatic renal insufficiency and vascular injuries" was assembled and dispatched to Korea on December 7, 1951. Davis, with his connections to Simeone and Artz, was one of just twenty-three surgeons selected to participate after he accepted the Armys invitation to enlist. The Team was stationed at the 11th Evacuation Hospital, 80 miles to the rear of the Eastern Front. Davis later rotated through the 8209th MASH (which was only ten miles from the notorious "Punch Bowl") for nine months, the 8076th, and the Vascular Surgical Unit of the 8055th MASH.[23]

One of the Team's first projects was to prevent renal failure through improved fluid resuscitation. Careful evaluation of the 11th Evac's vital signs and urine output records demonstrat-

FIGURE 29-7. Dialysis being performed in 11th Evacuation Hospital in Korea. R.S. Post supervises.

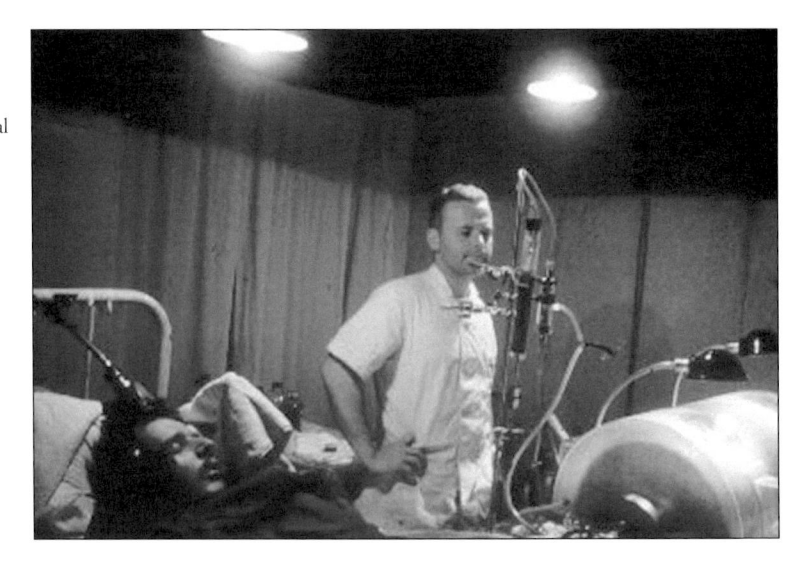

ed basic principles that have since become tenets of trauma care, namely that resuscitation begins at the scene of the injury, and continues at the pre-op, intra-op, and post-op levels. Blood or Dextran (crystalloids were not yet in widespread use) should be given through large bore, peripheral vein IVs. Urine output greater than 30 cc an hour, not normal blood pressure, indicated adequate volume replacement.[24]

Soldiers that had lapsed into persistent renal failure were tackled next. Walter Reed's only Kolff-Brigham artificial kidney was shipped to Korea and put into service at the 11th Evac's Renal Insufficiency Center. Anuric individuals were dialyzed for eight hours, resulting in a turnover rate of just three patients a day. Five days of dialysis, though, were lifesaving.[25] Davis, as one of the unit's researchers, occasionally tended to the washing machine-like device. The practice remained unique to the Korean Conflict, as the timely administration of fluid in the field rendered it obsolete in later wars.

Having honed his vascular skills placing hemodialysis catheters, Davis performed one of the war's first "approved" arterial injury repairs a short time later (surgeons at the 8076th had done unsanctioned procedures earlier).[26] He eventually crossed paths with surgeon H. Richard Hornberger of the 8055th MASH who, under the penname of Richard Hooker, wrote the book "M*A*S*H." Rumors have flown ever since then that Davis was at least in

FIGURE 29-8. John Davis posing as a model for Hawkeye in Korea.

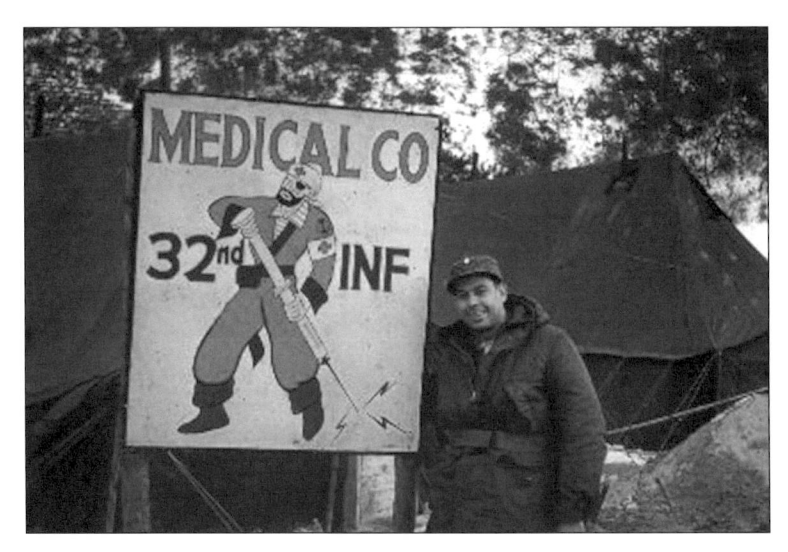

part the model for Hawkeye. Those who read the book and knew Davis certainly agreed. Davis has maintained that Hornberger "used a combination of all of our idiosyncrasies" for the character but admits that Hawkeye's surgical prowess was remarkably similar to his own. He has noted, however, that he never saw the degree of drinking that was depicted among the surgeons. "I've looked at 'M*A*S*H' and those guys are mixing martinis every night. And if you notice, none of them ever got drunk. It's a good story."[27]

Davis returned to Brooke Army Hospital at the end of his eighteen-month deployment, worked another two years on burn physiology with Artz, and then completed his University Hospital of Cleveland residency. The MASH units were renamed yet again, becoming "Surgical Hospitals (Mobile Army)" in the process. Many remained in service long after the armistice, treating the occupying American forces, prisoners of war, and civilian casualties.

David B. Pilcher: 48th Medical Detachment (KA Team): Vietnam, 1967-68

I (DBP) went to Vietnam fresh out of my UVM residency in June of 1967. Upon arriving, I was assigned command of the 48th Medical Detachment (KA Team), a mobile surgical unit at the forward base camp of the 502nd Division of the 101st Airborne in Duc Phô. Although K series teams were hospital augmentation detachments, the 48th was the only one in Vietnam to my knowledge that was not directly attached to a larger hospital. Each team consisted of two surgeons (I was the only one in mine), an anesthesiologist, an operating room

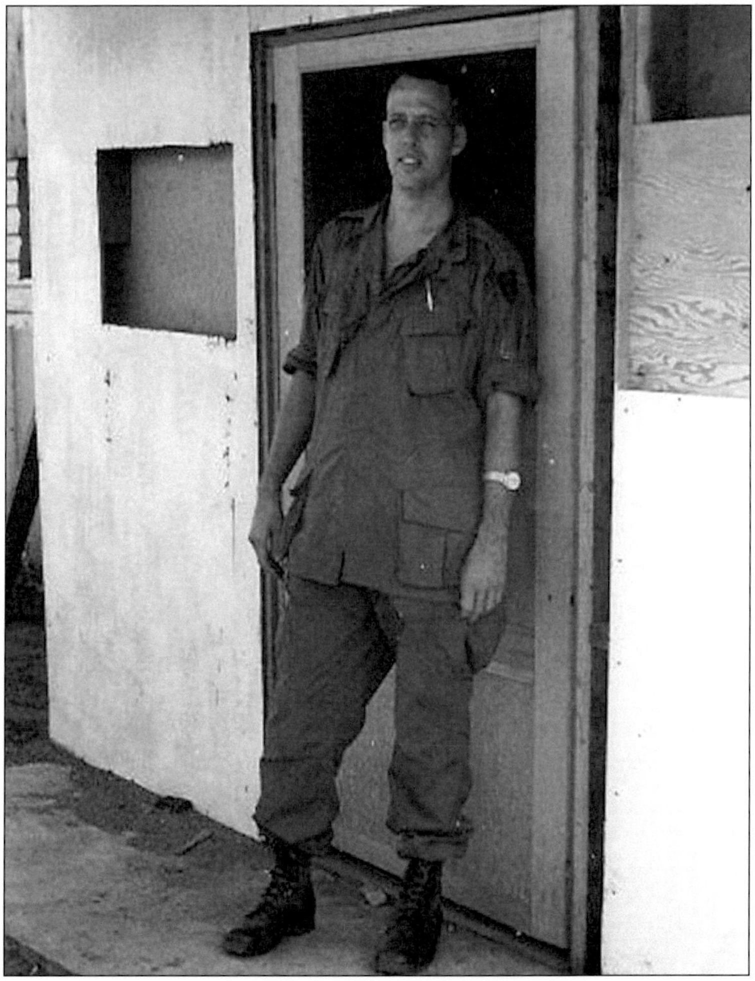

FIGURE 29-9. The author (DBP) in Vietnam ready to deploy with the 101st airborne.

FIGURE 29-10. The road to Montezuma here viewed from the receiving tent of the 48th KA team, was mined nightly by the Vietcong.

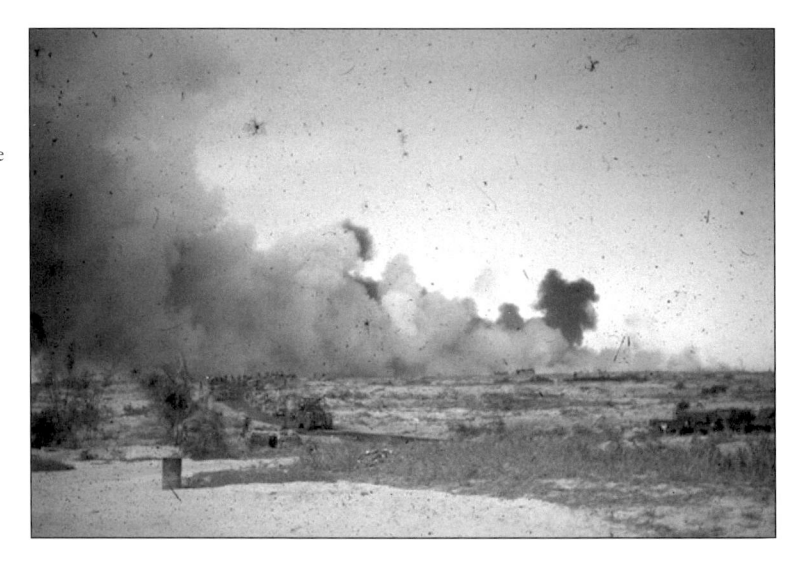

nurse, and three operating room technicians. Unbelievably, the anesthesiologist assigned to my unit was former UVM Anesthesia resident Gary Roman!

The two-bed surgical hospital's equipment was designed to fit within a jeep and a small truck. Fully mobile, it could be quickly assembled in a medical clearing company tent. The concept was reminiscent of Shea's PSH and Crandall's Airborne Team. Our function was to treat soldiers that could not wait to be transported to the nearest surgical hospital, which was only 20 kilometers away by helicopter. The 101st Airborne received the toughest assignments and were sent to the areas with the worst fighting. Although its members were all trained parachutists, their assaults were mostly by land or helicopter.

The 101st's forward base camp was linked to the 4th Infantry and its airstrip by a two-mile long road. Mined nightly by the Vietcong, it was considered safe for travel each morning only after several minesweepers and convoys had driven over it. The homemade mines contained very little metal, so the minesweepers usually did not detect them. In order to find them, a "deuce-and-a half" truck loaded with sand bags was backed down the road. The trucks were destroyed as the mines detonated, but the drivers remained unharmed!

There were no real front lines due to the war's guerilla nature. Nonetheless, the border between the Vietcong and the base camp at which we were stationed was measured in yards.

FIGURE 29-11. The author (L) operating in a tent in Duc Pho, RVN with UVM anesthesiologist Gary Roman (in khaki) giving anesthesia.

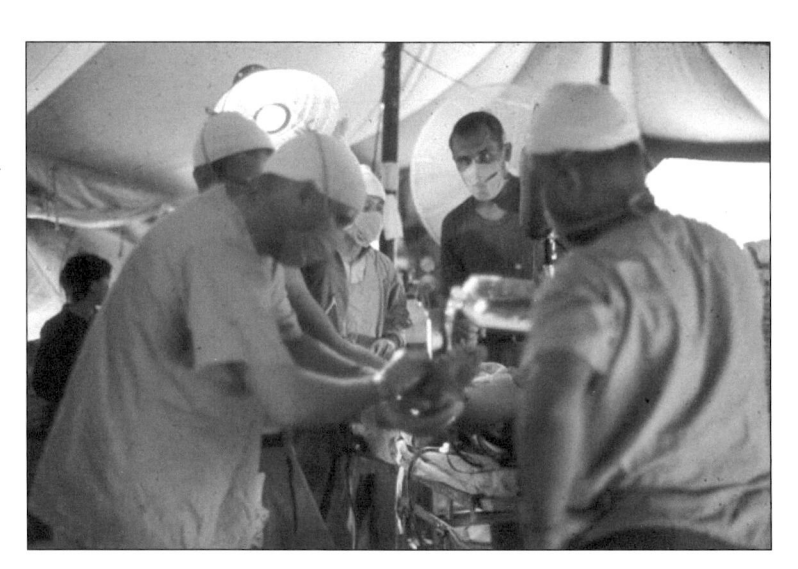

Incoming mortars and automatic weapons rounds were routinely met with return fire from within the physical boundaries of our unit. We lived and worked in tents similar to those depicted in the movie M*A*S*H. As the only surgeon in the area, I decided to forsake the plentiful supply of beer and alcohol on hand for the duration of my deployment.

Our fully equipped surgical unit was constantly busy, operating on injured soldiers, civilians, and enemy militia. The 101st Airborne kept the latter for thorough interrogation once treatment was completed. The civilian medical facilities were terribly inadequate, so we also performed a considerable number of elective surgeries while we waited for casualties. Among these were cleft lip repairs, partial gastrectomies, and herniorrhaphies.

After three months, our KA Team was integrated into the 2nd Surgical Hospital (Mobile Army). The 60-bed fixed facility was nestled behind an airstrip at the Chu Lai naval base. A Quonset hut held the operating rooms, while soldiers recovered in wooden wards. Several mortars hit the 2nd MASH despite the security afforded by our location. One totally destroyed the dental clinic building. While there, we saw the most active service of the Vietnam campaign, supporting the 101st and 82nd Airborne, the Americal Division, and the Marines. Nearly every casualty came to us by helicopter.

I remained with the 48th KA Team at the 2nd MASH for the final nine months of my tour. By the summer of 1968, I had returned to be a vascular surgery fellow at UCLA. I subsequently received the Bronze Star.

A Patient From Vietnam Reconnects

It is rare that a patient thanks or reconnects with his surgeon. Fred Downs wrote two books about his Vietnam experiences before and after I cared for his severe injuries including an amputated arm. He writes:

> *"There were two doctors standing on each side of my shoulders. They were talking to each other. The one on the left said, 'Who the hell tied this God Damn tourniquet. I watched in amazement as he used a scalpel to cut through the flesh on my stump down to a blood vessel, which he tied off. I thought, Jesus Christ I didn't even feel that. I must be in really bad shape.' ... I remembered something that was important. 'Tell my brother Mike I have been wounded. He is on the USS ...' I lost consciousness as my heart stopped."*
>
> *Later I would be known as the Lieutenant they brought back from the dead when they used closed heart massage ...*
>
> *"Fourteen years after that fateful day when I was brought into a combat surgical unit in Vietnam, I met Dr Dave Pilcher, the surgeon who asked 'Who tied this God Damn tourniquet?'. He had asked me to lecture to his class of residents where he taught surgery at the Medical School at the University of Vermont. The residents laughed when I related the incident, because he is famous for his outbursts when people tied a bad tourniquet. I thought how lucky I had been to have had Dr. Pilcher on duty the day I lost my arm. His skill and surgical techniques in the operating room saved my life and contributed to the salvage of my right arm [the other arm] and both my legs."* [28]

Downs revisited me again many years later to consult on updating amputation techniques at UVM in his role as Chief Consultant to the Prosthetics and Sensory Aids Service, Department of Veterans Affairs, Washington DC. His "disabilities" have not held him back from turning his life into a success story.

Matthew A. Conway: 947th Forward Surgical Team: Afghanistan, 2002 and Iraq, 2003

Concepts pioneered by MASH units, such as timely fluid resuscitation and rapid hospital transportation, found their way into civilian trauma centers over the years. The book, film, and television versions of M*A*S*H worked their way into the public consciousness as well. At the same time, the real MASH was at a crossroads. It had become too large to remain "mobile" in the modern military sense. It wasn't quite big enough to function as a fixed, stand-alone field hospital. The Gulf War of 1991, therefore, saw the deployment of two new types of casualty surgical hospitals.

The first was the Combat Support Hospital (CSH), a larger but less portable affair. The CSH was developed in the 1980s during an operational shift from division to brigade level medical support. Improving structurally on the MASH, each hospital was assembled from standardized modules. The operating rooms, intensive care units, and other critical departments were housed in rigid climate-controlled aluminum shelters, while auxiliary services were placed in modular tents. Capacity ranged anywhere from 16 to 256 beds due to the uniform design, with an average of 84.

The second, more compact entity was the Forward Surgical Team (FST). Staffed by four surgeons (one of whom was an orthopedist), two nurse anesthetists, and sixteen nurses and medics, the 6-8 bed FST was equipped to perform 30 lifesaving operations over a 72-hour span in a "far forward" environment. Post-op intensive care and holding capability were intentionally limited since casualties could be readily airlifted to a CSH or evacuation hospital once stabilized. The FST was not intended to be a self-sustaining entity; rather it was to be supported by a medical holding company or larger hospital.

The MASH units had largely been decommissioned by the time former UVM resident and current Clinical Assistant Professor of Surgery Matt Conway joined the Army Reserve. The benefits were helpful, and the one weekend a month, two weeks a year commitment appeared reasonable. Originally assigned to the 405th CSH, Conway elected to transfer to the 947th FST out of Hartford, Connecticut realizing that he would be of more use in a forward position. Although the FST was still a new concept, the group impressed the brass with its skill during a field exercise inspection. The strong showing placed the company at the top of the Army's readiness list after 9/11.

The 947th was thus the first reserve (and third overall) FST in Afghanistan when it arrived in April 2002. Conway and crew were deposited at Bagram Air Force Base, a Soviet-era compound choked with "dust, dirt, and diesel." Conway grew accustomed to the frequent mine detonation, but never got over having to carry a loaded 9mm pistol. Although "the only surgical asset of any consequence in the area" saw its fair share of action, boredom occasionally set in. When reading, working out, and sick call failed to relieve the tedium, the group decided to x-ray a dog with pneumonia. The patient recovered without incident, even though no one knew how to interpret the film.

The members of the 947th went "down range" after a proper CSH came to Bagram. The unit soon found itself at Forward Operating Base Orgun-E on the Pakistani border, home to an artillery range and a company of soldiers. The base had been nicknamed "Camp Harriman" in honor of the first casualty of Operation Anaconda, Chief Warrant Officer Stanley Harriman, who coincidentally also had ties to Bristol, Vermont. While there, Conway performed a substantial number of index cases in what amounted to a sophisticated tent. Among the procedures were two successful lower extremity revascularizations.

Reminiscent of Crandall's forward hospital set up preceding D-Day landings in 1944, The 250th FST parachuted into Northern Iraq with the 173rd Airborne Brigade on March 26, 2003 supporting Operation Iraqi Freedom. The FST was loaded onto four Humvees which were dropped with parachutes.[29]

Conway was redeployed with the Worcester, Massachusetts-based 912th FST, and was sent to a huge base at the outskirts of Baghdad International Airport in October of 2003. The parachute drop of an FST was not to be repeated. For Conway, the high velocity wounds of Bagram were replaced by the blast injuries of Bagdad, while the leisurely strolls through the Afghani village of Orgun-e Kalan were traded for fully-armed, high-speed convoys into the heart of the Green Zone. Conway and the 912th remained on base in support of a nearby CSH for his entire three-month stay. Conway's military service was later recognized with a Combat Medic Badge and an Army Commendation Medal.[30]

Gino T. Trevisani: 691st Forward Surgical Team: Afghanistan, 2003-04 and Iraq, 2008

UVM colorectal surgeon Gino Trevisani had also signed on with the Army Reserve as a resident. Upon completing his training, the Utica, New York native returned to his birthplace and settled into private practice. As it turned out, Utica was also the home of the 691st FST, a unit to which Trevisani was soon attached. The arrangement worked out well until Trevisani came back to Burlington in 2002. By then, however, the Global War on Terror was well underway. Trevisani was successful in maintaining his ties to the 691st rather than face reassignment.

Attention soon turned to ensuring the unit's combat preparedness. Trevisani and the rest of the FST were sent to Miami's Ryder Trauma Center during February of 2003 for some "real world" trauma exposure. While there, the 691st took an active part in the care of Ryder's emergency room patients. It was the first time that many of the soldiers had experienced the chaos, bloodshed, and futility associated with major penetrating injuries. At the end of the two-week exercise, the group was "validated" for mobilization.

The 691st was finally deployed in July of 2003. Trevisani arrived at the Reserve Center, ready for anything. Anything that is, except the Assumption of Command memo awaiting his signature. Taking it in stride, he signed his name and became the FST's commander with the stroke of a pen. The unit was equipped, organized, and drilled for another six weeks at Fort Drum before setting out for Afghanistan.

The team's final destination was Forward Operating Base Salerno, 90 miles to the south and east of Bagram. The intervening mountain range ensured that Salerno's dirt airstrip and helicopter pad were in constant use. As a result, the tent hospital was routinely caked with

FIGURE 29-12. Trevisani operating with his FST in Afghanistan in 2004.

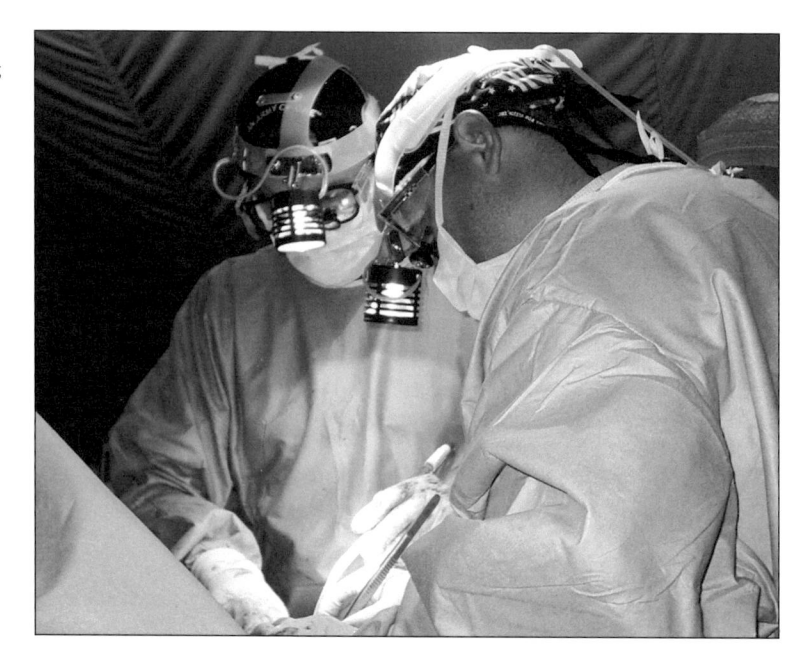

dust. Nonetheless, the 691st went on to perform over 100 life and limb salvage surgeries. In addition, the EMT section administered care to more than 2000 individuals. The group also provided a number of "un-doctrined" services for the base's 180 troops. Among these were preventative medicine check-ups, sick call, medical holding, combat stress relief, and moral support. During the down time, the staff trained field medics in Basic Life Support and Advanced Trauma Life Support.

Nearby villagers benefited from the 691st's expertise through a series of Civil Affairs Unit missions. Appalled that the locals had to purchase their own medical supplies prior to treatment, Trevisani took action, eventually securing over $15,000 in humanitarian aid from the Army. The funds were used to refurbish a former Taliban hospital with such basics as medicine, fuel, a generator, an ambulance, and even fresh water. In addition, Trevisani took it upon himself to teach the hospital's nurses and lone doctor basic surgical skills.

Minimal troop movement led to the rapid expansion of FOB Salerno's population during the first six months of the 691st's mission. A more "permanent" medical facility was built to accommodate the base's 1200 soldiers soon thereafter. The overworked 691st, of course, was not augmented until it was replaced by a 35-member FST-plus (or CSH-minus) three months later. The 691st was, however, one of the first Army Reserve Medical Units to receive a Meritorious Unit Citation for its achievements. Trevisani, in turn, was awarded the Bronze Star, while the old Taliban military clinic that he had assisted renamed itself the 691st Hospital.[31]

Trevasani found himself redeployed to Iraq assigned to the 325th CSH in Tikrit, in 2008. This hospital was the only "tent" set up hospital in Iraq and consisted of 140 beds. He performed over 115 surgical cases himself during his three and a half month deployment.

Michael A. Ricci: 158th Medical Group: Iraq, 2006-07

The nature of the conflict and the character of the countryside made the battle lines of Iraq even more stationary than those of Afghanistan. The flat terrain, however, exposed helicopters to attacks from rocket launchers and high-powered rifles. Ground transport, meanwhile,

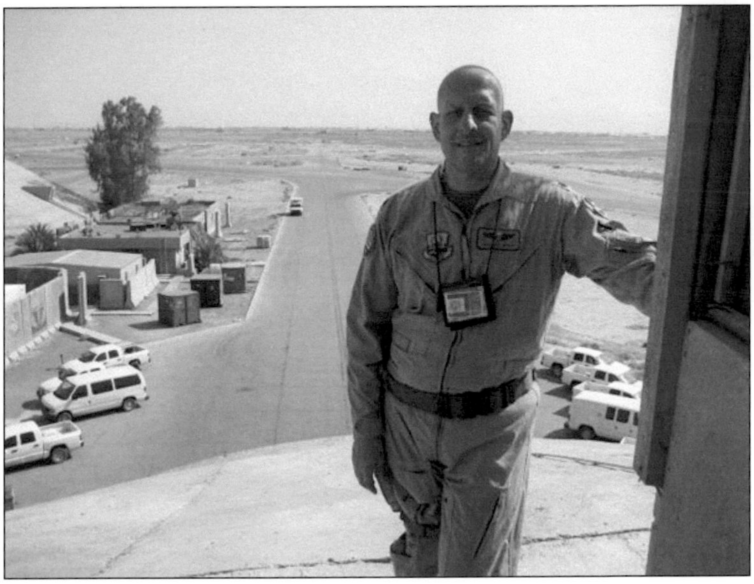

FIGURE 29-13. Ricci at Balad in Iraq in 2006.

was stymied by roadside bombs and other improvised explosives. Stable casualties were thus evacuated from forward units to larger hospitals by air at night in order to gain the maximum amount of cover. The Air Force found itself playing a much larger transfer and treatment role than it had initially anticipated.

Michael Ricci also took on a role that few would have predicted. Having already established himself as one of UVM's most durable vascular surgeons, he got into shape and joined the Vermont Air National Guard following 9/11. After extensive training, Ricci and other members of the Air Force's 158th Medical Group were deployed to Iraq in the spring of 2006. The unit was stationed at Balad Air Base and Logistics Support Area Anaconda, an immense military installment forty miles north of Baghdad. Ricci served as a flight surgeon, essentially providing primary care for F-16 aircrews. He also clocked more than 80 hours of airtime carrying out medical evacuation missions. He was subsequently awarded an Air Medal for flying more than twenty combat flights.

Ricci additionally worked as a trauma surgeon at the Air Force Theater Hospital (AFTH). The AFTH, described as a "MASH on steroids" by some, consisted of three operating room trailers and three-dozen support system and ward tents. It was notable for being the first such large-scale facility since the Vietnam era. The enlarged CSH's staff of 350 treated wounded coalition forces as well as large numbers of Iraqi civilians. The AFTH was also the central point for the aero-evacuation of all injured American soldiers to hospitals in Ramstein, Germany and the States, making it the busiest medical center in Iraq.[32]

Ricci returned to the AFTH as a full-time trauma surgeon in the summer of 2007. Temperatures frequently reached 120 degrees inside the base's "climate-controlled" tents, which were attacked by mortars and rockets on a daily basis. Despite the conditions, the facility achieved a greater than 95 percent survival rate for its multiply injured patients. As Ricci put it, "The Air Force's surgeons were excellent about passing on 'lessons learned' to each successive group. Surgical principles were adhered to at all times, in spite of rotating new surgeons every four months." Ricci and the other members of the 158th Medical Group went on to receive the Meritorious Unit Award for their efforts.[33]

A Legacy of Service to Vermont

The history of front line surgery confirms the military adage that a man dies over a period of time, not a period of miles. There is no question that the care administered by UVM's combat surgeons saved thousands of lives across the world. And there is no doubt that the work was grueling, to say the least, even under the best of circumstances. That it was done in extreme conditions with limited equipment is a testament to the skill and dedication of every one of these individuals.

That skill and dedication continued long after each returned to Vermont. Shea prepared UVM residents for the reality of community surgery. Crandall instilled the Fanny Allen's staff with a strong sense of awareness of their responsibility to patients. Abajian, Donaghy, and Wallman, returned to UVM as role models and leaders in their specialties and surgery overall. Davis maintained his commitment to trauma research, bringing UVM to national prominence through his efforts. I developed the EMT training program, and initiated the revolution in ambulance service, the modern UVM Emergency Room, and brought ATLS course instruction to Vermont. Conway and Trevisani employ the latest surgical techniques and engage in local outreach programs, while Ricci improves telecommunication among the State's far flung hospitals.

John Pomeroy's spirit of community service lives on in these actions. I think he would be proud.

Chapter 1

1. Duncan LC. Medical men in the American Revolution 1775-1783. (Carlisle, PA: Army Medical Bulletin No. 25, Medical Field Service School, 1931): 46-82.
2. Ibid: 406.
3. Thayer SW, The New England historical and genealogical register. (Boston: Samuel G. Drake, 1848): 279.
4. Reade P. Massachusetts at Valley Forge. The Magazine of History, with Notes and Queries 1916; 23 (June): 150.
5. Miller G, "Medical apprenticeship in the American colonies," Ciba Symposia 1947; 8 (January): 502-10.
6. Thayer SW, p. 279.
7. Hemenway AM (ed), The Vermont Historical Gazetteer 1868; 1: 611.
8. Chapin WAR, Allen L. History of the University of Vermont College of Medicine. (Hanover, NH: Dartmouth Printing Co. 1951): 17.
9. Ibid : 113.
10. Grinnell AP, History of the Medical Department of the University of Vermont, an introductory address delivered before the Medical Class, March 4, 1880.(Burlington VT: The Free Press Association, 1880): 4-5.
11. Ibid: 5.
12. Thompson Z. History of Vermont, natural, civil, and statistical, vol. 2. (Burlington VT: Chauncey Goodrich, 1842): 144-5.
13. Benedict GW. History of the University of Vermont. American Quarterly Register 1841; 13: 400-401.
14. Hemenway: 539.
15. Ibid: 522.
16. Benedict: 401-2.
17. Grinnell: 7.
18. UVM trustee minutes, August 13-14, 1804, UVM Archives, quoted in Kaufman M. The University of Vermont College of Medicine (Hanover,NH: UVM College of Medicine, 1979): 4.
19. House Journal, October 18, 1811: 63ff , quoted in Kaufman: 6.
20. Kaufman: 4.
21. Minutes of the Third Medical Society, December 29, 1803, January 3, 1804. Special Collections, Bailey/Howe Library, University of Vermont. quoted in Kaufman: 7.
22. Kaufman: 7.
23. Vermont State Medical Society Minutes, November 13, 1813, July 9, 1814, October 17, 1814, Special Collections, Bailey/Howe Library, University of Vermont, quoted in Kaufman: 9-10.
24. Vermont Centinel, August 18, 1809: 3, quoted in Kaufman: 9.
25. UVM Trustee Minutes, August 15-17, 1809, UVM Archives, quoted in Kaufman: 7, 9.
26. Schachner A. Ephraim McDowell "father of ovariotomy" and founder of abdominal surgery. (Philadelphia PA: J.B. Lippincott, 1921): 87.
27. Myer JS. Life and letters of Dr. William Beaumont. (St Louis MO: CV Mosby Co, 1912): 18-32.
28. Ibid: 34-73.
29. Ibid: 212.
30. Duffy J. From humors to medical science: A history of American medicine. (Urbana and Chicago, IL: University of Illinois Press, 1993): 107-110.
31. Millard JP. Burlington, Vermont during the War of 1812," America's historic lakes, May 13, 2007: 1-3.
32. Hemenway: 630-2.
33. Kaufman: 9-10.
34. Root E, A journal of the most remarkable proceedings, studies and observations kept by Erastus Root, October 1, 1815 - February 10, 1816: 20. Special Collections, Bailey/Howe Library, University of Vermont.
35. Thompson: 145.
36. Grinnell: 4-5.
37. UVM Trustee minutes, July 27, 1815, UVM Archives, quoted in Kaufman: 12.
38. Root:.
39. Root: 25-72.
40. Burlington Gazette, December 29, 1815: 3. January 19, 1816: 3, quoted in Kaufman: 12.
41. Northern Sentinel, January 2, 1818: 3 quoted in Kaufman: 13.
42. Kaufman: 13.
43. Kaufman: 13-14.
44. Allen L. A sketch of Vermont's early surgical history. NEJM 1933; 209 (October 16): 795.

Chapter 2

1. Kaufman M. University of Vermont College of Medicine, (Burlington,VT: UVM College of Medicine, 1979) : 16.
2. Alan Gregg to John Sloan Dickey, President of Dartmouth College, April 1948, quoted in Hayward OS and Putnam CE. Improve, perfect & perpetuate, Dr. Nathan Smith and early American medical education, (Hanover, NH: University Press of New England, 1998): 263.
3. Williams SW. American medical biography: Memoirs of eminent physicians. (Greenfield, MA: L. Merriam, 1845): 203.
4. Hayward OS. A search for the real Nathan Smith. Journal of the History of Medicine, 1960; 15: 271-2.
5. Child WH, History of the Town of Cornish, New Hampshire, vol. 2, (Concord, NH:Rumford Press, 1911): 335.
6. Hayward and Putnam : 19-23.
7. Ibid: 193.
8. Ibid.: 36-7.
9. Ibid: 39, 42, 48, 50, 136.
10. Ibid: 187.
11. Ellis H. Operations that made history. (Cambridge, MA: Cambridge University Press, 1996): 11-13.

12. Smith N. Case of ovarian dropsy, successfully removed by a surgical operation. American Medical Recorder 1822; 5: 124-6.
13. McDowell E. Three cases of extirpation of diseased ovaria. Eclectic Repertory & Analytical Review 1817; (April): 242-4.
14. Benedict WA, Tracy WAB, History of the Town of Sutton, Massachusetts, from 1704 to 1876. (Worcester MA, Sanford & Company, 1878): 413.
15. Wirthlin LS. Nathan Smith (1762-1829) surgical consultant to Joseph Smith. Brigham Young University Studies, Spring 1977: 337.
16. Hayward and Putnam: 183-4.
17. Ibid: 132, 199-200.
18. Smith EA. Life and letters. (New Haven, CT: Yale University Press, 1914): 126.
19. Ibid: 51-2.
20. Hayward and Putnam: 198, 201.
21. Smith EA: 94.
22. Hayward and Putnam: 100, 204.
23. Nathan Smith to Ezekiel Dodge Cushing, June 28, 1819, Ezekiel Dodge Cushing Papers, Manuscripts & Archives, Yale University Library, quoted in Hayward and Putnam: 206.
24. Hayward and Putnam: 210-14.
25. Kaufman: 16-17.
26. Nathan Smith to Parker Cleveland, August 13, 1822, Manuscript 822473, Dartmouth College Archives, Baker Library, quoted in Hayward and Putnam: 225.
27. Nathan Smith to George C. Shattuck, Brunswick, Maine, April 18, 1823, Yale University Library, quoted in Smith EA: 122.
28. Kaufman: 16.
29. UVM Trustee Minutes, August 15, 1822, UVM Archives, quoted in Kaufman: 17.
30. Ibid.
31. Spooner's Vermont Journal, July 27, 1822.
32. Northern Sentinel, June 20, 1823, p. 3, June 27, 1823, p. 3, July 4, 1823, p. 2, quoted in Kaufman: 19.
33. Kaufman: 19.
34. Thayer SW. The New England Historical and Genealogical Register. (Boston: New England Historic Genealogic Society, 1848): 279.
35. Visser T, Gearhart T. History of Pomeroy Hall, UVM Historic Preservation Program, Burlington, 1991: 8.
36. Nathan Smith to Mills Olcott, Burlington, September 29, 1822, Dartmouth College Archives, quoted in Hayward and Putnam: 225.
37. Fitch WL. Extracts from lectures on surgery. Delivered at the Medical Institution at New Haven by Nathan Smith 1824.: 178-79, Manuscripts and Archives, Yale University Library, quoted in Hayward and Putnam: 174.
38. Ibid: 319, quoted in Hayward and Putnam: 177.
39. Ibid: 323-24, quoted in Hayward and Putnam: 178.
40. Ibid: 394, 399, quoted in Hayward and Putnam:181.
41. Ibid: 6-7, 78-79, quoted in Hayward and Putnam: 172-73.
42. Kaufman: 19.
43. Cutter WR (ed.). Genealogical and family history of northern New York, vol. 2 & 3. (New York, Lewis Historical Publishing Company, 1910).
44. Pearson TS. Catalogue of the Graduates of Middlebury College. (Windsor, VT: Vermont Chronicle Press, 1853): 31.
45. College of Physicians and Surgeons in the city of New York, Catalogue of the Alumni, Officers, and Fellows, 1807-1880. (New York: Bradstreet Press, , 1880): 54.
46. Ellis: 17-25.
47. Bigelow HS (ed.). The American Monthly Magazine and Critical Review, vol. 1, Kirk & Mercein, 1817: 444-5.
48. Ibid.
49. Cooper AP, Travers B. Surgical essays, Parts 1 and 2. (Philadelphia: James Webster, 1821): 83-103.
50. Beck JB.Necrology. The New York Monthly Chronicle of Medicine and Surgery 1824; 1: 182-3.
51. Smith to Shattuck, April 18, 1823, quoted in Smith EA: 122.
52. Beck: 183.
53. Northern Sentinel. May 29, 1824: 3, quoted in Kaufman: 20.
54. Kaufman: 21.
55. Triennial Catalogue of the University of Vermont. (Burlington, VT: Free Press Printers, 1854): 10.
56. Heitman FB. Historical Register of the Officers of the Continental Army during the War of the Revolution. (Washington, DC: The Rare Book Shop Publishing Co, 1914): 574-5.
57. Austin JD, Mayflower Families through five generations, Vol. 6: Stephen Hopkins (3rd ed.). (Plymouth, MA: General Society of Mayflower Descendants, 2001): 123.
58. Smith HP (ed.), History of Addison County Vermont. (New York: D. Smith & Co., 1881): 178.
59. Hastings H (ed.). Military minutes of the Council of Appointment of the State of New York, 1783-1821. (New York: J.B. Lyon, 1910): 2136.
60. Triennial Catalogue of the University of Vermont: 45.
61. "Review of Chapman's Philadelphia Journal," The New York Monthly Chronicle of Medicine and Surgery 1824; 1: 113.
62. Tindall HL. Florida Keys Sea Heritage Journal 1995; 5 (Spring): 7.
63. Ibid: 8.
64. Triennial Catalogue of the University of Vermont: 11-12.
65. Smith to Shattuck, April 18, 1823, quoted in Smith EA: 122.
66. Longcope WT. "Smith, Nathan Ryno," in Dictionary of American biography, vol. 17. Dumas Malone,ed. (New York: Charles Scribner's Sons, 1935): 328.

Chapter 3
1. Wallman LJ. "Benjamin Lincoln MD, Vermont medical educator," Vermont History 1961; 29 (October):. 202-203.
2. Kaufman M, The University of Vermont College of Medicine, (Hanover, New Hampshire: UVM College of Medicine,1979: 25-26.

3 Chapin WAR, Allen L. History University of Vermont College of Medicine (Hanover, New Hampshire: Dartmouth Printing Co, 1951): 23.
4 Kaufman: 27, 48.
5 Crockett WH, "George Wyllys Benedict," Vermont Alumni Weekly. 1926; 266 (February) quoted in Wallman: 201-202.
6 Visser T, Gearhart T, History of Pomeroy Hall, UVM Historic Preservation Program, Burlington, 1991: 1.
7 Northern Sentinel, January 27, 1826: 3, as quoted in Visser: 1.
8 Visser: 1.
9 Hemenway AM (ed), The Vermont Historical Gazetteer 1868; 1: 648.
10 Ibid.
11 Hayward OS, Putnam CE, Improve, perfect, and perpetuate: Dr. Nathan Smith and early American medical education. (Hanover, New Hampshire: University Press of New England: 116.
12 Class of 1823, Box 28, Folder 22, George J. Mitchell Department of Special Collections & Archives, Bowdoin Library.
13 Wheeler J, A historical discourse delivered on the occasion of the semi-centennial anniversary of the University of Vermont, Burlington: 27.
14 Hemenway: 648.
15 Medical Society of the University of Vermont, Records, September 30, 1828, UVM Archives, as quoted in Kaufman: 28.
16 Hemenway: 648.
17 Wallman: 198: 204.
18 Grob GN, Edward Jarvis and the Medical World of Nineteenth Century America (Knoxville, Tennessee:The University of Tennessee Press, 1978): 42.
19 Waite FC, "Grave robbing in New England," Bulletin of the Medical Library Associatio.1945; 33 (July): 274-75.
20 Ibid: 286-87.
21 Burlington Sentinel. February 5, 1830: 2, February 12, 1830: 2, February 19, 1830: 2-3, as quoted in Kaufman: 47.
22 Ibid., March 5, 1830: 3, March 19, 1830: 3, quoted in Kaufman: 47.
23 Marshall JD, The inquest (Lebanon, New Hampshire: University of Vermont Press,, 2006): 151.
24 Hemenway: 648-49.
25 Kaufman: 33.
26 Benjamin Lincoln to George C. Shattuck, Burlington, April 6, 1831, Shattuck Papers, Massachusetts Historical Society, Boston, quoted in Kaufman: 32.
27 Lincoln to Shattuck, May 1, 1831, Shattuck Papers, quoted in Kaufman: 32-33.
28 Wallman: 196-97.
29 Hayward and Putnam: 218.
30 Wallman: 196-97.
31 Kaufman: 33-34.
32 George C. Shattuck, Jr. to George C. Shattuck, Burlington, August 19, 1832, Shattuck Papers, Massachusetts Historical Society, Boston, quoted in Kaufman: 34.
33 Ibid., August 28, 1832, October 14, 1832, Shattuck Papers, quoted in Kaufman: 34.
34 Lincoln to Shattuck, September 30, 1832, Shattuck Papers, quoted in Kaufman: 35.
35 Wallman: 197.
36 Lincoln B, Hints on the present state of medical education and the influence of medical schools in New England. (Burlington, Vermont:Printed for the Author, 1833) appendix, p. vi-viii, quoted in Kaufman: 35-36.
37 Kaufman: 36.
38 Lincoln, Hints on the present state of medical education : 13-15, quoted in Wallman: 206-207.
39 Ibid, quoted in Wallman: 207-208.
40 Kaufman: 36-37.
41 Wheeler: 27.
42 George C. Shattuck, Jr. to Miss E. Shattuck, May 6, 1834, Shattuck Papers, Massachusetts Historical Society, Boston, quoted in Kaufman: 37.
43 Benjamin Lincoln to the UVM Corporation, Dennysville, Maine, June 23, 1834, Pomeroy Papers, Special Collections, Bailey/Howe Library, University of Vermont, quoted in Kaufman: 37.
44 Wheeler: 27.
45 Kaufman: 38.
46 George W. Benedict to Benjamin Lincoln, Burlington, January 24, 1835, Lincoln Papers.
47 UVM Trustee Minutes, September 3, 1835, UVM Archives, quoted in Kaufman: 39.
48 Phelps OS, Servin AT, The Phelps family of America and their English ancestors, vol. 1. (Pittsfield, Massachusetts: Eagle Publishing Company, 1899): 204.
49 Child H, Gazetteer and Business Directory of Windsor County, VT, For 1883-84, Journal Office, Syracuse, 1884: 280.
50 Ibid: 39.
51 Ibid: 49.
52 Macmillan M, "Phineas Gage: A case for all reasons," classic cases in neuropsychology, Christopher Code (ed.). (New York: Psychology Press, 1996): 243-48.
53 Ibid.
54 Blackington AH, More Yankee yarns. (New York, New York: Dodd, Mead, and Company, 1956): 80.
55 Macmillan: 247.
56 Blackington: 78-80.
57 Triennial Catalogue of the University of Vermont, Free Press Printers, Burlington, 1854: 17-27, 43-51.

Chapter 4
1 Fishbein M, Lawrence W. A History of the American Medical Association. (Philadelphia: WB Saunders & Co,,1947).

2. Pullen JJ. Gentlemen, this is no humbug. American Heritage Magazine 1979; 30 (August/September).
3. Ibid.
4. Ibid.
5. Rutkow IM. Surgery, an illustrated history, (St. Louis, Missouri: Mosby Year Book Inc,1993): 341-2.
6. Cartwright FF. The Development of modern surgery from 1830. (New York, New York: Thomas Y Crowell Co, 1968).
7. Kaufman M. University of Vermont College of Medicine (Hanover, New Hampshire: UVM College of Medicine, 1979): 50.
8. UVM Trustee Minutes, March 29, 1853, UVM Archives, quoted in Kaufman: 51.
9. ibid: 51.
10. UVM Medical Department, Announcement, Session of 1854, in Nelson's American Lancet. 1853-1854; 8 : unnumbered back pages.
11. Borthwick JD. History and biographical gazetteer of Montreal to the year 1892 (Montreal, P.Q. Canada: John Lovell & Son, 1892): 248.
12. Brown GW, Hayne DM, Trudel M (ed.). Dictionary of Canadian biography, Vol. IX. (Toronto, Canada: University of Toronto Press, 1976): 596.
13. Grinnell AP. History of the Medical Department of the University of Vermont, An introductory address delivered before the medical class, Thursday March 4, 1880, (Burlington Vermont: Free Press Association, 1880): 11-12.
14. Kaufman: 53.
15. Grinnell: 12.
16. Nelson's American Lancet. 1856; 11 (April to October): 1.
17. "Necrology," Transactions of the Minnesota State Medical Association, 1884: 187.
18. Wheeler JB. Memoirs of a small town surgeon. (Garden City, New York: Garden City Publishing Co, 1935): 289.
19. "Necrology,": 187.
20. Wheeler: 285.
21. Stearns JB. A Note on Dr. Thayer, Vermont Alumnus, vol. 20 (April 1941), quoted in Chapin WAR, Allen L, History of the University of Vermont College of Medicine. (Hanover, NH: Dartmouth Printing Co,1951): 124.
22. Kaufman: 53, 57.
23. Bibbins WB. A Biographical sketch of David S. Conant, M.D., read before the New York County Medical Society, March 5th, 1866 in: Transactions of the Medical Society of the State of New York, for the Year 1866, (Albany, NY: C. Wendell, 1866):336-338.
24. Kaufman: 60.
25. Ibid: 339.
26. Crosby AB. Memorial address, Prof. David S. Conant, M.D., delivered to the graduating class, in the Medical Department of the University of Vermont, Times Book and Job Office, Burlington: 11.
27. Kaufman: 55-56.
28. Visser T, Gearhart T. History of Pomeroy Hall, UVM Historic Preservation Program, Burlington, 1991: 2-3.
29. Kaufman: 60.
30. Peck TS. Revised roster of Vermont Volunteers: Lists of Vermonters who served in the Army and Navy of the United States during the War of the Rebellion 1861-66. (Montpelier, VT: Watchman Press, 1892). Searched via VermontCivilWar.org.
31. Ibid: 746.
32. Benedict GG, Vermont in the Civil War, Vol. 2, (Burlington,VT: Vermont:Free Press Association, 1888): 784.
33. Richmond Sentinel, June 18, 1863.
34. Crosby, Memorial Address: 12.
35. Bibbins: 336, 339-40.
36. The National CyclopÊdia of American Biography, vol. 9, (New York,:James T. White & Co, 1899): 98.
37. Ibid.
38. Crosby AB. A lost art in surgery. Transactions of the New Hampshire Medical Society. (Concord, NH:Charles C. Pearson & Company, 1876): 134.
39. Ibid: 133.
40. Ibid: 135.
41. Ibid: 135-136.
42. Ibid: 136.
43. Conant DS. Crosby AB: Memorial address, UVM Dana library archives,1866: 9.
44. National CyclopÊdia: 98.
45. Ibid.
46. St. Louis Clinical Record, 1877-8;4 (April): 193.
47. King J. Civil War medicine. VermontCivilWar.org.
48. Boone NE, Sherman M. Designed to cure: Civil War hospitals in Vermont Vermont History 2001; 69 (Winter/Spring): 192.
49. Dodge PC (ed.). Encyclopedia, Vermont Biography: A series of authentic biographical sketches of the representative men of Vermont and sons of Vermont in other states (Burlington Vermont: Ullery Publishing Co, 1912): 235-236.
50. Janes H. Notes of some of the gunshot injuries treated under the charge of Henry Janes surgeon USA. Special Collections, Bailey/Howe Library, University of Vermont.
51. Ibid.
52. Transactions of the Vermont Medical Society for the years 1867 and 1868, Vermont Medical Society, Burlington VT, 1869: 14.
53. Dodge: 236.
54. UVM Medical Department, Catalogue and Forty-Sixth Annual Announcement, 1886.
55. Wheeler: 302-305.
56. Howard BD. Prisoners of Russia: A personal study of convict life in Sakhalin and Siberia. (New York: D. Appleton and Co, 1902): v-x.
57. Howard B. Plain rules for the restoration of persons apparently dead from drowning. (New York: E.B. Treat & Co,1869).
58. The Sanitary Commission Bulletin, vol.1, (New York: Sanitary Commission, 1866): 981-994.
59. Howard B. An improvised tracheal cannula. The Medical Record, November 1871: 391.

60 Howard. Prisoners: xi-xii.
61 Howard B. On the application of sutures to bone in recent gunshot fractures, with cases. Medico-Chirurgical Transactions 1865; 48: 245.
62 Howard B. A case of trephining and removal of a miniÈ bullet which had passed into the brain through a trap-door fracture of the os frontis, followed by recovery. The American Journal of the Medical Sciences. 1871; 62 (Oct.): 385-389.
63 Berry FB. Medical Department, United States Army, surgery in World War II. Office of the Surgeon General, Department of the Army, Washington D.C. Thoracic Surgery 1963; 1: 5-6.
64 Nay WS. quoted in Chapin WAR, Allen L, History of the University of Vermont College of Medicine, (Hanover, NH:Dartmouth Printing Co, 1951): 99.
65 Howard. Prisoners: xii-xix.

Chapter 5
1 Orton V. Mary Fletcher Comes Back: a brief account of the History, Progress & Future of Vermont's First General Hospital (Burlington, VT: Board of Directors of the Mary Fletcher Hospital,1941): 19-20.
2 Orton: 20.
3 Wheeler JB, Memoirs of a small town surgeon. (Garden City, NY: Garden City Publishing Co, 1935): 22.
4 Wheeler: 22-23.
5 Rutkow IM. The history of surgery in the United States 1775-1900. (San Francisco: Norman Publishing, 1988): 342-344.
6 Wheeler: 16-17.
7 Lister JR. On the antiseptic principles of the practice of surgery. British Med Journal 1867 (August 9).
8 Ibid: 23.
9 Bishop WJ. The early history of surgery. (New York: Barnes & Noble Books, 1995): 168.
10 Walker K. Joseph Lister. (London: Hutchinson & Co,1956): 50.
11 St. John Roosa DB. A sketch of the life of James Lawrence Little, M.D., and of the twenty-five years in which he practiced surgery in New York. The Medical Record 1885; 28 (November 7, 1885): 506.
12 Ibid: 506-508.
13 Little JL. A report on the use of plaster of paris in surgery. Transactions of the American Medical Association 1867.
14 St. John Roosa: 508-509.
15 Allen L, "Old Burlington," A talk delivered before the Faculty Club of UVM, Feb. 3,1950.
16 Shaughnessy J. The Rutland road. (Berkeley, California: Howell North Books, 1964): 11-12.
17 Wheeler: 171.
18 St. John Roosa: 509.
19 Ibid: 508.
20 UVM Medical Department, Catalogue and twenty-ninth session, 1882: 1-2.
21 St. John Roosa: 509-510.
22 Little JL. A hitherto undescribed lesion as a cause of epistaxis, with four cases. New York Hospital Gazette 1879; 6 (March -Dec.): 5-6.
23 Rainey JJ. James Lawrence Little, a forgotten pioneer. AMA Archives of Otolarygology 1952; 55 (April): 451-452.
24 Nelson CW. Early New York surgeons and Dr. William J. Mayo. Mayo Clinic Proceedings 1996; 71: 728.
25 St. John Roosa: 509.
26 Boone NE, Sherman M. Designed to Cure: Civil War hospitals in Vermont. Vermont History 2001; 69 (Winter/Spring): 176-178.
27 Kaufman M. University of Vermont College of Medicine. (Hanover, NH:UVM College of Medicine, 1979): 60.
28 Orton: 9.
29 Allen: 3.
30 Orton: 9-13.
31 Ibid: 13.
32 Hemenway AM (ed). The Vermont Historical Gazetteer, Vol. 1. (Burlington, VT: Abby Maria Hemenway, 1868): 593-594.
33 Kaufman: 89-90.
34 Ibid: 90.
35 St. John Roosa: 509.
36 Mary Fletcher Hospital Report for Jan 1926. MFH archives.
37 Casebook #2, Mary Fletcher Hospital, Special Collections, Dana Medical Library, University of Vermont.
38 Ibid.
39 Kaufman: 87.
40 Williams HC (ed). Biographical encyclopedia of Vermont of the nineteenth century. (Boston: Metropolitan Publishing and Engraving Co, 1885): 290-295.
41 Kaufman:. 87-88.
42 Chapin WAR, Allen L. History, University of Vermont College of Medicine. (Hanover, NH: Dartmouth Printing Co, 1951): 37.
43 Wheeler: 1-4.
44 Ibid: 3-4.
45 Ibid: 2-3.
46 Ibid: 180-181.
47 Ibid: 168.
48 UVM Medical Department, 32nd annual announcement and catalogue, 1885: 16.
49 St. John Roosa: 510-511.
50 Kaufman: 69.
51 The University Cynic, June 10,1885:32, quoted in Kaufman: 69.
52 Kaufman: 69.
53 Ibid.

54 Chaffee G (ed). Transactions of the New York and New England Association of Railway Surgeons, (New York: Surgery Publishing Co, 1912): 112-113.
55 Ibid.: 70-72.
56 Chaffee: 113.
57 Kaufman: 72.
58 Wheeler: 198.
59 Chi Phi Fraternity, The Chi Phi Quarterly, 1877; 1 (January): 169.
60 Wheeler: 198.
61 Atkinson WB. The Physicians and Surgeons of the United States. (Philadelphia: Charles Robson, 1878): 392.
62 College of Physicians and Surgeons, Catalogue of the Alumni, Officers, and Fellows, 1807-1880. (New York: Bradstreet Press, 1880): 112.
63 Wheeler: 198.
64 Wright JL. Lectures on diseases of the rectum. (New York: Bermingham & Co, 1884).
65 Rutkow IM. The history of surgery in the United States 1775-1900. (San Francisco: Norman Publishing, 1988): 373.
66 Wright JW. Possible danger incident to the application of cocaine about the head: Local anesthesia in general medicine and surgery. (New York: D. Appleton and Co, 1886): 78.
67 Wright JW. Congenital cyst of the tongue: Medical analectic. A monthly epitome of progress in all divisions of medico-chirurgical practice 1885; 2: 253.
68 Wright JW. Treatment of compound fracture by wiring the fragments. New York Medical Journal 1885; 42.
69 George Tiemann & Co., American armamentarium Chirurgicum. (New York: C.H. Ludwig, 1889): 73.
70 Wheeler: 199-200.
71 Vermont State Medical Society, Proceedings of the Vermont State Medical Society 1887. (Montpelier,VT: Vermont State Medical Society, 1888): 8-9.
72 The Ohio State University Monthly. 1912; 4: 1952.
73 Kaufman: 74.
74 Keating JW (ed. Necrology,. The physician and surgeon, a professional medical journal 1902; 24 : 520-522.
75 Wheeler: 204.
76 Keating: 522.
77 Ibid: 522
78 "Death list of a day," New York Times, October 7, 1902.
79 Phelps AM. The present status of the open incision method for talipes varo-equinus. Medical Record 1890; 38: 593-598.
80 Kaufman: 109-112.
81 Ibid: 75, 111.
82 Wheeler: 206-207.
83 Noyo G, Phelps AM. N.E. Medical Monthly 1895 (Nov) (reprint in the Dana Medical Library, UVM).
84 Mayer L. Orthopaedic surgery in the United States of America. Journal of Bone and Joint Surgery 1950; 32 B: 461-462.
85 Kaufman: 76-83.
86 Keating: 520.

Chapter 6
1 Kaufman M. University of Vermont College of Medicine. (Hanover, NH:UVM College of Medicine, 1979): 84.
2 Wheeler JB. Memoirs of a small town surgeon. (Garden City, NY: Garden City Publishing Co, 1935): 1, 50.
3 Bell B. A system of surgery. 1st American Ed. Corrected. (Boston: Isiah Thomas and Ebenezer T. Andrews, 1791.
4 Wheeler: 127-158.
5 Ibid: 175-179.
6 Ibid: 179, 217-218.
7 Ibid: 263-266.
8 Ibid: 220-221.
9 Wheeler JB, "An incident in country surgery," The Ariel, 1924. (Burlington, VT: UVM, 1924): 169-170.
10 Ibid.
11 Debré P (Translated by E Forster) Louis Pasteur (Baltimore, MD: Johns Hopkins University Press, 2000): 288.
12 Wheeler. Memoirs: 30.
13 Rutkow IM. Surgery, an illustrated history. (St. Louis, MO: Mosby Year Book Inc., 1993): 349.
14 Pilcher LS. The treatment of wounds, its principles and practice, general and special. (New York: William Wood & Co, 1883): 60.
15 Wheeler. Memoirs: 9-12.
16 Wheeler JB Modifications in antiseptics. Transactions of the Vermont Medical Society 1881. (St. Albans, VT: The Vermont Medical Society Society, 1882): 113-123.
17 Wheeler JB. Cocaine in general surgery, Transactions of the Vermont Medical Society 1886. (Montpelier, VT:Vermont State Medical Society, Montpelier VT, 1887): 6.
18 Wheeler JB. The necessity of prompt operative treatment in appendicitis. New York Medical Journal 1894; 60: 7.
19 Wheeler JB. Radical cure of hernia; Halsted's operation. Vermont Medical Monthly 1895; 1: 103-108.
20 Wheeler JB. Surgery in its relations to the female pelvic organ. Annals of Gynecology and Pediatrics 1899; 13: 6.
21 Wheeler JB. Modern treatment of prostatic hypertrophy. Vermont Medical Monthly 1902; 8: 261-265.
22 Wheeler JB. Medical education in America at present day. Vermont Medical Monthly 1907; 13: 183-185.
23 Billroth CAT. Clinical surgery. (London: New Syndenham Society, 1881): 140.
24 Wheeler. Memoirs: 188-194.
25 Wheeler JB. Use of the O'Dwyer tube in diphtheria. New York Medical Journal 1887: 53.
26 Wheeler. Memoirs: 211, 221-222.
27 Ibid. 183.

28 Pridmore J. Northwestern University, celebrating 150 years,. (Chicago: Northwestern University Press, 2000): 72.
29 Chapin WAR. Allen L. History of the University of Vermont College of Medicine. (Hanover NH: Dartmouth Printing Co, 1951): 48-49.
30 Wheeler. Memoirs: 184.
31 Kaufman: 96.
32 Wheeler. Memoirs: 185.
33 Kaufman: 96-100.
34 Chapin: 49.
35 Wheeler, Memoirs: 212.
36 Carleton H (ed). Genealogical and family history of the State of Vermont. (New York: The Lewis Publishing Co, 1903): 289-290.
37 Wheeler. Memoirs: 211-212.
38 Tinkham HC. Cancer of the uterus. Vermont Medical Monthly 1900; 6: 157-160.
39 Tinkham HC. The care of surgical cases; their preparation for operation and their care after operation; with specific reference to abdominal surgery. Vermont Medical Monthly 1907; 13: 131-136.
40 Tinkham HC. The surgical aspect of inflammation of the biliary tract whether accompanied or not by gall stone. Vermont Medical Monthly 1909; 15: 27-32.
41 Tinkham HC. The differential diagnosis of some of the more common pathological conditions in the right side of the abdomen. Vermont Medical Monthly 1909; 15 : 157-160.
42 Tinkham HC. Chronic arterio-mesenteric obstruction of the duodenum. Boston Medical & Surgical Journal, 1923; 188: 397-401.
43 Kaufman: 130-133.
44 Beck AH. The Flexner Report and the standardization of American medical education JAMA 2004 ; 291: 2139-2140.
45 Bierring WL. Medical licensure after forty years. Federation Bulletin 1956; 43: 101-102.
46 Third annual conference of council on medical education of the AMA, 29 April 1907. JAMA 1907; 48: 1701-1707.
47 Flexner A. Medical education in the United States and Canada. (Boston :The Merrymount Press, 1910): viii.
48 Ibid: vii-xvi.
49 Ibid: 19, 127, 154.
50 Ibid: 313-314.
51 Ibid: 15, 31, 313-314.
52 Ibid: 147.
53 Kaufman: 135.
54 Editorial, Vermont Medical Monthly 1910;16: 173 quoted in Kaufman: 136-137.
55 Wheeler. Memoirs: 185-186.
56 Kaufman: 137-141.
57 Kaufman: 148.
58 Ibid: 143-145.
59 Vermont Cynic, October 25, 1913: 6, quoted in Kaufman: 145
60 Wheeler. Memoirs: 185-186.
61 Ibid: 149.
62 Healy MJ. Walking in the spirit: Fanny Allen Hospital 1894-1994 (Colchester, VT:Fanny Allen Hospital, 1993): 16-21, 30-41.
63 DeGoesbriand L. Catholic memoirs of Vermont and New Hampshire, with sketches of the lives of Rev. L. DeGoesbriand and Fanny Allen (Burlington VT: Wm. Henry Hoyt, 1886): 12-19.
64 Ibid: 19-23.
65 McLaughlin J. The Limerick lad, the Burlington lady, and the founding of Saint Michael's College. A talk presented at the 3rd Burlington Irish Heritage Festival on March, 16, 1998: 22-24.
66 Ibid.: 15, 20-24.
67 Healy: 39-41.
68 Burlington Free Press, May 1,1898.
69 Ibid.
70 Healy : 52-53.
71 Fanny Allen Hospital record of surgical operations, 1905-1908. Box 3 Archives of Fanny Allen Hospital, St Michaels Archives Library: 142-143.
72 UVM Medical Faculty Minutes, May 20, 1914, quoted in Kaufman: 149.
73 Kaufman: 150.
74 Putnam CE. The science we have loved and taught (Hanover NH: University Press of New England , 2004): 241-250.
75 Wheeler. Memoirs: 216.
76 Kaufman: 152-153.
77 "Obituary, Tinkham (Henry Crain) (1856-1925)" JAMA 1926; 86(4): 54.

Chapter Seven
1 Allen L, "Old Burlington," a talk delivered before the Faculty Club of the University of Vermont on February 3, 1950, Manuscript from the archives of E.D. McSweeney Jr.
2 University of Vermont, Athletic hall of fame inductees. Brief bios, 2007: 1.
3 UVM Medical Faculty Minutes, June 21, 1894, quoted in Kaufman M. University of Vermont College of Medicine. (Hanover NH: UVM College of Medicine, 1979): 125.
4 Wheeler JB. Memoirs of a small town surgeon. (Garden City NY: Garden City Publishing Co, 1935): 236-237.
5 Ibid: 237-238.
6 Dodge PC (ed.),. Encyclopedia, Vermont biography: A series of authentic biographical sketches of the representative men of Vermont and sons of Vermont in other states. (Burlington VT: Ullery Publishing Co, 1912): 100.

7. Davies P, American road: The story of an epic transcontinental journey at the dawn of the motor age. (New York: Henry Holt and Co, 2002): 14.
8. UVM Catalogue 1914/1915. (Burlington VT: University of Vermont, 1914): 21.
9. UVM Catalogue 1922/1923. (Burlington VT: University of Vermont, 1922): 18.
10. Allen L. The temperature as a guide to the existence of suppuration. Vermont Medical Monthly 1903; 9: 298-301.
11. Allen L. The use of bismuth vaseline paste in suppurating tracts. Vermont Medical Monthly 1911; 17: 9-12.
12. Allen L. Lacerated wound into knee joint, treated by complete closure and immediate active mobilization. Boston Medical & Surgical Journal 1921; 184: 167-170.
13. Allen L. The significance of the blood count in appendicitis. New England Journal of Medicine 1931; 205: 1105-1107.
14. Allen L,. Primary torsion of the great omentum. New England Journal of Medicine 1933; 209: 235.
15. Ferguson JA, Allen L. Complete medial dislocation of the knee joint with division of the common peroneal nerve. Journal of Bone & Joint Surgery 1939; 21: 1012-1014.
16. Allen L. Head injuries. New England Journal of Medicine 1932; 209: 1011-1014.
17. Transactions of the Vermont Medical Society for the Year 1904. (Rutland VT: The Tuttle Co, 1905): 30.
18. Past Presidents. Vermont Medical Society 2005 Annual Report, VMS, 2005: 29.
19. Davis LL, Thomas CC. Fellowship of surgeons, a history of the American College of Surgeons. (Springfield IL: Charles C. Thomas, 1960): 45, 266.
20. Crombie HD. The beginnings of the New England Surgical Society. Archives of Surgery1998; 133: 351-353.
21. Mackay AG. Some recollections of Dr Albert G. Mackay. University of Vermont College of Medicine Oral History Collection ,1964-1974. Special Collections, Bailey-Howe Library, University of Vermont, 1968:24.
22. Ibid: 154.
23. Ibid: 25-25a.
24. Ibid: 154-155.
25. McSweeney ED, Jr., UVM Surgery Newsletter.
26. Kaufman: 151.
27. Meehan TF. "Burlington" The Catholic Encyclopedia, Vol. III (New York: Robert Appleton Co, 1908).
28. McLaughlin J. "The limerick lad, the burlington lady, and the founding of Saint Michael's College. Talk presented at the 3rd Burlington Irish Heritage Festival on March 16, 1998 ED McSweeney, Jr. archives. p. 24.
29. Durick JK (ed.). 1853-1953, 100 years of achievement. (Burlington VT: Diocese of Burlington, 1953).
30. McSweeney ED, Jr., UVM Surgery Newsletter.
31. Mackay AG. Some recollections. (Oral History)
32. Wheeler JB. An incident in country surgery The Ariel (UVM Yearbook). (Burlington VT: UVM, 1924): 169-170.
33. Healy MJ,. Walking in the spirit: Fanny Allen Hospital 1894-1994. (Colchester VT: Fanny Allen Hospital, 1993): 76.
34. Rutkow IM. Surgery, an illustrated history. (St. Louis: Mosby-Year Book Inc, 1993): 506, 510.
35. Dodge : 283.
36. Cushing JT, Sheldon HP. Vermont in the World War, 1917-1919. (Burlington VT: Free Press Printing Co., 1928): 713.
37. Pease CA. Tetanus, with special reference to Fourth of July injuries. Vermont Medical Monthly 1906: 244-248.
38. Pease CA,. The comparative value of local anesthesia and nerve blocking in major & minor surgery. Vermont Medical Monthly 1913; 19: 213-215.
39. Pease CA. The Dakin-Carrel method of treating wounds. Vermont Medicine 1918: 291-296.
40. UVM Catalogue 1926/1927. (Burlington VT: University of Vermont, 1926): 20.
41. Marquis AN (ed.). Who's who in New England, a biographical dictionary of leading men and women of the states of Maine, New Hampshire, Vermont, Massachusetts, Rhode Island and Connecticut, 2nd ed. (Chicago IL: A.N. Marquis & Co, 1916): 936.
42. Sabin GM. Double extra-uterine pregnancy. Vermont Medical Monthly 1914: 20: 532.
43. UVM Catalogue 1926/1927: 20.
44. UVM Catalogue 1935/1936 (Burlington VT: University of Vermont, 1935): 14.
45. Mackay. Oral history.
46. Mackay. Oral History.
47. American Ancestry. Baltimore MD. Genealogical Publishing Co. 1968; 9 : 37.
48. Mackay. Oral History: 46
49. UVM Catalogue 1914/1915, (Burlington VT: University of Vermont, 1914): 24, 266.
50. University of Vermont Notes, University of Vermont, vol. 5 October 1917-July 1920
51. UVM Catalogue 1926/1927: 21.
52. UVM Catalogue 1935/1936: 18.
53. Maloney M. Adams Building to Close Fletcher Allen Health Care Sun. 2001; 7: 1.
54. Gladstone AA, Kirkness E. Beyond the scalpel, reflections of a Vermont surgeon. (Shelburne VT: The New England Press, 1979): 38.
55. Ibid: 68-69.
56. Mackay, Oral History.
57. Page HG. Interview 2006.
58. Page Interview, 2006.
59. Hill RN, Carlisle LB. The story of the Shelburne Museum,. (Shelburne VT: Shelburne Museum Publishing, , 1955): 60.
60. Maloney: 1-2.
61. Page. Interview. 2006
62. Maloney: 1-2.
63. Mackay, AG. Some recollections: 23.
64. AMA Council on Medical Education and Hospitals, inspection of UVM, October 16-18, 1935. Medical College Reorganization Box, UVM Archives. quoted in Kaufman: 157.
65. Kaufman: 155-157.

66 AMA, Inspection of UVM:16-18, quoted in Kaufman: 157.
67 WD Cutter to JN Jenne, Chicago, October 21, 1936, Medical College Reorganization Box, UVM Archives, quoted in Kaufman: 158.
68 FC Zapffe to JN Jenne, Chicago, November 16, 1936, Medical College Reorganization Box, UVM Archives, quoted in Kaufman: 158.
69 Kaufman: 159-162.
70 UVM Medical Faculty Minutes, May 18, 1937, UVM Archives, quoted in Kaufman: 162.
71 Mackay. Some recollections: 26.
72 Kaufman: 162-163.
73 Ibid: 164.
74 Orton V. Mary Fletcher comes back, a brief account of the history, progress & future of Vermont's first general hospital, Board of Directors of the Mary Fletcher Hospital, Burlington VT, 1941: 67.
75 UVM Medical Faculty Minutes, May 18, 1937, UVM Archives.
76 Davis: 340-343.
77 Kaufman: 162.
78 FC Zapffe to AB Soule, Chicago, October 31, 1938, Medical College Reorganization Box, UVM Archives, quoted in Kaufman: 165.
79 Kaufman: 165-167.
80 FC Zapffe to HA Kemp, Chicago, November 1, 1940, AAMC Folder, Dean's Office Papers, UVM Archives, quoted in Kaufman: 168.

Chapter 8

1 Orton V, Mary Fletcher Comes Back, A Brief Account of the History, Progress & Future of Vermont's First General Hospital, Board of Directors of the Mary Fletcher Hospital, Burlington VT, 1941, pp. 30-35.
2 Ibid., p. 35.
3 Ibid, fold out insert.
4 Chapin WAR, Allen L, History, University of Vermont College of Medicine, Dartmouth Printing Co, Hanover NH, 1951, p. 135.
5 Rees WT, "Cutaneous Anthrax, With Report of Case," Bulletin of the Mary Fletcher Hospital, vol. 1 (1933), p. 3.
6 Rees WT, "Use of Iodine in the Treatment of Goiter," Bulletin of the Mary Fletcher Hospital, vol. 3 (1935), p. 1.
7 Mackay AG, "Some Recollections of Dr. Albert G. Mackay, Dictated 26 October, 1968," University of Vermont College of Medicine Oral History Collection, 1964-1974, Special Collections, Bailey/Howe Library, University of Vermont, p. 23.
8 Meet your doctor. Gauzette. Dec. 1958 .Pub Mary Fletcher Hosp. p3
9 Chapin, p. 137.
10 Truax KF, "The treatment of burns with especial reference to the use of gentian violet," Bulletin of the Mary Fletcher Hospital, vol. 2 (1934), pp. 2-4.
11 Truax KF, "Prepubertal malignant melanoma," Annals of Surgery, vol. 137 (February 1953), pp. 255-260.
12 Marquis AN (ed.), Who's Who in New England, A biographical dictionary of leading men and women of the States of Maine, New Hampshire, Vermont, Massachusetts, Rhode Island and Connecticut, 2nd ed., A.N. Marquis & Co., Chicago IL, 1916, p. 705.
13 "Recent deaths," University of Vermont Notes, v. 11-13 (1914-1917), p. ?
14 Mackay, Oral History, p. 5.
15 Ibid., p. 15.
16 Ibid., pp. 30-31, 34-35.
17 Ibid., pp. 17-19.
18 Chapin, p. 78.
19 Mackay, Oral History, p. 37.
20 Press JC (ed.), American Men & Women of Science, The Physical and Biological Sciences, 14th ed., vol. 5, Bowker, New York, 1986, p. 3122.
21 Meet your doctor. Mary Fletcher Hospital "Gauzette" June 1965 p 2.
22 Chapin, p. 137.
23 Mackay, Oral History, pp. 48-49.
24 Healy MJ, Walking in the spirit: Fanny Allen Hospital 1894-1994, Fanny Allen Hospital, Colchester VT, 1993, pp. 122-123.
25 Ibid., p. 123.
26 Ibid., pp. 101-102.
27 Crandall AJ, Curriculum Vitae, Fanny Allen Hospital Archives, Staff Records Subseries (1909-1909), Archives-Collections, St. Michael's College Library, p. 1.
28 Fanny Allen Newsletter, October 1982, quoted in Healy, pp. 103-104.
29 Gladstone AA, Kirkness E, Beyond the scalpel, reflections of a Vermont Surgeon, The New England Press, Shelburne VT, 1979, pp. 24-25, 38, 127.
30 Ibid., pp. 38-39.
31 Kaufman, p. 172.
32 Chapin, pp. 59-60.
33 Ibid., p. 60.
34 Ibid.
35 Ibid.
36 Vermont Cynic, January 5, 1943, p. 1, quoted in Kaufman, p. 173.
37 Chapin, p. 150.
38 Kreutz JM, "The Abajian Scales: The Untold History of John Abajian, Ed Brazell, and the University of Vermont's 1956 to 1959 Halothane Research," Manuscript presented at the Anesthesia History Association 2007 Annual Meeting, May 3-5, 2007, p. 62.
39 Chapin, pp. 151-152.
40 Mackay, Oral History, pp. 42-43.
41 Ibid., p. 43.
42 Ibid.
43 Obituary, Burlington Free Press, September 26, 1974.

44 Ibid., pp. 13-14.
45 Hedin J, "Guns, Planes, and Surgery," Vermont Quarterly, November 1989, p. 25.
46 Crrandall AJ, Office of the Surgeon General. Report of Medical Activities in European Theater of Operations. (See: http://history.amedd.army.mil/booksdocs/wwii/Crandall.html)
47 Crandall, Curriculum Vitae, pp. 7-8.
48 Chapin, pp. 132, 137.
49 Mackay, Oral History, p. 44.
50 AMA Investigation of UVM Medical College, 1944, p. 32, Dean's Office Papers, UVM Archives, quoted in Kaufman, p. 176.
51 Kaufman, pp. 176-177.
52 Ibid., pp. 177-178.
53 Thompson JC, "The Stomach and Duodenum," Textbook of Surgery: The Biological Basis of Modern Surgical Practice, DC Sabiston Jr. (ed.), 14th ed., W.B. Saunders Co., Philadelphia PA, 1991, p. 775.
54 Page HG, Interview with DB Pilcher, 2006.
55 Ibid.
56 Mackay, Oral History, pp. 37, 44.
57 Keller JE, Interview with DB Pilcher, 2006.
58 Ibid.
59 Meet your doctor. Progress and Care Nov 1970. p2.
60 Interview.
61 Ibid.

Chapter 9
1 Our history: A timeline. Fletcher Allen Health Care Sun 2005; 11: 3.
2 Kaufman M. University of Vermont College of Medicine. (Hanover NH: UVM College of Medicine, 1979): 160, 182.
3 UVM Bulletins 1945 and 1953.
4 Mackay AG. Some recollections of Dr. Albert G. Mackay, dictated 26 October, 1968," University of Vermont College of Medicine oral history collection, 1964-1974. Special Collections, Bailey/Howe Library, University of Vermont: 52.
5 Physician profiles, Board of Medical Practice, Vermont Department of Health, State of Vermont.
6 Progress and care 1965;May.
7 Obituary. Burlington Free Press, October 21, 1997.
8 Shea WI. Doc Shea remembers. December 23, 1987, video kindly supplied by the Shea family with their permission to excerpt.
9 Abair L Interview 2008.
10 Ibid. and personal recollections of the author (DBP)
11 Ibid.
12 Haines CR, Interviews, 2006 and 2008.
13 Haines CR, Curriculum Vitae:1 kindly supplied by CR Haines with his permission to excerpt.
14 Ibid.
15 McGill BF. Interview 2006.
16 Obituary, Burlington Free Press, October 17, 2007.
17 Personal recollections of the author (DBP).
18 Page HG, Interviews, 2006 and 2007.
19 Ibid.
20 Ibid.
21 Ibid.
22 Ibid.
23 Ibid.
24 Ibid.
25 Ibid.
26 Ibid.
27 Ibid.
28 Pilcher DB, recollections.
31 Overholt RH, Pilcher LS II. Changes in venous pressure after thoracoplasty: Its significance in relation to the extent of rib removal. Presentation at the 1934 annual meeting of the American Association for Thoracic Surgery.
32 Obituaries, Boston Globe, August 11, 1996.
33 Eisendrath DN, Wolbarst AM, Smith EO, et al. A tribute to the memory of Paul M. Pilcher. Annals of Surgery 1917; 65: 529-533.
34 Jennings JE. Memoir, Lewis Stephen Pilcher 1845-1934. Annals of Surgery 1935; 102: 793-797.
35 Pilcher JE. Life and labors of Elijah H. Pilcher of Michigan. (New York: Hunt and Eaton, 1892): 102.
36 Billroth T. Clinical surgery. (London: New Syndenham Society, 1881): 140.
37 The Mary Fletcher ...your Hospital. (Burlington, VT: Mary Fletcher Hospital Board of Trustees): 15.
38 Pilcher DB personal recollection and experiences.
39 Howe HE. Interview 2007.
40 Ibid.
41 Ibid.
42 Ittleman FP, UVM Surgery Newsletter. 2001; 8(2): 4.
43 Medline Search, February 2008.
44 Ibid.
45 Jacobson JH, 2nd, Address to North Eastern Society of Plastic Surgeons, Washington, DC, November 4, 2005, transcript kindly supplied by the author with his permission to excerpt.
46 Ibid.

47 Ibid.
48 Ibid.
49 Jacobson JH, 2nd, The early days of microsurgery in Vermont. Mt. Sinai Journal of Medicine, 1997; 64: 160-161.
50 Ibid. : 161.
51 Ibid.
52 Jacobson JH, 2nd. Address to NE Society
53 Jacobson JH, 2nd. Early Days of Microsurgery: 161.
54 Jacobson JH,2nd, Suarez EL. Microsurgery in anastamosis of small vessels. Surgical Forum 1960; 11: 243-247.
55 Jacobson, Early Days of Microsurgery: 162.
56 Jacobson, Address to NE Society.
57 Jacobson, Early Days of Microsurgery: 162.
58 Jacobson, Address to NE Society.
59 Jacobson JH,2nd, Wallman LJ, Schumacher GA, Flanagan M, Suarez EL, Donaghy RMP, Microsurgery as an aid to middle cerebral artery endarterectomy. Journal of Neurosurgery 1962; 19: 108-114.
60 Yasargil MG, ed. Anastomosis between the superficial temporal artery and a branch of the middle cerebral artery. Microsurgery applied to neurosurgery. (Stuttgart, Germany: George Thieme, 1969): 105-115.
61 Jacobson JH, 2nd. Early Days of Microsurgery: 162.
62 Ibid: 160-161.
63 Jacobson JH,2nd, Suarez EL Microvascular surgery. Chest 1962; 41: 224.
64 Surgeon aids profession through gifts, global technology. Headlines@Hopkins, Office of News and Information (Baltimore MD: Johns Hopkins University, April 21, 2003).
65 Jacobson JH, 2nd. The classical music experience. (Naperville, IN: Soucebooks Inc, 2002).
66 Stahl WM, Jr. Supportive care of the surgical patient. (New York: Grune & Stratton, 1972.)
67 Medline Search, February 2008.
68 Obituary, Burlington Free Press, February 26, 2002.
69 McSweeney ED Jr., Interviews with Suzanne Ferland, 1993, transcript kindly supplied by Marilyn McSweeney with her permission to excerpt.
70 Obituary 2002
71 News Release, "Emeritus Status Approvals," Chironian, New York Medical College, Fall, 1999.
72 Mackay: 53.
73 Medline Search, February 2008.
74 Erickson DR, Blair E, Davis JH, Dwyer E. Pathodynamics of blunt chest trauma: A preliminary report. American Surgeon 1970; 36: 717-720.
75 Mackay: 53.
76 Obituary, Cortez Journal, December 8, 2006.
77 Karatepe M, Tomatir E, Bozkurt P. The resuscitation greats. Cemil Topuzlu Pasha: One of the forgotten pioneers in the history of open chest cardiac massage. Resuscitation 2006; 68: 179-183.
78 Barrows HS, Tamblyn RM. Problem-based learning: An approach to medical education (New York: Springer Publishing Company, 1980.)
79 Bunker CE. Interview 2007.
80 Mackay: 54.

Chapter 10

1 Kaufman M. University of Vermont College of Medicine. (Hanover NH: UVM College of Medicine, 1979); 193: 203-204.
2 Our history: A timeline. Fletcher Allen Health Care Sun 2005; 11: 3.
3 Kaufman: 191-200, 206-209.
4 Davis JH. Interviews with DB Pilcher, 2005-2008.
5 Ibid.
6 Pulaski EJ, Artz CP, Reiss E, Davis JH, Huckabee WE. Evaluation of the exposure method in the treatment of burns. Surgical Forum 1951: 518-523.
7 Davis Interviews.
8 Reiss E, Stirman JA, Artz CP, Davis JH, Amsapacher WH. Fluid and electrolyte balance in burns. JAMA 1953; 152: 1309-1313.
9 Artz CP, Reiss E. Calculator for estimating early fluid requirement in burns. JAMA 1954; 155: 1156-1158.
10 Davis Interviews.
11 Ibid.
12 Ibid.
13 Ibid.
14 Abrams JS. A hard look at colonoscopy. American Journal of Surgery 1977; 133: 111-115.
15 Abrams JS, Willard CJ. Aftercare of the patient with an ileostomy. Primary Care 1974; 1: 691-706.
16 Abrams JS. Surgical treatment of inflammatory bowel disease of the colon. Ulcerative colitis and granulomatous (Crohn's) colitis. American Journal of Surgery 1975; 130: 528-531.
17 Abrams JS, Reines HD. Increasing incidence of right-sided lesions in colorectal cancer. American Journal of Surgery 1979; 137: 522-526.
18 Abrams JS. Elective resection for colorectal cancer in Vermont: 1971-1975. American Journal of Surgery 1979; 139: 78-83.
19 Abrams JS. A second look at colonoscopy: Indications, failures, and costs. Archives of Surgery 1980; 117: 913-917.
20 Foster RS, Jr. Interviews with DB Pilcher, 2005-2008.
21 Foster RS Jr, Metcalf D, Kirchmyer R. Induction of bone marrow colony-stimulating activity by a filterable agent in leukemic and normal mouse serum. Journal of Experimental Medicine 1968; 127: 853-866.

22 Foster RS Jr, Metcalf D, Robinson WA, Bradley TR. Bone marrow colony stimulating activity in human sera. Results of two independent surveys in Buffalo and Melbourne. British Journal of Haematology 1968; 15: 147-159.
23 Foster Interviews
24 Ibid.
25 Crile GW Jr. The way it was: sex, surgery, treasure, and travel, 1907-1987. (Kent, OH: Kent State University Press, 1992): 360.
26 Foster Interviews
27 Fisher B, Redmond C, Elias EG, Evans J, Foster R, et al. Adjuvant chemotherapy for breast cancer: An overview of NSABP findings. International Advances in Surgical Oncology 1982; 5: 65-90.
28 Foster RS Jr., Lang SP, Costanza MC, Worden JK, Haines CR, Yates JW. Breast self-examination practices and breast-cancer stage. New England Journal of Medicine 1978; 299: 265-70.
29 Foster RS Jr. Effect of Corynebacterium Parvum on the proliferative rate of granulocyte-macrophage progenitor cells and the toxicity of chemotherapy. Cancer Research 1978; 38: 2666-2672.
30 Foster Interviews.
31 Davis JH. Rough draft of the history of the department of surgery. Department of Surgery archives. 1992.
32 Page HG & Davis JH. Interviews with DB Pilcher, 2005-2008.
33 Davis Interviews.
34 Curley JE, Cronin JCJ, Frymoyer JW, et al. Fletcher Allen Health Care: A future built on a proud past (New York: Newcomen Society of the United States, 1995): 15-16.
35 Davis Interviews.
36 Davis JH. Rough draft.
37 Ibid.
38 Healy MJ. Walking in the spirit: Fanny Allen Hospital 1894-1994 (Colchester, VT: Fanny Allen Hospital, 1993): 134-135.
39 Ibid: 103, 133, 139, 146, 150.
40 Healy: 124-125.
41 Bunker CE. Interview with DB Pilcher, 2008.
42 Koplewitz M. Interview with DB Pilcher, 2006.
43 Morrow M. "John Davis Lecture" at UVM, October 2004.
44 Ittleman FP. UVM Surgery Newsletter 2001;VII (2): 4.
45 AAST website, accessed April 2008.
46 Coil JA, Dickerman JD, Boulton E. Increased susceptibility of splenectomized mice to infection after exposure to an aerosolized suspension of type III Streptococcus Pneumonia. Infection and Immunity 1978; 21: 412-416.
47 Colorado College Class Notes, Fall 1998 & April 2001.
48 Loyola University Health System & Loyola University Medical Board of Directors Biographies, April 5, 2007.
49 Medline Search, April 2008.
50 Hebert JC. Immunization with heat-killed pneumococci, but not pneumococcal capsular polysaccharides, improves survival in splenectomized mice. J of Surgical Research 1987; 42: 19-23.
51 Hebert JC, Coil JA, Jr. Increased susceptibility to pulmonary infection in alloxan diabetic mice. Journal of Surgical Research 1981; 31: 337-342.
52 Hebert JC, Gamelli RL, Dickerman JD, et al. Lack of protection by pneumococcal vaccine after splenectomy in mice challenged with aerosolized pneumococci. J of Trauma 1983; 23: 1-6.
53 Hebert, James C. The History of Surgery in Vermont. Arch Surg 2001; 36: 467-472.
54 Payne SR. Personal communication, 2008.
55 Davis Interviews
56 Davis JH, Sheldon GF, Drucker WR, Foster RS Jr, Gamelli RL, Gann DS, Pruitt BA Jr (eds). Clinical Surgery: Concepts and Processes (St Louis, MO: Mosby-Year Book Inc, 1987).

Chapter 11
1 Shackford SR. Interviews with DB Pilcher, 2005-2008.
2 Ibid.
3 Shackford SR, Mackersie RC, Hoyt DB, et al. Impact of a trauma system on outcome of severely injured patients. Archives of Surgery 1987; 122: 523-527.
4 Shackford SR, Hollingsworth-Fridlund P, McArdle M, Eastman AB. Assuring quality in a trauma system—the medical audit committee: Composition, cost, and results. Journal of Trauma 1987; 27: 866-875.
5 Shackford interviews.
6 Shackford SR. Chairman's Column. UVM Surgery Newsletter. 1990; 1.
7 Hyman NH. Interviews with DB Pilcher, 2005-2008.
8 Ibid.
9 Shackford interviews.
10 Shackford, Chairman's Column.
11 Schmoker JD, Zhuang J, Shackford SR. Hypertonic fluid resuscitation improves cerebral oxygen delivery and reduces intracranial pressure after hemorrhagic shock. Journal of Trauma 1991; 31: 1607-1613.
12 Shackford SR, Zhuang J, Schmoker JD. Intravenous fluid tonicity: Effect on intracranial pressure, cerebral blood flow, and cerebral oxygen delivery in focal brain injury. Journal of Neurosurgery 1992; 76: 91-98.
13 Shackford SR, Bourguignon PR, Wald SL, et al. Hypertonic saline resuscitation of patients with head injury: A prospective randomized clinical trial. Journal of Trauma 1998; 44: 50-58.
14 Wald SL, Shackford SR, Fenwick J. The effect of secondary insults on mortality and long-term disability after severe head injury in a rural region without a trauma system. Journal of Trauma 1993; 34: 377-381.
15 Stevens SA, Thakore NJ, Lakin WD, Penar PL, Tranmer BI. A modeling study of idiopathic intracranial hypertension: Etiology and diagnosis. Neurological Research 2007; 29: 777-786.

16 Khoshyomn S, Nathan D, Manske GC, Osler TM, Penar PL. Synergistic effect of genistein and BCNU on growth inhibition and cytotoxicity of glioblastoma cells. Journal of Neurooncology 2002; 57: 193-200.
17 Hebert JC. Pulmonary anitpneumococcal defenses after hemi-splenectomy. Journal of Trauma 1989; 29: 1217-1220.
18 Graham AM, Baffour R, Burdon T, et al. A demonstration of vascular proliferation in response to arteriovenous reversal in the ischemic canine hind limb. Journal of Surgical Research 1989; 47: 341-347.
19 Gadowski GR, Pilcher DB, Ricci MA. Abdominal aortic aneurysm expansion rate: Effect of size and beta-adrenergic blockade. Journal of Vascular Surgery 1994; 19: 727-731.
20 Ricci MA, Strindberg G, Slaiby JM, et al. Anti-CD 10 monoclonal antibody slows experimental aortic aneurysm expansion. Journal of Vascular Surgery 1996; 23: 301-307.
21 Ricci MA, Callas PW, Montgomery WL. The Vermont telemedicine project: Initial implementation phases. Telemedicine Journal 1997; 3: 197-205.
22 Rogers FB, Ricci MA, Caputo MP, et al. The use of telemedicine for real-time video consultation between trauma center and community hospital in a rural setting improves early trauma care: Preliminary results. Journal of Trauma 2001; 51: 1037-1041.
23 Krag DN, Weaver DL, Alex JC, Fairbank JT. Surgical resection and radiolocalization of the sentinel lymph node in breast cancer using a gamma probe. Surgical Oncology 1993; 2: 335-339.
24 Kaufman M, University of Vermont College of Medicine. (Hanover NH, UVM College of Medicine, 1979): 244-245.
25 UVM College of Medicine website, accessed June 2008.
26 Frymoyer JW. Interviews with DB Pilcher, 2005-2008.
27 Koplewitz MJ. Interviews with DB Pilcher, 2005-2008.
28 Codman EA. The product of a hospital. Surgery, Gynecology & Obstetrics1914; 18: 491-496.
29 Healey MA, Shackford SR, Osler TM, et al. Complications in surgical patients. Archives of Surgery 2002; 137: 611-617.
30 Bertges DJ, Shackford SR, Cloud AK, et al. Toward optimal recording of surgical complications: Concurrent tracking compared to the discharge data set. Surgery 2007; 14: 19-31.
31 Ibid.
32 Barna E. Fletcher Allen enters the renaissance era. Vermont Business Magazine 2005; 33.
33 ACGME website, accessed June 2008.
34 Esposito, et al, UVM Surgery Newsletter. 2006; 15(2).
35 Rogers FB, Shackford SR, Daniel S, et al. Workload redistribution: A new approach to the 80-Hour workweek. Journal of Trauma 2005; 58: 911-916.
36 Esposito, et al.
37 Sartorelli KS, Interviews with DB Pilcher, 2008.
38 Ibid.
39 Osborne E. Institute for Quality & Operational Effectiveness established. FAHC Sun 2004; 10: 1.
40 News Round-Up. FAHC Sun. 2005; 11: 2.
41 Shackford SR. How then shall we change? Journal of Trauma. 2006; 60: 1-7.
42 Shackford interview.

Chapter 13

1 Wheeler JB. Memoirs of a Small Town Surgeon. (Garden City, NY; Garden City Publishing Co., 1935) : 201-3.
2 Kreutz, JM, John Hazen Dodds, MD, UVM Anesthesia News, Summer 2007, 2: 3.
3 Wells B, Anesthesia History: Now and Then . 1990. Unpublished manuscript from the UVM Department of Anesthesia archives.
4 Mackay AG. Some recollections of Dr. Albert G Mackay. UVM Library Wilbur Collection, Dictated October 26,1968. (For the Medical History Committee of the Century Club), p. 45
5 Healey MJ. Walking in the Spirit. (Colchester, VT: The Fanny Allen Hospital, 1993): 104-5.
6 Ibid.
7 Abajian J, Jr. Oral history from anesthesia archives.
8 Wells. Anesthesia History.
9 Kreutz JM, The Abajian Scales, John Abajian, Ed Brazell, and the University of Vermont's 1956 to 1959 halothane research, Bulletin of Anesthesia History, vol. 26 (April 2008), pp. 1-7.
10 Abajian. Oral history.
11 Ibid.
12 Ibid.
13 Meet Your Doctor: John Abajian MD, Mary Fletcher Gauzette, August 1958, UVM Department of Anesthesiology Archives.
14 Mackay. Oral History, pp. 52-53.
15 Dente GA. Interview 2005.
16 Abajian. Oral history.
17 Dente. Interview.
18 Mary Fletcher Hospital Records. "Anesthesia" folder 24. UVM Archives, Dana Medical Library.
19 Dente. Interview.
20 Abajian J et al. Fluothane: A clinical appraisal. Presented at the New England Assembly of Nurse Anesthetists March 24,1958. Quoted by Kreutz : 3.
21 Abajian J et al. Experience with halothane (fluothane) in more than five thousand cases. JAMA 1959; 171: 535-540.
22 Kreutz, Abajian Scales.
23 Meet your doctor. Progress and Care 1960; January : 2.
24 Mazuzan JE. Interview 2006.
25 Ibid.
26 Ibid.
27 Ibid.
28 Abajian JC, Interview 2005.

29 Abajian JC, Spinal anesthesia in infants. J Anaesthesia 1980.
30 Abajian JC, Mellish RWP, Browne AF et al. Spinal anesthesia for surgery in the high risk infant. Anesth Analg 1984; 63: 359-362.
31 Jacobson JH, II, The Classical Music Experience, Sourcebooks, Inc., Naperville, IL, 2002, p. 42.
32 Mazuzen. Interview.
33 Bierstein, K. False Claims Act Lawsuit Settles for $3.2 Million. American Society of Anesthesiologists Newsletter 63: 11 (Nov 1999).

Chapter 14

1 Frymoyer JW ed. The Adult Spine Ed 2 (Philadelphia: Lippicott-Raven, 1997).
2 Frymoyer JW personal communication.
3 Roberts MJ. The electro-osteotome. A new instrument for the performance of the operation for osteotomy. Medical Record, New York, Oct 27,1883.
4 Phelps AM. The present status of the open incision method for talipes varo equines. N.E. Med Fron. 1801; 10: 217.
5 Wheeler, JB. Memoirs of a Small Town Surgeon. (Garden City,NY:Garden City Pub, 1935): 206-8.
6 Albee FH. Transplantation of a portion of the tibia into the spine for Pott's disease. JAMA 1911; 57(11): 885-6.
7 Hibbs RA. An operation for progressive spinal deformities. New York Med Jour. May 27, 1911.
8 Albee, F.H. Bone-graft surgery. (New York:W.B.Saunders Co,1915).
9 Soule AB, Personal communication to JW Frymoyer.
10 Bell J and Rust CB. Personal communication to JW Frymoyer.
11 Rust CB. Personal communication to J W Frymoyer.
12 Ishizuka T. Dr Japan. (Tokyo; T Ishizuka, pub, 1987). (English translation 2004)
13 Frymoyer JF recollections 2007.
14 Lovett RW. The treatment of infantile paralysis (Philadelphia: Blakiston, 1916).
15 Mixter WJ, Barr JS. Rupture of the intervertebral disk with involvement of the spinal canal. N Engl J Med 1934; 211:210-215.
16 Frymoyer JW, Donaghy RMP. The ruptured intervertebral disc: Follow-up report on the first case fifty years after recognition of the syndrome and its surgical significance. J Bone Joint Surg (Am) 1985; 67:1113-1116.
17 University of Vermont Bulletins 1947-1954.
18 Personal communication J W Frymoyer.
19 Ibid.
20 Mackay, AG. Oral history in the Wilbur Special Collections, UVM Library.
21 FrymoyerJW, Hanley E, Howe J et al. Disc excision and spine fusion in the management of lumbar disc disease. A minimum ten-year followup. Spine 1978; 3: 1-6.
22 Frymoyer JW, Matteri RE, Hanley EN et al. Failed lumbar disc surgery requiring second operation. A long term follow-up study. Spine 1978; 3: 7-11.
23 Personal communication, J W Frymoyer.
24 Johnson RJ. personal communication.
25 Johnson RJ, Pope MH, and Ettlinger C. Ski injuries and equipment function. 1974; Sports Medicine 1975; 2: 299-307.
26 Deibert MC, Aronsson DD, Johnson RJ et al. Skiing injuries in Children, Adolescents, and adults. JBJS 1998; 80-A; 25-31.
27 Ettlinger CF, Johnson RJ and Shealy JE. A method to help reduce the risk of serious knee sprains incurred in alpine skiing. American Journal of Sports Medicine 1995; 23: 531-537.
28 Stokes I A F , Aronsson DD, Dimock AN et al. Endochondral growth in growth plates of three species at two anatomical locations modulated by mechanical compression and tension. J of Orthopaedic Research 2006; 24: 1327-1334.
29 Krag MH, Bennyon BD, Pope MH et al. An internal fixator for posterior application to short segments of the thoracic, lumbar, or lumbosacral spine: Design and testing. Clinical Orthopaedics 1986; 203: 75-98.
30 Frymoyer JW ed . The Adult Spine (ref 1).
31 Pope MH, Andersson GBJ, Frymoyer JW, and Chaffiin DB. Occupational low back pain. Assessment, treatment, and prevention. (St. Louis:Mosby Year Book).
32 Kristiansen TK, Fleming B, Pope M et al. A comparative study of fracture gap motion in external fixation. Clin Biomechanics 1987; 2: 191-5.
33 Kristiansen TK. The effect of low power specifically programmed ultrasound on the healing time of fresh fractures using a Colled' model. J Orthop Trauma 1990; 4: 227-8.
34 Krag MH, Beynnon BD. A new halo-vest: Rationale, design and biomechanical comparison to standard halo-vest designs. Spine 1988;13: 228-235.

Chapter 15

1 Berry FB. Medical Department, United States Army, Surgery in World War II, Thoracic Surgery, Vol. 1, (Washington DC: Office of the Surgeon General, Department of the Army,1963) : 5-6.
2 UVM Catalogue 1943/1944: 15.
3 Berger RL, Dunton RF, Ashraf MM, et al. Thoracic surgery and the war against smoking: Richard H. Overholt, MD. Annals of Thoracic Surgery 1992; 53: 719-25.
4 Ibid.
5 Chapin WAR, Allen L, History of the University of Vermont College of Medicine. (Hanover, NH:Dartmouth Printing Co. 1951): 138.
6 Gauzette, Meet Your Doctor, December 1954: 3.
7 Miller GW. King of hearts. (NY: Crown Publishers, 2000): 79-82, and 151-164.
8 Gauzette, Mary Fletcher Hospital Newsletter, November 1956: 2.
9 Obituary, Burlington Free Press, May 15, 2004.
10 Burlington Free Press, August 7, 1959
11 Cooley DA, Christie SG. An implantable cardiac pacemaker in the management of complete heart block. Texas Medicine 1963; 59: 31-35.
12 Progress and Care, January 1964: 2.

13　Kay E (ed.), International Who's who in Medicine. (Cambridge, England: International Biographical Centre. 1987): 257.
14　Kay E (ed.), Men of Achievement. (Raleigh, NC: American Biographical Institute. 1978): 51.
15　Coffin LH Jr, Interview with DB Pilcher, 2003.
16　Spector AA, Coffin LH Jr, Pauli WA, Myocardial oxidative metabolism and alkali cation content following burn trauma. Research Reports. U.S. Naval Medical Field Research Laboratory, Vol. 13 (October 1963: 1-11.
17　Ittleman FP, Eulogy for James DeMeules, August 1988.
18　Browdie DA, Deane R, Shinozaki T, Morgan J, DeMeules JE, Coffin LH Jr, Davis JH. Adult respiratory distress syndrome (ARDS), sepsis, and extracorporeal membrane oxygenation (ECMO). Journal of Trauma 1977; 17: 579-586.
19　Beaty HN, Miller AA, Broome CV, et al. Legionnaires' Disease in Vermont, May to October 1977. JAMA. 1978; 240: 127-131.
20　Leavitt BJ, "Editor's Corner," New England Surgical Society Newsletter, Vol. 8 (August 2006): 1,6.
21　Mulieri LA, Barnes W, Leavitt BJ et al. Alterations of myocardial stiffness implicating abnormal crossbridge function in human mitral regurgitation heart failure," Circulation Research. 2002; 90 : 66-72.
22　Leavitt BJ, Olmstead EM, Plume SK, et al. Use of internal mammary artery graft in northern New England. Circulation, 1997; 96 , Suppl. II: II-32-II-37.
23　Leavitt BJ, Sheppard L, Maloney C, et al. Effect of diabetes and associated conditions on long-term survival after coronary artery bypass graft surgery. Circulation. 2004; 110, Suppl. II: II-41-II-44.
24　Leavitt BJ, Ross CS, Spence B, et al. Long-term survival of patients with chronic obstructive pulmonary disease undergoing coronary artery bypass surgery. Circulation, 2006; 114, Suppl. I: I-430-I-434.
25　Schmoker JD, Zhuang J, Shackford SR. Hypertonic fluid resuscitation improves cerebral oxygen delivery and reduces intracranial pressure after hemorrhagic shock. Journal of Trauma. 1991; 131: 1607-1613.
26　Schmoker JD, Lee CH, Taylor RG, et al. A novel model of blunt thoracic aortic injury: A mechanism confirmed? Journal of Trauma. 2008; 64: 923-931.

Chapter 16
1　Connolly TW, Danielson PA, and Farnham JE. Interviews 2007-2008.

Chapter 17
1　Orton V. Mary Fletcher Comes Back, A Brief Account of the History, Progress & Future of Vermont's First General Hospital. Board of Directors of the Mary Fletcher Hospital (Burlington VT: 1941).
2　Consolidation of emergency rooms. Progress and Care 1969: 19 (8): 1.
3　Farrington JD. Death in a ditch. Bulletin Amer Coll Surgeons 1967: 1-10.
4　Waller, JA, Jacobs, L. Ambulance Service in Vermont (Burlington VT: 1970).
5　Perrine MW, Waller JA, Harris LS. Alcohol and highway safety: Behavioral and medical aspects, Final report to the Department of Transportation, Project ABETS, Psychology Dept., UVM, Burlington, 1971.
6　New focus on emergency service. Progress and Care 1972: 21(12): 1.
7　Pilcher DB, Gettinger CE, Jr, Seligson D. Recurrent themes in ambulance critique review sessions over eight years. Journal of Trauma 1979; 19 (5): 324-328.
8　Uphold R. Emergency Department history. Supplied by R. Uphold 2006.
9　Payne SR. Personal communication 2008.
10　Burnett J. National Transportation Safety Board, Safety Recommendation R-85-129, January 15, 1986.
11　Uphold R. Emergency Department history.
12　Staren ED, Knudson MM, Rozycki GS, Harness JK, Wherry FC, Shackford SR. An evaluation of the American College of Surgeons' ultrasound education program. Am J Surg 2006; 191: 489-496.

Chapter 18
1　Wright JW. Lectures on diseases of the rectum (New York: Bermingham & Co., 1884).
2　Gladstone, AA. Beyond the Scalpel. Reflections of a Vermont surgeon (Shelburne VT: The New England Press, 1979): 38.
3　Ibid: 39.
4　Ibid: 104-105.
5　Wolff WL, Shinya H. Colonofiberoscopy. JAMA 1971; 217 (11): 1509-12.
6　Koplewitz MJ. Interview with DB Pilcher, 2006.
7　Hyman NH, Ko CY, Cataldo PA, et al. The New England colorectal cancer quality project: A prospective multi-institutional feasibility study. J Am Coll Surg 2006; 202: 36-44.
8　Cataldo PA, MacKeigan JM. Intestinal stomas. Principles, techniques and management 2nd edition (New York: Marcel Dekker Inc, 2004).
9　Cataldo PA. Transanal endoscopic microsurgery. Surg Clin N America 2006. 86 (4): 915-925.
10　Sugerman HJ, Starkey JV, Birkenhauer R. A randomized prospective trial of gastric bypass versus vertical banded gastroplasty for morbid obesity and their effects on sweets versus non-sweets eaters. Ann. Surg. 1987; 205: 613-624.
11　Forgione PM. Interview with DB Pilcher, 2008.

Chapter 19
1　Kaufman M. The University of Vermont College of Medicine (Hanover, NH: University Press of New England, 1979): 5.
2　Fitch WL. Extracts From Lectures on Surgery Delivered at the Medical Institution at New Haven by Nathan Smith 1824: 311. Quoted in Hayward OS, Putnam CE. Improve, Perfect, & Perpetuate (Hanover, NH: University Press of New England, 1998): 177.
3　Haines CR, Wallace HJ, Jr, Nevinny HB, Hall TC. Clinical evaluation of estrogen-androgen combination in advanced breast cancer. Am J Surg 1969; 117(4): 589-94.
4　Costanza MC, Foster RS, Jr. Relationship between breast self-examination and death from breast cancer by age groups. Cancer Detect Prov 1984; 7(2): 103-8.

5 Morton DL, Wen DR, Wong JH, et al. Technical details of intraoperative lymphatic mapping for early stage melanoma. Arch Surg 1992; 127(4): 392-9.
6 Alex JC, Krag DN. Gamma probe guided localization of lymph nodes. Surg Oncol 1993; 2(3): 137-43.
7 Krag DN, Weaver D, Ashikaga T, et al. The sentinel node in breast cancer: a multicenter validation study. NEJM 1998; 339(14): 941-46.
8 Harlow SP, Krag DN, Julian TB, et al. Pre-randomization surgical training for the National Surgical Adjuvant Breast and Bowel Project (NSABP) B-32 trial: a randomized phase III clinical trial to compare sentinel node resection to conventional axillary dissection in clinically node-negative breast cancer. Ann Surg 2005; 241(1): 48-54.
9 Harlow SP, Krag DN, Ames SE, Weaver DL. Intraoperative ultrasound localization to guide surgical excision of non-palpable breast carcinoma. J Amer Coll Surg 1999; 189(3): 241-46.
10 Kenny, H. Improving patient quality of life. Innovations Winter 2008: 1-2.
11 McCahill LE, Privette AR, Hart MR, James TA. Are mastectomy rates a reasonable quality measure of breast cancer surgery? Amer J Surg 2009; 197(2): 216-21.
12 James TA. Measuring individual surgeon performance in breast cancer surgery. Presentation Society of Surgical Oncology Cancer Symposium; Washington DC, March 2007.

Chapter 20
1 Wheeler JB Memoirs of a small town surgeon. (Garden City, NY: Garden City Publishing Co.1935): 265-6.
2 Davis JH. Interview with DB Pilcher, 2007.
3 Lindberg RB, Moncrief JA, Switzer WE, Mason AD, Jr. Control of bacterial infection in severe burns with a topical sulfonamide burn cream. Antimicrobial Agents and Chemotherapy 1964; 10: 708-716.
4 Krizek TJ, Davis JH, Desprez JD, Kiehn CL. Topical therapy of burns: Experimental evaluation. Plastic and Reconstructive Surgery 1967; 39: 248-255.
5 Krizek TJ, Davis JH. Experimental pseudomonas burn sepsis - Evaluation of topical therapy. Journal of Trauma 1967; 7: 433-442.
6 Coil JA, Dickerman JD, Boulton E. Increased susceptibility of splenectomized mice to infection after exposure to an aerosolized suspension of type III Streptococcus pneumoniae. Infect Immun. 1978 Aug; 21(2): 412-6.
7 Pories SE, Gamelli RL, Vacek P, et al. Predicting hospital charges for trauma care. Arch Surg 1988; 123: 579-82.
8 Foley RW, Harris LSD, Pilcher DB. Abdominal injuries in automobile accidents: Review of care of fatally injured patients. J Trauma 1977; 17: 611-615.
9 Pilcher DB. Penetrating injuries of the liver in Vietnam. Ann Surg 1969; 17: 793-800.
10 Schrock T, Blaisdell FW, Mathewson C, Jr. Management of blunt trauma to the liver and hepatic veins. Arch Surgery 1968; 96: 698-704.
11 Pilcher DB, Harman PK, Moore EE, Jr. Retrohepatic vena cava shunt introduced via the sapheno-femoral junction. J Trauma 1977; 17: 873-41.
12 Vane D. Teaching the method of ATLS. UVM Surgery 2005; 4: 7.
13 Mazuzan J. Interview with DB Pilcher, 2006.
14 Ibid.
15 Certo TF, Pilcher DB, Rogers FB. Review of care of fatally injured patients in a rural state: 5 year follow-up. J Trauma 1983; 23:7: 559-565.
16 Charash WE, Rogers FB, Crookes BA. The utility of near-infrared spectroscopy during resuscitation from hemorrhagic shock. Int Jour Int Care, in press.

Chapter 21
1 Chapin WAR, Allen L, History of the University of Vermont College of Medicine. (Hanover, NH: Dartmouth Printing Co. 1951): 129.
2 Kaufman M. University of Vermont College of Medicine. (Hanover NH: UVM College of Medicine, 1979); 183.
3 Donaghy, RMP. 1969 Oral History, Wilbur Collection, UVM Special Collections.
4 Gross CE. Video Interview with Lester J. Wallman.
5 Donaghy, Oral History.
6 Jacobson JH, II, Wallman LJ, Schumacher GA, Flanagan M, Suarez EL, and Donaghy RMP. Microsurgery as an aid to middle cerebral artery endarterectomy. J of Neurosurgery 1961; 19: 108-115.
7 Jacobson JH, II, Personal communication.
8 Donaghy RMP. The History of Microsurgery in neurosurgery. Clinical Neurology 1979; 26: 617-625.
9 EC/IC Bypass study group. Failure of extracranial-intracranial arterial bypass to reduce the risk of ischemic stroke: results of an international randomized trial. NEJM 1985; 313: 1191-1200.
10 Yasargil MG. A legacy of microneurosurgery. Neurosurgery 1999; 45 (5): 1025-1037.
11 Inscription on memorial to Dr. Donaghy in the Neurosurgery offices of UVM.
12 Donaghy RMP. Interview with DB Pilcher during the 1970s.
13 Ibid.
14 Lookout Column. People Magazine 1975; 3 (10): 39.
15 Schmidek HH, Roberts DW. Schmidek and Sweet's Operative Neurosurgical Techniques, 5th Edition. (Philadelphia: WB Saunders, 2005).
16 Ishiguro M, Honda A, Russell SR, Tranmer BI, Wellman GC. Emergence of a dihydropyridine-Insensitive R-type Ca 2+ Channel (CaV2.3) contributes to cerebral artery constriction following sub-arachnoid hemorrhage. Circ. Res. 2005; 96 (4): 419-426.
17 Jewell RP. Interview with DB Pilcher 2008.

18 Wallman LJ, Schmidek HH, Wald SL, Penar PL, Tranmer BI, Horgan MA, and Jewell RP contributed material to this text.

Chapter 22

1. Bell,B. A System of Surgery. Worcester, MA, Isaiah Thomas pub, 1796 ed.
2. Hayward OS, Putnam CE. Improve, Perfect, & Perpetuate (Hanover, NH: University Press of New England, 1998): 176.
3. Emerson JB. Dr. Daniel Bennett St. John Roosa, necrology. Transactions American Ophthalmological Society 1909: 14-15.
4. Obituary. New York Times, July 30,1916: 15.
5. Mackay, AG. Oral History, Special Collections Bailey Howe Library. 1968: 50.
6. Ibid: 29.
7. Jaffe NS. Thirty years of intraocular lens implantation: The way it was and the way it is. ASCRS 1999; 25.
8. Irwin AE. Interview with DB Pilcher, 2006
9. Millay RH, Aitken PA. Interviews with DB Pilcher, 2008.
10. Millay interview.
11. Ibid.
12. Tabin GC. Blind corners. (Guilford CT: Globe Pequot Press, 2002): xvii.
13. Ibid: 81-85.
14. Ibid: 192-193.
15. Irwin ES, Aitken PA, Irwin AE, and Millay RH contributed material to this text.

Chapter 23

1. Kelly HA, Burrage WL. A cyclopedia of American medical biography. (Baltimore; The Norman Remington Company 1920): 457-59.
2. Pierpont JR. Letters. MSS, New York Academy of Medicine, New York, 1850.
3. Kelly. Cyclopedia.
4. New York Academy of Medicine Notes. Medical News 1901; 78 (10): 361.
5. Obituary. New York Times, November 26, 1914.
6. Mackay, AG. Oral History, Special Collections Bailey Howe Library. 1968: 22, 36.
7. McGinnis JM. Interview with DB Pilcher, 2007.
8. Meet your doctor. Gauzette: The Mary Fletcher Hospital newsletter, July 1958: 2.
9. Maurice M. Rufus and Dorothy Morrow honored by St. Michael's. Burlington Free Press. May 30, 1975: 12.
10. Morrow RC. Medical education on the SS Hope. JAMA 1970; 211 (2): 257-60.
11. McGinnis Interview.
12. Sofferman RA. Interview with DB Pilcher, 2006.
13. Hubbell RN. Interview with DB Pilcher, 2008.
14. Sofferman Interview.
15. Ibid.
16. Sofferman RA. Sphenoethmoid approach to the optic nerve. Laryngoscope. 1981 Feb; 91(2): 184-96.
17. Sofferman RA. Surgical management of primary hyperparathyroidism: review of my experience at the University of Vermont. Arch Otolaryngol Head Neck Surg. 1998 Sep; 124(9): 1056.
18. Communication from Sofferman, 2007.
19. McGinnis JM, Sofferman RA, Hubbell RN, and Brundage WJ contributed material to this text.

Chapter 24

1. Mellish RWP. Interview with DB Pilcher 2007.
2. Meet your doctor. Progress and Care. 1963; October: 2.
3. Koop CE, Mellish RWP. Some aspects of nutrition in pediatric surgical patients. Am J Clin Nutr. 1955; 3(6): 487-493.
4. Mellish RWP, Koop CE. Clinical manifestations of duplication of the bowel. Pediatrics. 1961; 27(3): 397-407.
5. Mellish RWP. Preparation of a child for hospitalization and surgery. Pediatr Clin North Am. 1969; 16(3): 543-53.
6. Abajian JC, Mellish RWP, Browne AF, Perkins FM, Lambert DH, Mazuzan JE, Jr. Spinal anesthesia for surgery in the high-risk infant. Anesth Analg. 1984; 63(3): 359-62.
7. Mellish interview.
8. Browne AF: Interview with DB Pilcher 2007-2008.
9. Browne AF. ibid.
10. Vane DW. Interview with DB Pilcher, 2007.
11. Sartorelli KH. Interview with DB Pilcher, 2006-2007.
12. Curran MG. Anecdote recollected by Curran 2009.

Chapter 25

1. Hayward OS, Putnam CE. Improve, Perfect, and Perpetuate. (Hanover, NH: University Press of New England, 1998): 168.
2. Progress and Care. MCHV, Burlington VT.
3. Leitner DW. Interview with DB Pilcher, 2006-7.
4. Linton PN. Interview with DB Pilcher, 2006-7.
5. Leitner interview.
6. Ibid.
7. Linton interview.
8. Mathes SJ, Nahai F. Clinical atlas of muscle and musculocutaneous flaps. (St Louis MO: CV Mosby, 1979).
9. Linton interview.
10. Leitner interview.
11. Hamm JC, Stevenson TR, Mathes SJ. Knee joint salvage utilizing a plantar musculocutaneous island pedicle flap. Br J Plast Surg 1986; 39: 249-54.
12. Bohjalian C. Avery's golden hour ticks away. Burlington Free Press, Sept 2, 1997: 1a, 4a, 5a.
13. www.treehouses.org.

14 Trabulsy PP. Interview with DB Pilcher, 2006-7.
15 Laub DR, Sr, Laub DR, Jr., Lebovic GS. Rectosigmoid neocolpopiesis for male to female transsexuals. Ann Plast Surg. 1996; 36 (6): 662.
16 Laub D, Jr. Interview with DB Pilcher 2006-7.
17 www.healthfinder.gov. In reversal FDA panel backs return of silicone breast implants.
18 www.pbs.org/wgbh/pages/frontline/implants/cron.html.
19 Mitchell P. No syndrome linked to breast implants says Institute of Medicine. Lancet. 1999; 353 (9171): 2215.

Chapter 26
1 Davis JH, Interviews with DB Pilcher, 2005-7.
2 Foster RS, Interviews with DB Pilcher, 2005.
3 Ad hoc committee of the Harvard Medical School. A definition of irreversible coma; a report of the Ad Hoc Committee of the Harvard Medical School to examine the definition of brain death. JAMA. 1968; 205: 337-340.
4 Yamaguchi JS. Interview with DB Pilcher, 2008.
5 Broome CV, Goings SA, Thacker SB, Vogt RL, Beaty HN, Fraser DW. The Vermont epidemic of Legionnaires' disease. Ann Intern Med. 1979; 90(4): 573-7.
6 Marshall W, Foster RS Jr., Winn W. Legionnaire's disease in renal transplant patients. Am J. Surg 1981; 141(4): 423-429.
7 Klaucke DN, Vogt RL, LaRue D, et al. Legionnaires' disease: the epidemiology of two outbreaks in Burlington, Vermont, 1980. Am J Epidemiol 1984; 119 (3): 382-91.
8 Di Carlo A. Personal communication.
9 Fernandez LA, Di Carlo A, Odorico JS, et al. Simultaneous pancreas-kidney transplantation from donation after cardiac death: Successful long-term outcomes. Ann Surg 2005; 242: 716-723.
10 Davis JH, Foster RS, Jr, Gamelli RL, Haisch CE, Di Carlo A, and Yamaguchi JS contributed material to this text.

Chapter 27
1 Hayward OS, Putnam CE. Improve, Perfect, & Perpetuate (Hanover, NH: University Press of New England, 1998): 173.
2 Pilcher PM. Practical cystoscopy. (Philadelphia: W B Saunders Co, 1911).
3 Rutkow IM. American surgery. (New York: Lippincott-Raven, 1998): 586.
4 Young HH. Hugh Young: A surgeon's autobiography. (New York: Harcourt, Brace and Co, 1940): 76.
5 Chapin WAR, Allen L, History of the University of Vermont College of Medicine. (Hanover, NH: Dartmouth Printing Co. 1951): 130-133.
6 Mackay, AG. Oral History, Special Collections Bailey Howe Library. 1968: 29.
7 Leadbetter GW, Jr. Urology at the University of Vermont Medical School, unpublished manuscript.
8 Meet your doctor. Mary Fletcher gauzette. 1956; May : 3.
9 Powell PR. Interview with DB Pilcher, 2006.
10 Fagan WT. Interview with DB Pilcher, 2007.
11 Leadbetter GW, Jr. Interview with DB Pilcher, 2007.
12 Morrisseau PM. Interview with DB Pilcher, 2006.
13 Ibid.
14 Morrisseau PM, Trotter SJ. Interviews with DB Pilcher, 2006-2007.
15 Ibid.
16 Ibid.
17 Zvara P, Karpman E, Plante MK. Ablation of canine prostate using transurethral intraprostatic absolute ethanol injection. Urology 1999; 54: 411-15.
18 Plante MK, Marks R, Anderson C. et al. Phase I/II trial to examine the safety of transurethral ethanol ablation of the prostate for the treatment of benign prostatic hyperplasia (IND #61337) Accepted for Publication March 2007, J Urology.
19 Powell PR, Fagan WT, Leadbetter GW, Jr., Morrisseau PM, Trotter SJ, Jackson TL, and Plante MK contributed material to this text.

Chapter 28
1 Friedman SG. A history of vascular surgery. (Mount Kisco, NY: Futura Publishing Co., 1989): 15-18.
2 Murphy JB. Resection of arteries and veins injured in continuity - End-to-end suture - Experimental and Clinical Research. Med Rec. 1897; 51: 73.
3 Carrel A. Les anastamoses vasculaires et leur technique operatoire. Union Med Can 1904; 33: 521.
4 Friedman: 99.
5 Wheeler JB. Memoirs of a small town surgeon. (Garden City NY: Garden City Publishing Co., 1935): 96-97.
6 Blakemore AH. Progressive constrictive occlusion of the aorta with wiring and electrothermic coagulation for the treatment of atherosclerotic aneurysms of the abdominal aorta. Ann Surg 1953; 137(5): 760-77.
7 Keller J. Interview with DB Pilcher 2007.
8 Friedman: 134-136.
9 Pilcher DB recollections of events and conversations with H G Page.
10 Robicsek F, Daugherty HK, Mullen DC, et al. Long-range observations with external aortic grafts. Coll Works Cardiopulm Dis 1975; 20: 5-12.
11 Keller interview.
12 Howard EK, Bouchard RE, Jacobson JH, 2nd. Repair of ruptured abdominal aortic aneurysm in the aged. Am J. Med Sci. 1962; 243: 86-91.
13 Humphries AW, DeWolfe VG, Lefevre FA. Reversibility of pre-gangrene in the severely ischaemic limb. J Bone Joint Surg Am 1958; 40-A(5): 983-993.
14 Davis JH. Interviews with DB Pilcher 2005 & 2006.

15. Davis JH, Benson JW, Miller RC. Thoracoabdominal aneurysm involving celiac, superior mesenteric and renal arteries. Arch Surgery 1957; 75(6): 871-76.
16. Davis interviews.
17. Blakemore AH. The portal-caval shunt for the correction of portal hypertension. Trans Conf Liver Inj 1948; 24(7th Conf): 41.
18. Darling RC, Raines JK, Brener BJ, Austen WG. Quantitative segmental pulse volume recorder: a clinical tool. Surgery 1972; 72(6): 873-7.
19. Finley DH, Pilcher DB. A simplified instrument for noninvasive vascular assessment. Arch Surg 1978; 113(8): 936-9.
20. Pilcher DB, Davis JH, Ashikaga T et al. Treatment of abdominal aortic aneurysm in an entire state over 7 1/2 years. Am J Surg 1980; 139(4): 487-494.
21. Graham AM, Baffour R, Burdon T, DeVarennes B, Ricci MA, et al. A demonstration of vascular proliferation in response to arteriovenous reversal in the ischemic canine hind limb. J Surg Res 1989; 47(4): 341-7.
22. Ricci MA, Strindberg G, Slaiby JM, et al. Anti-CD 18 monoclonal antibody slows experimental aneurysm expansion. J Vasc Surg 1996; 23(2): 301-307.
23. Ricci MA, Slaiby JM, Gadowski GR, et al. Effects of hypertension and propanolol upon aneurysm expansion in the Andijat/Dobrin aneurysm model. Ann NY Acad Sci 1996; 800: 89-96.
24. Ricci MA, Waters MA, Peate D. In: Rutherford RB, ed. Vascular Surgery, 6th Ed, (Philadelphia: WB Saunders Co. 2005). Chapter 137: The role of noninvasive studies in the diagnosis and management of cerebrovascular disease.
25. Ricci MA. Intravascular ultrasound and angioscopy. Downstate endovascular symposium. 1996 to 2000.
26. Pilcher DB. In: Machi J, Staren ED. Ultrasound for surgeons. (Philadelphia: Lippincott Williams and Wilkins, 2004) Chapter 8: Vascular Ultrasound: 143-166.
27. Sarnow MR, Interview with DB Pilcher, 2008.
28. Tarry WC, Walsh DB, Birkmeyer NJ, et al. Fate of the contralateral leg after infrainguinal bypass. J Vasc Surg 1998; 27: 1039-47.
29. Cronenwett JL, Likosky DS, Russell MT, et al. A regional registry for quality assurance and improvement: The Vascular Study Group of Northern New England (VSGNNE). J Vasc Surg 2007; 46: 1093-1101.
30. Vascular Study Group of Northern New England. Operations Manual: Confidentiality Policies and Procedures for Data Management. 2003: 1.

Chapter 29

1. Walton C. History of the British standing army. A.D. 1660-1700 (London: Harrison and Sons, 1894): 849.
2. Ortiz JM. The Revolutionary Flying Ambulance of Napoleon's Surgeon. US Army Medical Department Journal, Oct-Dec 1998: 17-25.
3. Lam, DM. The Aerochir: The first flying hospital. Aviat Space Environ Med. 2005; 76(2): 1174-9.
4. Shea WI. Doc Shea Remembers, Dec 23, 1987. Video supplied to the author by the family.
5. Cannon MH. United States Army in World War II, the War in the Pacific, Leyte: The Return to the Philippines. (Washington, DC: Office of the Chief of Military History, Department of the Army, 1993): 195.
6. King B, Jatoi I. The Mobile Army Surgical Hospital (MASH): A Military and Surgical Legacy. Journal of the National Medical Association, May 2005, 97: 648-656.
7. Link TE, Bisson E, Horgan MA, Tranmer BI. Raymond M.P. Donaghy: a pioneer in microneurosurgery. Journal of Neurosurgery, September 11, 2009, ePub: 1-6.
8. Crandall AJ. Curriculum Vitae with narrative of 2nd World War. Archives of FAH. St Michaels College Archives. Box 14, File 13.
9. Ibid.
10. Crandall AJ Curriculum Vitae.
11. Hedin J. Guns, planes and surgery. Vermont Quarterly Nov 1989. (Burlington, VT: UVM, 1989): .22-23.
12. Crandall AJ. Report of Medical Department : 4.
13. Crandall AJ. Curriculum Vitae: 3 - 4.
14. Crandall AJ. Report of the Medical Department :6.
15. Ibid: 7.
16. ibid: 4.
17. ibid: 5.
18. Ibid: 8-13.
19. Ibid: 13-14.
20. Crandall Curriculum Vitae.
21. Davis JH. Interviews with DB Pilcher, 2006-8.
22. Howard JM, "Introduction-Historical Background and Development," Battle Casualties in Korea: Studies of the Surgical Research Team, Vol. I: The Systemic Response to Injury, Army Medical Service Graduate School (Washington, DC: Walter Reed Army Medical Center, 1954): 3.
23. Davis interviews.
24. Teschan PE, Post RS, Smith LH, Jr. et al. "Post-traumatic renal insufficiency in military casualties: I: Clinical characteristics. American Journal of Medicine 1955; 18: 172-186.
25. Teschan PE, Post RS, Smith LH, Jr. et al. Post-traumatic renal insufficiency in military casualties: II: Management, use of an artificial kidney, prognosis. American Journal of Medicine 1955; 18: 187-198.
26. Moore EE, Feliciano DV, Mattox K (eds). Trauma, 5th ed. (New York: McGraw-Hill Medical Publishing Division, 2003): 9.
27. Pollak S. Locals: The Myth of Hawkeye. Burlington Free Press, April 14, 1996: D1.
28. Downs F Jr. A Veterans Perspective in Traumatic Amputation and Prosthetics. (Washington DC: Department of Veterans Affairs, 2002): 2-8.
29. Peoples GE, Jezior JR and Shriver CD. Caring for the Wounded in Iraq - A Photo Essay. NEJM 351; 24 Dec 9, 2004.
30. Conway MA. Personal communication, 2002-2009.
31. Trevisani GT. Personal communication, 2008 and 2009.
32. Zucchino D. The Journey Through Trauma. Los Angeles Times, April 3, 2006: 1.
33. Ricci MA. Personal communication, 2008.

APPENDIX A: Chiefs[1] of Surgery at UVM College of Medicine

Lecturer in Surgery
1804-1809   John Pomeroy

Chief of Surgery / Professor of Surgery
1809-1822   John Pomeroy
1823-1824   James Kent Platt
1825-1827   Henry Stevens Waterhouse
1828-1834   Benjamin Lincoln "lecturer in 1828"
1835-1837   Edward Elisha Phelps

1837-1853   Medical School Closed

1853-1854   Horace Henry Nelson
1854-1855   Samuel White Thayer
1855-1865   David Sloan Conant
1866-1872   Alpheus Benning Crosby
1873-1875   Benjamin Howard
1875-1885   James Lawrence Little
1885   Joel Williston Wright (Interim)
1886   LeRoy Monroe Brigham
1887-1889   Joel Williston Wright
1890-1900   Abel Mix Phelps
1900-1924   John Brooks Wheeler
1924-1942   Lyman Allen
1942-1969   Albert George Mackay (Associate Professor and Chief 1942-45)
1969-1989   John Herschel Davis
1989-2006   Steven R. Shackford
2006   Frank Paul Ittleman (Interim)
2007-present   David Wayne McFadden

Chief of Surgery, Bishop DeGoesbriand Hospital
1941-1967   Arthur A. Gladstone

Chief of Surgery, Fanny Allen Hospital
1957-1974   Louis George Thabault
1974-1982   Clarence Edward Bunker
1982-1995   Donald Anthony Majercik

1 From 1809 to 1969 there was only one full time "professor of surgery" which makes him considered as ipso facto "Chief of Surgery" at UVM. There were other "special professors" such as Daniel St. John Roosa and Edward Sprague in eye and ear in 1876, Henry Janes in Military surgery in 1886, Marshall Twitchell in ENT in 1899, and Aurelius Shands, Orthopaedics in 1901. There were Clinical Professors of Surgery in 1937 such as George Sabin. Some were termed "Visiting Professors" such as Frank Ober, and David Bosworth in Orthopaedics. There were also "professors of clinical surgery" such as Tinkham, and Rees.

APPENDIX B 1: UVM General Surgery Residents

NAME	COMPLETED	LOCATION & SPECIALTY
Mackay, Albert G.	1935	UVM; "It happened that Ells Amidon and I were the first...double residents at the Mary Fletcher Hospital; Amidon in medicine, and Mackay in surgery. The year before there had been one general resident...who was actually medical as well as surgical. So that makes me the first surgical resident." (AGM oral hx)
Bottamini, Joseph T.	1942	Vergennes, VT; Family Practice
Wiedeman, Geoffrey P.	1942	San Antonio, TX; Aviation Medicine
Moorehead, Matthew T.	1946	Ridgecrest, CA; General, Pathology
Holm, Benton A.	1947	Enfield, NH; General
Rubino, Bernard C.	1947	Athol, MA; Family Practice
Collins, Ray W. Jr.	1948	Middlebury, VT; General
Woodruff, Frank E.	1948	Barre, VT; General, ER
Pache, Henri L.	1949	UVM; Academic General
Haines, Carleton R.	1950	UVM; Academic General/Surgical Oncology
Derham, Robert J.	1950	Upper Darby, PA; General
Murphy, Clarence J.	1951	Worcester, MA; General
Kavouksorian, John K.	1951	Utica, NY; General
McGill, J. Bishop	1952	UVM; Academic General/Hand
Page, H. Gordon	1952	UVM; Academic General/Vascular
Caccavo, F. Arnold	1954	UVM; Academic General Surgery
Dwyre, William R.	1955	USAF, Aiken, SC; Pathology
Minot, Henry D. Jr.	1955	Cardiac, CT
Howe, Harry E.	1957	Potsdam, NY; General
Hewson, James S.	1958	Beverly, MA; Orthopedics
Koplewitz, Martin J.	1959	St Albans, VT/UVM; Academic General
Thomas, Launey J. Jr.	1959	Sarasota, FL; General
McCauley, Robert W.	1960	St. Johnsbury, VT; General
Hindawi, Ruhi K.	1961	Trenton, NJ; Thoracic
Lambert, Kenton Chickering	1962	Goderich, ONT; General
Pois, Allen J.	1962	Cleveland, OH; Academic Cardiothoracic
Sullivan, Richard A.	1963	Brighton, MA; General
Bush, Hubert S. Jr.	1964	Manchester, CT; General
Frohman, Boris	1964	Sikeston, MO; Academic General
Lavell, Thomas E. Jr.	1965	Walton, NY; General
Abadier, Abdalla G.	1965	East Greenwich, RI; General
Pilcher, David B.	1966	UVM; Academic General/Trauma/Vascular
Dewitt, Robert J.	1966	Marinette, WI; General
Howe, Gerald E.	1967	Cortez, CO; General
Topuzlu, Cemalettin	1967	Istanbul, Turkey; Academic General
Hegarty, James C.	1968	Chelmsford, MA; General
Andrews, Willard E.	1969	Hailey, ID; General
West, Robert S.	1969	Coeur D'Alene, ID; General
Hassinger, John T.	1970	Decatur, GA; General
Soeter, John R.	1970	Green Bay, WI; Cardiothoracic
Wise, Arthur J. Jr.	1970	Manhasset, NY; Plastics
Bostrom, Paul D.	1971	Montezuma City, CO; Family Practice
Elo, Denis R.	1971	Loveland, CO; General
Browdie, David A.	1971	Scranton, PA; Academic Pediatric Cardiothoracic
Longstreth, George B. III	1971	Fairfield, CT; General
Erikson, Daryl R.	1972	Nashua, NH; General
Hixson, Edward G.	1972	Saranac Lake, NY; General
Leone, Michael R.	1972	Greensboro, NC; General
Detraglia, John J.	1973	Utica, NY; General/Vascular

Rankin, Jerry D.	1973	St. Johnsbury, VT; General
Cramer, Frederick S.	1974	USAF, San Francisco, CA; Hyperbaric Medicine
Leadbetter, Allen W.	1974	Westerly, RI; General
Majercik, Donald A.	1975	Colchester, VT; General
Palmer, Edward C.	1975	Marble Falls, TX; Anesthesiology
Zarrett, Robert	1975	Fargo, ND ; General
Coletti, David C.	1976	Troy, NY; General
Linta, James M.	1976	Dayton, OH; Academic General
Moore, Ernest E. Jr.	1976	Denver, CO; Academic General/Trauma
Butler, Paul W.	1977	Dover, NH; General
Ittleman, Francis P.	1977	UVM; Academic Cardiothoracic
Reines, Howard David	1977	Falls Church, VA; Academic General/Bariatric
Douglas, Peter R.	1978	San Francisco, CA; General
Finley, David H.	1978	White Plains, NY; General
Gould, Steven A.	1978	Chicago, IL; Academic General
Bonello, Julius C.	1979	Urbana, IL; General/Colorectal
Gamelli, Richard A.	1979	Maywood, IL; Academic Burn/Trauma
Sargent, William A.	1979	St. Johnsbury, VT; General, ER
Eberly, Donald A.	1980	New London, NH; General
Jackson, Richard S.	1980	UVM; Academic Cardiothoracic
Peetz, Dwaine J.	1980	Omaha, NE; Academic Cardiothoracic
Flynn, James Bryan	1981	Marinette, WI; Vascular
Mason, Michael H.	1981	Berlin, VT; General
Morrow, Monica D.	1981	New York, NY; Surgical Oncology
Hebert, James C.	1982	UVM; Academic General
Yeaton, Howard L.	1982	Saratoga Springs, NY; General
Manjoney, Deborah L.	1983	Waukesha, WI; Cardiothoracic, Vein
Marshall, Wendy J.	1983	Maywood, IL; Academic General/Trauma
Wait, Richard B.	1983	Springfield, MA; Academic General
Schwarcz, Thomas H.	1984	Lexington, KY; Academic Vascular
Shorr, Robert M.	1984	Inglewood, CA; General
Stevens-Jaqua, Patricia I.	1984	Morrisville, VT; General
Duda, Rosemary B.	1985	Boston, MA; Academic Surgical Oncology
Grube, Baiba J.	1985	New Haven, CT; Academic Surgical Oncology
Zeiler, David Z.	1985	Suffolk, VA; General
Cioffi, William G. Jr.	1986	Providence, RI; Academic Burn/Trauma
Gartside, Roberta L.	1986	Reston, VA; Plastics
Greenhalgh, David G.	1986	Sacramento, CA; Academic Burn/Trauma
Fuller, Bradbury	1987	Middlebury, VT; General
Kispert, Paul H.	1987	Dartmouth, NH; Academic General/Critical Care
Wilson, William R. Jr.	1987	El Dorado, AR; Academic Pediatric Cardiothoracic
Lafleur, Joel D.	1988	Rockport, ME; General
Newman, Jan B.	1988	Clinton, MT; General
Payne, Stephen R.	1988	St. Albans, VT; General
Kaplan, Jeffrey H.	1989	San Jose, CA; General/Vascular/Thoracic
O'Gorman, Michael C.	1989	Greenfield, MA; General
Pories, Susan E.	1989	Boston, MA; Academic Surgical Oncology
Cobean, Roy A.	1990	Portland, ME; Academic General/Minimal Access
Hong, Andrew R.	1990	New Hyde Park, NY; Academic Pediatric
Trabulsy, Philip P.	1990	UVM; Academic Plastics/Hand
Dostal, Gregory H.	1991	Juneau, AK; Plastics
Mooney, David P.	1991	Boston, MA; Academic Pediatric
Spaulding, Laurie	1991	UVM; Academic General/Bariatric
Kelley, John M.	1992	Albany, NY; Academic Cardiothoracic
Mueller, Michael C.	1992	Austin, TX; Cardiothoracic
Silver, Geoffrey M.	1992	Maywood, IL; Academic Burn/Trauma
Murphy, Edward T.	1993	Grand Rapids, MI; Academic Cardiothoracic

Popovich, Joseph F.	1993	Jersey City, NJ; General/Vascular
Sartorelli, Kennith H.	1993	UVM; Academic Pediatric
Norotsky, Mitchell C.	1994	UVM; Academic Cardiothoracic
Pietropaoli, John A. Jr.	1994	Owings, MD; Vascular
Pigula, Frank A.	1994	Boston, MA; Academic Pediatric Cardiothoracic
Butler, Michael D.	1995	Erie, PA; Cardiothoracic
Gadowski, Gregory R.	1995	Brattleboro, VT; General
Schmoker, Joseph D.	1995	UVM; Academic Cardiothoracic
Conklin, Elizabeth	1996	Wakefield, RI; General
Keller, Martin S.	1996	St. Louis, MO; Academic Pediatric
Miles, Wandra K.	1996	Seattle, WA; Plastics/Breast
Jensen, Peter E.	1997	Salt Lake City, UT; Cardiothoracic, Vein
Trevisani, Gino T.	1997	UVM; Academic Colorectal/Bariatric
Yoder, Douglas W.	1997	Findlay, OH; General/Colorectal
McBride, Whitney J.	1998	Valhalla, NY; Academic Pediatric
Schmieder, Frank A.	1998	Philadelphia, PA; Academic Vascular
Strindberg, Gail	1998	Tooele, UT; Cardiothoracic, General
Camp, Phillip C.	1999	Boston, MA; Academic Cardiothoracic Transplant
Conway, Matthew A.	1999	Rutland, VT; General
Curran, Michael G.	1999	Cincinnati, OH; General
Bourguignon, Paul R.	2000	Ledyard, CT; General
Dicker, Rochelle A.	2000	San Francisco, CA; Academic General/Trauma
Patel, Manisha A.	2000	Cincinnati, OH; Cardiothoracic
Dhudshia, Neel V.	2001	Las Vegas, NV; Cardiothoracic
Frumiento, Carmine O.	2001	Lewiston, ME; Cardiothoracic
Novak, Lawrence M.	2001	Hyannis, MA; General
Alspaugh, Dahlia	2002	Sacramento, CA; Cardiothoracic, Vascular
Jimmo, Brad L.	2002	Rutland, VT; General
Okum, Eric J.	2002	Cincinnati, OH; Cardiothoracic
Adams, Julie E.	2003	UVM; Academic Vascular
Cavanaugh, Megan M.	2003	Portland, OR; Colorectal
Ziedens, Eduards G.	2003	Berlin, VT; General
Deross, Anthony L.	2004	Worcester, MA; Academic Pediatric
Fellinger, Erika K.	2004	Cambridge, MA; Academic General/Min Access
Forgione, Patrick M.	2004	UVM; Academic General/Min Access/Bariatric
Daniel, Subashini R.	2005	San Francisco, CA; Academic Cardiothoracic
Healey, Christopher T.	2005	Portland, ME; Academic Vascular
Juviler, Adam H.	2005	Seattle, WA; Colorectal
Boyum, Jon D.	2006	US Army, Fairbanks, AK; General
Fernandez, Nathanial N.	2006	US Navy, Philadelphia, PA; Vascular
McPartland, Kenneth J.	2006	Springfield, MA; Academic Hepatic/Transplant
Azizian, Maria	2007	Nashua, NH; General
Fisk, Peter E.	2007	Schenectady, NY; Pediatric
Cook, Alan D.	2007	Dallas, TX; Trauma/Critical Care
Chung, Arnold D.	2008	Chapel Hill, NC; Cardiothoracic
Floyd, Lisa A.	2008	Baltimore, MD; Vascular
Alizadeh, Kayvon	2008	Seattle, WA; Minimal Access
Costedio, Meagan	2009	Cleveland, OH Colorectal
Freiburg, Carter	2009	New Haven, CT, Vascular
Therrien, Christopher III	2009	New Haven, CT, Cardiothoracic

Appendix B 2: UVM Anesthesiology Residents

NAME	COMPLETED	LOCATION
Bayuk, Anthony J.	1947	Youngstown, OH
Mills, Ernest L.	1947	UVM
Egbert, Clarence H.	1948	Hamilton, OH
Harwood, Donald H.	1949	Columbia, SC
Dente, Gino A.	1950	UVM
Jacobs, Howard H.	1951	St. Albans, VT
Woodruff, Charlotte S.	1951	Burlington, VT
Buber, Luther W.	1952	Berlin, NH
Cox, Charles V.	1953	Barrington, RI
Deos, Harland M.	1953	Sacramento, CA
Fukuda, Minoru David	1953	Barre, VT
Glover, Nathan	1954	Miami, FL
Jones, Allen T.	1955	Saratoga Springs, NY
Brazell, Edward H.	1956	UVM/Sacramento, CA
Gauthier, Jerome L.	1956	Columbus, OH
Peppard, Raymond W.	1956	Phoenix, AZ
Pycental-Bellini, Raymon	1957	
Sen, Dilip K.	1958	London, ENG
Emerson, Philip E.	1959	Sacramento, CA
deGerman, Francesca	1958	
Ho, Ching-Hsin	1958	
Kosaka, Futami	1958	
Pease, Richard E.	1958	Jericho, VT
Telemaque, Fritz Gerald	1960	Barre, VT
Cetin, Avedis	1960	Woodbury, NY
Pena, Emilio F.	1960	Clearwater, FL
Aubry, Ubald	1960	Montreal, QB
Sanchez, Eduardo A.	1960	Corpus Christi, TX
Jamharian, Jan	1961	Southington, CT
Lew, Sanghwan J.	1961	Windermere, FL
Hazaryan, Antranik	1961	Lutz, FL
Wehling, Donald W.	1961	Barberton, OH
Browne, Anthony B.	1961	Redmond, WA
Guttman, Donald I.	1962	San Diego, CA
Lucia, George E., Jr.	1962	Lake Placid, NY
Mareno, Marco T.	1962	Tampa, FL
Naveria, Jose	1962	
Street, William C.	1962	Brockton, MA
Bell, Roy	1963	UVM
Van Vliet, Jetse	1964	Patchogue, NY
Vedamanikam, Devanandam	1964	
Deane, Robert S.	1964	UVM
McKeever, Robert W.	1965	St. John's, NFLD
Cestone, Kenneth J.	1965	Bennington, VT
Roaf, Edward R.	1966	Boston, MA
Charles, Rodrigue T.	1966	Guilderland, NY
Shinozaki, Tamotsu	1967	UVM
Furman, Eric B.	1967	Seattle, WA
Chryn, Richard H.	1967	Louisville, KY
Lemmer, Lodewyk Arlo	1968	Tampa, FL
Duguid, Margaret G.	1968	Plainfield, NJ
Crowe, James A.	1968	Noblesville, IN
Falkenberg, Gisela	1969	Athens, PA
Beauregard, Joseph R.	1969	Northampton, MA
Hartford, John E.	1969	Franklin, NH

Newton, Neil A.	1969	Augusta, ME (Radiology)
Roman, Denis Garry	1969	Westlake Village, CA
Garcia, Jose E.	1969	Santurce, PR
Holm, Peter J.	1969	Middlebury, VT (Radiology)
Perkins, David L.	1970	North Hero, VT
Hong, Songho	1970	North Hero, VT
White, Joseph R.	1971	Fall River, MA
Zimmerman, Carol E.	1971	Summit, NJ
Barnes, Stephanie A.	1972	Wolfeboro, NH
Ikeda, Shigemasa	1972	St. Louis, MO
Perry, Frederick T.	1972	Pawtucket, RI
Tyson, Judith	1972	Lebanon, NH (OB/GYN)
White, Ronald L.	1972	Washington, DC
Rubins, Talivaldies	1972	Gorham, ME
Degerli, Osman	1973	Bayreuth, Germany
Dempsey, William J. (Gus)	1973	Clarks Summit, PA (E.R.)
McQuade, James S.	1973	Lillington, NC
Khalil, Rosaly Saba	1973	West Orange, NJ
Gadowski, Walter	1974	Hyannis, MA
Johnpulle, Camillus J.R.	1974	Tampa, FL
Park, Choo-Oong	1974	Poughkeepsie, NY (F.P.)
Bauzys, Raymond J.	1975	Tampa, FL
Shear, Elliott S.	1975	Bethlehem, PA (D.D.S)
Barnett, Daniel L.	1976	New Vineyard, ME
Paul, Marie M.	1976	Monroe, WI
Smail, David F.	1976	UVM
Beasley, Ralph D.	1977	Manchester, NH
Chase, Christopher R.	1977	UVM
Kennedy, Ronald C.	1977	Manchester, NH
Sewall, Douglas M.	1977	Bangor, ME
Shapiro, Jeryl R.	1977	UVM
Rogers, Paul M.	1978	Johnson, VT (F.P.)
Vacanti, Charles A.	1978	Lexington, MA
Halfar, Wayne P.	1979	Englewood, CO
Johnson, David L.	1979	UVM
Kristensen, Eva A. (Heidi)	1979	UVM
Leung, Mabel L.	1979	Mercer Island, WA
Lorenz, Dieter	1979	Chatham, MA
Wasdyke, Wesley R.	1979	Manchester, NH
Elliott, Riley A.	1980	UVM
Fishleder, Rand I.	1980	Cedar Rapids, IA
McElfresh, Peter A.	1980	Oceanside, CA
Nicholson, Robert M.	1980	Kalamazoo, MI
Martin, Douglas J.	1980	Pittsburgh, PA
Betit, Mary Ellen	1981	Ridgefield, CT
Johnson, Steven P.	1981	Las Vegas, NV
Lambert, Donald H.	1981	Westwood, MA
Mah, Trudabeth Q.	1981	
Gomes, Ligia B.	1982	Tampa, FL
Walton, Karen Cook	1982	Concord, NH
Fingard, David H.	1982	Milwaukee, WI
Langdon, James Russell	1983	Knoxville, TN
Sherman, Elden P.	1983	Charleston, SC
Hust, William P.	1983	Atlanta, GA
Ianacone, David C.	1983	Moreno Valley, CA
Mack, Maria J.	1983	Tacoma, WA
Peachman, Frederick A.	1983	Youngstown, OH
Hood, Linda A. Strang	1983	Bedford, NH
Chaffee, William H. III	1984	Las Vegas, NM
Lewis, Gloria L.	1984	Knoxville, TN

Appendicies

Steinberg, Robert B.	1984	Springfield, MA
Tweedie, Eric L.	1984	Montgomery, AL
Spaulding, Richard P.	1985	Bedford, NH
Stern, Peter	1985	Shelburne, VT
Bevacqua, Brian K.	1985	Madison, WI
Johnsrud, Eric P.	1985	Gillette, WY
Schapiro, Howard M.	1985	UVM
White, Jerry L.	1985	Bedford, NH
Knisely, Geoffrey R.	1985	Middlebury, VT
Briggs, Dana G.	1986	Orrington, ME
Viani, Bruce A.	1986	UVM
Limanek, James S.	1986	UVM
Boerman, Paul G.	1986	S. Burlington, VT (D.D.S.)
Burt, Ronald E.	1986	Hartford, CT
Ianni, Kevin L.	1987	Middlebury, VT
Kennedy, Thomas M.	1987	Latham, NY
Perz, Robert R.	1987	Cincinnati, OH
Quamme, Bradley D.	1987	Lancaster, OH
Tonrey, Frank G.	1987	Albuquerque, NM (E.R.)
Ullman, David A.	1987	Rochester, NY
Whalen, Thomas J.	1987	Albuquerque, NM
Torbicki, Edward A.	1987	Kitchener, ONT
Kreutz, Joseph M.	1988	UVM
Mote, Thomas R.	1988	Indianapolis, IN
Clark, E. Richard	1988	Philomath, OR
Ryterband, Sarah	1988	Bloomington, IN
Caruso, Louis	1989	Zephyrhills, FL (Cardiology)
Fisher, John Matthew	1989	UVM
Ginsberg, Martin L.	1989	Manchester, NH
Nitzsche, David D.	1989	Lexington, OH
Oberding, Michael J.	1989	Saranac Lake, NY
Pero, Barbara A.	1989	Santa Fe, NM
Sharp, Nina A.	1989	Randolph, VT
Astorian, Donald G.	1990	Zanesville, OH
Bauss, Lawrence A.	1990	Kalamazoo, MI
Brackett, Rebecca P.	1990	Augusta, ME
Cuda, Michael P.	1990	Utica, NY
Johnston, Michael D.	1990	Lihue, HI
Lerner, Guy M.	1990	Louisville, KY
Oliner, Charles J.	1990	Bethesda, MD
Richey, John M.	1990	Concord, NH
Stein, Susan K.	1990	Brattleboro, VT
Williams, Robert K.	1990	UVM
Roberts, William A.	1991	Fairfield, VT
Krane, Barry D.	1991	Brooklyn, NY
Thompson, Peter W.	1991	Bangor, ME
Zagroba, Marie L.	1991	Berlin, VT
Dowsett, Paul A.	1992	Augusta, MI
Giustozzi, John J. Jr.	1992	Salisbury, MD
LaRue, Denise	1992	Albuquerque, NM
Love, Wendy	1992	West Bath, ME
Viapiano, James	1992	UVM
Aragon, Charles A.	1992	Billings, MT
Glynn, Christopher P.	1992	Salisbury, MD
Hovland, Michael P.	1992	Billings, MT
Rubinfeld, Julie A. Broome	1992	Morristown, NJ
Blickensderfer, E. David	1993	Sioux Falls, SD
Harris, Craig R.	1993	Vacaville, CA
Pinn, Elke	1993	Berlin, VT
Resop, Daniel J.	1993	Berlin, WI

Samson, Jose M.	1993	Falmouth, MA
Irwin, Louis J.	1993	Roanoke, VA
Chan, Gregory C.	1994	S. Burlington, VT (D.D.S.)
Eaton, Michael P.	1994	Fairport, NY
Malik, Christopher J.	1994	Eagle Rock, VA
Maron, Jonathan S.	1994	Seattle, WA
Neil, Jay L.	1994	Asheville, NC
O'Reilly, Michael O.	1994	Ann Arbor, MI
Tobi, Patricia Kuncheff	1994	Gillette, WY
Aladjem, Eva V.	1994	UVM
Aveni, Maria C.	1995	Berlin, VT
Garahan, Margaret B. (Mitzi)	1995	San Diego, CA
Letourneau, L. Scott	1995	Bend, OR
Roth, Jeremy B.	1995	Baltimore, MD
Russell, Richard J.	1995	Rapid City, SD
Swanson, David E.	1995	Berlin, WI
Adams, Jeffrey A.	1995	Statesville, NC
Mason, Stephen B.	1995	St. Albans, VT
Burzynski, Norbert J., Jr.	1996	Louisville, KY (Radiology)
Johnson, Timothy A.	1996	Cadillac, MI
Sankel, Jordan H.	1996	Santa Fe, NM
Transtrom, Debra A.	1996	Sacramento, CA
Burns, Sean	1996	Elmira, NY
Simmons, Eric L.	1996	Colorado Springs, CO
Evelti, David J.	1997	Decatur, IL
Freilich, Erin M.	1997	Potomac, MD
Gutierrez, Carl J.	1997	Morrisville, VT
Kelly, Sean L.	1997	Brunswick, ME
Silfer, Cynthia R.	1997	Utica, NY
Woodring, Phyllis M.	1997	Hilo, HI
Traul, John B.	1998	Pocatello, ID
Borchardt, Jeffrey A.	1998	Metairie, LA
Kanan, Fadi	1999	Essex Junction, VT (D.D.S.)
Li, Paul X.	2000	Northville, MI (Int Med)
Torian, Dikran	2000	Rancho Mirage, CA
Bilge, Aykut	2001	Boston, MA
Qi, Jin	2001	Watertown, NY
Lenkovsky, Fima	2001	Dallas, TX
Torbin, Olga I.	2001	Hollywood, FL
Memon, Zarina G.	2001	Westerly, RI
Carney, Timothy H.	2002	Bend, OR
Pomciter, Edward T.	2002	St. Albans, VT
George, Gordon P.	2002	Orem, UT
Benedetti, Esther M.	2003	Iowa City, IA
Sears, Jeffrey S.	2003	Muskegon, MI
Khoshyomn, Mani	2003	Albuquerque, NM
Loutzenheiser, Todd D.	2004	Bremerton, WA
Fazzone, Anthony B.	2004	Springfield, VT
Abnet, Kevin R.	2004	UVM
Choate, Laurance W. (Lric)	2004	Hamburg, IA (G.P.)
Daigle, Richard A.	2004	West Lafayette, IN
McCormack, Mirjam Kotar	2004	Morrisville, VT
Lair, Timothy R.	2004	Overland Park, KS
Nauman, Bushra	2004	Needham Heights, MA
Ivie, Clarence S. III (Sonny)	2005	UVM
Franowicz, Lawrence M.	2005	Burlington, MA
Grondin, Lydia S.	2005	UVM
Ketcham, John P.	2005	Portland, OR
Kyper, Robert J.	2005	Vancouver, WA
Megdal, William H.	2005	Athens, GA

Name	Completed	Location
Paffendorf, Paul Jeffrey	2005	Aspen, CO
Brown, Blaine W.	2006	San Bernardino, CA
Pino, Carlos A.	2006	UVM
Hofsess, Craig P.	2006	Plattsburgh, NY
Schaefer, Sara M. Nesler	2006	Springfield, VT
Tsai, Mitchell H.	2006	UVM
Borgoy, John A.	2006	Atlanta, GA
Breth, John J.	2006	Kansas City, KS
Hill, Bradley C.	2006	Antioch, TN
Leduc, Laura H.	2006	Boston, MA
Reed, Kelly J. Doerzbacher	2007	Chapel Hill, NC
Martin, Jacob A.	2007	UVM
McNally, Walter E.	2007	Rutland, VT
Miller, Vincent J.	2007	UVM
Murphy, Todd L.	2007	Savannah, GA
Parker, Colleen M.	2007	Springfield, VT
Reed, James Taylor	2007	Boston, MA
Torbin, Valery	2007	Hollywood, FL
Eastwood, Charles B.	2008	Cincinnati, OH
MacDonald, Kathleen S.	2008	Lebanon, NH
Sutherland, Michael A.	2008	UVM
Waring, John Timothy	2008	Cambridge, MA
Watson, Nicholas C.	2008	Boston, MA

Appendix B 3: UVM Orthopaedic Surgery Residents

NAME	COMPLETED	LOCATION
Frymoyer, John W.	1969	UVM
Lippert, Frederick G.	1970	Seattle, WA
Holmes, Edgar M.	1970	Rutland, VT
Jennings, Charles D.	1971	Great Falls, MT
Chan, Donald P.K.	1971	Charlottesville, VA
Moreland, Morey S.	1972	Pittsburgh, PA
Pepe, Albert J.	1973	Oakland, ME
Renne, James W.	1973	Evansville, IN
Goodnough, Charles Peter	1974	Elmira, NY
Henkel, Charles Edward	1974	Norfolk, NE
Matteri, Richard E.	1974	Eugene, OR
Munk, Richard L.	1975	Toledo, OH
Cancro, J. Chriss	1976	Auburn, WA
Grossman, Robert B.	1976	Tinton Falls, NJ
Lipke, Robert W.	1977	Anchorage, AK
McCutcheon, Michael E.	1977	Albuquerque, NM
Melkonian, Gregory J.	1977	Concord, NH
Brown, Douglas W.	1978	Portland, ME
Howe, James G.	1978	UVM
Thomas, Herbert J. III	1978	Englewood, CO
Leung, Kenneth Y.K.	1979	Seattle, WA
Mogan, James V.	1979	South Burlington, VT
Jones, Gary S.	1979	Concord, NH
Blute, John W.	1980	Concord, MA
Wagner, Leonard Y.	1981	Springfield, MA
White, Raymond R.	1981	Portland, ME
Jenkins, Raeburn M.	1983	Billings, MT
Kristiansen, Thomas K.	1983	UVM
Blitzer, Charles M.	1984	Somersworth, NH

Kuhn, Douglas A.	1984	Carmel, IN
Gassman, Jeffrey I.	1984	Norwood, MA
Carr, Daniel E.	1985	Williamsburg, VA
DeCoster, Thomas A.	1985	Albuquerque, NM
Jung, Charles F.	1985	Seattle, WA
Flick, Arthur Bartholomew	1986	Clayton, GA
Fischer, Richard A.	1986	Hilliard, OH
Byrt, William T.	1987	Saratoga Springs, NY
Wertz, Michael P.	1987	Boulder, CO
Stein, Ann C.	1988	Rutland, VT
Incavo, Stephen J.	1988	UVM
Saltzman, Andrew T.	1989	Evansville, IN
Amrani, Jacob	1989	Wichita, KS
Dohring, Edward J.	1990	Phoenix, AZ
Wertheimer, Clay M.	1990	Everett, WA
Halsey, David A.	1990	Springfield, VT
Monsey, Robert D.	1991	UVM
George, Daniel C.	1991	Sharon, CT
Neale, S. Glen	1991	Morrisville, VT
Kaplan, Michael J.	1992	Middlebury, CT
Ninomiya, James T.	1992	Milwaukee, WI
Landvater, Stephanie J.	1992	Williston, VT
Pyne, John I. B.	1993	Bangor, ME
DiFazio, Frank A.	1993	Overland, KS
Hurlbut, Patrick T.	1993	Lincoln, NE
Baumhauer, Judith F.	1994	Rochester, NY
Rudd, Eric W.	1994	Aberdeen, WA
Muller, David L.	1994	Springfield, VT
Dirks, Marco P.	1995	Pawtucket, RI
Meriam, Christopher M.	1995	Berlin, VT
Samani, John E.	1995	Rochester, MI
Deibert, Mark C.	1996	Bozeman, MT
Lynch, Scott A.	1996	Hershey, PA
Sandmeier, Robert H.	1996	Portland, OR
Beard, David M.	1997	Fargo, ND
Huber, Bryan M.	1997	Morrisville, VT
Reid, James G.	1997	Louisville, CO
Fehnel, David J.	1998	Peabody, MA
Levine, Benjamin P.	1998	Woburn, MA
Schwender, James D.	1998	Minneapolis, MN
Jones, Marci D.	1999	Worcester, MA
Lemos, Stephen E.	1999	Detroit, MI
Woolley, C. Todd	1999	Portland, OR
Barker, Howard B.	2000	Everett, WA
Jones, Pamela L.	2000	North Andover, MA
Macy, John C.	2000	South Burlington, VT
Ames, S. Elizabeth	2001	UVM
Blackmon, Darnell E.	2001	Tulsa, OK
Uroskie, Jonathan A.	2001	Peabody, MA
Dayton, Michael R.	2002	Denver, CO
Devanny, Patrick D.	2002	Colorado Springs, CO
Uh, Benjamin S.	2002	Long Beach, NY
Braun, Stuart V.	2003	Boston, MA
Havener, Todd H.	2003	Everett, WA
Mullaney, Kevin J.	2003	Bloomington, MN
Mullins, Eric R.	2004	Morrisville, VT
Risinger, Randall J.	2004	Wakefield, RI
Tuttle, Harrison G.	2004	Raleigh, NC
Kelly, Stephen J.	2005	Portland, ME
Mihalich, Robert M.	2005	Brighton, MI

Wisotsky, Scott M.	2005	Tampa Bay, FL
Durant, Denise M.	2006	Bennington, VT
Endres, Nathan K.	2006	UVM
Frenzen, Seth W.	2006	South Burlington, VT
Doohen, Robert R.	2007	Cambridge, MN
Hennig, Alexander C.	2007	Gilford, NH
Kelleher, Peter M.	2007	Bozeman, MT
Noud, Patrick H.	2008	San Diego, CA (fellow)
Putnam, Ryan M.	2008	St. Louis, MO (fellow)
Wild, John J. III	2008	Tucson, AZ

Appendix B 4: UVM Neurosurgery Residents

NAME	COMPLETED	LOCATION
Flanagan, Martin E.	1962	UVM
Chaffee, Bruce A.	1965	Lewiston, ME
Slater, John P.	1966	Fresno, CA
Moody, Robert A.	1967	Swampscott, MA
Upton, Peter D.	1969	Rutland, VT
Keranen, Victor J.	1970	Fayetteville, NC
Inoa, Abelardo D.	1971	Dover, NJ
Kumar, Vasantha A.	1972	Chambersburg, PA
Fagelman, Frederic I.	1973	Glens Falls, NY
Limcaco, Oscar G.	1974	Terre Haute, IN
Wright, Sanford J., Jr.	1975	Everett, WA
Ivamoto, Henrique Seiji	1976	Santos, Brazil
Karumbaya, Romola	1978	Scranton, PA
Mortara, Ronald W.	1978	Framingham, MA
Guthikonda, Murali	1980	Detroit, MI
Gomes, Francisco B.	1981	Sarasota, FL
Olin, Michael S.	1981	North Smithfield, RI
Smith, Donald A.	1983	Tampa, FL
Cutler, Scott G	1986	Tampa, FL
Binter, Nancy E.	1987	Burlington, VT
Duckworth, John W.	1988	Bangor, ME
Gelbard, Steven D.	1991	Pompano Beach, FL
Bednar, Martin M.	1992	Groton, CT
Leivy, Sander W.	1993	Roanoke, VA
Johnson, Stephen H.	1994	South Weymouth, MA
Adey, Geoffrey R.	1995	Walnut Creek, CA
Wilson, James T.	1996	Scarborough, ME
Ordonez, B. Joe	1997	Norfolk, VA
Maurin, Edward E., III	1998	Farmington, NM
Gates, Marilyn L.	1999	Detroit, MI
Kohut, James J.	2000	Santa Cruz, CA
Florman, Jeffrey E.	2001	Scarborough, ME
Lew, Sean M.	2002	Milwaukee, WI
Berryhill, Philip C.	2003	Santa Fe, NM
Khoshyomn, Sami	2004	Springfield, MO
Nathan, David J.	2005	Salt Lake City, UT
Jewell, Ryan P.	2006	UVM
Bisson, Erica F.	2007	Burlington, MA
Walsh, Michael T.	2008	Salt Lake City, UT (fellow)

Appendix B 5: UVM Otolaryngology Residents

NAME	COMPLETED	LOCATION
Lyons, Richard C.	1976	Winooski, VT
Pender, Daniel J.	1978	New York, NY
Karabachev, Ivan D.	1980	Las Vegas, NV
Spinella, Martin J.	1983	Waterbury, CT
Hubbell, Richard N.	1985	UVM
Larrivey, Roberto A.	1986	Owosso, MI
Schneiderman, Terrence S.	1987	Dayton, OH
Ehlert, Tamara K.	1988	St. Louis, MO
Stone, Gwen E.	1989	Marshfield, WI
Freije, James E.	1990	Hershey, PA
Pyle, Paula B.	1991	Pensacola, FL
Brundage, William J.	1992	UVM
Righi, Paul D.	1993	Indianapolis, IN
Gonzalez, Debra A.	1994	Memphis, TN
Keller, Christopher J.	1995	Manitowoc, WI
Alex, James C.	1996	New Haven, CT
Dray, Todd G.	1997	Seattle, WA
Rankin, Brett S.	1998	Kittery, ME
Gourin, Christine G.	1999	Baltimore, MD
Rankin, Deane E.	2000	Littleton, NH
Ihm, Peter S.	2001	Exeter, NH
Krakovitz, Paul R.	2002	Cleveland, OH
Davies, Louise	2003	White River Junction, VT
Fahrner, Kristen S.	2004	Biddeford, ME
Zavod, Matthew B.	2005	Woodland, CA
Anderson, Eric R.	2006	Exeter, NH
Rimash, Tamara	2007	UVM
Danielson, Gregory P.	2008	Exeter, NH

Appendix B 6: UVM Urology Residents

NAME	COMPLETED	LOCATION
Powell, Platt R.	1948	UVM
White, Fletcher H.	1949	Exeter, NH
Larner, Paul Kingston	1950	Palatine Bridge, NY
Tulip, Henry T.	1951	St. Albans, VT
Fagan, William T.	1952	Stowe, VT
Pearson, Albert M.	1953	Westminster, MA
Zagroba, John A.	1957	Barre, VT
Murphy, Patrick		
Ross, James E.	1963	Redlands, CA
Kosse, Karl H.K.	1963	Aberdeen, SD
Pelkey, Wesley J.	1964	Wevertown, NY
Antiles, Leonard	1966	Glen Ridge, NJ
Hamlin, Paul S.	1966	Presque Isle, ME
Morrisseau, Paul M.	1969	Jensen Beach, FL
Clark, Curtis W.	1970	Ames, IA
Allison, Ronald C.	1970	Stockton, CA
Richardson, John R.	1971	Hanover, NH
Caponegro, Peter J.	1972	Brooklyn, NY
Vickers, Martyn A.	1973	Boston, MA
King, Brian H.	1974	Glens Falls, NY

DeCenzo, J. Michael	1975	Springfield, MA
Maddocks, Raymond A.	1976	Glens Falls, NY
Zickerman, Philip M.	1977	Wausau, WI
Bisson, John A.	1978	Burlington, VT
Leffke, David W.	1979	Lynchburg, VA
Kutscher, Harlan A.	1980	Reading, PA
Noyes, David T.	1981	Pittsfield, MA
Broaddus, Samuel B.	1982	South Portland, ME
Fleischer, Alan N.	1983	Wyomissing, PA
Steinbock, Greg S.	1984	Louisville, KY
Isen, Jeffrey S.	1985	Worcester, MA
Trotter, Samuel J.	1986	UVM
Agee, Lawrence Carter	1987	Auburn, CA
Jumper, Brian M.	1988	South Portland, ME
Jackson, Thomas L.	1989	UVM
Thompson, David E.	1990	Grand Rapids, MI
Cadoff, Robert E.	1991	Billings, MT
Distefano, Anthony J.	1992	Vernon Rockville, CT
Schow, Douglas A.	1993	San Antonio, TX
Ortiz, G. Michael	1994	Saratoga Springs, NY
Phelps, Rick D.	1995	Manchester, NH

Appendix C: General Surgery Teacher of the Year as Selected by the Residents

1976	David B. Pilcher		1993	Martin J. Koplewitz
1977	James E. DeMeules		1994	Steven R. Shackford
1978	John H. Davis		1995	David B. Pilcher
1979	Jerome S. Abrams		1996	Robert S. Deane and Tamotsu Shinozaki
1980	H. Gordon Page		1997	Laurie Spaulding
1981	Roger S. Foster		1998	David B. Pilcher
1982	David B. Pilcher		1999	David B. Pilcher
1983	Richard L. Gamelli		2000	Peter A. Cataldo
1984	David B. Pilcher		2001	Wallace C. Tarry
1985	Richard L. Gamelli		2002	Dennis W. Vane
1986	Richard L. Gamelli		2003	Steven R. Shackford
1987	Richard L. Gamelli		2004	Kennith H. Sartorelli
1988	Richard L. Gamelli		2005	Kennith H. Sartorelli
1989	David B. Pilcher		2006	Kennith H. Sartorelli
1990	Richard L. Gamelli		2007	Neil H. Hyman
1991	Neil H. Hyman		2008	Julie E. Adams
1992	James C. Hebert		2009	Neil H. Hyman

Appendix D: Orthopaedic Teacher of the Year as Selected by the Residents

1988	John W. Frymoyer		1999	Joseph A. Abate, III
1989	Morey S. Moreland		2000	Craig S. Bartlett, III
1990	Claude E. Nichols, III		2001	Thomas K. Kristiansen
1991	Martin H. Krag		2002	Robert J. Johnson
1992	Saul G. Trevino		2003	Robert D. Monsey
1993	David D. Aronsson		2004	David D. Aronsson
1994	Robert J. Johnson		2005	S. Elizabeth Ames
1995	Robert D. Monsey		2006	Martin H. Krag
1996	David D. Aronsson		2007	James G. Howe
1997	Claude E. Nichols, III		2008	Thomas K. Kristiansen
1998	Claude E. Nichols, III & Robert D. Monsey			

University of Vermont College of Medicine
Fletcher Allen Health Care
Department of Surgery Endowments & Funds

Endowments provide perpetual support for the core missions of the Department of Surgery, especially scholarly activities that often struggle for sufficient funding. Endowments also carry forward the legacies of surgical leaders into future generations, ensuring that the values of these role models endure.

The establishment of funds to meet the immediate needs of physicians, faculty and students is critical for the ongoing advancement of the delivery of clinical care, research and education.

The University of Vermont College of Medicine and Fletcher Allen Health Care Department of Surgery are both proud and grateful to steward the following named Chairs, Professors, Lectures and Funds.

Name	*Established*	*Appointee (where applicable)*
Elliot W. Shipman Professor in Ophthalmology	1934	Vacant
Jerome S. Abrams Memorial Fund	1985	
Dr. Lewis S. & Eleanor Bogart Pilcher Endowed Scholarship	1998	
S.D. Ireland Family Professorship in Surgical Oncology	1999	David N. Krag, MD 1999
Arnold H. Colodny, MD Lectureship in Pediatric Surgery	2000	
The Madison Jaurigue Endowed Lectureship in Neurosurgery ("Madi's Fund")	2000	
Roger H. Allbee, MD'31 Professor	2000	Vacant
Harry Howe, MD'52 and Theo Howe Endowed Scholarship and Surgical Excellence Prize	2000	
UVM Thoracic Surgery Prize Fund	2000	
Stanley S. Fieber, MD'48 Chair in Surgery	2002	David W. McFadden, MD 2007
The Urology Research Development Fund	2002	
Duncan W. Persons, MD'34 Green & Gold Professor	2003	Brian Y. Kim, MD 2008
Samuel B. and Michelle D. Labow Green & Gold Professor of Colon & Rectal Surgery	2005	Neil Hyman, MD
Samuel B. and Michelle D. Labow Endowed Lecture	2005	
Cordell E. Gross, MD Green & Gold Professor in Neurosurgery	2005	Bruce Tranmer, MD 2005
Albert G. Mackay, MD'32 and H. Gordon Page, MD'45 Professor in Surgery	2005	James Hebert, MD 2005
John H. Davis, MD Endowed Lecture	2006	
Steven R. Shackford, MD / Samuel B. Labow, MD Endowed Lecture in Quality	2007	
Martin H. Wennar, MD Endowed Lecture in Professionalism	2008	
The Irene and John LaPorte Scholarship Fund	1970	
Fletcher Allen Health Care Organ Transplant Fund	1998	
Emergency Department Endowed Fund	2008	

CATAMOUNT SURGEONS

ILLUSTRATION SOURCES AND ACKNOWLEDGEMENTS

Courtesy of UVM Special Collections and the Wilbur Collection 1-1, 1-2, 3-3, 3-4, 4-3, 4-7, 4-8, 4-9, 4-10 (4-7 - 4-10 are photographs loose or pasted in Henry Janes' Journal), 6-7, 8-8 (from Progress and Care Sept, 1959), 22-1, 22-3

Courtesy of UVM College of Medicine Dana Library Historical Collection 1-3, 22-2

Courtesy of Yale University, Harvey Cushing/John Hay Whitney Medical Library, New Haven Connecticut 2-1, 2-2

From the authors collection (DBP) 3-1, 5-7, 5-8, 5-11, 6-3, 6-5, 8-3, 9-10, 9-14, 9-15, 9-19, 10-13, 11-8, 11-11, 14-1, 14-16, 16-2, 17-2, 17-4, 17-13, 18-2, 20-7, 20-8, 20-9, 22-15, 25-10, 25-11, 26-4, 27-2, 28-8, 28-9, 28-10, 28-11, 28-14, 29-9, 29-10, 29-11

Courtesy of Bowdoin College Archives, Brunswick, Maine 3-2

Courtesy of the Hood Museum of Art, Dartmouth College, Hanover, New Hampshire; gift of Edwin W. Stoughton, Class of 1862H 3-5

From the public domain (internet) 3-6, 23-1, 25-1, 29-5, 29-6

UVM College of Medicine Archives 4-1, 4-2, 4-4, 4-12, 5-4, 5-5, 5-6, 5-9, 5-10, 5-12, 5-13, 6-1, 6-4, 6-6, 6-11, 6-15, 7-1, 7-2, 7-3, 7-6, 7-7, 7-9, 8-4, 9-16, 9-17, 14-18

Courtesy of Michael Curran 4-5

Courtesy of Waterbury Historical Society, Waterbury, VT. 4-6, 4-11, 5-3

Illustration in Memoirs of a Small Town Surgeon, Wheeler, JB. 5-1

Courtesy of Stan Malcolm, Marlborough, Connecticut 5-2

Insert in book; Tracheostomy, by Lewis Stephen Pilcher, in collection of the author. 6-2

Courtesy of Fanny Allen Hospital Archives (at St Michael's College) 6-8, 6-9, 6-10, 6-12, 6-13, 6-14, 6-16, 7-4, 7-5, 8-5, 8-6, 17-1, 29-2, 29-3, 29-4

Courtesy of Fletcher Allen Health Care (MCHV) Archives 7-1, 7-10, 8-1, 8-2 (published in Gauzette Dec, 1958), 8-7, 8-9, 8-10 (P&C 1968), 9-1, 9-2, 9-3, 9-6, 9-11, 9-12, 9-18 (P&C 1962), 9-21, 10-1, 10-2, 10-3, 10-4, 10-5, 10-6, 10-7,10-9, 10-10, 10-12,10-14, 11-1, 11-2, 11-3, 11-4, 11-12, 13-6, 13-10, 13-11, 13-12, 13-13, 14-6, 14-19, 14-22, 15-1, 15-2, 15-9, 15-10, 15-11, 15-15, 15-19, 15-20, 16-1, 17-3, 17-5, 17-6, 17-7, 17-8, 17-9, 17-10, 17-11, 17-12, 17-14, 17-15, 18-1, 18-3, 18-5, 18-9, 18-10, 19-1, 19-2, 19-4, 19-5, 19-6, 20-1, 20-2, 20-5, 20-6, 20-10, 20-11, 20-12, 20-13, 20-14, 20-15, 21-2, 21-3, 21-4, 21-5, 21-7, 21-8, 21-12, 21-13, 21-14, 22-5, 22-6, 22-8, 22-9, 22-10, 23-2, 23-3, 23-4, 23-5, 23-7, 23-8, 23-9, 24-1, 24-3, 24-4, 25-2, 25-3, 25-4, 25-5, 25-13, 25-15, 26-1, 26-2, 26-5, 27-1, 27-3, 27-7, 27-8, 27-9, 28-1, 28-2, 28-12, 28-13, 28-15

Courtesy of Anesthesia Archives and Joseph Kreutz, MD 7-8, 13-2, 13-3, 13-4, 13-5, 13-7, 13-8, 13-9, 13-14

Courtesy of Robert Cain 9-4,10-15

Courtesy of Lucy Abair (Daughter of W I Shea, MD) 9-5, 29-1

Courtesy of Betty McGill 9-7, 9-8

Courtesy of H G Page, MD 9-9, 9-13

Courtesy of Marilyn McSweeney 9-20, 28-3

Courtesy of John H Davis, MD 10-8, 29-7, 29-8

Courtesy of Roger Foster, Jr, MD 10-11, 26-3

Courtesy of Martin Koplewitz, MD 10-16

Courtesy of James T. Ninomiya, MD 10-17, 10-18, 10-19, 10-20, 10-21, 18-4, 28-4

Courtesy of Bruce Leavitt, MD 11-5, 11-6, 11-7, 15-16, 15-17, 15-18, 19-7, 22-7, 24-2, 28-16

Courtesy of John Schneider, MD 11-9

Courtesy of Steven R Shackford, MD 11-10, 12-9, 12-11

Courtesy of David McFadden, MD 12-1

Courtesy of Peter Upton, MD and Joseph Kreutz MD 13-1

Courtesy of John W. Frymoyer, MD 14-2, 14-3, 14-4, 14-7, 14-8, 14-9, 14-10, 14-11, 14-12, 14-13, 14-14, 14-17

Courtesy of Orthopaedic Archives, UVM College of Medicine 14-5

Courtesy of Robert Johnson, MD 14-15

Courtesy of Martin Krag, MD 14-20, 19-3

Courtesy of UVM, medical photography division 14-21, 15-12, 18-8, 20-3, 21-11, 23-6, 28-7

Courtesy of James Micheslon, MD 14-23

Courtesy of Miriam Parkinson, RN and Cardiac Surgery Division Archives, FAHC, Burlington, VT 15-3, 15-4, 15-5, 15-7, 15-8, 15-13, 15-14, 15-21

Courtesy of Laurence Coffin, MD 15-6

Courtesy of Paul Danielson, MD 16-3

Courtesy of Peter Cataldo, MD 18-6, 18-7

Courtesy of David Krag, MD 19-3

Courtesy of James Hebert, MD 20-4

Courtesy of Neurosurgery Archives, FAHC and UVM College of Medicine 21-1, 21-6, 21-9

Courtesy of Linda Gross 21-10

Courtesy of Ryan Jewell, MD 21-15

Courtesy of Geoffrey Tabin, MD 22-11, 22-12, 22-13

Courtesy of Alan Irwin, MD 22-4, 22-14

Courtesy of Philip Trabulsy, MD 25-6, 25-7, 25-12

Courtesy of Linda Horn 25-8, 25-9,

Courtesy of Donald Laub, MD 25-14

Courtesy of Jon Yamaguchi, MD 26-6, 26-7

Courtesy of Samuel Trotter, MD 27-4, 27-5, 27-6

Courtesy of Michael Ricci, MD 28-6, 29-13

Courtesy of Gino Trevisani, MD 29-12

Courtesy of Douglas Halporn, MD 28-5